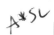
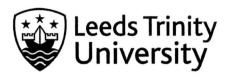
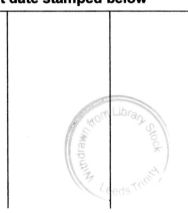
The Witch

Notions of witchcraf   turies.
At the height of w   entury
Europe, some 50,000 people were executed. They were accused of acts including
murder, cannibalism, black magic, and Devil worshipping.

The Witchcraft Reader offers a selection of the best historical writing on witchcraft, exploring how belief in witchcraft began, and the social and cultural context
in which this belief flourished. A whole range of historical perspectives is collected
here, including recent research on the role of gender in witch trials, ideas about
the Devil and demonic possession, and reasons for the decline of witch trials.

The major themes and debates in the study of witchcraft are brought together
in a general introduction, which places the extracts in a critical context. Bringing
together a wide range of important work in a single, accessible volume, *The
Witchcraft Reader* is essential reading for anyone intrigued by this complex and
fascinating subject.

Darren Oldridge is Lecturer in History at University College Worcester.

The
Witchcraft
Reader

Edited by

Darren Oldridge

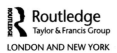

Routledge
Taylor & Francis Group

LONDON AND NEW YORK

First published 2002 by Routledge
11 New Fetter Lane, London EC4P 4EE

Simultaneously published in the USA and Canada
by Routledge
29 West 35th Street, New York, NY 10001

Reprinted 2004

Routledge is an imprint of the Taylor & Francis Group

Individual chapters © the original copyright holders
Selection and editorial matter ©2002 Darren Oldridge

Typeset in Perpetua and Bell Gothic
by Florence Production Ltd, Stoodleigh, Devon
Printed and bound in Great Britain by
TJ International Ltd, Padstow, Cornwall

British Library Cataloguing in Publication Data
A catalogue record for this book is available from the British Library

Library of Congress Cataloging in Publication Data
The Witchcraft Reader / [edited by] Darren Oldridge.
    p. cm.
    Includes bibliographical references and index.
    1. Witchcraft — History.   I. Oldridge Darren, 1966–

BF1566 .W7395 2001
133.4'3'09 — dc21   2001048166

ISBN 0–415–21492–0 (hbk)
ISBN 0–415–21493–9 (pbk)

For Meg

Contents

Acknowledgements   xi

General Introduction
Darren Oldridge   1

PART ONE
Mediaeval Origins   21

1   Richard Kieckhefer
     WITCH TRIALS IN MEDIAEVAL EUROPE   25

2   Norman Cohn
     THE DEMONIZATION OF MEDIAEVAL HERETICS   36

PART TWO
Witchcraft, Magic and Culture   53

3   Robin Briggs
     THE EXPERIENCE OF BEWITCHMENT   57

4   Wolfgang Behringer
     WEATHER, HUNGER AND FEAR: ORIGINS OF THE EUROPEAN
     WITCH-HUNTS IN CLIMATE, SOCIETY AND MENTALITY   69

5   E. William Monter
     THE SOCIOLOGY OF JURA WITCHCRAFT   87

6   David Gentilcore
     WITCHCRAFT NARRATIVES AND FOLKLORE MOTIFS
     IN SOUTHERN ITALY   97

PART THREE
The Idea of a Witch Cult   109

7   H.C. Erik Midelfort
     HEARTLAND OF THE WITCHCRAZE   113

8   Carlo Ginzburg
     DECIPHERING THE WITCHES' SABBAT   120

9   Éva Pócs
     THE ALTERNATIVE WORLD OF THE WITCHES' SABBAT   129

10 Robert Muchembled
     SATANIC MYTHS AND CULTURAL REALITIES   136

11 Stuart Clark
     INVERSION, MISRULE AND THE MEANING OF WITCHCRAFT   149

PART FOUR
Witchcraft and the Reformation   161

12 Stuart Clark
     PROTESTANT WITCHCRAFT, CATHOLIC WITCHCRAFT   165

13 Edmund Kern
     CONFESSIONAL IDENTITY AND MAGIC IN THE LATE
     SIXTEENTH CENTURY: JAKOB BITHNER AND WITCHCRAFT
     IN STYRIA   180

14 Gary K. Waite
     BETWEEN THE DEVIL AND THE INQUISITOR: ANABAPTISTS,
     DIABOLICAL CONSPIRACIES AND MAGICAL BELIEFS   189

PART FIVE
Witchcraft, the State and Social Control   201

15 Christina Larner
     THE CRIME OF WITCHCRAFT IN EARLY MODERN EUROPE   205

16 Brian Levack
    STATE-BUILDING AND WITCH HUNTING IN EARLY
    MODERN EUROPE   213

PART SIX
Witchcraft, Possession and the Devil   227

17 David Nicholls
    THE DEVIL IN RENAISSANCE FRANCE   233

18 H.C. Erik Midelfort
    THE DEVIL AND THE GERMAN PEOPLE   240

19 Moshe Sluhovsky
    A DIVINE APPARITION OR DEMONIC POSSESSION?   254

PART SEVEN
Witchcraft and Gender   267

20 Christina Larner
    WAS WITCH-HUNTING WOMAN-HUNTING?   273

21 Marianne Hester
    PATRIARCHAL RECONSTRUCTION AND WITCH-HUNTING   276

22 Jim Sharpe
    WOMEN, WITCHCRAFT AND THE LEGAL PROCESS   289

23 Clive Holmes
    WOMEN: WITCHES AND WITNESSES   303

PART EIGHT
Reading Confessions   323

24 Lyndal Roper
    OEDIPUS AND THE DEVIL   329

25 Malcolm Gaskill
    WITCHCRAFT AND POWER IN EARLY MODERN ENGLAND:
    THE CASE OF MARGARET MOORE   343

26 Louise Jackson
WITCHES, WIVES AND MOTHERS: WITCHCRAFT PERSECUTION
AND WOMEN'S CONFESSIONS IN SEVENTEENTH-CENTURY
ENGLAND   353

PART NINE
The Decline of Witchcraft   367

27 Brian Levack
THE END OF WITCH TRIALS   373

28 Gábor Klaniczay
THE DECLINE OF WITCHES AND THE RISE OF VAMPIRES   387

29 Owen Davies
URBANIZATION AND THE DECLINE OF WITCHCRAFT:
AN EXAMINATION OF LONDON   399

PART TEN
A New Witch-Hunt?   413

30 Philip Jenkins and Daniel Maier-Katkin
OCCULT SURVIVORS: THE MAKING OF A MYTH   419

31 Patrick Casement
THE WISH NOT TO KNOW   433

    Index   437

Acknowledgements

The author and publishers wish to thank the following for their permission to reproduce copyright material:

'Witch Trials in Mediaeval Europe' from *European Witch Trials: Their Foundations in Popular and Learned Culture 1300–1500* by Richard Kieckhefer (Routledge & Kegan Paul 1976), pp. 10–26, by permission of Taylor & Francis; 'The Demonization of Mediaeval Heretics' reproduced from *Europe's Inner Demons* by Norman Cohn (copyright © Norman Cohn 1975, 1993), pp. 51–78, published by Pimlico and reprinted by permission of The Random House Group Ltd and PFD on behalf of Professor Norman Cohn; 'The Experience of Bewitchment' from *Witches and Neighbours* by Robin Briggs (HarperCollins 1996), pp. 63–95, reproduced by permission of HarperCollins Publishers Ltd, Felicity Bryan and the author; 'Weather, Hunger and Fear' by Wolfgang Behringer from *German History*, 13 (1995), pp. 1–27, by permission of The German History Society; 'The Sociology of Jura Witchcraft' reprinted from *Witchcraft in France and Switzerland: The Borderlands during the Reformation* by E. William Monter (copyright © 1976 Cornell University), pp. 115–41, used by permission of the publisher Cornell University Press; 'Witchcraft Narratives and Folklore Motifs in Southern Italy' from *From Bishop to Witch* by David Gentilcore (Manchester University Press 1992), pp. 238–58, by permission of the author; 'Heartland of the Witchcraze' by H. C. Erik Midelfort from *History Today*, 31 (February 1981), pp. 27–36, by permission of *History Today*; 'Deciphering the Witches' Sabbat' by Carlo Ginzburg from *Early Modern European Witchcraft*, edited by Bengt Ankaloo and Gustav Henningsen (Oxford University Press 1993), pp. 121–35, originally published in 1987 by Institutet för Rättshistorisk Forskning under the title *Häxornas Europa 1400–1700*, by permission of Oxford University Press and the Institutet för Rättshistorisk Forskning; 'The Alternative World of the Witches' Sabbat' from *Between the Living and the Dead* by Éva Pócs (1999), pp. 73–105, by permission of the Central European University Press; 'Satanic Myths and Cultural Realities' by Robert Muchembled from *Early Modern European Witchcraft*, edited by Bengt Ankaloo and Gustav Henningsen (Oxford University Press 1993), pp. 139–60, originally published in 1987 by Institutet för Rättshistorisk Forskning under the title *Häxomas Europa 1400–1700*, by permission of Oxford University Press and the Institutet för Rättshistorisk Forskning; 'Inversion, Misrule and the Meaning of Witchcraft' by Stuart Clark from *Past and Present*, 87 (1980), pp. 98–127, by permission of Oxford University Press; 'Protestant Witchcraft, Catholic Witchcraft', copyright © Stuart Clark 1997, reprinted from *Thinking with Demons: The Idea of Witchcraft in Early Modern Europe* by Stuart Clark (1997) by permission of Oxford University Press; 'Confessional Identity and Magic in the Late Sixteenth Century' by Edmund Kern from *The Sixteenth Century Journal*, 25(2) (1994), pp. 323–40, copyright © 1994 by The Sixteenth Century Journal Publishers, Inc., reproduced by permission; 'Between the Devil and the Inquisitor' by Gary K. Waite from *Radical Reformation Studies*, edited by Werner O. Packull and Geoffrey L. Dipple (Ashgate 1999), ch. 8, pp. 120–40; 'The Crime of Witchcraft in Early Modern Europe' and 'Was Witch-Hunting Woman-Hunting?' from *Witchcraft and Religion* by Christina Larner (Blackwell 1984), pp. 35–67 and 79–91 by permission of Blackwell Publishers Ltd; 'State-Building and Witch Hunting in Early Modern Europe' by Brian Levack from *Witchcraft in Early Modern Europe: Studies in Culture and Belief*, edited by Jonathan Barry, Marianne Hester and Gareth Roberts (Cambridge University Press 1996) by permission of Cambridge University Press and Brian Levack; 'The Devil in Renaissance France' by David Nicholls from *History Today*, 30 (November 1980), pp. 25–30, by permission of *History Today*; 'The Devil and the German People' by H. C. Erik Midelfort from *Religion and Culture in the Renaissance and Reformation*, vol. 11 of *Sixteenth Century Essays and Studies*, edited by Steven Ozment (Sixteenth Century Journal Publishers 1989), pp. 99–119, by permission of Truman State University Press; 'A Divine Apparition or Demonic Possession?' by Moshe Sluhovsky from *The Sixteenth Century Journal*, 27(4) (1996), pp. 1039–55, copyright © 1996 by The Sixteenth Century Journal Publishers, Inc., reproduced by permission; 'Patriarchal Reconstruction and Witch-Hunting' by Marianne Hester from *Witchcraft in Early Modern Europe: Studies in Culture and Belief*, edited by Jonathan Barry, Marianne Hester and Gareth Roberts (Cambridge University Press 1996), pp. 288–308, by permission of Cambridge University Press and Marianne Hester; 'Women, Witchcraft and the Legal Process' by Jim Sharpe from *Women, Crime and the Courts*, edited by Jenny Kermode and Garthine Walker (UCL Press 1994), pp. 106–24, by permission of Taylor & Francis; 'Women: Witches and Witnesses' by Clive Holmes from *Past and Present*, 140 (1993), pp. 45–78, by permission of Oxford University Press; 'Oedipus and the Devil' from *Oedipus and the Devil* by Lyndal Roper (Routledge 1994), ch. 10, pp. 226–48, by permission of Taylor & Francis; 'Witchcraft and Power in Early Modern England' by Malcolm Gaskill from *Women, Crime and the Courts*, edited by Jenny Kermode and Garthine Walker (UCL Press 1994), ch. 6, by permission of Taylor & Francis; 'Witches, Wives and Mothers' by Louise Jackson from *Women's History Review*, 4(1) (1995), by permission of Louise Jackson; 'The End of Witch Trials' by Brian Levack from *The Witch Hunt in Early Modern Europe* (2nd edition copyright © Longman Group Ltd 1995), reprinted by permission of Pearson Education Ltd; 'The Decline of Witches and the Rise of Vampires' from *The Uses of Supernatural Power* by Gábor Klaniczay (copyright © 1990 Princeton University Press), reprinted by permission of Princeton University Press; 'Urbanization and the Decline of Witchcraft' by Owen Davies from *Journal of Social History*, 30 (1997), pp. 597–617, reproduced by permission of the *Journal of Social History*; 'Occult Survivors: The Making of a Myth' by Philip Jenkins and Daniel Maier-Katkin from *The Satanism Scare*, edited by James T. Richardson, Joel Best and David G. Bromley (Aldine De Gruyter 1991), ch. 8, reproduced by permission of Aldine De Gruyter, New York; 'The Wish Not to Know' by Patrick Casement from *Treating Survivors of Satanist Abuse*, edited by Valerie Sinason (Routledge 1994), ch. 2, pp. 22–5, by permission of Taylor & Francis.

Every effort has been made to obtain permission to reproduce copyright material. If any proper acknowledgement has not been made, we would invite copyright holders to inform us of the oversight.

General Introduction

MOST PEOPLE INTERESTED in witchcraft are first attracted to the subject by stories and images from popular culture. Witches enjoy a high profile in children's books and TV; they populate innumerable films, from the canon of Walt Disney to *The Blair Witch Project*; and they are the subject of an eclectic and colourful sub-genre of popular literature. If you visit the 'Mind, Body and Spirit' department of any large bookshop, you will normally find a disparate collection of publications under the heading of 'Witchcraft'. The texts displayed will cover a range of topics loosely related to the history and practice of magic, including works by the neo-pagan movement, academic texts, modern editions of much older books like the *Malleus Maleficarum*, and reprints of eccentric but still popular publications like Montague Summers' *History of Witchcraft*. This mixture reflects the extremely diverse range of interests that converge on the subject, and indicates its fascination for a wide audience. It is also significant, perhaps, that books on the subject are commonly displayed in a section of their own. Rather like Jack the Ripper, the Kennedy assassination and the search for the Holy Grail, the topic has established itself as a genre in its own right, combining elements of history, myth, and religious speculation.

The widespread interest in witchcraft is nothing new. At the time of the most intense witch persecutions in the sixteenth and seventeenth centuries, there was already a large market for publications on the subject, ranging from learned treatises on the problem of satanic magic to ballads recounting the activities of individuals accused of the crime. In some instances, demand was so great that entirely fictitious accounts were created.[1] Popular tales of witchcraft continued to circulate in the eighteenth and nineteenth centuries, while academic works on the subject generally assumed a more sceptical tone. These texts attributed magical beliefs to the folly and superstition of the 'vulgar' masses, and viewed the persecution of witches as a token of a less enlightened age. By the early years of the twentieth century, a more romantic view of the subject had emerged in some quarters. Championed by the English Egyptologist Margaret Murray, the idea that witchcraft was an ancient fertility cult suppressed by the Christian church attracted considerable publicity and some academic support.[2] By the 1950s, when the phrase 'witch-hunting' was coined in America, witch persecutions were associated with the suppression of deviant groups by political elites. This view was exemplified in Arthur Miller's play *The Crucible*, which was based loosely on the Salem witch trials of 1692. All these interpretations of witchcraft have survived into the present age, and are represented in the various books that compete for the attention of readers drawn to the topic.

Pagan cults, hysteria, and evil witch finders

Despite the diversity of popular writing on witchcraft, a number of general themes occur frequently in the genre. One common assumption, derived partly from the work of Murray, is that witchcraft was a pagan cult driven underground by the Christian authorities. Unsurprisingly, this claim features most often in the work of neo-pagans and self-proclaimed 'witches', who wish to trace the lineage of their beliefs back to the ancient world. This aspiration is summed up neatly in the title of a book by Vivianne Crowley, *Wicca: The Old Religion in the New Age* (1989).[3] In a variation of this idea, some feminist writers have stressed the female-centred nature of the 'old religion', which was brutally suppressed by the male-dominated Christian church.[4] Another theme in popular accounts is the credulity and 'superstition' of those men and women who accepted the existence of harmful magic in the past, and reacted 'hysterically' to the non-existent threat of a witch cult. This notion is linked to the tendency to assume that most witch trials took place in the Middle Ages, when western society was somehow less rational than it is today. These ideas are combined in the common English phrase, 'If I'd lived in the Middle Ages they'd have burnt me as a witch'. A third common assumption is the belief that witch-hunts were pursued by ruthless and sadistic men who stopped at nothing to secure convictions for the crime. In this version, allegations of witchcraft led inevitably to torture, enforced confession and death.

It would be tempting at this point to explode these popular conceptions. The views described above are, undoubtedly, oversimplifications of the history of witchcraft, and some of them are simply untrue. Relatively few witch trials occurred in the Middle Ages. There was nothing inherently irrational about witchcraft beliefs, and the most extreme of these beliefs – involving the idea of secret assemblies of Devil-worshipping cannibals – were developed by the most educated men in European society. If any fertility cults existed in the sixteenth century, they have no historical or intellectual connection to the twentieth-century witchcraft movement, which was invented in the 1950s by a retired civil servant from England named Gerard Gardner.[5] Nonetheless, it would be wrong to dismiss these popular assumptions entirely. Despite their obvious shortcomings, they do encapsulate some serious issues in the history of witchcraft. While it is easy to discredit the claims of Murray and

Gardner, it is altogether less simple to discount the idea that non-Christian religious practices existed in the early modern period, and were sometimes implicated in accusations of witchcraft. Even Murray's idea of a pagan fertility cult has survived – in modified form – in the work of historians like Carlo Ginzburg and Gábor Klaniczay. Equally, the popular image of the cruel witch finder who imposed his obsessions on the victims of torture raises profound questions about the origins of witch trials. While those responsible for prosecutions were normally sincere in their motives, it appears that they sometimes imposed their own views of the crime in the course of interrogations. Some confessions were entirely false. In 1628 the mayor of Bamburg, Johannes Junius, smuggled a tragic letter to his daughter from his cell in the town's 'witch prison', declaring that his confession to the crime was 'sheer lies and made-up things . . . For all this I was forced to say through fear of the torture which was threatened, beyond what I had already endured'.[6] In this instance, the willingness of the authorities to use torture was sufficient to ensure a conviction, whatever the other circumstances of the case. The fact that this was possible presents historians with some awkward problems. Is it necessary to assume that anything 'real' lay behind allegations of witchcraft? Did witch trials depend on popular support, since the authorities were capable of securing convictions through the use of torture alone?

The popular stereotypes of pagan cults and evil witch finders can be viewed as simplified versions of positions available to academic historians. For many scholars, the best way to explain allegations of witchcraft is to assume that some of the practices described by early modern demonologists were based on real activities or aspects of folk religion. This principle is often used to account for allegations of harmful magic, but can be extended to explain details of the witches' sabbat. Thus Carlo Ginzburg and Éva Pócs argue in this book that the origins of the sabbat can be found in folk beliefs. On the opposite extreme, some historians have argued that *all* the elements in witchcraft accusations should be regarded as learned fantasies. There is no reason to assume that any charges against witches were based on folk traditions, according to M. J. Kephart, 'when we already know that it was perfectly easy to fabricate accusations of sorcery, heresy and sundry disgusting behaviours against any group or person whom authorities wanted to get rid of for any reason'.[7] None of the writers in this collection go quite so far, but the extracts from Muchembled and Larner emphasise the role of the fantasies of educated men in witch persecutions. The majority of historians occupy ground somewhere in between. In other words, they try to strike a balance between the evidence suggesting that witch trials reflected the real activities and beliefs of ordinary people, and the possibility that prosecutions were simply imposed by elite groups. The attempt to find the most appropriate position between these two interpretations is one of the underlying themes of witchcraft research, and recurs in different contexts throughout this book. This introduction will explore some of the problems involved in getting the balance right. It will also consider the popular image of witchcraft as an 'irrational' belief, which has attracted the attention of historians and philosophers in recent years. Before considering these issues in detail, however, it is necessary to provide a brief survey of what is known about witch persecutions in Europe.

European witch trials, *c.* 1400–1750

Thanks to the work of Richard Kieckhefer and Norman Cohn, the chronology of European witch persecutions is now fairly well established. The earliest known prosecution occurred in Kilkenny in Ireland in 1324, when an aristocratic lady, Alice Kyteler, was accused of practising harmful magic and participating in diabolical rites with a small group of associates. This case involved many of the key elements found in later allegations of witchcraft, though some of them – notably the idea of a pact with the Devil – were only implied in the surviving documents. The idea of a secret society of Devil worshippers appears to have developed slowly in the later fourteenth century, and resurfaced in 1437 in a letter from Pope Eugenius IV 'to all inquisitors of heretical depravity'. This expressed the concept of witchcraft more fully, and deserves to be quoted at length:

> They sacrifice to demons, adore them, seek out and accept responses from them, do homage to them, and make with them a written agreement or another kind of pact through which, by a single word, touch or sign, they may perform whatever evil deeds or sorcery they wish and be transported to or away from wherever they wish ... In their sorcery they are not afraid to use the materials of baptism, the eucharist, and other sacraments. They make images of wax or other materials, which by their invocations they baptise or cause to be baptised. Sometimes they make a reversal of the holy cross, upon which our saviour hanged for us. Not honouring the mysteries, they sometimes inflict upon the representations and other signs of the cross various shameful things by execrable means.[8]

This account lacks the idea of infanticide and cannibalism that featured prominently in later descriptions of the crime, but includes most of the other ingredients of the Renaissance concept of witchcraft. In 1486 these ingredients were combined by the German inquisitors Heinrich Kramer and Jacob Sprenger in the *Malleus Maleficarum*. The publication of the *Malleus* occurred during the first wave of major witch panics in France and Germany, which lasted until the early years of the sixteenth century. Prosecutions then declined until around 1560, when a second wave of trials began, this time extending beyond Germany and France to Switzerland and England. Another outbreak occurred towards the end of the century, extending to Flanders and Scotland. After a period of respite in the early 1600s, a final wave of severe persecutions began around 1620 and continued in much of Europe until the last quarter of the seventeenth century. Subsequently, witch trials declined in number and intensity. In 1692 the famous episode in Salem, New England, was one of the last witch panics in the western world.

   It is important to note that there were considerable regional variations within this pattern. There were relatively few trials in Italy, the Netherlands and Spain throughout the whole period, and English trials tended to be small-scale affairs until a spectacular eruption of persecution in 1645. In contrast, Germany suffered particularly savage panics, as did Scotland after 1620. While witch trials had ended in much of Europe by the eighteenth century, they reached their peak in Poland and Hungary in the same period. These variations have thwarted most attempts to impose a single-cause explanation for the tragedy. Protestant states like England and the Netherlands suffered relatively few persecutions, but the same can be said for Catholic Italy and Spain. Equally, the ferocity of some witch panics in Catholic France was matched by events in Presbyterian Scotland. Intense persecutions occurred in regions suffering sustained warfare in the seventeenth century, like the principalities of Germany; but major witch panics also took place in relatively peaceful regions like Scandinavia.

As well as these regional variations, there were differences between social groups about the meaning of witchcraft itself. All those who acknowledged the existence of witches accepted their ability to perform harmful magic, or *maleficium*, most often involving disease, the destruction of crops or disturbances in the weather. Allegations of this kind made up the bulk of the accusations levelled by ordinary people against suspected witches. The emphasis in these allegations was overwhelmingly on the harm caused by the witch, rather than the origins of their power. In contrast, university-trained lawyers and churchmen tended to stress the satanic nature of the witch's magic, and insisted that their abilities derived from a pact with the Devil. There is some evidence that folk traditions linked *maleficium* with the Devil, particularly in English witchcraft and cases involving demonic possession; but even in these cases, the victims of witchcraft were far more concerned with the effects of *maleficium* than the supposed pact between Satan and the witch. Primary allegations also tended to focus on individuals rather than groups. The idea that witchcraft was a collective enterprise involving nocturnal gatherings for Devil worship, desecration and murder was generally confined to the higher ranks of European society. This idea played a central role in the works of learned demonologists like Henri Boguet, Jean Bodin and King James VI of Scotland, but was mostly absent from the allegations brought by European villagers against their neighbours. During the course of a trial, however, it was easy for these disparate elements to merge together, particularly when the legal authorities were more interested in the satanic aspects of witchcraft than simple *maleficium*.

The confession of Françoise Secretain

The conflation of these various ideas, and the problem it presents for the interpretation of witchcraft confessions, can be illustrated by the testimony of Françoise Secretain, a French woman convicted in 1598. According to Henri Boguet's account of her interrogation, she was imprisoned for three days before making her initial admission of guilt. Subsequently, she added new details to this statement 'from day to day'. Eventually, he was able to present the 'principal points' of her confession as follows:

> First, that she had wished five devils on Loyse Maillat.
>
> Second, that she had long since given herself to the Devil, who at that time had the likeness of a big black man.

Third, that the Devil had four or five times known her carnally, in the form sometimes of a dog, sometimes of a cat, and sometimes of a fowl; and that his semen was very cold.

Fourth, that she had countless times been to the sabbat and assembly of witches near the village of Coyrieres in a place called Combes by the water; and that she went there on a white staff which she placed between her legs.

Fifth, that at the sabbat she had danced, and had beaten water to cause hail.

Sixth, that she and Groz-Jacques Bocquet had caused Loys Monneret to die by making her eat a piece of bread which they had dusted with a powder given to them by the Devil.

Seventh, that she had caused several cows to die, and that she did so by touching them with her hand or with a wand while saying certain words.[9]

It is impossible to know for certain the origin of these bizarre disclosures. As Louise Jackson points out in Chapter 26, a confession text is 'a palimpsest made of different layers of detail and interpretation, added one on top of another as different people became involved in the process of accusation and confession'.[10] At least two layers of meaning appear to be present in Boguet's document. First, there are specific acts of *maleficium* against named individuals, which probably constituted the initial allegations against Secretain. She was accused of causing the death of cattle, poisoning a woman to death and sending devils into the body of a young girl. Second, she claimed to have attended the sabbat and indulged in sex with the Devil. The allegations of poisoning and killing livestock were common in cases of suspected bewitchment in sixteenth-century France, and much of contemporary Europe. The claim that Secretain was responsible for a demonic possession was a little more unusual; but possession was closely associated with witchcraft in the folklore of France, Germany and England. In this particular case, Boguet reported that the first allegation against Secretain came from 8-year-old Loyse Maillat, whose parents suspected possession when she was struck by a mysterious sickness. In contrast to these acts of malicious magic, the references to the sabbat were probably not part of the original allegations. If they were introduced in the course of Secretain's interrogation, this would certainly reflect Boguet's own preoccupation with the subject, which he described at length elsewhere in his text. Similarly, the sexual relationship between the accused woman and the Devil owed much to learned stereotypes. Even the lurid detail that his semen was cold reflected the theological assumption that Satan's earthly body was composed of lifeless matter, since he possessed no physical body of his own.[11]

While many aspects of Secretain's final confession were probably added to the initial claims of *maleficium*, it appears that the words of her testimony were not simply imposed on her by the authorities. Lyndal Roper argues in Chapter 24 that witchcraft confessions could involve a process of negotiation between the accused and her questioners, even though the relationship between them was deeply unequal.

This process allowed suspects to weave their own fantasies and beliefs into the outline narrative provided by officials of the courts. In this case, it appears that Secretain mixed details from local folklore into her story. The image of Satan as 'a big black man', or as a dog or cat, was reminiscent of popular tales about the Devil. The tendency of witches to craft stories of demonic encounters from folklore is noted by David Gentilcore in Chapter 6. While we can do no more than speculate on the surviving evidence, it is possible that Secretain's fantasy derived from some event in her own life, like the confessions discussed by Roper and Malcolm Gaskill in Chapters 24 and 25. Thus the confession combined ideas from learned demonology with more widely held concepts of *maleficium*, and possibly incorporated more personal elements as well. This combination of diverse beliefs – each appealing to different social actors in the drama of a prosecution – was typical of witch trials in the early modern period, and makes it even harder to explain the phenomenon in terms of a single cause that shaped the behaviour of all the groups involved. With this note of caution in mind, it is now time to consider some of the elements that contributed to European witch persecutions. The first theme to explore is the possibility that witch beliefs were inspired by some kind of real cultic activity.

Did a witch cult exist?

In Margaret Murray's original formulation, the 'witch cult' suppressed in the sixteenth century was a folk religion practised widely in Europe to ensure the fertility of harvests. Men and women would gather at sacred sites to offer devotion to 'ancient gods' which had survived the advent of Christianity, and been partially assimilated by the mediaeval church. The relative tolerance of the authorities towards this practice ended in the late Middle Ages, when the old gods were condemned as demons and their worshippers were redefined as witches. This interpretation is now unsustainable. As Norman Cohn pointed out in *Europe's Inner Demons* (1975), Murray's evidence was drawn entirely from witchcraft confessions which she edited selectively to create the impression that they described real events. When these confessions are read in full, complete with details of witches flying at night and transforming themselves into animals, it becomes obvious that they are not straightforward accounts of actual happenings. Moreover, Cohn observed that allegations similar to those made against witches had been levelled at dissenting groups since antiquity, when Christians themselves were accused of nocturnal gatherings involving cannibalism and murder.[12] Apart from the allegations themselves – and occasional confessions extracted by force – there is no evidence that such meetings ever took place. Cohn's arguments have achieved general acceptance since the mid-1970s, and have been reinforced by much new research. Most strikingly, Gustav Henningsen's work on Alfonso Salazar, an inquisitor in the Basque region of Spain in the early seventeenth century, has shown that contemporaries were unable to find physical evidence of alleged sabbats when they carefully searched for it. After a group of young women confessed to attending a sabbat in 1610,

Salazar conducted an exhaustive investigation of their supposed activities, and concluded that they could be regarded only as delusions.[13]

Agrarian cults and fairies

While Murray's concept of a witch cult can be safely disgarded, a more subtle and persuasive version of the theory has been developed by other historians. The principal architect of this interpretation is Carlo Ginzburg, whose work is based largely on the Friuli region of northern Italy. From 1580 onwards, a series of extraordinary testimonies were recorded there by the Roman Inquisition. These related to a local cult known as the *benandante*, whose beliefs were described as follows by one of its members:

> I am a *benandante* because I go with the others to fight four times a year, that is during the ember days, at night; I go invisibly in spirit and the body remains behind; we go forth in the service of Christ, and the witches [go forth] in the name of the Devil; we fight each other, we with bundles of fennel and they with sorghum stalks.[14]

On the basis of this rich body of material, Ginzburg has reconstructed the belief-system of the *benandante*. Membership of the group was determined at birth, when certain individuals were born with their 'cauls', or amniotic sacs, still intact around their bodies. As adults, the *benandante* travelled in spirit on certain nights of the year – the 'ember days' in December – to meet with assemblies of evil spirits they described as witches. Their purpose was to fight the witches, armed with the bunches of fennel mentioned in the deposition, with the outcome of this combat deciding the fate of the next harvest. None of these testimonies were obtained through torture, and their details were remarkably consistent over a period of several decades. It appears that Ginzburg has uncovered an agrarian cult related to witchcraft, whose members perceived themselves and their nocturnal foes in very different terms from those understood by the men responsible for their prosecution. Moreover, he demonstrates that the *benandante* were gradually redefined by the inquisition as sabbat-attending witches, and this new definition of their activities was eventually accepted by the communities in which they lived.

At a regional level, then, Ginzburg's work reveals that a fertility cult did exist, and its activities provoked accusations of witchcraft from the authorities. His interpretation becomes more controversial, however, when he tries to extend this model to other areas of Europe. His argument is presented in Chapter 8. Support for Ginzburg's thesis has come from the Hungarian historian, Gábor Klaniczay, who has identified similar beliefs in the confessions of witches in that country. In this version, cult members, or *táltos*, travelled in spirit to fight rival *táltos* for control of the weather.[15] For those sympathetic to Ginzburg's case, the most compelling evidence comes from details in witchcraft confessions that contradicted the assumptions of demonologists, and were generally rejected by eductated writers on the subject. It is difficult to see how these details could have been imposed from above, and it is quite possible that they originated in popular culture. Boguet, for example, repudiated the idea that 'for the most part it is only in spirit that witches go to the sabbat', despite the fact that one of the witches accused alongside Françoise Secretain claimed it was 'quite possible' to do so. He provided another example of the belief, which suggests that it was accepted in French folklore in the late sixteenth century:

> Some little time ago, there was a man of Orgelet who brought his wife to this place and accused her of being a witch, saying among other things that when they were in bed together one Thursday night he noticed that his wife was absolutely still, without even breathing; whereupon he began to shake her, but could not waken her . . . This lasted for two or three hours until the cock crowed; and then his wife suddenly awoke, and when he asked her what was amiss, she answered that she was so tired from the work she had done the day before that she was weighed down with sleep and felt nothing of what her husband had done to her. The man then supposed that she had been to the sabbat, for he had already had some suspicion of her because the cattle of some of their neighbours, whom she had threatened, had been dying.[16]

James VI of Scotland noted very similar claims in 1597, despite his conviction that they were merely delusions.[17] Reports that the spirits of witches left their bodies at night were also recorded in Germany in the late seventeenth century, though little credence was given to this idea in the region's demonological literature.[18]

As well as these intriguing details, Ginzburg's thesis receives indirect support from another body of evidence. This relates to so-called 'fairy cults' in early modern Europe. Like the belief that witches could travel at night in spirit form, references to fairies occur quite frequently in connection to witchcraft cases, despite the fact that they had no place in the learned stereotype of the witch. Again, it is unlikely that these details were imposed by lawyers or theologians, who often appear to have found them incomprehensible. An early example of fairy beliefs was preserved in the register of the archdeacon's court of Norwich in England in 1499. Three members of the Clerk family from Suffolk were convicted of 'heretical depravity' for consorting with spirits they described as 'gracious fairies'. These creatures performed various feats on the family's behalf, helping them to cure diseases and locate hidden treasure, as well as transporting Marion Clerk through the air to Canterbury cathedral.[19] Fairies continued to figure in English witch trials until the seventeenth century.[20] In Scotland, James VI noted that 'sundry witches have gone to death with the confession that they have been transported with the fairies to such a hill, which opening, they went in, and there saw a fair queen'. He could only explain such claims by assuming they were satanic delusions.[21] On the other side of Europe, Gustav Henningsen has shown that fairy beliefs were well established in Sicily during the sixteenth century. Here, men and women from humble backgrounds were organised into 'companies', whose members believed they were conveyed through the air to attend joyful gatherings with fairies, and travelled with the creatures as they performed good deeds in the homes of their neighbours. These events were reinterpreted by the inquisition as sabbats.[22] The role of fairy beliefs in European witchcraft is a subject that awaits fuller investigation, but it is possible that such popular ideas provided the raw material from which the learned notion of a witch cult was formed.

There are, however, some serious weaknesses in this interpretation. First of all, it appears that the kind of fully developed belief-systems that could have inspired the idea of the sabbat were confined to a relatively small area of Europe. Ideas similar to those held by the Italian *benandante* can be found in Germany, Scotland and France, but there is little evidence that they were integrated into a coherent body of religious beliefs. As Richard Muchembled points out in Chapter 10, there is a danger that historians can take fragments from popular tradition and infer from them a composite belief-system that never existed as a whole. Such an approach can ignore the specific cultural circumstances in which the persecution of witches occurred. Second, critics of Ginzburg have argued that the learned concept of witchcraft could have arisen without any reference to popular beliefs. Norman Cohn shows in Chapter 2 that the major ingredients of the sabbat were present in mediaeval descriptions of heretics. In the early modern period, some of the ideas associated with the witches' gathering, like the practice of Devil-worship and infanticide, were occasionally attributed to entirely unrelated groups. Thus William Gouge asserted in 1626 that American tribesmen 'excelled in unnatural cruelty, sacrificing their children and offering them to devils'.[23] Many elements of the sabbat could have derived from the fantasy of an 'anti-society' which inverted the conventions of official religion, as Stuart Clark argues in Chapter 11. It is striking that scholarly accounts of witchcraft tended to reverse their authors' most cherished religious beliefs, down to specific details of confessional practice. Thus the Catholic Boguet emphasised the desecration of the mass in the sabbat, alleging that a black turnip and urine were offered as the body and blood of Christ.[24] James VI, in contrast, claimed that a blasphemous parody of a sermon was the centre-piece of the witches' assembly, which seemed to resemble a demonic version of a Scots Protestant service.[25] These imaginary reversals of accepted behaviour provide a plausible, alternative source for the myth of the sabbat.

At a more basic level, it is problematic to argue that the existence of fertility cults gave rise to witch persecutions. Even if such cults existed in Renaissance Europe, this in itself could not explain the development of a witch panic. It would be necessary to explain why official attitudes changed from indifference to intolerance, and why popular beliefs were demonised at this particular time. A similar objection can be made to other attempts to explain witch trials in terms of popular beliefs. If, for example, one argues that the persecutions were caused by fears of *maleficium* among the European population, it would be necessary to show that these fears increased from the late fifteenth century onwards, or that the authorities were prepared to take them more seriously for some reason. These points relate to the much wider question of whether witchcraft prosecutions were imposed 'from above' or should be regarded as a response to popular concerns. We can now turn to that question.

Social and political contexts

It is instructive at this point to return to the case of Françoise Secretain. According to Boguet's account, the events leading to her apprehension began when she visited the house of Humberte and Claude Maillat to ask for overnight lodgings. With her husband away, Humberte first refused and asked her to leave, then relented in the face of her visitor's persistence. The next morning, her young daughter Loyse was afflicted with a strange illness that weakened her limbs and twisted her mouth 'in a very strange manner'. Some days later, her parents began to suspect bewitchment and took her to a priest, who confirmed the diagnosis of possession. It was during the girl's exorcism that she named Secretain as the person responsible for her suffering.[26] The dynamics of this story were fairly typical of village-level cases of witchcraft. A dispute between two women was followed by the illness of a child, subsequently ascribed to *maleficium*. In this particular instance, the belief that the girl was possessed with demons encouraged an allegation of witchcraft, since the condition was often attributed to witches. But in common with most other accusations of harmful magic, it appears that the case of Françoise Secretain served two major functions for the people involved: it provided an outlet for anger in a situation of social conflict, and it offered an explanation, and possibly a remedy, for a misfortune that was otherwise hard to understand. These themes of social conflict and the explanation of suffering have played a prominent role in attempts to explain witchcraft 'from below'.

The view that witch trials were a response to increased social tensions during the sixteenth century is most closely associated with English research. In the early 1970s, the studies of Keith Thomas and Alan Macfarlane suggested that accusations typically occurred when a relatively wealthy villager felt obliged to refuse charity to a less fortunate neighbour. One consequence of this was a feeling of guilt, which could easily be transferred to the person who had been turned away. In Macfarlane's view, the tensions associated with inequality were created largely by economic transitions – principally the growth in population and the beginnings of capitalism – which were not accompanied by an adequate system of provision for those who lost out.[27] The strength of this approach is that it provides a plausible account of the circumstances of local accusations, which is consistent with much of the surviving evidence; its principal weakness is that it is less applicable to large-scale witch panics such as those in East Anglia in 1645, and in Scotland and central Europe during the seventeenth century. Moreover, the economic changes experienced in England were not mirrored in other countries, like Scotland, which suffered more intense persecutions. The other kind of explanation for witch trials 'from below' – based on the need of early modern societies to make sense of natural calamities – has been advanced most persuasively by the German historian Wolfgang Behringer. In Chapter 4, Behringer points out that the most savage period of witch persecutions from 1560 coincided with the climatic phenomenon known as the 'little ice age', which caused crop failures across much of Europe until the middle years of the seventeenth century. This weather pattern was correctly perceived as abnormal by contemporaries, who found it easy to attribute to witches intent on destroying whole communities. The popular clamour for action caused the political elites of central Europe to move against those believed to be responsible. As Behringer acknowledges, however, the hardships induced by the 'little ice age' cannot provide a complete explanation for Europe's witch trials. For a start, the first wave of panics commenced some eighty years earlier. Furthermore, large-scale witch-hunts often occurred when the learned concept of collective witchcraft was involved, since the idea of a witch cult encouraged the courts to pursue the alleged confederates of convicted witches. Regions where this concept was absent from learned witch beliefs experienced relatively few trials, despite the effects of climatic change. This was the case in Denmark and England until the 1640s. In the latter case, the notion of the sabbat achieved prominence for the first time during the East Anglian trials of 1645, which constituted by far the largest witch persecution in England.[28]

While Behringer's work shows the major role played by popular concerns in some witch persecutions, it is hard to see how trials could have spread without the active support of ruling elites. This impression is supported by the pattern of decline in prosecutions from around 1680. At the level of rural communities, allegations of *maleficium* continued to be made in England throughout the eighteenth century, and it appears that similar beliefs persisted in much of mainland Europe. Indeed, witch beliefs were flourishing in parts of Denmark and Spain as late as the 1960s.[29] In the same period, however, educated Europeans were increasingly reluctant to accept the reality of satanic witchcraft, and the courts in most countries ceased to recognise it as a crime. Broadly speaking, it appears that major panics ended when local authorities ceased to regard witchcraft as a problem. By the same token, prosecutions ended earlier in regions like Spain where elites were sceptical about satanic witchcraft. This does not mean, of course, that popular anxieties about *maleficium* could not sometimes provoke judicial action, as happened in sixteenth-century Bavaria and Trier; but it suggests that the response of elite groups to such anxieties helped to determine the extent and severity of panics. The learned concept of a satanic 'anti-society' was particularly important here, and it is necessary to consider the political and religious circumstances in which this idea came to be accepted by a section of Europe's governing class.

The effects of religious division

From the 1520s onwards, one major factor that encouraged belief in a satanic conspiracy was the division of Europe into Catholic and Protestant factions. The doctrines of Protestantism did not, in themselves, induce witch persecutions, despite Martin Luther's firm belief in the existence of witches and his insistence on Satan's great earthly power.[30] Rather, the importance of the Reformation lay in the many indirect consequences of religious division. One result of the split in the mediaeval church was that political elites across Europe were forced to identify with one denominational faction against another. This increased the political importance of maintaining religious orthodoxy, and the political threat posed by religious dissent. At the same time, conflict between Catholics and Protestants recast European politics as a crusade between the forces of God and His enemies. In the context of these developments campaigns against satanic witchcraft could confirm their agents as the champions of true religion. Indeed, the very existence of witches was sometimes viewed as a hellish endorsement of the authority of ruling groups. As the Catholic demonologist Nicholas Rémy explained, witches had a special hatred of the pious magistrate, who should strike against them 'with confidence, knowing he is pursuing a vocation in which he will always have God as his champion and defender'.[31] The same argument was advanced in Protestant Scotland, where the deliverance of James VI from a plot to destroy him by witchcraft in 1591 was presented as a vindication of his faith and a tacit endorsement of his ecclesiastical policies.[32]

The politics of religious division not only affected the political elites of early modern Europe, but also helped shape the behaviour of Protestant and Catholic clergy. This was evident in cases of demonic possession. Lyndal Roper has shown that German Jesuits in the later sixteenth century used exorcisms to validate the power of the Roman church.[33] Similarly, Moshe Sluhovsky notes in Chapter 19 that high-profile dispossessions were a powerful tool of confessional propaganda in France. In one instance, Boguet told the story of a Huguenot gentleman whose son was possessed by a demon but found that his local pastor 'had no power against devils'. He 'secretly sent for a Catholic priest, who used the accustomed exorcisms of the Roman church with such sincerity that the possessed was soon delivered'.[34] During a visit to the possessed convent of Loudon in 1634, the Duke of Lauderdale was asked by a priest if the power of the Jesuit exorcists could persuade him to convert to Catholicism.[35] Puritan exorcists in England were caught in a two-way conflict between their Catholic rivals and the hierarchy of the established church, which feared that successful dispossessions could bolster the authority of nonconforming ministers. This conflict was epitomised in the 1590s by the exorcist John Darrel, who claimed that papists and their 'secret friends' – including some English bishops – 'do what they can [so] that the true church of Christ may not have credit by casting out devils'.[36] The relevance of these propaganda battles was that possession was often attributed to witchcraft in popular belief, and exorcisms were frequently attended by allegations of the crime. This was the case in Germany, France and England, where Darrel's activities led to a series of witch trials and at least two executions.

Another consequence of the Reformation was the attempt by local elites, both Catholic and Protestant, to impose Christian beliefs on the population at large. As Edmund Kern remarks in Chapter 13, this entailed an attack on folk ideas and practices as part of 'an overall missionary effort to reform the common people of Europe'.[37] As part of this process, traditional beliefs about ghosts, fairies and saints, and popular expressions of piety like prophetic visions, were subjected to reinterpretation. If they could not be incorporated within the framework of orthodox religion, or appeared to threaten the authority of the official church, they were readily explained in terms of demonic activity. Several of the contributors to this book describe this process, which occurred in a great variety of different contexts: the redefinition of a ghost as the Devil in 1560s France (Chapter 19); the condemnation of the *benandante* (Chapter 8); the denunciation of folk magic as diabolism in sixteenth-century Austria (Chapter 13); and the suppression of 'visionary' women in Italy (Chapter 6). Such events were symptoms of a general climate of anxiety about the Devil's power in the world, and in some cases they led directly to accusations of witchcraft. One such instance was recorded in 1688 when a group of devout Protestants wrote to the English divine, Richard Baxter, concerning an outbreak of witchcraft in Exeter. When a local apprentice named Nathan Crab was afflicted with epilepsy, his parents took him for treatment to one Mr Gibs, who gave him 'a bag to hang about his neck' with instructions to remove it after a week. A few days later, however, this medication aroused the suspicion of the boy's God-fearing master, who believed that it might be a charm. He made the boy remove the bag so he could inspect its contents, which turned out to be a paper inscribed with magical words. Once it was established that Gibs was a 'cunning man' rather than a legitimate physician, Crab's master and parents began to suspect witchcraft. As a result, they accused the healer of *maleficium* when the boy's fits returned.[38]

The desire of Protestants and Catholics to reform popular religion was accompanied by anxieties about sexual conduct. In part, this arose from the abolition of monasticism and priestly celibacy in Protestant regions, which meant that households became the focus for religious devotion; this, in turn, encouraged new standards of 'God-fearing' behaviour within the family. More generally, the desire to enforce sexual morality reflected the need to maintain social order in a time of political and religious change, since the stability of households was viewed as essential to the welfare of society as a whole. In sixteenth-century Augsburg, Lyndal Roper has chronicled the rise of 'the holy household', in which parents assumed new responsibilities for the religious education of their children and servants. This development was paralleled by official intolerance towards perceived threats to family life, such as prostitutes, and increased regulation of marriage.[39] Similar trends have been identified in other parts of Germany, as well as France and England.[40] As Christina Larner points out in Chapter 15, this trend was accompanied by a rise in prosecutions for 'secret crimes' like infanticide, which represented an attack on the family. In the context of these wider concerns, it is easy to see how the idea of satanic witchcraft – which involved a secret cult devoted to illicit sexuality and the murder of infants – was able to gain support among educated Europeans. It is also relevant, perhaps, that women were the principal targets of witch persecutions. In a patriarchal culture, disorderly women were perceived as the main danger to family life, and the attack on witches might be viewed as an adjunct to the prosecution of other female enemies of the 'holy household', such as prostitutes, unmarried mothers and women accused of infanticide.

While the impact of religious division offers an attractive explanation for European witch trials, it is helpful to remember Robin Briggs' warning that 'any attempt to suggest that there is a single cause, or even a dominant one, a hidden key to the mystery, should be treated with great suspicion'. As Briggs points out, the most plausible interpretations of witchcraft involve the interaction of numerous causes.[41] The learned fantasy of the sabbat, the various consequences of the Reformation, and the social and environmental changes that encouraged fears of *maleficium* in some parts of Europe: all contributed to witch persecutions in the sixteenth and seventeenth centuries. The challenge to historians is to explain how these various factors interacted in particular regions at particular moments, while resisting the temptation to impose a single theory to explain the tragedy as a whole. Whatever the local circumstances of witch persecutions, however, they all depended on the general acceptance of the existence of harmful magic, an idea that is widely regarded as untenable in western societies today. The last section of this introduction will consider the social context in which this belief operated, and make a case for the essential rationality of such thinking in the early modern period.

The rational basis for witch beliefs

At the level of village communities, it appears that witchcraft functioned essentially as a theory of causation. When the daughter of Humberte and Claude Maillat fell ill, *maleficium* was one of the possible explanations available to them; and the identification of Françoise Secretain as the person responsible also provided an opportunity to relieve their child's suffering by acting against her. In this respect, allegations of witchcraft played a similar role to the less common practice of prosecuting animals for crimes against people and their property, which occurred sporadically in early modern Germany and France.[42] They supplied an explanation for an otherwise arbitrary event, and allowed those whom it affected to assume some control over the situation. Such mechanisms were important in rural communities whose livelihoods depended largely on forces beyond human control, such as the weather, physical illness, and the health of livestock and crops. The tendency to attribute misfortune to one's neighbours was also encouraged by a social environment in which most people worked and lived in extended households comprising family members, servants or apprentices. Such arrangements created a profound sense of interdependency, and meant that good personal relationships were essential to emotional and physical wellbeing. The link between ill health and social friction was acknowledged by the English physician, Richard Napier, in the early seventeenth century. In 1634, for example, he noted that one of his patients, Joan Fellow, was afflicted with acute insomnia and 'light-headedness', adding that 'her mother in law hath used her very unkindly'. On other occasions, Napier attributed various physical symptoms to bad feelings between family members or neighbours.[43] It is reasonable to assume that such experiences were common in early modern communities, and sometimes provided the basis for witchcraft allegations. Equally, it is plausible to argue that the diagnosis of *maleficium* in such cases had a sound medical basis. Medical studies suggest that many adults living in traditional African societies have a high natural resistance to disease, since those lacking this quality often perish in infancy. As a result, sickness frequently arises from a weakening of the immune system, which can be triggered by stressful social situations.[44] If the same circumstances prevailed in pre-industrial Europe, many charges of witchcraft may well have reflected the real origin of the victim's symptoms in their strained relationship with another person.

The idea of witchcraft could also explain mental and physical experiences that were otherwise very hard to define or comprehend. This point is especially relevant to conditions later defined as psychological 'disorders', such as schizophrenia and depression. As Roy Porter has noted, successful explanations for these syndromes remain elusive, and the efforts of exorcists to relieve the symptoms of schizophrenics sometimes appear to have been as effective as those of psychiatrists today.[45] Witchcraft also provided an explanation for less severe hallucinatory experiences that are still very common. Malcolm Gaskill points out in Chapter 25 that bereaved people often have visions of the dead, an experience that was described in English witchcraft confessions in 1645. Another area of experience linked to witchcraft was sleep disturbance. The syndrome of 'sleep paralysis' − in which individuals awake to find themselves immobilised, and sometimes suffer hallucinations or extreme sensations of fear − was readily attributed to *maleficium*. Thus Henri Boguet described how a bewitched man was paralysed in his bed one night, and was even unable to call to his neighbours for help.[46] In 1592, a similar affliction was visited on Lady Cromwell of Huntingdonshire in England, who was 'strangely tormented in her sleep' by a witch's familiar in the shape of a cat.[47] As late as 1871, a man from Dorset was tried for assaulting an old woman whom he believed had sent spirits to attack him at night.[48] In these and similar cases, it appears that victims of witchcraft were attributing real experiences to malicious magic. Given that most of these conditions are still little understood, this can be regarded as a wholly reasonable response.

The fear of *maleficium* becomes still easier to understand when it is placed in the context of popular religion as a whole. Since the late 1960s, research from many parts of Europe has shown that magical beliefs and practices were widespread among the peasant population. Popular magic, often mixed with elements of official religion, was employed for a wide range of practical purposes. In 1594 the Lutheran inspectors of the province of Weisbaden in Germany noted the prevalence of such activities:

> The use of spells is so widespread among the people here that not a man or woman begins, undertakes, does or refrains from doing anything . . . without employing some particular blessing, incantation, spell, or other such heathenish means . . . Whenever an article of clothing has been mislaid and cannot be found, when someone feels sickly or a cow acts queer, they run at once to the soothsayer to ask who has stolen it or put a bad spell on it, and to fetch some charm to use against the enchanter . . . All the people hereabouts engage in superstitious practices with familiar and unfamiliar words, names, and rhymes, especially with the names of God, the Holy Trinity, certain angels, the Virgin Mary, the twelve apostles, the three kings, numerous saints, the wounds of Christ, his seven words on the cross [and] verses from the New Testament . . . These are spoken secretly or openly, they are written on scraps of paper, swallowed or worn as charms.[49]

Similar practices were recorded in France, Italy, England and Spain, and were probably typical of popular culture across western Europe.[50] The general acceptance of magical techniques, and the assumption that they could be used for both good and bad purposes, makes it likely that *maleficium* was sometimes attempted. In 1566, the English magician John Walsh described how the words of charms could be reversed to create harmful spells, though he denied ever doing such things.[51] Likewise, the visitors to Weisbaden claimed that spells were performed 'to work harm on others or to do good, to make things better or worse'.[52] With such activities in mind, the author of a recent study of popular culture in England has concluded that those accused of witchcraft were not chosen at random: 'they were those who had cultivated a reputation for witchcraft as a means of survival, who were linked to such people by blood or household ties, or who actually thought that they practised the art of black or white witchcraft'.[53] The reality of magic as a social practice makes it entirely understandable that men and women sometimes suspected their neighbours of witchcraft, whatever the actual consequences of magical acts.

The credibility of a witch cult

While it is relatively easy to accept the rational basis for fears of *maleficium* in early modern Europe, it is more difficult perhaps to understand the less common but important idea of a clandestine, Devil-worshipping cult. After all, there was no empirical evidence to support this belief, except the confessions of alleged cult members. Many of these were obtained through torture. Why, then, did the concept of a witch cult seem so credible to educated Europeans? In part, the answer lies in the conventions of scholarly debate in early modern Europe. As Sydney Anglo has observed, much of the evidence for satanic witchcraft was derived from scripture and the writings of the church fathers. These citations were generally regarded as authoritative, and carried at least as much weight as empirical investigations into the alleged activities of witches.[54] Viewed in this light, the *Malleus Maleficarum* made a very strong case for the existence of satanic witchcraft, since the genuineness of its classical sources was beyond question. It is striking that allegations of collective witchcraft did not lead to prosecutions on those occasions when the authorities sought corroborating evidence for confessions, as was the case in Spain in 1610, and across much of western Europe from around 1680. Once the citation of classical sources was no longer regarded as sufficent evidence, it was much harder for academics to prove the existence of the crime; but this emphasis on empirical inquiry was not widely accepted among scholars until the latter part of the seventeenth century. Belief in the witch cult was also encouraged by changes in information technology. The development of print from the late fifteenth century allowed information about witchcraft to spread quickly and widely among the literate minority of the European population. It also helped to consolidate the myth of a satanic cult, since accounts of trials were reproduced in demonologies that were subsequently used by those responsible for conducting further prosecutions. The result was a largely self-referential and self-perpetuating body of literature, which encouraged exactly the kind of confessions that could be fed back into the genre as 'evidence'. On occasions, scholarly writers referred explicitly to the consistency of confessions as proof of a satanic cult. In 1595, for example, Nicholas Rémy observed that witches often described how they smeared an ointment on their bodies to enable them to fly to the sabbat. He noted that 'they are even particular in describing its colour, which provides further evidence that the matter is no dream, but visible and perceptible to the eyes'.[55] With the benefit of hindsight, it is tempting to mock the apparent naivety of such claims; but we should remember that the potentially distorting effects of print culture were impossible to anticipate, much as the impact of the internet cannot be adequately predicted today.

This leads to one final point about the rationality of witch beliefs. During the late twentieth century, a set of strikingly similar ideas attracted the support of highly educated men and women in northern America and western Europe. The belief in secret satanic organisations devoted to the sexual abuse, murder and cannibalism of young children led to a series of legal proceedings in the United States and Great Britain between 1982 and 1990, most of which collapsed through lack of acceptable evidence. The issue of 'satanic abuse' continues to arouse intense controversy, and is examined in detail in Part 10. While it is possible that some satanic cults do exist, it is undeniable that many of the specific allegations about them have proved to be false, despite the passionate advocacy of some psychotherapists and social workers.[56] This has led historians like Robin Briggs and Robert Walinski-Keihl to suggest that satanic abuse is an updated version of the myth of a witch cult, while the anthropologist Philip Stevens has claimed that 'a demonology is flourishing, and variants of it have inspired some local witch-hunts among our contemporaries'.[57] If these claims are accurate, it appears that the capacity to believe in satanic witchcraft was not confined to the early modern period. Equally, the pursuit of satanic child abusers shows that the business of witch-finding can be conducted by perfectly reasonable and methodical people, motivated chiefly by their compassion for the apparent victims of a terrible crime. When the horrors they describe prove to be no more substantial than the imagined sabbats of the sixteenth century, it is a powerful reminder that the origins of witch beliefs are not to be found in superstition or hysteria. Rather, such beliefs were the products of social and political circumstances that can recur even today.

Notes

1   Fictitious accounts of English witchcraft included later editions of the story of Mother Shipton, such as *The Strange and Wonderful History of Mother Shipton* (1682).

2   Margaret Murray, *The Witch Cult in Western Europe* (Clarendon, Oxford 1921). Murray's theory of a witch cult was echoed in early editions of Christopher Hill's textbook *Reformation to Industrial Revolution* (2nd edn, Penguin, Harmondsworth 1969), 109. Her work was regarded as sufficiently important to merit a detailed critique in Norman Cohn's *Europe's Inner Demons* (2nd edn, Pimlico, London 1993), 152–60.

3   Crowley reminds modern-day witches that thousands of their fellows perished in the sixteenth and seventeenth centuries. Vivianne Crowley, *Wicca: The Old Religion in the New Age* (Aquarian, Wellingborough 1989), 51. See also Doreen Valiente, *An ABC*

of Witchcraft (Robert Hale, London 1984). For a non-religious work making similar claims, see Colin Wilson, *Witches* (Crescent, New York 1981).

4   See, for example, Mary Daly, *Gyn/Ecology: The Metaethics of Radical Feminism* (Women's Press, London 1978).

5   For a fascinating account of the origins and claims of the modern witchcraft movement, see T. H. Luhrmann, *Persuasions to the Witches' Craft* (Blackwell, Oxford 1989).

6   Alan Kors and Edward Peters, eds, *Witchcraft in Europe: A Documentary History* (University of Pennsylvania Press, Philadelphia 1972), 259.

7   M. J. Kephart, 'Rationalists vs. Romantics Among Scholars of Witchcraft', in Max Marwick, ed., *Witchcraft and Sorcery* (2nd edn, Penguin, Harmondworth 1982), 341.

8   Kors and Peters, *Witchcraft*, 101.

9   Henri Boguet, *An Examen of Witches*, trans. Montague Summers (John Rodker, London 1929), 5.

10   Louise Jackson, Chapter 26 in this collection.

11   The means by which the Devil, as a disembodied spirit, was able to copulate with witches was discussed at length in the *Malleus Maleficarum*. See Kors and Peters, *Witchcraft*, 136–45.

12   Cohn, *Europe's Inner Demons*, 152–60.

13   Gustav Henningsen, *The Witches' Advocate: Basque Witchcraft and the Spanish Inquisition* (University of Nevada Press, Reno 1980).

14   Carlo Ginzburg, *The Night Battles: Witchcraft and Agrarian Cults in the Sixteenth and Seventeenth Centuries*, trans. John and Anne Tedeschi (Routledge, London 1983), 6.

15   Gábor Klaniczay, *The Uses of Supernatural Power* (Princeton University Press, Princeton, NJ 1990), ch. 8.

16   Boguet, *Examen*, 46–7.

17   James, *Daemonologie*, 39.

18   Robert Walinski-Keihl, 'The Devil's Children: Child Witch Trials in Early Modern Germany', *Continuity and Change*, 11 (2), (1996), 177.

19   R. Seton-Watson, ed., *Tudor Studies* (London 1924), 72–4.

20   For a nice example, see *The Wonderfull Discoverie of the Witchcrafts of Margaret and Phillip Flower* (1619), reprinted in Barbara Rosen, ed., *Witchcraft in England, 1558–1618* (University of Massachusetts Press 1992), 377.

21   James, *Daemonologie*, 74–5.

22   Bengt Ankarloo and Gustav Henningsen, eds, *Early Modern European Witchcraft: Centres and Peripheries* (Clarendon, Oxford 1993), ch. 7.

23   William Gouge, *Of Domesticall Duties* (2nd edn, 1626), 282.

24   Boguet, *Examen*, 60.

25   James, *Daemonologie*, 36.

26   Boguet, *Examen*, 1–3.

27   Alan Macfarlane, *Witchcraft in Tudor and Stuart England* (2nd edn, Routledge, London 1999); Keith Thomas, *Religion and the Decline of Magic* (Weidenfeld and Nicolson, London 1971).

28   For Denmark, see Jens Christian Johansen's chapter in Ankarloo and Henningsen's *Early Modern European Witchcraft*, ch. 13; for the 1645–7 trials in England, see James Sharpe, *Instruments of Darkness: Witchcraft in England, 1550–1750* (Hamish Hamilton, London 1996), ch. 5.

29   Owen Davies, *Witchcraft, Magic and Culture, 1736–1951* (Manchester University Press 1999); Henningsen, *Witches' Advocate*, 12–13.

30   For Luther's views on witchcraft and the Devil, see Heiko Oberman, *Luther: Man Between God and the Devil* (Fontana, London 1993), 102–6.

31   Kors and Peters, *Witchcraft*, 242–3.

32   *Newes from Scotland* (Edinburgh 1592), 17, 29.

33   Lyndal Roper, *Oedipus and the Devil: Witchcraft, Sexuality and Religion in Early Modern Europe* (Routledge, London 1994), ch. 8.

34   Boguet, *Examen*, 181–2.

35   Lauderdale recounted this story in a letter to Richard Baxter, which he published in *The Certainty of the World of Spirits* (1691), 90–1.

36   John Darrel, *The Triall of Maist. Dorrell* (1599), 66.

37   Edmund Kern, Chapter 13 in this collection.

38   Lyndal Roper, *The Holy Household: Women and Morals in Reformation Augsburg* (Clarendon, Oxford 1989).

39   Thomas Robisheaux, 'Peasants and Pastors', *Social History*, 6 (1986), 281–300; Anthony Fletcher, *Gender, Sex and Subordination in England, 1500–1800* (Yale University Press, New Haven, Conn. 1995).

40   Baxter, *Certainty*, 47–52.

41   Robin Briggs, 'Many Reasons Why: Witchcraft and the Problem of Multiple Explanation', in Jonathan Barry, Marianne Hester and Gareth Roberts, eds, *Witchcraft in Early Modern Europe* (Cambridge University Press 1996), 51.

42   For a discussion of animal trials in mediaeval and early modern Europe, see Esther Cohen, 'Law, Folklore and Animal Lore', *Past and Present*, 110 (1986), 6–37.

43   Bodleian Library, Oxford, Ashmole MS 412, 131r, 150r, 150v.

44   R. Hopton, 'African Traditional Thought and Western Science', in M. Young, ed., *Knowledge and Control* (Addison Wesley, Cambridge, Mass. 1971).

45   Roy Porter, *A Social History of Madness* (2nd edn, Phoenix, London 1996), 82–93.

46   Boguet, *Examen*, 47.

47   Rosen, *Witchcraft*, 254.

48   Davies, *Witchcraft*, 41.

49   This report is taken from Gerald Strauss, 'Success and Failure in the German Reformation', *Past and Present*, 67 (1975), 62–3.

50   For an excellent collection of sources relating to popular and learned magic, see P. G. Maxwell-Stuart, *The Occult in Early Modern Europe: A Documentary History* (Macmillan, London 1999).

51   Rosen, *Witchcraft*, 70–1.

52   Strauss, 'Success and Failure', 63.

53   Barry Reay, *Popular Cultures in England, 1550–1750* (Longman, London 1998), 130.

54   Sydney Anglo, 'Evident Authority and Authoritative Evidence', in Anglo, ed., *The Damned Art* (Routledge and Kegan Paul, London 1976), 1–31.

55   Kors and Peters, *Witchcraft*, 245.

56   A Department of Health investigation into allegations in Britain was conducted by Jean La Fontaine in 1992. This found that elements of 'ritual' were involved in a small number of cases, but dismissed the idea of organised satanism.

57   Robin Briggs, *Witches and Neighbours* (HarperCollins, London 1996), 410–11; Philip Stevens, 'The Demonology of Satanism', in J. T. Richardson, J. Best and D. G. Bromley, eds, *The Satanism Scare* (Lexington Books, New York 1991), 35–6.

PART ONE

Mediaeval Origins

WRITING IN THE LAST QUARTER of the twelfth century, the chronicler Ralph of Coggeshall described the extraordinary climax of a heresy trial in the French town of Rheims. The trial ended with the burning of an unnamed young woman, who faced her death so 'steadfastly and eagerly' that it astonished even those responsible for her prosecution. The woman was a humble member of a heretical community whose alleged leader was tried alongside her, and was also sentenced to the flames. The older woman escaped her punishment, however, through the intervention of a demon:

> When the fire had been lighted in the city and the officials were about to drag them to the punishment decreed, that mistress of vile error exclaimed, 'Oh foolish and unjust judges, do you think now to burn me in your flames?' ... With these words, she suddenly pulled a ball of thread from her bosom and threw it out of a large window, but keeping the end of the thread in her hands; then in a loud voice, audible to all, she said 'Catch!' At the word, she was lifted from the earth right before everyone's eyes and followed the ball out [of] the window in rapid flight, sustained, we believe, by the ministry of the evil spirits who once caught Simon Magus up into the air. What became of that wicked woman or wither she was transported, the onlookers could in no wise discover.

This bizarre story underlined Ralph's conviction that the ultimate source of all heresy was the Devil. The link between religious dissent and Satan was reinforced in the conclusion of his account. Here he offered a brief exposition of the doctrines held by the two women, which conformed closely to the known beliefs of the Cathars, a heretical Christian sect that flourished in southern France in the late twelfth and early thirteenth centuries. At the end of this passage, Ralph added a dark rumour that was apparently circulating about the Cathars' practices: 'Some also say that in their subterranean haunts they perform execrable sacrifices to their Lucifer at stated times, and that there they enact certain sacrilegious infamies.'[1]

Ralph's account suggests that one of the key elements of the theory of witchcraft – the belief in a clandestine society of Devil-worshippers – was already known to some educated men in the High Middle Ages. Indeed, the charge of meeting in secret to perform 'sacrilegious infamies' had been made against dissenting groups since antiquity, when it was levelled against the early Christians.[2] It would be misleading, however, to assume that the threat of witchcraft was a major preoccupation in mediaeval Europe. While the heretics at Rheims were explicitly linked to the Devil in Ralph's chronicle, and rumoured to have participated in diabolical rites, they were formally accused of heresy rather than satanism; and his account makes no reference to the practice of harmful magic, which played a crucial role in the witch trials of the sixteenth and seventeenth centuries. Trials for witchcraft were uncommon at the time of the events in Rheims, and this remained the case for at least a hundred years. It was once believed that major witch persecutions took place in France in the early fourteenth century, but the documents supporting this claim have been exposed as forgeries.[3] This discovery has led to what one study has described as a 'chronological revolution' in the history of witchcraft, 'which has obliged us to withdraw the phenomenon from mediaeval history and redefine it as a Renaissance problem'.[4] In other words, it appears that the crime of witchcraft emerged in the early period of the modern age, and should not be regarded as a typical feature of the Middle Ages.

Richard Kieckhefer shows in Chapter 1 that the modern concept of witchcraft developed gradually in the course of the fifteenth century. It was in this period that the ideas of nocturnal Devil-worship, the satanic pact, and harmful magic were combined in a series of major trials, though he notes that such trials were still less common than prosecutions for simple sorcery. Before the Renaissance period, the various elements that would eventually coalesce into the witchcraft stereotype surfaced occasionally in the prosecution of magicians and heretics, and politically inspired actions like the suppression of the order of the Knights Templars in fourteenth-century France. These precedents provided the raw material from which jurists and theologians later composed the fantasy of satanic witchcraft. Kieckhefer's work was first published in 1976, shortly after the appearance of Norman Cohn's *Europe's Inner Demons* (1975), which also traced the origins of witchcraft in the late Middle Ages. Like Kieckhefer, Cohn identified the fifteenth century as the critical period, and argued that the first major persecutions were targeted against the Italian Fraticelli, dissident followers of St Francis of Assisi. In Chapter 2, Cohn reconstructs the demonisation of heretics in the late mediaeval period, and argues persuasively that the charges of magic and diabolism made against them were fictions imposed by their prosecutors, with no basis in the actual practices of the groups concerned.

The work of Kieckhefer and Cohn has made a lasting impression on witchcraft research, and one that extends well beyond the historical period with which they were directly concerned. First, they established a chronology of the early witch-hunts that has been accepted by all serious scholars in the field. Second, they under-mined the once-popular view that a pagan 'witch cult' existed in the Middle Ages, forcing academics to find other explanations for the appearance of witch trials during the Renaissance. If anxieties about a non-existent, clandestine sect of Devil-worshipping magicians slowly gathered momentum during the fifteenth century, then the source of these anxieties can presumably be found in the circumstances of that period. Kieckhefer and Cohn offer various possible explanations. In Chapter 1, Kieckhefer suggests that the introduction of inquisitorial procedures in the European courts, and the abolition of the principle of *talion*, whereby lay accusers faced serious penalties if their allegations could not be proven, made it much easier to bring successful prosecutions for secret crimes like witchcraft. Confessions were also much easier to obtain as the use of torture became more widely accepted. He also argues that the development of printing from the mid-1400s allowed news of trials to circulate quickly, encouraging prosecutions to spread. Norman Cohn has argued that fears of a satanic cult at the heart of Christian society might also have reflected wider concerns about the threat of social and political disorder. As the ultimate symbol of chaos, the Devil emerged as the natural leader of a secret plot to destroy Christendom. The attempt to eliminate witches was, therefore, 'an urge to purify the world through the annihilation of some category of human beings imagined as agents of corruption and incarnations of evil'.[5]

By the late fifteenth century, then, a body of learned theory had emerged that made possible the persecution of an imaginary sect of Devil-worshipping witches. This was one of the foundations of the European witch-hunt of the sixteenth and seventeenth centuries; but it did not make that event inevitable. Kieckhefer and Cohn have shown that elite groups were increasingly concerned with the threat of satanism at the close of the Middle Ages, and this concern was expressed in a series of witch trials; but the number of these trials was still relatively small, despite the lethal potential of the ideas promulgated by men like the authors of the *Malleus Maleficarum* (1486). The much greater persecutions that followed were possible only because of the social, religious and political circumstances of early modern Europe. It is only with the benefit of hindsight that the sufferings of late medi-aeval heretics – described so movingly here by Norman Cohn – can be viewed as part of a great European campaign to rid the world of witches.

Notes

1   Ralph's text is reproduced in Walter Wakefield and Austin Evans, *Heresies of the High Middle Ages* (Columbia University Press, New York 1969), 251–4.

2   See Norman Cohn, *Europe's Inner Demons* (2nd edn, Pimlico, London 1993), ch. 1.

3   See Chapter 1 by Richard Kieckhefer. Kieckhefer's conclusions were confirmed inde-pendently by Cohn in *Europe's Inner Demons*, 187–93.

4   Gustav Henningsen and Bengt Ankarloo, eds, *Early Modern European Witchcraft* (Clarendon, Oxford 1990), editors' introduction, 2.

5   Cohn, *Europe's Inner Demons*, preface xi.

Richard Kieckhefer

WITCH TRIALS IN MEDIAEVAL
EUROPE

I N COMPARISON WITH THE MASS PERSECUTION of following
centuries, the witch trials of the years 1300–1500 were few and sporadic. There
was seldom a sustained effort in any one community to exterminate witches, as
occurred frequently in the sixteenth and seventeenth centuries. Even in years when
there were multiple trials, they generally occurred in widely separate towns. Yet
historians have rightly viewed the fourteenth and fifteenth centuries as witnessing
the initial stages of the European witch craze. It was during this period that prosecution of witches first gained real momentum. And the intensified hunts of the
sixteenth and seventeenth centuries can be explained only as outgrowths of an
earlier obsession.

Even during the period 1300–1500, though, one must distinguish various stages
of prosecution. On the one hand, the rate of frequency changed sharply; on the
other, the nature of the accusations altered significantly. Bearing in mind both the
intensity and the form of witch-hunting, one can perceive four broad periods during
the fourteenth and fifteenth centuries, extending roughly from 1300 to 1330, from
1330 to 1375, from 1375 to 1435, and from 1435 to 1500.

During the first period, the rate of frequency was low indeed. For all of Europe,
the trials occurred on an average of roughly one each year. Slightly more than half
of these come from France; among other countries, only England and Germany
had significant numbers of witch-hunts.[1] Probably the most remarkable feature of
the trials during this first phase is their political character. Almost two-thirds of
them involved prominent ecclesiastical or secular figures, sometimes as suspects
but most commonly as sorcerers' victims. The political climate was ideal for foster-
ing the obsession that leaders everywhere were being attacked through the
surreptitious weapons of sorcery. In France, the Capetian dynasty had lost the
blessing of longevity which had favored its members for more than three centuries.
In the early fourteenth century the last four Capetian kings died, all within a space
of twelve years; it was easy to imagine that they had succumbed to bewitchment.
Suspicions of this kind had arisen earlier, as when the nephew of the bishop of

Bayeux went to his death in 1278 for allegedly attempting sorcery against Philip III. In the early years of the fourteenth century, however, the charge became virtually habitual as an explanation for deaths within the royal family, or as a credible excuse for prosecution among political rivals. The trial of the Templars no doubt helped to heighten fear of witchcraft, though the Templars were accused of diabolism rather than sorcery. It was during the course of their famous trial, in any event, that the bishop of Troyes stood trial for image magic and invocation of the Devil – practices which had supposedly succeeded in bringing the demise of the queen, though they had failed in their further objective of killing other members of the French court.[2] A few years later Enguerrand de Marigny was executed along with a female associate for using image magic against Louis X and Charles of Valois. And with the rapid succession of monarchs who fell ill and died young, the charge arose seven more times within the next few years.[3]

The papacy was not subject to the same difficulties. Pope Clement V was sickly for much of his pontificate, but he reigned from 1305 to 1314, which was a respectable length of time considering that he, like most popes, was elected at an advanced age. And many churchmen would have been gratified if his successor John XXII had lived less than his eighteen years after election to the papacy. Yet the papal court was ridden with factionalism, which generally followed national lines: the Italian cardinals, resentful of French domination in the Avignonese papacy, were openly hostile to the Frenchmen, while the latter group was divided by the formation of a specifically Gascon faction. It was the animosity of these groups that led to a two-year vacancy between the death of Clement V and the election of John XXII; no one faction was powerful enough to secure the election of its own candidate. Nor did hostilities between Italians and Frenchmen cease altogether when a French cardinal at last became John XXII. The atmosphere of contention fostered lasting suspicion. In addition, John appears to have been naturally superstitious, and given to such practices as keeping a magical snake-skin to detect poisoned food and drink.[4]

Through most of his pontificate John was active in prosecution of sorcerers and invokers of demons. The year after his election, Bishop Hugo Géraud of Cahors went to the stake for involvement in a conspiracy against the pope and certain cardinals. The bishop and his accomplices had allegedly employed wax images and other magical objects to bring about the pontiff's ruin; after the plot was detected, various clerics at the papal court confessed under torture that they had dabbled in sundry forms of witchcraft. Two years later, the Franciscan Bernard Delicieux, earlier a harsh critic of inquisitorial procedures was brought to trial on charges of witchcraft; he was acquitted of one charge, that of attempting to bewitch one of John XXII's predecessors through drinks and powders. But on the grounds of possession of magical books he was sentenced to life imprisonment. On three occasions – in 1318, 1320 and 1326 – Pope John took the initiative in the investigation of those persons in southern France who were forming pacts with the Devil, employing image magic, abusing the sacraments, and committing other such offences. In a trial with clear political implications, the archbishop of Milan and an inquisitor charged that Matteo and Galeazzo Visconti, two of John's main political adversaries, had entered a pact with the Devil, had invoked the Devil on numerous occasions, and had used sorcery against the pope. Meanwhile the pope issued commands to the bishop of Ancona and an inquisitor, directing them to prosecute other political enemies on the charges of idolatry, heresy, and diabolism. And on two occasions, the pope aided in investigation of sorcery directed against the French kings.

Likewise, the English monarch Edward II, whose weak hold on the throne led to deposition in 1327, found witches among his opponents. Even in the early years of his reign, a rebel was found who had allegedly made a pact with the Devil to obtain the crown.[5] Less directly affecting the throne was the trial of Edward I's treasurer and minister, Walter Langton, Bishop of Coventry. Charged before the pope of having formed a pact with the Devil and kissed him on the posterior, Langton received the king's support, and ultimately obtained acquittal.[6]

The best known political trials of the early fourteenth century are those of the Templars and of Dame Alice Kyteler. The Templars, tried on the urging of the French crown, were convicted of charges that were certainly exaggerated, if not wholly fabricated. In addition to sodomy, blasphemy, and other species of immorality, they are supposed to have venerated the Devil in the guise of an animal named Baphomet.[7] Whereas the motives in many political trials are only vaguely ascertainable, the desire of Philip IV to confiscate the Templars' abundant wealth is notorious. Almost as apparent were the political motives in the trial of Alice Kyteler, an aristocratic lady of Ireland. This woman had family relations with numerous political leaders, and the best accounts of her trial explain it as largely an outgrowth of feuds among these aristocratic families.[8] Her accusers charged that she had killed three husbands and reduced a fourth to debility through sorcery; she had furthermore maintained an imp named Robert Artisson, and engaged in diabolical rituals.

The prominence of the sorcerers and victims in these trials is of the utmost importance. Though in some instances the accusers may have raised the charges cynically as ways of undermining their opponents, in the majority of cases the charges were no doubt based on sincere belief in the reality of witchcraft. Yet the fact that these trials reflect concern with sorcery and invocation is less important in the long run than the likelihood that they intensified this concern throughout western Europe. The notoriety and suggestive force of these episodes may have been largely responsible for the gradual increase in witch prosecution through the following generations.

Apart from the political character of prosecution during the first phase, its most significant feature is the mildness of the allegations. Sorcery was by far the most common charge; invocation was not so frequent, but was known; diabolism, though, was extremely rare, and even when alleged it was usually not described in great detail. Even in the trials of Walter Langton, the Templars, and Alice Kyteler, the depictions of Devil-worship are less lurid than in later trials. Pope John XXII routinely spoke of pacts with the Devil, yet did not specify whether these agreements led to diabolism or merely to invocation of the Devil. One of the more elaborate cases was that of the Carmelite friar Peter Recordi, who was charged with a peculiar mixture of sorcery, invocation, and mild diabolism.[9] On various occasions, Recordi had made five wax images and performed conjurations and invocation of demons over them. He had poured over these images poisons and blood extracted 'in a terrible and horrible manner' from a toad. He had then placed the figures on a table, covered them with a cloth, and sprinkled them with blood from his own nostrils, mixed with saliva, as an immolation to the Devil. After this, he placed the images under the thresholds of women he wished to seduce. Through these means he had succeeded in seducing three women, and had he not been transferred to a new residence by his order he would have ensnared two more. After the images had accomplished their purpose, he cast them into the water, completing the ritual by sacrificing a butterfly to the Devil. He had believed that such figures had power not only to constrain women, but to bring afflictions upon them if they refused his advances. To test their magical properties, he had once stuck one of the figures in the stomach, and blood oozed out. Such, in any event, were the charges brought forth. Yet even here the classic elements of diabolism that later became important, the sabbat and all its attendant ceremonies, are absent.

Long before it appeared independently or in connection with sorcery, the charge of diabolism had been used in trials against heretics. No matter how rigorous their moral codes might be, mediaeval heretics such as the Cathars and Waldensians were believed to reject moral law entirely – a position known as antinomianism. They allegedly held nocturnal orgies, and in some instances were thought of as paying homage to the Devil. In a few trials of the early fourteenth century charges of diabolism seem to have been made against heretics, in the specific form of Luciferanism. The basic premise of Luciferanism, if indeed anyone actually subscribed to the doctrine, seems to have been that Lucifer would eventually attain salvation, and would even rule over creation in place of the Christian God. Churchmen accused Luciferans of venerating the Devil in underground assemblies. To be sure, in most instances the charge of Luciferanism is related only in chronicles, usually of questionable veracity. Thus it is not even fully certain that the accusation actually arose in the heresy trials, much less that it was accurate. In any case, the allegation was set forth a few times in the years 1300–30, though its importance was apparently minimal.

The second period, from around 1330 to about 1375, is like the first in that the accusations were still for the most part relatively tame, but unlike it in that trials connected with important public figures were virtually unknown. Changes in the political environment may have influenced the character of prosecution. Edward III and Philip VI brought stable government to England and France, and though there were two trials in 1331 for attempts to bewitch the French king the furor quickly subsided. John XXII died in 1334, and his successor Benedict XII turned his witch-hunting zeal toward unimportant suspects. This shift occurred in part, perhaps, because the charge of witchcraft had been overworked during the first thirty years of the century. The political trials of those years had aroused widespread attention, and may have aggravated general concern about witchcraft, but may also have made people skeptical about accusations that arose specifically from political or personal motives. Possibly also there were would-be assassins who, having witnessed the prosecutions of the early fourteenth century, were less inclined to view sorcery as a safe method for murder with impunity.

The fact that stands out is that, for whatever reason, known political trials cease abruptly shortly after the year 1330. Largely because of the decrease in political trials, the rate of prosecution in the second phase was slightly less than in the first. With a few exceptions, the trials occurred in France and Germany, with only a scattering of cases in England and Italy. Once again, apart from a few trials for Luciferanism, the charge of diabolism was rare and undeveloped.[10]

In short, until about 1375 the emphasis was mainly on sorcery, and to a lesser extent on invocation; diabolism seldom arose in the allegations, and when it came forth at all it took a vague or subdued form. One possible exception to this rule, however, is a series of trials at Toulouse and Carcassonne, in which diabolism is supposed to have figured prominently even in the mid-fourteenth century. The source for these trials is of some interest in itself. In 1829, Etienne-Léon de Lamothe-Langon published a three-volume history of the French Inquisition, including lengthy translations or paraphrases from inquisitorial records. By the late 1800s these documents were nowhere to be found, but at the turn of the century Joseph Hansen reprinted the relevant excerpts from Lamothe-Langon's work. Ever since then they have constituted perhaps the most important single body of sources for early European witch trials and as such have received the detailed attention of historians. Indeed, some scholars have built critical arguments upon them.

What historians have failed to recognize, however, is that there is serious reason to believe that Lamothe-Langon's texts are forgeries. The highly atypical nature of the allegations might reflect genuinely anomalous circumstances, and the mysterious disappearance of his documents would in itself prove nothing, though such losses were more common before and during the French Revolution. But when one couples these facts with certain inaccuracies and anachronisms in the reports, credibility is strained. In particular, Lamothe-Langon uses the word 'Sabbath' in rendering documents for fourteenth-century diabolical assemblies, though this word did not begin to displace the term 'synagogue' or 'synagogue of Satan' until well into the fifteenth century. A review of Lamothe-Langon's biography does little to reinforce one's confidence in the value of his account. He devised other known forgeries; to persuade his contemporaries that he came from a long-established noble family he concocted several genealogies showing his illustrious ancestors. His reputation was based mainly on his prolific authorship of popular novels, particularly romans noirs, dealing with such subjects as vampires and demons. In addition, his history of the Inquisition was one of a series of polemic works – all of them bitterly attacking agencies of repression – which had been sparked by the censorship he himself had encountered. Hence, he had motivation to embellish his account, and quite possibly to invent substantial portions of it. Lurid details of inquisitorial work against witches might indeed have stirred more widespread revulsion in nineteenth-century France than a less sensational recounting of anti-heretical proceedings. One further consideration is relevant: there were in fact inquisitorial documents from Carcassonne that survived into modern times, but were lost possibly during the French Revolution, if not earlier. By the mid-nineteenth century, in any event, only a summary inventory of these documents survived or had been uncovered; it was published in 1855. And there is no correspondence whatsoever between this inventory and the materials in Lamothe-Langon. In delineating the general pattern of early witch prosecution, it is important to note that Lamothe-Langon's evidence is at best highly questionable.[11]

It was during the third period, then, roughly 1375 to 1435, that a twofold change took place. Throughout these years there was first of all a steady increase in the number of trials for witchcraft in general, and second an intensification of concern for diabolism. The rise of prosecution during this period may in part be an optical illusion caused by the general increase in extant judicial records from these years. But it is surely not coincidental that the later part of the fourteenth century was the period when in many places municipal courts began to adopt inquisitorial procedure. Once such procedure was adopted, even if the judges were not yet familiar with theological notions of diabolism there would be machinery appropriate for handling sorcery charges that arose among the populace. Perhaps the most important feature of inquisitorial procedure, for present purposes, is that it did away with the earlier custom of judicial penalties for an accuser who failed to substantiate his charges. In trials for sorcery it would be particularly difficult for the accuser to prove his case, because the alleged culprit was not connected with the victim in the usual ways; the sorcerer might carry out his deed several blocks away from the scene of the crime. Prior to the development of inquisitorial justice, it must therefore have been particularly dangerous to accuse someone of sorcery or of witchcraft generally. In one peculiar case from Strasbourg in the mid-fifteenth century the earlier, accusatory procedure was revived: a man accused a woman of weather magic, and when he was unable to prove his claim he himself was drowned. If those judicial rules had been maintained throughout Europe, no doubt very few people would have raised accusations of this kind, difficult as they were to prove. After the introduction of inquisitorial procedure, one might expect a surge of prosecution such as in fact occurred. And to some degree the concern with trials for sorcery would be self-perpetuating; under appropriate circumstances the sensation aroused by one trial could generate a chain of further trials. Indirectly, the spurt of witch trials beginning around 1375 may also have been influenced by the plague. The long-term social effects of the plague, particularly in those areas where it brought migration from the countryside into the cities, may have stimulated social friction that could have aggravated the preoccupation with witchcraft.

It has also been suggested that inquisitors began prosecuting witches – or began prosecuting people *as* witches – when they had succeeded in exterminating Cathars and Waldensians.[12] It is true that in circumstances in which papal inquisitors faced a shortage of legitimate subjects they frequently tended to focus their attention on religious eccentrics, marginally heretical communities, political subjects, and alleged witches. This was true most of the time in Germany and Spain. But the chronology of witch trials does not suggest that this was a major factor in their development. Catharism was uprooted from southern France, and Waldensianism driven safely underground, by the early fourteenth century. But unless one accepts Lamothe-Langon's evidence, prosecution for sorcery did not gain full momentum until late in the century, and trials for diabolism were not widespread until the following century. The lessened threat from heresies may have been important as a factor which *allowed* ecclesiastical judges to attend to witchcraft, but not as a positive cause of the rise in witch trials. Even apart from the chronological gap between the decline of heresies and the acceleration of witch trials, it should be borne in mind that the trials of this third phase were not led exclusively by inquisitors or other ecclesiastical judges. The connection between the fate of earlier heresy and the intensified obsession with witchcraft is thus tenuous.

The overall acceleration can be traced most clearly for Switzerland, where conditions in modern times have favored the survival of documents that might have been

lost elsewhere. Prior to 1383 there
ritories. In the last decades of the f
each involving a single sorceress —
no judicial proceedings. Around the
in Simmenthal under the secular ju
ies to the Dominican John Nider. T
believe the much later account th
accused of diabolism as well as sor
to their 'little master', repudiated
thirteen infants. When the authori
their hands began to tremble unco
loathsome stench. Yet the judge wa
witches he managed to apprehend

Between the turn of the cen
twenty trials in various towns of Switzerland, notably Lucerne, Basel, and Fribourg.
In most, the charges were simple sorcery. In 1428 there was extensive persecution in Valais; whereas the fragmentary judicial documents speak only of sorcery,
the chronicler John Fründ gives abundant details about a Devil-worshipping cult in
southern Switzerland. According to Fründ, the Devil seeks out men who are in a
state of doubt or despair, and promises to make them rich, powerful, and successful,
and to punish those who have done them harm. First, though, they must dedicate
themselves to him, deny their former faith, and make some kind of sacrifice to him
— a black sheep, one of their bodily limbs (to be claimed after death), or some
other offering. Fründ tells of wild assemblies in which the Devil appeared in bestial
form and encouraged the witches to commit foul deeds; the witches are supposed
to have flown to orgies or elsewhere on chairs that they anointed with an unguent.
Though not typical of Swiss witch cases during this period, this chronicler's account
shows the kind of extravagant detail that was beginning to be associated with maleficent activities.

Italy, like Switzerland, joined with France and Germany in the forefront of
witch persecution during the third period. But there is another, more important
respect in which Italy took the lead at this time: with the exception of the trials in
Simmenthal and Valais, it is from Italy that the only definite instances of prosecution for diabolism come during this phase. Historians have long thought of southern
France as the area in which diabolism and sorcery were joined to form a composite
notion of witchcraft, chiefly because of the evidence proffered by Lamothe-Langon.
Judging from the most reliable records, though, the honor of priority goes instead
to Italy. This adjustment makes the development of witch beliefs more plausible:
instead of finding a thousand trials all at once, with full-blown diabolism prominent
in the charges, one finds gradual evolution and elaboration of witch prosecution. The
trials from Italy during the late fourteenth and early fifteenth centuries were still for
the most part restrained; the allegation of diabolism, though more common, was
still often vague and peripheral. Thus a Florentine subject named Niccolö Consigli
was accused primarily of sorcery, necromancy, and unlicensed exorcism, but an additional charge was that, while imprisoned, he dedicated himself to demons named
Lucifer, Satan and Beelzebub. No further elements of diabolism are mentioned in
the records of his proceedings.[13]

In a small minority of Italian trials, one finds a mixture of charges that cannot be categorized as either sorcery or typical diabolism. For example, a Milanese woman who went before an inquisitor in 1384 confessed that each Thursday evening she went to an assembly led by a woman named Oriente. There was every kind of animal at this meeting except the ass, which was excluded because of its role in Christ's passion. Oriente gave instruction to her followers, foretold future events and revealed occult matters. After their deaths, the followers' souls were received by the signora.

Perhaps the most important statement by the accused woman is that she had never confessed her involvement in these activities, because it had never occurred to her that they were sinful. The details of this case, which do not at all fit the stereotype of contemporary demonology, suggest that the woman was merely engaging in a popular festivity or ritual. The gatherings that she attended may have survived from before the conversion of the Italian countryside to Christianity; yet it would be misleading to speak of them as conscious and deliberate pagan survivals since the participants seem to have viewed themselves as Christians, despite the reservations that churchmen evidently held. In an age when notions of diabolism were becoming important, however, a sinister interpretation of these activities lay readily at hand. When this woman relapsed into her illicit activities she again fell prey to an inquisitor, and this time went to the stake for outright diabolism.[14]

Why did diabolism enter into witch trials during this period? The component elements of diabolism – veneration of Satan, nefarious assemblies, flight through the air, formation of a pact, and so forth – had been known for centuries. They had arisen in trials of heretics as early as the eleventh century. In the course of the thirteenth and fourteenth centuries, jurists and theologians tended increasingly to view witchcraft as a form of heresy. The theological faculty of the University of Paris deliberated in 1398 whether *maleficia,* or acts of sorcery, entailed idolatry and apostasy if they were accomplished through a tacit or express pact with the Devil. The conclusion reached was that such deeds did involve idolatry and apostasy, and were thus tantamount to heresy. This decision – which was merely the culmination of a series of writings to the same basic effect – was intended to justify the prosecution of witchcraft by inquisitors, whose main task was supposed to be the extirpation of heresy. A secondary result of this definition of witchcraft as heresy was that the stereotypes earlier found in heresy trials now increasingly transferred to witch trials.

The new obsession with diabolism was also related to developments in the theological literature of the late fourteenth and early fifteenth centuries, which set forth all the elements of diabolism in great, pornographic detail. The first of these writings were brief treatises, or sections in judicial manuals; for the most part they were technical works, yet they evidently circulated widely among the people engaged in prosecution. They both symptomized and augmented the concern with witchcraft among the educated elite. Whether this literature in itself was enough to stimulate the increase in witch trials is another question. For present purposes, it is sufficient to note the correlation between the literary and judicial correlation may be extended one step further: it is not surprising that the first well authenticated series of trials for diabolism occurred in Italy; it was there that legal scholarship was most developed, and it was in the Italian court that one might expect to find ideas of the literate elite reflected in the judicial practice.

The full force of the new composite notion of witchcraft came only in the fourth phase of witch prosecution, from around 1435 to 1500. This is the longest of the four stages, and in virtually every way the most important. Trials were particularly frequent during the years 1455–60 and 1480–5, while during the intervening years the rate of prosecution remained higher than it had been in any previous period. The intense witch-hunting of this stage anticipated, if it did not equal, the witch craze of the sixteenth and seventeenth centuries. Once again there is correlation between judicial and literary developments. Around the year 1435, an extended and non-technical account of Devil-worship was produced with the fifth book of John Nider's *Formicarius*. Further writings followed; the publication of Jacob Sprenger and Henry Institoris's *Malleus Maleficarum* in 1486 made available a fully developed manual for witch-hunters. Even if these writings were not solely responsible for the acceleration of trials, they surely must have contributed greatly towards that result.

By far the majority of cases during this final period occurred in France, Germany, and Switzerland. Only a few took place in England and Italy, and virtually none in further countries. Once again, the majority of trials were for sorcery alone, or for vaguely specified 'witchcraft', with no specific allegation of diabolism. Yet in addition there were now many trials throughout Europe in which diabolism was charged, and when it came forth at all it was usually the prominent allegation. Thus, more than any previous period, this fourth phase was a time of sensational trials. Some of the earlier political trials – those of the early fourteenth century, and especially that of Joan of Arc in 1431 had aroused widespread attention. But in the later fifteenth century the charge of diabolism or even sorcery by itself, regardless of political implications, was enough to produce a dramatic episode. In the mid-fifteenth century an epidemic that struck a French town resulted in vigilante prosecution of sorceresses thought to be culpable; the affair aroused such attention that the king himself intervened, and punished the local officials for failure to maintain order. A famous trial that began a few years later at Arras led to hearings before the parlement of Paris. By the end of the century, secular and ecclesiastical dignitaries commonly recognized a duty to purge their lands of the menace: examples such as Sigismund of Tirol or Innocent VIII are merely the best known. Nor was the concern limited to ruling circles. The above-mentioned case of vigilante justice, as well as other incidents, suggests that the people at large were keenly aware of the supposed problem.

Three examples may suffice to epitomize the witch persecutions of this period. In 1459, a woman named Catherine Simon went before the secular authorities at Andermatt, and confessed that one Jagli Jeger had taught her the art of witchcraft. He had given her a box with salve, with which she could turn herself into a fox, a cat, or a wolf. She also received instruction from a certain woman of Andermatt, and in turn she taught her own daughter Grete how to repay offenses with evil deeds. Catherine went to an assembly at Wallenboden, where she renounced God and the saints, and swore to do the Devil's will; her daughter did likewise at a later meeting. After they had formed this allegiance with the Devil, he accompanied them occasionally as they went about doing harm to their neighbors. On one occasion Catherine turned herself into a fox, and in the Devil's company went out to create an avalanche that killed a woman. Another time she transformed herself into a wolf, while the Devil rode along on another wolf, and together they caused another avalanche. She confessed to numerous further misdeeds: infliction of illnesses, killing of livestock, and still more avalanches. In some instances she was unable to carry out her maleficent desires. She wanted to afflict a man named Henri Krieg with a disease so severe that he would lie in bed for a month or two, but she was unable to approach him to impose the malady. On another occasion she wanted to poison her son-in-law (whether naturally or magically), but failed for lack of the requisite poison. More often than not, however, her sorcery took effect. On her conviction, the court declared that the local executioner shall take her to the place of execution and with his sword divide her into two pieces, of which one shall be her head and the other her body, which shall be so completely severed that a cart-wheel can be rolled between them. Both sections of her remains were then to be burned, and the ashes cast into the Reuss River, 'so that no further harm may ensue therefrom.'

In 1477, in the Savoyard town of Villars-Chabod, a woman called Antonia stubbornly refused to confess what the inquisitor Stephan Hugonodi demanded that she admit. After more than a month the imprisonment and torture to which she was subjected broke her resistance, and at last she gave a lengthy confession. About eleven years earlier, one Massetus Garini found her in a state of sorrow and discontent, and ascertained that she had fallen into financial embarrassment. He told her that she could solve her problems by going with him to a certain friend. Reluctantly she left her home and went to Giessbach, where a synagogue was being held, with a large number of people feasting and dancing. Allaying her apprehensions, Massetus introduced her to a demon named Robinet, in the form of a black man, and said that he was the master of the group. He explained that to obtain her desires she would have to pay homage to this demon by denying God, the Catholic faith, and the blessed Virgin, and taking Robinet as her lord and master. She hesitated. Robinet addressed her in a barely intelligible voice, promising her gold, silver, and other good things; others in attendance likewise encouraged her. Then she consented, kissed the demon's foot, received a 'sign' on her left little finger (which was deadened ever afterward), and trampled and broke a wooden crucifix. The demon gave her a purse full of gold and silver, a container full of unguent and a stick. When she rubbed the stick with the unguent and recited an appropriate incantation, the stick would transport her through the air to the synagogue.

After further feasting and dancing, the members of the sect paid homage to the demon who by now had changed into the form of a black dog by kissing on the posterior. Then the demon cried out 'Meclet! Meclet!' and the fire was put out, whereupon the participants in the festivity gave themselves 'over to each other sexually, in the manner of beasts'. When the meeting was over Antonia went home, only to find that the purse she thought was filled with gold and silver was in fact empty. In further confessions she told of the activities she engaged in as a member of the sect: further synagogues, consumption of human infants, manufacture of maleficent powders from the bones and intestines of these babies, use of such powders to inflict illness and death on men and animals, and desecration of the eucharist.[15]

The last example is a less involved episode, which occurred in Constance at the end of the century. The wife of a cobbler was apprehended for witchcraft, and at first the Devil kept her from confessing her guilt. The only item of information that the judges could extract from her was that the demon to whom she had dedicated herself was named Haintxle. After obtaining this lead, the judges dismissed the woman until the next day, detaining her in a tower prison for the interim. During the night, the Devil went to her in the tower, and confronted her so violently that the watchman thought twenty or thirty horses were loose in the building. At last, the fiend strangled her, and when the authorities entered the next morning they found her lying dead, crumpled over, with her head awry. They placed her body in a cask and floated it down the Rhine. In any event, these were the details furnished by a local chronicler.[16]

As already indicated, even during the years 1435–1500 cases of this kind were less common than trials for mere sorcery, yet the incidence of diabolism was far greater than in any previous period.

Notes

1   In this chapter the designation 'France' is used to apply to all French-speaking territories, and 'Germany' to all German-speaking lands, with the exception of Switzerland, which is treated separately.

2   For more information about this episode, see G. L. Kittredge, *Witchcraft in Old and New England* (Cambridge Mass. 1929), 76, 108 f, and Norman Cohn, *Europe's Inner Demons* (London 1975), 185–92.

3   Allegations of sorcery related to the French crown arose in 1316, 1317, 1319, 1326, 1327, and twice in 1331. For documents concerning some of these incidents, see Charles Henry Lea, *A History of the Inquisition of the Middle Ages*, vol. I (New York 1888), 230, vol. III, 458.

4   For the Avignon papacy generally, see Guillaume Mollat, *The Popes at Avignon* (London 1963).

5   Kittredge, *Witchcraft*, 51 f.

6   Lea, *History*, III, 451; Kittredge, *Witchcraft*, 241 f.

7   For the suppression of the Templars, see Martin Barber, *The Trial of the Templars* (Cambridge 1978).

8   See Norman Cohn, *Europe's Inner Demons* (London 1975), 198–204.

9   Charles Henry Lea, *A History of the Inquisition of the Middle Ages*, vol. III (New York 1888), 657–9.

10 One case from Novara in 1340 is discussed by Norman Cohn in Chapter 2 of this book.

11 Norman Cohn reached the same conclusion inidependently in *Europe's Inner Demons*, 128–38. The Lamothe-Langon texts are now generally regarded as fakes.

12 Hugh Trevor-Roper, *The European Witch-Craze of the Sixteenth and Seventeenth Centuries* (London 1978).

13 For a detailed account of this incident, see Gene A. Brucker, 'Sorcery in Renaissance Florence', *Studies in the Renaissance* 10 (1963), 13–16.

14 This episode is similar to those described by Ginzburg and Pócs in Chapters 8 and 9 of this collection.

15 For contemporary documents relating to this episode, see Charles Henry Lea, *Materials toward a History of Witchcraft* vol. I (Philadelphia, Pa 1939), 238–41.

16 Ibid., 257.

Chapter 2

Norman Cohn

THE DEMONIZATION OF
MEDIAEVAL HERETICS

I N 1173 A RICH MERCHANT OF LYONS called Valos or Valdos was
moved by a passionate craving for salvation. The words of Jesus, in the parable
of the rich young man, seemed to point the way: 'If thou wouldst be perfect, go,
sell that thou hast, and give to the poor'. Valdos disposed of all his possessions and
became a beggar. A group formed around him, intent on following the way of
absolute poverty, after the example of the apostles. And soon these men began to
preach.

So far the story exactly parallels the beginning of the Franciscan venture which
was to come a generation later. But whereas St Francis and his companions
succeeded, with some difficulty, in obtaining papal approbation for their way of
life, and with it permission to preach, Valdos and his followers failed: when they
appeared at the Lateran Council in Rome in 1179, the pope, though impressed by
their piety, imposed restrictions on their preaching. Faced with the alternatives of
giving up preaching or of disobeying the pope, 'the poor of Lyons' chose the latter
course, with the inevitable consequence that in 1181 they were excommunicated;
and in 1184 were formally condemned as heretics.

Persecuted, expelled from one diocese after another, sometimes burned at the
stake, the Waldensians (as they were now called) nevertheless multiplied.[1] The
original French movement spread north to Liege, east to Metz, but above all south,
to Provence, Languedoc, Catalonia, Aragon. And meanwhile new branches
appeared in Italy, where the stronghold was Milan; along the Rhine, at Strasbourg,
Trier and Mainz; in Bavaria and Austria.

The Waldensians were practically untouched by non-Christian influences. They
managed to get the Vulgate translated into their various vernaculars; and these
(often rather inaccurate) renderings of the Bible supplied the framework of their
faith. Though they were not learned people – being mostly peasants and artisans
– they devoted themselves to an intensive study of the Scriptures; even the totally
illiterate were often able to recite the four Gospels and the Book of Job by heart.
All the peculiarities of their doctrine arose simply from a one-sided interpretation

of the New Testament. For instance, they refused in any circumstances to take an oath; and they had an intense horror of any sort of lying, however trivial. They were opposed to capital punishment and also, it would seem, to military service. Passages to justify all these attitudes could easily be found in the New Testament.

Voluntary poverty remained the supreme value, and supplied the yardstick by which the Waldensians measured both themselves and their enemies, the Catholic clergy. As they saw it, in so far as the clergy failed to practise voluntary poverty, they could not really baptize, confirm, consecrate the Eucharist, ordain priests, hear confession or grant absolution. The power validly to administer these sacraments was reserved for the only true devotees of voluntary poverty, the Waldensians.

Such was the sect which, according to Conrad of Marburg and Pope Gregory IX, practised nameless orgies and worshipped the Devil. In the thirteenth century the discrepancy between the accusations and the reality was obvious to many even amongst the guardians of orthodoxy. The archbishop of Mainz, when he wrote to the pope after Conrad's assassination, was clearly unimpressed; and so was the cele-brated preacher David of Augsburg when, around 1265, he wrote his *Treatise on the heresy of the poor of Lyons*. In this systematic account of the sect and its doctrines, the charge of Devil-worship is flatly rejected, and the orgies are reduced to mere transgressions by individual Waldensian preachers who, having given up their wives for the sake of their vocation, found perpetual chastity too much for them. Nevertheless, the old defamatory stereotype survived in the German-speaking lands, and early in the fourteenth century it woke to new life.

From 1311 to 1315 Duke Frederick of Austria joined with the archbishop of Salzburg and the bishop of Passau in a drive to clear the Austrian lands of heretics who, again, were clearly Waldensians. As usual, those who would not recant were burned; and these seem to have been the great majority. A contemporary chroni-cler notes that 'all showed an incredible stubbornness, even to death; they went joyfully to execution'. The same chronicler summarizes the sect's doctrine – and amongst tenets which the Waldensians really hold he intersperses some which come straight from the bull *Vox in Rama*. These people, he says, believe that Lucifer and his demons were unjustly expelled from heaven, and in the end will find eternal blessedness; whereas Michael and his angels will be eternally damned. Meanwhile God neither punishes, nor even knows of, anything done under the earth; so the heretics hold their meetings in subterranean caverns, where they indulge in inces-tuous orgies – father with daughter, brother with sister, son with mother. Conveniently, this view of the doctrine and behaviour of the Waldensians was confirmed by the confession which Dominican inquisitors extracted from one Ulrich Wollar, of Krems.

Popes took these fantasies seriously and used their unique authority to dissem-inate them. Like Gregory IX before him, John XXII incorporated them into a bull; and in both cases the pope took this step under the influence of a single cleric in a distant country. Just as Pope Gregory in Rome took on trust the reports which Conrad of Marburg sent from Germany, so Pope John, resident at Avignon, accepted without question the tales concocted by a canon of Prague cathedral. The canon, Henry of Schonberg, was not even a genuine fanatic like Conrad but simply an intriguer, intent on ruining his bishop. Inspired by this man, the pope in 1318 issued a bull accusing the bishop of protecting heretics. Here, too, the heresy described is unmistakably Waldensian – but here, too, real Waldensian doctrine is blended with fantasies of Lucifer-worship and of nocturnal orgies in caverns.

Already in *Vox in Rama*, in 1233, the Devil is shown as presiding in corporeal form over the nocturnal assemblies of the Waldensians; and the same fantasy is found a century later. Under the year 1338 the Franciscan John of Winterthur, in Switzerland, tells of heretics who were being tortured to death or burned at the stake, in Austria and the neighbouring countries. These too must have been Waldensians; and the rituals ascribed to them are strange indeed. When they have assembled in a subterranean hide-out, the proceedings open with a sermon in which the head of the sect expounds its doctrine. Next four youths appear, bearing burning torches; and then there enters a king, clad in precious robes, with a sparkling crown and strangely shining sceptre, and surrounded by a brilliant retinue of knights.

The king announces that he is the king of heaven – which means that he is Lucifer. He confirms the doctrine that has just been expounded and commands, in virtue of his authority, that it be observed and obeyed forever. At once a grasshopper comes and settles on the mouth of each individual in turn; whereupon all are overwhelmed with such a joyous ecstasy that they lose all self-control. The moment has come for the customary orgy: the lights are extinguished and each has intercourse with his or her neighbour; often a man with a man, a woman with a woman. The chronicler ends with the comment that these sectarians are the special sons of Satan, for they imitate his words and works before other men.

That is what people believed about the Waldensians in the southernmost parts of the German-speaking world – but in the far north the picture was apparently just the same. Around 1336 rumours reached the bishop of Brandenburg that the town of Angermunde was infected with heresy. Inquisitors were sent to investigate, and not in vain. They found a number of people who were suspected of 'the heresy of the Luciferans'; and fourteen men and women, having refused to recant, were burned. Details of the charges are lacking, but a story which reached John of Winterthur at least suggests what was meant by 'the heresy of the Luciferans'.

According to the Swiss chronicler – who bases himself on 'a faithful report' – a schoolmaster in Brandenburg invited a Franciscan friend of his to come and see the Holy Trinity. Having obtained permission of his brethren, and armed himself with a consecrated wafer, the Franciscan accompanied the schoolmaster to what turned out to be an assembly of heretics. It was presided over by three strikingly handsome men, clad in shining robes, whom the schoolmaster identified as the Father, the Son and the Holy Spirit. Unimpressed, the Franciscan produced the Eucharist and held it aloft, crying: 'Then who is this?' John of Winterthur finishes his story:

> The spirits which, in the guise of the Trinity, had so long fooled people and made them mad, vanished at the sight of the Eucharist; leaving behind a most evil stink. The Franciscan returned thankfully to his brethren, and reported on God's power and its wondrous effects. But the heretics who had let themselves be mocked and deceived by the spirits were sent to the stake and burned. When they were warned to cast off the filth of superstitions and devilish deceit, to reflect, and to profess the true faith, as they ought to do, they persevered in their heretical perversity, being

too much ensnared and seduced. They preferred to perish in the fire, in the midst of their sins, to being saved by confession of the true faith. Indeed, they said that they saw in the flames golden chariots which would at once carry them over to the joys of heaven.

In 1384 a further group of 'Luciferans' was discovered in Brandenburg, and on this occasion we know what they were accused of. Like the Austrian heretics, and like Conrad of Marburg's victims, they were supposed to believe that Lucifer had been wrongfully expelled from heaven, and would in due course return there and take over from God. Meanwhile they worshipped Lucifer as their god, and also held promiscuous orgies in underground cellars. The rest of the doctrine ascribed to these people is purely Waldensian, and everything suggests that they too were Waldensians.

There is no reason to think that Waldensians were very numerous in the German lands at any time. Nor, after their earliest days, were they socially influential: by the fourteenth century they consisted almost entirely of artisans, modest tradesmen and peasants. Certainly when pitted against the massive structure and vast resources of the Catholic Church the sect was much too small, scattered and obscure to constitute any real threat. Yet in certain quarters it was felt not simply as a threat but as a destructive force of overwhelming, superhuman power. Again we may turn to the Franciscan John of Winterthur to discover not indeed how things were, but how they were imagined to be. In his view, only the most strenuous efforts of Catholic preachers – including of course Franciscan preachers – prevented the Church from being altogether overwhelmed and obliterated:

> These people would overthrow the faith of Peter, if the teachers did not each day fortify it with the word of truth. So Peter's little boat, which sails on the billows of the sea of this world, is battered by the blows of the tempest; but it does not sink, because it is sustained by the strong hands of the teachers.

The persistent efforts to defame the sect are inseparable from this fantastic overestimation of its power. The Waldensians were imagined as Devil-worshippers, and as themselves quasi-demonic. This meant that they must be almost irresistible in their work of undermining and destroying the Christian religion, identified with the Catholic Church. It also meant that whatever was felt to be most anti-human, such as blindly promiscuous orgies and incest between parent and offspring, must be an essential part of their world. And during the fourteenth century this stereotype came to be widely accepted even by professional inquisitors. The account of the Waldensians which the inquisitor for Aragon, Nicolas Eymeric, gave in his manual, the *Directorium Inquisitorum*, around 1368, is on the whole well informed and objective – yet even here the following turns up, as one of the Waldensian articles of faith:

> It is better to satisfy one's lust by any kind of evil act than to be harassed by the goadings of the flesh. In the dark it is lawful for any man to mate with any woman, without distinction, whenever and as often as they are moved by carnal desires. This they both say and do.[2]

In France and Italy the Waldensians were originally a more considerable force than in Germany; but there too they were persecuted so fiercely that their heyday was already over by the fourteeth century. By that time, most of the survivors had withdrawn into the Cottian Alps, which straddle the French–Italian border, roughly between Gap and Turin. There they formed a solid colony, under Italian leadership. Inquisitors penetrated into those remote valleys at their peril; two are known to have been killed by the embattled Waldensians. Nevertheless, from time to time a few Waldensians were caught, and at some of the resulting trials mention was made of the same fantastic beliefs and deeds as had been ascribed to the German Waldensians generations earlier.

Early in 1387 a Dominican inquisitor called Antonio di Setto, of Savigliano, began investigations in the area around Pinerolo, in the Italian foothills of the Cottian Alps. The results were meagre until, some time in the same year, he laid hands on a religious layman, a member of the Third Order of Saint Francis, called Antonio Galosna of Monte San Raffaello. He kept the man in prison for many months, until May 1388, when he produced him before the tribunal which he had set up in Turin. It now appeared that this Tertiary was really a Waldensian. He had often attended nocturnal meetings of the sect, and was able to give most detailed accounts of what went on.

The meetings were commonly held at the home of a Waldensian, or else at an inn, at an hour when the neighbours were safely asleep. The company consisted of artisans and small tradesmen – innkeepers, bankers, cobblers, tailors, haberdashers, fruiterers. It could vary in size from a mere dozen to forty or so; but it always included both sexes. The proceedings opened with a sort of Eucharist. The preacher would distribute bread, explaining that it was worth more than the Catholic faith, and indeed more than God's grace. An old woman would pour out drink from a special flask in her keeping. This drink was a foul beverage which, if taken in any large quantity, made the body swell up and could even lead to death; but even a sip of it would bind a person to the sect for ever. It was said to contain the excrement of a huge toad which the woman kept for that purpose under her bed; and it was always brewed on the eve of Epiphany. Unappetizing though the fare might be, those present banqueted 'with great joy'. So fortified, they promised to obey the preacher in all things, and never to reveal what happened at the meetings. They also promised to worship the dragon which wages war on God and his angels (meaning the dragon in the Book of Revelation, which is Lucifer or Satan). Thereupon the lights were extinguished and the cry went up: 'Let him who has, keep hold.' The orgy began, and continued until dawn; and here too it is particularly mentioned that the closest relatives had intercourse. But sometimes things were arranged in more orderly fashion: the men drew lots for the women.

Antonio Galosna named more than a dozen villages around Turin where these performances were supposed to take place – and not just occasionally but once or twice in each month (except, he added, when the weather was wet). He also named dozens of men and women who were supposed to participate in them. But, circumstantial though his confession was, in the end it helped him not at all. At one point the secular authorities intervened to remove him from the inquisitor's power – whereupon he promptly denied everything, as having been extracted by fear of torture. But the inquisitor reasserted his claims; and though Antonio reverted to his original confession, he was burned nevertheless. And in 1451 another Dominican inquisitor, also at Pinerolo, induced another Waldensian to confirm that the sect did indeed indulge in promiscuous and incestuous orgies.

Meanwhile, the French Waldensians were a constant source of vexation to the archbishops of Embrun, in whose see they were concentrated. Not that they ever were a power in the land – on the contrary, they were mostly poor peasants and shepherds, living in small compact communities in the high, remote valleys of Fressiniere, Argentiere, Valpute and Valcluson, and seldom venturing outside. But the very fact that such communities existed and persisted was felt by successive archbishops and inquisitors as an intolerable offence – and not by them alone. The example set by Emperor Frederick II in 1231, when he joined forces with Pope Gregory IX in an effort to stamp out heresy within the Empire, had since been imitated by many rulers; and from 1365 onwards the governor of Dauphine and the council of Dauphine (later the parlement of Grenoble) repeatedly sent armed expeditions against the mountain villages. In effect it was an intermittent crusade; and like other crusades it enjoyed papal blessing. Desiderated already by John XXII and Benedict XII, the campaign against the Waldensians of Dauphine was actively supported by Clement VI, Alexander V, Eugenius IV and Innocent VIII.

It reached its height in the years after 1486, when a particularly resolute archbishop, Jean Baile, made a supreme effort to extirpate the sect. He appealed to the Waldensians to return to the Church; and as not a single Waldensian came forward, turned to Pope Innocent VIII for help. The pope responded by replacing the regular inquisitor for Dauphine, who was elderly, by an Italian called Alberto Cattaneo, who seems to have been only twenty-two years old. Normally an inquisitor was appointed by the provincial of his order, Dominican or Franciscan as the case might be, and was chosen largely for his familiarity with local conditions. Cattaneo, however, was an extraordinary commissioner, appointed directly by the pope; and he proved a bad choice. Though not lacking in attainments – he was archdeacon of Cremona and a doctor of canon and of civil law – he was quite unequipped to act as a judicious inquisitor. Knowing not a word of French, wholly ignorant of conditions in Dauphine, he was unable to control the secular officials who were his assistants. During his time torture and threats of torture were used far more freely than was usual; Waldensians are known to have died while being tortured by the officials of Embrun.

Cattaneo's first step was moderate enough: like the archbishop before him, he summoned the inhabitants of the valleys to give themselves up, to accept absolution, to be reconciled with the Church. But when he in his turn met with no response, he pressed for a military invasion of the valleys where the Waldensians had their stronghold; and his request was granted. By order of the parlement of Grenoble, and under the command of the lieutenant of the governor of Dauphine, an expeditionary force set out in March 1488. Those who took part in it could look forward both to a plenary indulgence – which was promised by the pope – and to a share in the property of the heretics; and they were correspondingly zealous. The Waldensians were forced back to the icy mountain peaks, where after a gallant resistance they were overwhelmed. Scores were put to the sword or thrown from the rocks.

Many more were taken prisoner or gave themselves up; and while a few were burned as impenitent or relapsed heretics, the majority were received into the

Church. Some fifty of these were interrogated by Cattaneo with the assistance of secular lawyers, including the chief magistrate of Briancon. Doctrinally these Waldensians turned out to be as close to Catholicism as their precursors two and three centuries earlier – professing all the principal Catholic dogmas, including the real presence in the Eucharist, and rejecting only the hierarchy of the Roman Church. Nevertheless the old slanders against the sect not only persisted but were reinforced. Already before the expedition some captured Waldensians, under interrogation, had talked of nocturnal orgies; and some amongst the new batch of prisoners spoke in similar vein. While many indignantly denied that such things occurred at all, others were more forthcoming. In particular, they had much to say about the Waldensian preachers, or 'barbes' (so called from the Piedmontese word for 'uncle'). They stated that the 'barbe' would commonly launch the orgy by crying out, 'Let him who has, have. Let him who holds, hold. Whoever puts the light out shall have life eternal.' This curious notion was not new – Antonio Galosna had produced it a century earlier – and its factual basis is known: at the end of a Waldensian service the preacher would say, 'Let him who has grasped (the meaning), retain it'; after which the congregation would meditate for a few minutes in darkness before dispersing.

The 'barbes' were simple, uneducated men, mostly of Italian origin. They functioned not as resident priests but – like Catholic friars – as itinerant preachers. Disguised as merchants or pedlars, they were constantly on the move and covered vast distances on foot. It was a dangerous, nerve-racking existence; and though the Waldensian communities sheltered them loyally, from time to time one of them would be captured. It seems that four perished at Grenoble in 1492; and in the same year two more were caught in the mountains north of Briancon. One of these, an Italian from Spoleto called Francis of Girundino, otherwise known as the 'barbe' Martin, was tried at Oulx (now on the Italian side of the frontier). His interrogation, which was carried out not by an inquisitor but by a canon of the abbey of Oulx, assisted by a councillor of the governor of Dauphine and the chief magistrate of Embrun, provided new and picturesque details concerning the imaginary orgies.[3] Now it appeared that the orgy or 'synagogue' was held only once a year, always in a different region; but it was very incestuous indeed. If the presiding 'barbe' was not a local man, he had to withdraw after delivering his sermon, before the orgy began; for only a local man would have relatives available to mate with. Martin added that a male child conceived at this incestuous orgy was regarded as pre-eminently suited to become a 'barbe' in due course. As for Martin's companion, the 'barbe' Pietro de Jacopo, he was interrogated separately, by the episcopal commissary at Valence. He agreed about the orgies – and added that at these gatherings the Waldensians worshipped an idol called Bacchus!

Incredibly, the very transcript of Martin's interrogation contains a phrase which makes nonsense of the whole story: in the Waldensian view the Catholic clergy, from the pope downwards, were no true clergy precisely because they broke their vows of virginity and chastity. Other prisoners, interrogated in other places, are recorded as maintaining that the sacrament of matrimony is to be faithfully and firmly kept. And indeed the moral strictness of the Waldensians, even at this late stage, is beyond all doubt.

The statements about orgies nevertheless served their purpose. Widely publicized, they brought the Waldensians into general disrepute, so that the sectarians came to be regarded as the worst enemies of society, against whom fresh pursuits could be launched with general approval. Moreover, as so often, economic motives contributed to the dynamism of the persecution. A Waldensian who recanted and was absolved could still see anything up to a third of his property confiscated; a Waldensian who refused to recant was either burned or imprisoned for life – and in either case all his property was confiscated. The total confiscations were massive – in some valleys the land confiscated amounted to a third of all taxable land. It is not surprising that the beneficiaries – the archbishop of Embrun in the first place, but also the various local lords – did everything possible to keep their gains.

Viewed from Paris things looked different. When Louis XII succeeded to the throne in 1499 he was not convinced that small groups of Waldensians in remote Alpine valleys really constituted a threat to French society; and with the pope's agreement he sent his own confessor, the bishop of Sisteron, Laurent Bureau, to carry out an enquiry on the spot. It was the beginning of a gradual rehabilitation. In 1509 the grand council, sitting in Paris, annulled all the sentences passed by the late archbishop, Jean Baile, the inquisitor Alberto Cattaneo and his successor Franqois Plouvier, and restored all confiscated properties to the original owners or their heirs. This came about not because the persecuted were able to prove their orthodoxy – most of them certainly were Waldensians, not Catholics – but because the king had an overriding interest in establishing peace and unity within the kingdom, and was unimpressed by an inquisitorial institution which had lost almost all the power and prestige it had once possessed. Thereafter no more was heard of Waldensian 'synagogues'.

For at least two and a half centuries tales of promiscuous and incestuous orgies and of Devil-worship had pursued this purely – indeed naively – Christian sect. Yet it so happens that in no single instance can one fill in all the details – who first voiced the charges, what sources he drew on, how much pressure was needed to obtain substantiation. However, the lacuna can be filled: one has only to examine the case of another group of poverty-loving Christians, the Fraticelli 'de opinione' in fourteenth-century Italy.

The Fraticelli can be understood only in terms of the Franciscan movement and its development.[4] The original confraternity which St Francis gathered around him, from 1209 onwards, was wholly unworldly and lived in absolute poverty. Members had to dispose of all their possessions before joining; they aimed to own nothing but the barest necessities of life; they earned their bread from day to day, by manual work; they were not permitted to receive or to handle money. All the energies of these first Franciscans were devoted to nomadic preaching amongst the poor, and to caring for lepers and outcasts. But within a few years the little confraternity grew until it numbered thousands of members; and in 1220 a papal bull constituted it as a monastic order.

Francis died in 1226, and by the 1230s the Franciscan Order had already departed far from his ideal. It was now a great organization extending throughout western Christendom; seeking and wielding influence in church and state; active in teaching theology and canon law in the universities; and – like other monastic orders – owning vast properties in land and buildings. But many Franciscans could not reconcile themselves to these transformations and strove to restore the hard, simple way of life that had prevailed in the earliest years. At first these zealots –

or Spirituals, as they called themselves – formed a minority within the order; and at times they were even able to set the tone for the order as a whole. The most extreme amongst them, however, chose another course. Already in the thirteenth century some of the Spiritual party left first the official order and then the Church itself. The Fraticelli were the successors, in the fourteenth and fifteenth centuries, of these heretical Spirituals.

The most radical of the Fraticelli were known as the Fraticelli 'de opinione', a term which requires some elucidation. At one time, very many Franciscans had believed that Christ and the apostles had lived in absolute poverty, owning no property at all, whether as individuals or in common. But in 1323 John XXII declared that to affirm the absolute poverty of Christ and the apostles was to fall into heresy; and this view of the matter was maintained by subsequent popes. It was also accepted, however reluctantly, by the Franciscan order as such. For the Fraticelli 'de opinione', on the other hand, the absolute poverty of Christ and the apostles was an article of faith. In response to papal condemnations they retorted that John XXII and all popes following him were themselves heretics; that the Catholic clergy, in so far as they obeyed the popes, had forfeited all authority; and that sacraments administered by such clergy were worthless.

The Fraticelli 'de opinione' were never very numerous, nor did they evolve a unified organization. By the middle of the fifteenth century the sect had been reduced to a few obscure, clandestine groups, and the heresy had lost most of its importance. The papal onslaught of 1466 was directed against an already defeated foe.

The pope at that time, Paul II, was a man whose enthusiasm was more easily engaged by his magnificent collection of antiquities and works of art, and by the jewels which he assembled for his personal adornment, than by the ideal of absolute poverty. In 1466 it came to his ears that many Fraticelli 'de opinione' would be making their way to Assisi, to attend the festival of Portiuncula that was to be held there in July. The little chapel of St Mary of the Angels, known as the Portiuncula, was the place where St Francis had received the revelation which determined his vocation; now it had become a favourite place of pilgrimage for the Fraticelli – and also a place where, amongst the crowds of pilgrims, they could meet without attracting notice. Not so, however, on this occasion: investigators sent specially by the pope seized a score of them, of both sexes and the most various ages.

It turned out that the prisoners had come a long way to Assisi: some from the area around Poli, not far from Rome; others from the area around Maiolati, in the mountainous, inland part of the March of Ancona. All were obscure inhabitants of obscure villages; but despite this, it was thought worthwhile to transport them all the way to Rome and to incarcerate them in the papal fortress itself. Moreover, the ecclesiastics who interrogated them there included an archbishop and two bishops, as well as the commandant of the fortress; and torture was used freely. Clearly, great expectations were attached to this mass interrogation and the confessions it might produce. They were not disappointed.

The first prisoner to be interrogated was a 'priest' of the sect, called Bernard of Bergamo. His answers give a lively and convincing picture of Fraticelli life. Bernard had spent his noviciate in Greece; for the Fraticelli, in flight from persecution in Italy, had established monasteries across the water, outside the bounds of Latin Christendom. After ordination Bernard had returned to Italy, to teach the doctrine of the Fraticelli at Poli: preaching against the errors of John XXII, condemning the Catholic clergy, exalting absolute poverty. Though his activity was clandestine, it evidently found some response. Even great nobles were favourably disposed. The overlord of the village, Count Stefano de Conti, protected the Fraticelli and treated Bernard as his father confessor – and in due course was imprisoned by the pope in the fortress of Sant' Angelo for so doing. Bernard recalled, too, how a great lady of the Colonna family summoned him to her castle, so that she could make her confession to him instead of to a Catholic priest; she has been identified as Sueva, the mother of Stefano Colonna, count of Palestrina.

The first confession made at the Castel Sant' Angelo yields a perfectly coherent picture, but the second reveals some strangely incongruous features. For the statements by the next prisoner, Francis of Maiolati, include the following:

> Interrogated concerning the matter of the barilotto, he said that when he was young, ten or twelve years of age, he twice found himself in the crypt of a church which has since been destroyed, at a spot near Maiolati. After mass had been celebrated at night, just before dawn, the lights were put out and the people cried, 'Put out the light, let us go to eternal life, alleluia, alleluia; and let each man take hold of his woman.' Asked what he did himself, and whether he had sexual intercourse with any woman, he replied that he was young at that time, and the young people left the church; the adults stayed behind and had intercourse with the women present. They made a stamping noise, like the noise on the holy day of Venus.
>
> Interrogated concerning the powders, he replied that, from the babies born, they take one little boy as a sacrifice. They make a fire, around which they stand in a circle. They pass the little boy from hand to hand until he is quite dried up. Later they make powders from the body. They put these powders in a flask of wine. After the end of mass they give some of this wine to all taking part; each drinks once from the flask, by way of communion. And he, Francis, was there twice, and drank twice, when attending mass. He also said that for thirty years he had not belonged to the sect, because he had had no occasion. He joined again after the arrival of Brother Bernard, who brought him back to it by his preaching; and he had made confession four times to the same Bernard.

Such was the story told by Francis of Maiolati. To understand it, two facts have to be borne in mind. As in all inquisitorial trials, the tribunal was empowered to use torture; and again and again the record of the enquiry expressly states that torture was in fact used. Francis may not have been tortured, but he certainly knew that he could be. Secondly, the prisoners incarcerated in the Castel Sant' Angelo included a Fraticelli 'bishop', Nicholas of Massaro. This man did not figure at all in the first series of interrogations; but there are strong indications that Francis's statement was intended to prepare the way for his appearance later. Interrogated afresh, Francis stated that he knew of the ritual infanticide only from senior members of the sect. Another prisoner, Angelo of Poli, was more precise: the first time he had ever heard of the barilotto was now, in prison, when the 'bishop' Nicholas had told him of it. It is impossible to tell whether these laymen were forced to incriminate their 'bishop' or whether, on the contrary, the 'bishop' was forced to mislead his followers; but it is also immaterial. By whatever means, the scene was set for a dramatic confession by a leader of the Fraticelli.

The enquiry began in August 1466, and in October the commission laid its report before Pope Paul. The pope insisted that the enquiry should be resumed forthwith, and the prisoners interrogated afresh. This time Nicholas of Massaro was at the head of the line; a venerable figure, it would seem, for he had been a bishop for some forty years. He had once confessed to everything – to taking part in the orgies and in the infanticides; also to handing out the wine with the ashes of the incinerated baby 'nine or ten times'. He had only one correction to make: the orgies were not wholly promiscuous, the men usually chose women they knew, and he himself usually took Catherine of Palumbaria. Catherine, being summoned, failed to confirm this – she could recall having intercourse with the elderly Nicholas only once or twice. On the other hand, she knew all about the infanticides and the making of the powders; indeed, these things were frequently done in her very house.

This is the sum total of evidence concerning orgies, infanticides and cannibalistic beverages amongst the Fraticelli: for the rest, the records of the interrogations, which are unusually full and vivid, show only how utterly strange these stories seemed to the ordinary lay members of the sect. The reaction of one exceptionally strong character, Antonio of Sacco, is revealing. In August and again in October this man stood by his faith. He refused to abjure, and he refused to kneel before the tribunal. Told that the 'bishop' Nicholas himself had abjured, he remained unshaken; in that case, he replied, he would subordinate himself not to a heretical pope but to God alone. He admitted, and gloried in, every article of faith of the Fraticelli. At the same time he denied all knowledge of the barilotto. So, at the renewed enquiry in October, Antonio de Sacco was tortured in the usual way; being hauled up by a rope around his wrists, which were tied behind him, and then suddenly dropped – a proceeding calculated to tear the muscles and dislocate the joints. After several applications of this torture Antonio admitted to taking part in the barilotto – but as soon as he was taken off the rope, he denied it. Tortured again, he confirmed his first statement – but when he was brought before the tribunal, he again denied everything.

In the end Antonio capitulated, like all the other accused, to the extent of abjuring his faith, asking to be received back into the Church, and promising to accept the pope as the true vicar of God on earth. Coming close up to the commissioners he said humbly: 'My lords, forgive me.' But he also said: 'My lords, you saw how yesterday, when I was being tortured, I said I had twice attended the barilotto. It's not true. I have a young wife and a beautiful daughter, who are detained here in the prisons of Sant' Angelo. I would never have permitted such things.'

The rest of the accused were no more helpful. Unlike Antonio of Sacco they all abjured very quickly, during the first series of interrogations – but even so, nobody supported Francis of Maiolati in his allegations. It was not simply that nobody confessed to taking part in such sinister practices – nobody knew anything at all about them. And the same happened when the interrogations were resumed in October. Apart from Nicholas, Catherine and Francis, nobody could throw any light on the matter — and Francis himself insisted that he had never seen any of these things himself. Indeed, as the proceedings continued he could no longer even recall the age at which he had heard, from outside a church, what he thought was a barilotto — perhaps it was ten, but then again perhaps it was fifteen.

The final picture, then, is paradoxical in the extreme. The tribunal really had investigated two groups of Fraticelli 'de opinione'. It had found them to hold all those views — on the all-importance of absolute poverty, on the sublime merits of the Fraticelli, on the depravity of the Church of Rome — which were commonly attributed to them. That much can be regarded as established; and it was enough, by itself, to get the prisoners condemned as heretics. But beyond that point the case is submerged in a welter of implausibilities and contradictions. In the end the tribunal was left with two leading personalities — the 'bishops' Nicholas of Massaro and his friend Catherine of Palumbaria — who admitted to organizing orgies and infanticides and cannibalistic communions on a massive scale; but not one member of the rank and file who had ever taken part in, or even witnessed, any of these activities. A couple of generals, in short, with no troops at all.

Moreover, the behaviour of the tribunal itself was full of paradoxes. With the means at its disposal, it certainly could have extracted confessions from the other prisoners, some of whom were adolescent boys and girls; but it did not insist. And when it came to sentence the prisoners, it revealed a similar uncertainty. It sentenced them for their real beliefs — banishing some for seven years, imprisoning others for life; but it also described them collectively as 'murderers, adulterous, incestuous'. The explanation must surely be that the tribunal had a double task. In the first place it was concerned, as the Inquisition normally was, to reclaim repentant heretics for the Church and to punish the impenitent or relapsed. But it was also concerned to establish that the movement of the Fraticelli was a monstrous, anti-human conspiracy.

Yet it does not follow that the commission was a mere pack of cynics. It is quite possible that the eminent ecclesiastics who guided the interrogation believed that they were simply uncovering the truth. For by the time of the trial in 1466 these particular accusations formed part of the clergy's stereotype of the Fraticelli. The activities described by Francis of Maiolati include one very curious feature. The Fraticelli were said not simply to kill babies but to do so in a particularly bizarre manner — by passing them from hand to hand until they died. Now this strange fantasy had a long history behind it. As early as the eighth century the head of the Armenian church, John of Ojun, had described how the Paulician heretics killed the fruit of their orgies in just that way. And in the twelfth century the French chronicler Guibert de Nogent had said of the heretics of Soissons almost exactly what Francis of Maiolati said of the Fraticelli: 'They light a great fire and all sit around it. They pass the child from hand to hand and finally throw it on the fire, and leave it there until it is entirely consumed. Later, when the child is burned to ashes, they make those ashes into a sort of bread; each eats a piece by way of communion'. So, behind the grim and solemn procedures of interrogation and torture, we discover a literary tradition. More precisely, we discover an age-old fantasy enshrined in theological tracts and monastic chronicles.

The defamation of the Fraticelli, then, was the work of intellectuals in positions of authority. Also, it was carried out at a time when the Fraticelli no longer had any appreciable influence or importance. We have met this pattern before, and we shall be meeting it again. Again and again, over a period of many centuries, heretical sects were accused of holding promiscuous and incestuous orgies in the dark; of killing infants and devouring their remains; of worshipping the Devil. Is it conceivable that no sect ever did such things at all? In the past, historians have diverged over that question. But here the matter must be settled once and for all; for otherwise my whole argument hangs in the air.

One of the charges can be dismissed without more ado. Normally, when heretics were tried and interrogated by inquisitors, transcripts of the proceedings were kept. Hundreds of these transcripts have survived, and they offer no evidence for the killing and eating of babies or children. Indeed, only one sect ever seems to have been formally charged with such offences – the Fraticelli 'de opinione' at Fabriano and Rome; and as we have seen, the 'evidence' produced even in that belated instance turns out to have been taken almost *verbatim* from polemical tracts and monastic chronicles, written centuries before. All the other accounts of child-eating derive from the same literary tradition. Weighed against the silence of the inquisitors, they have no authority whatever.

At first glance, the charge of holding promiscuous and incestuous orgies might seem to have rather more basis in real happenings. It is certain, for instance, that some of the heretical mystics known as the Brethren of the Free Spirit did claim to have attained a state of total oneness with God, in which all things were permitted to them; and it was widely believed at the time that they gave expression to this conviction by practising free love amongst themselves. There is also the case of the dualist heretics known as Cathars. According to Catharist doctrine, all matter was evil, and human bodies were prisons from which human souls were struggling to escape; whence it followed that procreation was an abomination. Catholic polemics pointed out the logical consequences of such a view. If all procreation was utterly evil, no form of sexual intercourse was more reprehensible than any other; incest between mother and son was no worse than intercourse between man and wife. So long as no more souls were incarcerated in flesh, no harm was done; and to avoid that, abortion or even infanticide were legitimate.

However, on closer examination none of this really provides an explanation for the tales of promiscuous and incestuous orgies. There is no firm evidence that in practice Cathars ever drew libertine consequences from their hatred of the flesh. Catharist morality was only meant to be followed by the elite of the sect, the *perfecti*; and in general even the Catholic clergy, while attacking Catharist doctrine, paid tribute to the chastity of these people. Nor is there any reason to think that the Brethren of the Free Spirit indulged in collective orgies; if any of them did indeed practise free love, they did it in private. Indeed, of all the innumerable stories of nocturnal orgies only one, concerning an incident which is supposed to have taken place in Cologne in 1326, could possibly refer to the heretical mystics of the Free Spirit; and even that has now been shown to be mythical.[5]

Above all, there are the brute facts of chronology. Stories of heretics and their orgies were circulating in France already in the eleventh century – but there were no Cathars in the west before the middle of the twelfth century, and the Brethren of the Free Spirit are first heard of in the thirteenth. The beliefs and activities of these sectarians can no more account for the defamation of the Waldensians or the Fraticelli than the activities of the Carpocratians can account for the very similar tales told of the early Christians.

And of course it is to those ancient tales that we must look for an explanation. After all, both the accusations of promiscuous orgies and the accusations of child-eating belong to a tradition dating back to the second century. The Fathers who first defended the Christians against these accusations also, by the very act of putting them in writing, perpetuated the accusations. Embedded in theological works which were preserved in monastic libraries and which, moreover, were frequently recopied, these tales must have been familiar to many monks. It was only to be expected that, when it came to discrediting some new religious out-group, monks would draw on this traditional stock of defamatory clichés. Moreover, it is known that by the fourteenth century certain chroniclers deliberately inserted such stories into their narratives in order to provide preachers with materials for their sermons against heresy.

More serious consideration has to be given to the idea that heretics worshipped the Devil. This charge cannot simply be derived from what pagan Romans said about the Christian minority in their midst. Did it, then, reflect what some group or sect of *mediaeval* heretics really believed or practised? Few people nowadays are likely to accept that demonic cats descended miraculously from on high – but perhaps some reality lurks behind these fantasies, perhaps there really was a cult of Lucifer or Satan? Even so sceptical (and anticlerical) a historian as Henry Charles Lea thought so, and today it is still widely assumed that such a cult must have existed.[6]

Three arguments have been advanced in support of this view. It has been pointed out that some *mediaeval* sources describe a coherent and conceivable doctrine, which they attribute to a sect of 'Luciferans'. It has been suggested that the Dualist religion, pushed to its logical conclusion, could very well lead to Devil-worship. And it has also been said that the intelligent, educated and devout men – including some popes – who accepted that a cult of Satan existed, would not have done so without solid evidence. These arguments have to be examined.

It is true that accounts of a Luciferan doctrine are to be found not only in the bull which Pope Gregory IX issued at the prompting of Conrad of Marburg in 1233, but in half a dozen other German and Italian sources. The Luciferan doctrine, it appears, taught that Lucifer and his demons were unjustly expelled from heaven, but will return there in the end, to resume their rightful places and to cast God, Michael and his angels into hell for all eternity. Meanwhile the Luciferans must serve their master by doing everything in their power to offend God; their reward will be everlasting blessedness with Lucifer. The accounts agree with one another and are not, on the face of it, implausible. But how reliable are they?

Internal evidence shows them to be wholly unreliable. Each one is accompanied by statements which are anything but plausible. In one case we hear of demons who vanish into thin air when the Luciferan rite is interrupted by the appearance of the Eucharist. Another source blithely states that in Austria, Bohemia and the neighbouring territories alone the worshippers of Lucifer number 80,000. Another – a confession attributed to a heretic called Lepzet, of Cologne – proclaims that the man himself, in his zeal to serve Lucifer and offend God, has committed more than thirty murders! Yet another speaks of a magic potion containing the excrement of a gigantic toad; while in the bull *Vox in Rama* both a demonic toad and a demonic cat receive kisses of homage. Moreover, most of the sources contain references to those promiscuous and incestuous orgies which we have just shown to be unreliable.

In any case, these accounts of a particular Luciferan doctrine are simply very belated additions to the traditional tales about a Devil-worshipping sect, which can be traced back some four centuries earlier; and it is the tales themselves that present the problem. Is it possible that a Devil-worshipping sect really did develop out of the dualist religion?

One has only to examine the stories one by one to see how groundless this supposition is. Until recently it was thought that the Paulicians of Armenia, whom John of Ojun accused of Devil-worship in the eighth century, were Dualists; but the latest research has shown that at that date they were nothing of the kind.[7] The Bogomiles accused in the eleventh century were indeed Dualists – but not a word, in the couple of paragraphs allocated to them, suggests that Psellos was aware of the fact. Psellos was in Constantinople, the Bogomiles were in Thrace, and he knew so little about them that he even got their name wrong. And in the West too accusations of Devil-worship were hurled at sects which knew nothing of Dualism. Already the heretical group discovered at Orleans in 1022 was so accused; and the stereotype of the Devil-worshipping sect was fully developed, in every detail, by 1100. But historians are generally agreed that the Dualist religion was unknown in the West before 1140 at the earliest.[8]

Between the middle of the twelfth and the middle of the thirteenth century that form of the Dualist religion known as Catharism did flourish in the West, and it was widely interpreted as a cult of Satan. Is it possible that Catharism, at least, sometimes involved Devil-worship? Towards the close of the twelfth century a French monk called Rudolf Ardent summarized the belief of the Cathars. According to him, they held that, whereas God created all invisible things, the Devil created all visible ones; so they worshipped the Devil as the creator of their bodies. About the same time, a French chronicler recorded the confession which two Catharist leaders were supposed to have made after spending some months as captives of the papal legate: they said that Satan and Lucifer is the creator of heaven and earth, of all things visible and invisible. No doubt it was such reports as these that gave rise to the notion of a Luciferan doctrine. They must also have lent fresh credibility to the age-old tales of a Devil-worshipping sect. But as evidence for the existence of a Luciferan doctrine or a Devil-worshipping sect they are valueless, for they grossly distort what Cathars really believed.

We have reliable information concerning the real beliefs of the Cathars – including some Catharist writings. Like other Dualists, they were convinced that the material universe was created by an evil spirit – in effect, the Devil – who still dominated it. But so far from worshipping the Devil they were passionately concerned to escape from his clutches. That aspiration was the very heart of their religion. For souls were not created by the Devil but by God. Indeed, in the Catharist view, souls are the angels who fell from heaven; they have been imprisoned in one body after another, and they yearn to escape from the material world and re-enter the heaven of pure spirituality. The morality of the Catharist *perfecti*

– their condemnation of marriage, their horror of procreation, their vegetarianism and fasting – reflects their total rejection of the material world, imagined as a demonic creation. To come to terms with the flesh, to accept the world of matter – that is to reveal oneself as a servant of the Devil; and to be a servant of the Devil is to be incapable of salvation.

There is, then, no reason to think that, even in the twelfth and thirteenth centuries, tales of a Devil-worshipping sect reflected something that really existed amongst the Cathars. Moreover in the fifteenth century, long after the Cathars had been exterminated, those Bible-studying Christians the Waldensians were still being persecuted as 'Luciferans'.

Finally, we must ask ourselves whether intelligent, educated and devout men could have accepted that a cult of Satan existed, if they had not had good grounds for thinking so. Several modern historians have argued, and have convinced many readers, that such a thing is inconceivable. But they are in error. The same people who accepted that a cult of Satan existed, also accepted that Satan miraculously materialized at the celebration of his cult, usually in the form of a gigantic animal. The two beliefs were practically inseparable, and if the one seems to lack evidential value, so should the other.

There is in fact no serious evidence for the existence of such a sect of Devil-worshippers anywhere in mediaeval Europe. One can go further: there is serious evidence to the contrary. Very few inquisitors claimed to have come across these Devil-worshippers, and most of those few are known to have been fanatical amateurs, of the stamp of Conrad of Marburg. We may be sure that if any sect really had held such beliefs, it would have figured in one or other of the two standard manuals for inquisitors: that by Bernard Gui or that by Nicolas Eymeric, both dating from the fourteenth century, when the Luciferans are supposed to have been at the height of their influence. But it does not. The only kind of 'demonolatry' known to Eymeric lay in the efforts of individual practitioners of ritual or ceremonial magic to induce demons to do their will – which is a different matter altogether. Gui's comments have even less bearing on the matter. In fact, neither Eymeric nor Gui even hint at the existence of a sect of Devil-worshippers; and that should settle the question.

To understand why the stereotype of a Devil-worshipping sect emerged at all, why it exercised such fascination and why it survived so long, one must look not at the belief or behaviour of heretics, Dualist or other, but into the minds of the orthodox themselves. Many people, and particularly many priests and monks, were becoming more and more obsessed by the overwhelming power of the Devil and his demons. That is why their idea of the absolutely evil and anti-human came to include Devil-worship, alongside incest, infanticide and cannibalism.

Notes

1   For an introduction to the Waldensian movement, see Gabriel Audisio, *The Waldensian Dissent*, trans. Claire Davison (Cambridge 1999). A fine collection of texts on this as on other movements, in English translation, is contained in W. L. Wakefield and A. P. Evans, *Heresies of the High Middle Ages* (New York and London 1969).

2   Nicolas Eymeric, *Directorium Inquisitorum* (Rome 1578), 206. A translated extract from this work can be found in Alan Kors and Edward Peters, *Witchcraft in Europe: A Documentary History* (Philadelphia, Pa 1972), 84–92.

3   A transcript of the interrogation is in the Morland collection of Waldensian manuscripts in Cambridge University Library: Dd. 111. 26 (c) H 6. It is printed in Peter Allix, *Ancient Churches of Piedmont* (London 1690), 30717.

4   On the Fraticelli see D. L. Douie, *The Nature and the Effect of the Heresy of the Fraticelli* (Manchester 1932), and the briefer accounts in M. Reeves, *The Influence of Prophecy in the Later Middle Ages* (Oxford 1969), 212–28, and G. Leff, *Heresy in the Later Middle Ages* (Manchester and New York 1967), vol. I, 23–55. The particular group of Fraticelli considered here figures only in Douie, 243–6.

5   On the Free Spirit see Robert E. Lerner, *The Heresy of the Free Spirit in the Later Middle Ages* (Berkeley, Calif. 1972), which is not only the most recent but also the most thorough survey of this difficult field. Lerner doubts whether the Brethren ever practised free love at all. In view of what is known about the English Ranters of the seventeenth century, who professed very similar doctrines, this scepticism seems excessive. But however that may be, Lerner demonstrates conclusively (pp. 29–31) that the orgy at Cologne was imaginary.

6   C. H. Lea, *The Inquisition of the Middle Ages,* Vol. II (New York 1888), 358.

7   See N. G. Garsolan, *The Paulician Heresy: A Study of the Origin and Development of Paulicianism in Armenia and the Eastern Provinces of the Byzantine Empire* (The Hague and Paris 1967), esp. 232–3.

8   See J. B. Russell, *Dissent and Reform in the Early Middle Ages* (Berkeley and Los Angeles 1965), 205–15.

PART TWO

Witchcraft, Magic and Culture

THE EXISTENCE OF WITCHCRAFT DEPENDED on a complex set of cultural assumptions. These assumptions established the possibility of the crime, identified the motives behind it, and determined the kind of people who were most likely to be its perpetrators. It can be argued, of course, that similar assumptions underlie the perception of *all* crimes; indeed, some thinkers have argued that the concept of 'crime' itself should be viewed as a social construction, shaped entirely by ethnic and historical circumstances.[1] In the case of witchcraft, the role of cultural factors is particularly obvious to modern observers, since many of the assumptions which made it possible – notably the existence of harmful magic – are no longer taken seriously in western industrial societies. As Christina Larner has noted, the refusal of most westerners to accept the existence of magic *per se* makes it difficult for witch trials to take place in the modern age: even if individuals attempt to cast harmful spells, most of their contemporaries will simply ignore them or regard them as mad. The willingness of most people in pre-industrial Europe to accept the reality of witchcraft, therefore, illustrates the gulf between their view of the world and our own. The nature of early modern witch beliefs, and the wider cultural assumptions and social experiences which sustained them, are the subject of the chapters in this section.

The cultural context of accusations of witchcraft is considered in depth in the first contribution by Robin Briggs. Briggs notes that cases of witchcraft normally centred on experiences of illness or misfortune, and allegations of *maleficium* provided an explanation for such occurrences. But he also notes that very few types of disease or hardship were connected exclusively with the crime. In other words, witchcraft could be linked to a wide range of very different experiences; this meant that it could, in principle, be used to explain practically any form of human suffering. It is striking, however, that relatively few unpleasant experiences were understood in this way. Indeed, the villages of pre-industrial Europe 'were not populated by a race of credulous half-wits who attributed any and every misfortune to witchcraft'. Why, then, were some events ascribed to hurtful magic when many others were not? Briggs suggests that a key factor was the existence of a plausible suspect, who appeared to possess both a motive for wishing harm on the afflicted individual and the requisite magical skills. When such a person was identified, the principal motive of those accusing them was often to have the spell lifted. This could be accomplished in many cases without recourse to the courts: informal contacts between the alleged witch and their victim could restore neighbourly relations and provide an ostensible 'cure'. Briggs' work challenges several modern assumptions about witchcraft: it suggests that many allegations might have been resolved peacefully, and therefore escaped the written record; and it reverses the normal priorities in witchcraft research by asking why trials did not occur *more frequently* than they actually did. Briggs also focuses attention on the social and physical reality of *maleficium*. With reference to modern phenomena like 'voodoo death' and the placebo effect in medicine, he shows that belief in magic could have produced some of the effects attributed to witchcraft in early modern Europe. This in turn suggests that fear of such effects was in no way irrational or 'superstitious'.

While Briggs concentrates on allegations of witchcraft against individuals, Chapter 4 by Wolfgang Behringer focuses on acts of collective *maleficium* that fuelled the large-scale witch panics in Germany in the late sixteenth and early seventeenth centuries. The consequences of these episodes were more terrible than those described by Briggs, but Behringer's approach to them is similar in important respects. First, he views fears of collective witchcraft as an explanation for human suffering, and efforts to deal with witches as a means to counteract this suffering. During the major German panics, he argues that ordinary people tended to ascribe bad weather to the activity of witches. This was an understandable response since the idea that groups of witches could maliciously alter the climate was already well established; and it made sense to attribute an attack on a whole community, such as the blighting of harvests by unseasonal weather, to the actions of more than one individual. Popular anxieties about weather magic forced local authorities to act against those who were believed to be responsible, despite the general reluctance of political elites to take the initiative in such matters. Second, Behringer suggests that fears of witchcraft were provoked by real phenomena. There *was* a severe decline in the climate in the period of the major panics, and this abnormal circumstance could be reasonably explained in terms of witchcraft. The exceptional weather patterns of the late sixteenth century encouraged the exceptional response of large-scale witch persecutions. While Behringer is careful to avoid attributing witchcraft trials solely to climatic phenomena, he convincingly explores the role of weather, hunger and fear in promoting popular concerns about the crime.

The work of Briggs and Behringer provides a general framework for understanding allegations of harmful magic in early modern Europe. It is helpful to supplement this approach with more detailed studies of particular regions, which can fill in the fine details of witchcraft prosecutions. This method is adopted in Chapters 5 and 6. E. William Monter presents in Chapter 5 an account of the sociology of witchcraft in the Jura region on the border between France and

Switzerland. Like Behringer, Monter concentrates on accusations of collective *maleficium*. He seeks first to identify the kind of people most frequently accused of the crime, then to describe the social dynamics behind a series of particular allegations. In pursuit of the first goal, he offers a breakdown of the known occupations and gender of individuals convicted in the Genevan panic of 1571–2, which resulted in the execution of thirty-six people and the banishment of many others. These figures suggest that Genevan witches were drawn largely from the poor, and that women were far more likely to be convicted than men. Monter's research indicates that local stereotypes of witches could make some groups much more vulnerable to accusations than others. But while his profile of a typical suspect has been shown to apply in many other European regions, it is important to note that it was not universally accepted: in some parts of France, for example, men were as likely as women to be accused of the crime.[2] Later in the chapter, Monter shows that allegations of collective witchcraft in the Jura often spread in directions determined by kinship and geography. After an initial accusation of *maleficium* was received by a local court, those most likely to be drawn into further investigations were the relatives of the accused and those living in their immediate vicinity. Since allegations of destructive magic depended largely on the availability of a plausible culprit, the identification of new witchcraft suspects could in turn provoke fresh accusations of *maleficium*.

One fascinating aspect of Monter's work is the light that it sheds on the attitudes of witchcraft suspects themselves. He suggests that the beliefs of the accused can sometimes reveal as much about the local context of witch trials as the depositions of those who testified against them. In several cases, it appears that Jura witches were guilty of unneighbourly or criminal behaviour, and were probably burdened by a guilty conscience. For Monter, this reflects the wider point that witches in the region were in a position of 'moral inferiority' to their accusers: they were often regarded as bad neighbours, whose use of evil magic was only one aspect of their generally antisocial personalities. David Gentilcore makes a similar point in Chapter 6. In the context of the Italian region of Terra d'Otranto, he shows that those accused of witchcraft often possessed a bad reputation among their neighbours, and charges of *maleficium* were often combined with allegations of blasphemy, religious deviance or 'filthy behaviour'. Thus suspects were not chosen at random, but accusations arose from reputations and social relationships built up over time. Like Monter, Gentilcore examines the confessions of alleged witches for evidence of popular beliefs: he finds that they sometimes incorporated aspects of local folklore, and witches' accounts of their meetings with the Devil resembled contemporary fables. When cases of witchcraft came before the courts, the final charges represented a complex interaction between different levels of local culture. The initial accusations of harmful magic were combined with more learned notions of the satanic pact; and this latter idea was understood by the accused in folkloric terms.

In common with the other contributors to this section, Gentilcore views witchcraft as one aspect of a much wider system of beliefs. The diagnosis of *maleficium* was one option among many for explaining and dealing with misfortune. The power of the saints or the Catholic clergy could be invoked to overcome disease, as could the services of *magara* – laymen and women who were skilled in the practice of magic. Such practitioners were condemned by the church hierarchy but were rarely punished with severity. Since the *magara* incorporated words from the Roman liturgy in their rituals, the boundaries between 'official' and 'unofficial' healing were decidedly blurred. In practice, it seems that most people were eclectic in their use of these resources: they were happy to seek assistance from a broad range of supernatural agencies as long as they appeared to meet their practical needs.[3]

By locating witch beliefs in their cultural context, the chapters in this section indicate the pitfalls of applying modern systems of classification to past societies. In the same way that anthropologists can read their own expectations into the practices of so-called 'primitive' societies, historians are prone to interpreting the beliefs and actions of early modern people according to their own, quite inappropriate assumptions about 'elite' and 'popular' culture, or the distinction between 'religion' and 'magic'. Equally, we are often tempted to isolate one particular set of social practices – like those surrounding the persecution of witches – and examine them outside the wider context of beliefs to which they belonged. It is only by considering the belief system of early modern people as a whole that we can start to understand the meaning of witchcraft. Ironically, it may be that one consequence of this approach is the discovery that modern historians are more preoccupied with witchcraft than were people in the pre-industrial age, to whom acts of *maleficia* were just one aspect of the vast 'economy of the sacred'.

Notes

1   For an overview of social constructionist thought, see Vivien Burr, *An Introduction to Social Constructionism* (Routledge, London 1995).

2   See Robin Briggs, *Witches and Neighbours* (HarperCollins, London 1996), ch. 7.

3   For the wider context of popular healing in the region, see David Gentilcore, *From Bishop to Witch: The System of the Sacred in Early Modern Terra d'Ontranto* (Manchester University Press 1992), chs 4 and 5.

Chapter 3

Robin Briggs

THE EXPERIENCE OF BEWITCHMENT

WHEN THE DEVIL PROMISED WITCHES prosperity and freedom from want he inevitably proved to have deceived them. It was very much otherwise with the power to harm others. His money might turn into leaves, but the powder or the familiars remained with his new servants and were all too efficacious. As far as other people were concerned, witchcraft was about power. To be bewitched was to suffer the effects of the witch's power; it was the defining experience of what this meant in the real world. In most cases a person or an animal fell ill; later they possibly died. There was general agreement that the affliction itself must be strange or unnatural, so known illnesses were almost never ascribed to witchcraft. Given the modest state of medical knowledge in early modern Europe, this still left a vast field open for argument.

The most clear-cut cases were those of sick people who were convinced they had been bewitched and named the witch responsible. They might demonstrate alarming symptoms if the suspect approached, or even at the mention of their name. The violence of some of these episodes is quite startling. The possessed London girl Mary Glover, having seen her alleged persecutor Elizabeth Jackson in church, went home and

> fell into a grievous fit, which was through repetitions of the witch's view, increased both in strength and in strangeness daily. In so much as now, she was turned round as a hoop, with her head backward to her hips; and in that position rolled and tumbled, with such violence, and swiftness, as that their pains in keeping her from receiving hurt against the bedstead, and posts, caused two or three women to sweat; she being all over cold and stiff as a frozen thing.

We may well see this particular instance as a hysterical attack, with the additional motive of gaining power and revenge, for when later the old woman was brought before her during such fits, a strange voice apparently coming from the girl's nostrils repeatedly said 'Hang her'.[1] There is every reason to suppose that such conviction could be an illness itself and that in some circumstances it might kill, either on its own or in conjunction with another complaint. The phenomenon of 'Voodoo death' sees the level of anxiety rise to a traumatic state, so that normal body functions collapse, and death may follow.[2] In effect those who are cursed or believe themselves to be the target of witchcraft go into shock; in most cases the result is some kind of pain or neurosis, which may well redouble in the presence of the suspect. Such phenomena have long been remarked on by observers of primitive societies, while more recently doctors have come to recognize how the immune system is affected by emotional states. The current trend towards less mechanistic ways of understanding the causes of sickness is very apposite here. In certain circumstances, it would appear, people can effectively be scared to death; more commonly, their normal social functioning and sense of well-being can be seriously impaired. While Haiti may be an extreme case, where impressive rituals reinforce the process, there is a very striking example from rural France as recently as 1968. In this instance a nocturnal session of counter-magic was followed the next day by the hospitalization of a neighbour suspected of witchcraft, who would presumably have been well aware of what was going on, and that the magic was intended to send the evil back to its alleged source. The woman concerned baffled the doctors; she would only repeat endlessly 'I'm afraid', and was too terrified to eat properly, dying seven months later.[3]

In societies where people believe in witchcraft their own fears usually function in this way, so that curses, threats and other expressions of ill-will have genuine power against the suggestible. The crime itself may be imaginary, but the imagination can be an immensely strong force. It is not surprising that children and adolescents seem to have been particularly prone to such disorders. While it would appear that most cases did not involve the most intense forms of witchcraft paranoia, a much larger number included claims that one or more of the alleged victims had blamed the accused for their fatal sickness. This was usually explicit, but might be expressed in a more oblique fashion, particularly if it was in a face-to-face encounter with the suspect. Margueritte Liegey, known as la Geline ('the hen'), had allegedly been a much feared beggar in the villages around Mirecourt in southern Lorraine for twenty years. After Claude George refused her alms one day she fell ill with her mouth twisted; when Margueritte returned she told her she had been very ill since the refusal. The suspect had no difficulty understanding the subtext of this remark, retorting 'so she wanted to say that she had given her the illness'; Claude still thought herself bewitched when she died three months later. This was just one of numerous allegations in this case from 1624, which ended with the confession and execution of the sixty-year-old widow. Eighteen months before the trial, Humbert Journal's wife had died after a violent illness lasting six days, during which she named Margueritte as the cause. Humbert chased after the suspect to beat her but she took refuge in the house of Didier Mongenot; Mongenot's wife had at first tried to keep her out and now believed she was bewitched, because several rat-sized animals seemed to be running about inside her body.[4]

Witnesses undoubtedly liked stories about blame attributed by past victims because they placed responsibility for the charges on persons who were safely dead. When it came to their own suspicions they were often more evasive, making use of various equivocations. Their testimony was commonly structured as a narrative, in which the causal links were by inference rather than direct statement. Isabel Bordon of Charmes, testifying against Claudon la Romaine, told how when the latter was ill she had asked the witness to visit her twice a day. She kept this up for some time, but finally stopped. After her recovery, Claudon came to Isabel's house to complain that the latter had begun her visits well, but finished badly. She then told Isabel that she did not like the plate of cabbage she was given, throwing it and the bread away. Isabel was angry, telling her she should not throw away such gifts in the name of God, when others might like them better than she did. This caused Claudon to leave 'angry and grumbling', at which the witness felt a sharp pain in her leg, which became so swollen she could only walk with a stick. A week later the suspect returned asking to sit by the fire, only for Isabel to tell her she could hardly make a fire for herself because of the bad leg she had since her last visit, adding 'I don't know what Devil has given it to me, but if it is not taken away some people will have to be put to death.' Claudon responded by advising her to rub it well with butter, a treatment which succeeded. Such statements arranged events in a sequence which strongly implied that one thing caused another without the need to state this explicitly. Some witnesses were prepared to affirm their belief directly; most limited themselves to suspicion or even a rather unconvincing pose of neutrality. Wherever possible the diagnosis of witchcraft was attributed to a third party. Jennon Napnuel might well have felt nervous when summoned as a witness against Georgeatte Herteman, since the latter, asked if she were not very vindictive, admitted she had a very quick temper. Jennon told of a quarrel at the mill and the subsequent death of a cow, whose flesh was rotting and coming away, so that the slaughterman 'gave it as his opinion that it was witchcraft'. These devices can be seen as evidence for the reluctance with which villagers testified at all, and their desire to leave a way open for reconciliation in case of an acquittal. They may also reveal the genuine uncertainty most people felt about witchcraft as an explanation, an awareness that there was something fragile and unreliable about it.

There is some evidence that the kin of sufferers were inclined to discourage ideas of bewitchment, and might show reluctance at any proposal they should summon the suspect. When Catherine Ancel was tried in 1614, Bastienne Morel testified about an incident, around 1600, when her late husband suspected Catherine over the illness of a bullock and wanted Bastienne to fetch her. In the end she agreed, and Catherine gave it some salt to lick, after which it recovered; Bastienne and her husband continued to dispute over the matter, as he suggested the cure showed it had been witchcraft, while she insisted one should not think ill of anyone and they did not know she was the cause. Most witnesses in this case used formulae to the effect that they were not sure, one saying rather pointlessly that he did not suspect her unless she was a witch. Catherine herself responded to questioning with the sensible comment that 'other people became ill just as she did, without anyone making them so'. In this case it seems that the accused had not given many real grounds for complaint to her neighbours, and that the suspicions owed a good deal to her mother's previous execution as a witch; in the event she withstood the torture to win her release, nearly two months after her arrest. Early modern European villages were not populated by a race of credulous half-wits who attributed any and every misfortune to witchcraft. Such people existed, but enjoyed little credit among neighbours who usually held more sophisticated views about causation and understood that sick people might be more desperate than wise. When Claudon Grand Demenge was on his deathbed he said a woman had caused his death; his brother thought he referred to his wife Jennon, but his sister-in-law thought it wrong to take any notice of what he said because he seemed to be out of his mind at the time. Since this was the most serious charge in a rather poorly supported accusation, these doubts may have been important in the subsequent decision to release Jennon without taking proceedings any further.

Religion, medicine and misfortune

Misfortune has always been a difficult concept, both intellectually and emotionally. Very few people are content to accept that blind chance plays a large part in their lives; they seek reasons in logical connections even where these do not really exist. In early modern Europe there were two large-scale systems which claimed to offer general explanations for success and failure, health and sickness, life and death. To the modern observer both appear almost wholly false, with their genuine power to explain being as meagre as their claims were grandiose. The first was religious or providential: God was an active force in the world, rewarding the faithful and punishing the impious, showing his hand in the issue of battles or the infliction of famine and plague. Some clever sleights of hand were necessary in order to deal with the more obvious cases in which the divine verdict was patently unjust; the almighty perforce became a very crafty operator, lulling some into a false sense of security while others endured tribulations designed to test or consolidate their faith. Although the resulting system was a supreme example of circular reasoning, it underlay a vast network of spiritual and therapeutic agencies that provided real comfort for many. Just as witchcraft could kill those who believed in it, so faith in divine power might well cure or succour them. The Devil himself was part of this way of thinking, and a particularly intractable one. Theologians wrestled none too successfully with the problem of evil and the reasons why God either inflicted it himself or allowed the Devil to do so in his stead.

The other, parallel system was that of natural philosophy, largely borrowed from Greek antiquity and imperfectly merged with the Christian tradition. This was the world of the elements and the humours, fictitious categories which supposedly governed everything from meteorology to medicine. Balance and harmony were the keys to peace in the skies, the state and the body alike. A whole arsenal of powerful imagery, still present in modern language and magnificently expressed by such authors as Shakespeare and Racine, was deployed to support these commonplaces. These literary glories cannot disguise the fact that the theory was little more than sonorous nonsense, which a few bold spirits were beginning to undermine, and would finally start replacing, in the later seventeenth century.

The intellectual leaders among clerics and doctors may have been ensnared in defective systems of thought, but they were quite capable of sharp perception on specific questions. For various reasons, they were never won over to support for the stronger versions of witchcraft theory, some isolated individuals apart. More importantly in the present context, these world views were far from being unknown at the popular level. It was the business of the clergy to disseminate Christian teachings, while almanacs and local medical practitioners were among the agencies which put about a rather fragmented version of natural philosophy. For all their weaknesses, these schemes had a very powerful effect on the way people at all levels of society apprehended their world. Explanations in terms of divine purpose and natural forces were normal; they did not exclude witchcraft, but both had a tendency to push it to the margins.

It was a commonplace among critics of persecution to ridicule the way medical failure was explained away by alleging witchcraft. There is no need to suppose this was merely cynical, for baffled doctors might have perfectly reasonable grounds for deciding on a supernatural explanation. At other times, university trained physicians could behave like any local wizard, identifying witchcraft on the basis of a sample of urine without even seeing the patient. The 1597 case of Alice Gooderidge, from Stapenhill near Burton-upon-Trent, shows how a diagnosis could evolve progressively. An aunt to a sick boy, Thomas Darling, took his urine to a physician, who suggested worms, then suspected witchcraft when the illness worsened. The aunt rejected the idea, but the possibility was then discussed in the boy's presence after which he came up with the story of his meeting with Alice Gooderidge and her anger against him. He had farted in front of her, after which she angrily said 'Gyp with a mischiefe, and fart with a bell: I will go to heaven, and thou shalt go to hell', then stooped ominously to the ground. At a later stage in this case a cunning man was called in who subjected the wretched old woman to a form of torture, putting her close to the fire with new shoes on her feet. This totally irregular (and indeed illegal) procedure was apparently carried out before an assembly of 'many worshipful personages'. Although she did not make a proper confession on this occasion, Alice finally agreed that she had been angry because the boy called her witch, then caused the Devil, in the form of a small dog, to afflict him; according to the pamphlet record she was convicted, only to die in prison.[5] Yet in the areas on which we have detailed information such episodes are relatively rare; it seems likely that a diagnosis of bewitchment was made only in a tiny fraction of all cases. This is particularly striking when one considers how much medical expertise was relatively amateurish and local. If practitioners had resorted to this technique to explain every failure, or those cases they did not understand, then accusations would have proliferated dramatically, far above the levels of which we know. In the absence of direct evidence one cannot know for sure why they were so restrained. They may have been so committed to their own approaches and methods that they preferred to seek explanations within the system rather than outside it; often they blamed the patient for not following the prescribed treatment.

Nothing in most of the illnesses seems to mark them off, apart from the reiterated claim that they were strange and unfamiliar, at best a highly subjective judgement. Sudden fatality and lingering decline might both be attributed to witchcraft, as might anything from eye trouble to a bad foot. People who felt sudden weights on their chest at night, so that they could not breathe, reported seeing other persons in the room who might attack them physically. Jacotte Simon told a complicated story about how she had remained in bed after her husband rose before dawn to work, then she felt something press down on her. Although she could not move, she managed to make the sign of the cross with her tongue, calling out to her husband for help. Finally managing to raise her head a little she saw Penthecoste Miette at the foot of her bed, but there was no reply when she spoke to her. Her husband then rushed in, at which two cats, both 'marvellously big and ugly', left with a great noise. She suspected that Mengeatte Lienard had been the other cat. On other occasions the cats spoke and might even hold a debate. Mesenne Vannier was ill in bed when three cats appeared and discussed whether to kill her, but decided that she was to be spared on account of her youth and recent marriage; their voices identified them as Jennon Zabey, the widow Rudepoil and Claudon Marchal's wife. This sounds like a typical hallucination brought on by a high fever. Other incidents where the sufferer felt paralysed in bed probably resulted from the quite common phenomenon of regaining partial consciousness while in a deep sleep. In addition, the various panic attacks may well have had a strong psychosomatic component, making them particularly suited for witchcraft explanations.

Angry exchanges and suspicions of bewitchment were much commoner than criminal prosecutions. A very powerful motive for accusing someone was the hope that they might offer a cure. This was likeliest if the charge were made indirectly, often in the form of an invitation to visit the sick person. There must have been a complex code in operation here, full of implicit understandings which are all too likely to escape the modern eye. In the negotiations which followed the witch was really being invited to accept responsibility, then secure pardon and immunity by removing the evil. Cures might be effected by touching, by bringing or preparing food, by more formal medical treatment with herbs or charms, or by pilgrimages and rituals. In the Labourd, according to de Lancre, it was customary to ask the suspect to wash their hands in a basin, then give the water to the sufferer to drink, a ritual with multiple resonances.[6] The display of good-will involved cancelled out the negative charge of the original ill-will; in many cases it must have made the sufferer feel much better. A good many of the witnesses in court cases were talking about episodes of this kind, which would have been regarded as closed until legal action started. The notion that illness might be related to the breakdown of inter-personal relations, also contained within this pattern of behaviour, was far from absurd. If the sickness resulted from a broken relationship with the witch, then the natural inference was that a formal display of reconciliation was a necessary part of a cure. When William Luckisone of Stirling was ill around 1653 he consulted Magdalen Blair, herself a suspect, who asked him 'if there was any enmitie or discord between Issobel Bennet and him'. When he replied that he sometimes threw stones at her chickens to drive them off his father's property, she advised him to 'go to Issobel Bennet and take a grip of her coat tail and drink a pint of ale with her. And crave his health from her thrie tymes for the Lords sake and he would be well'. William claimed he had not followed the advice, which is understandable, for such a confrontation required a degree of nerve.[7] Demands for signs of amity or neighbourliness further constituted a warning to the suspected witch, particularly in relation to the victim's family, with whom it would be wise to avoid further disputes. It was not unknown for the witch to make formal promises to cause them no further trouble. Claudon Renauldin was returning home with Didelon and Bietrix l'Hullier whom he believed to have caused him extensive losses; when he thought of this he went to beat Didelon, who reacted with the highly unwise statement 'that he would never harm him, nor cause him further losses or damage'.

Parents, children and witchcraft

Whereas illness was unpredictable, the dangers of childbirth were the opposite. Women had every reason to be nervous about the risks to themselves and their babies, against which they sought to mobilize help and protection. The presence of neighbours and relatives offered moral as well as practical support at a moment of great danger and stress. Failure to summon a neighbour with a reputation as a witch to either the birth or the christening was to keep them at a safe distance, while running the risk of giving offence that might provoke hostile action. This scenario appeared frequently in the trials as the explanation of a bad outcome for mother, child or both. Jacquotte Tixerand refused to attend the baptism of George Guyart's son, since she had not been asked to the childbed, but when she visited the house a week later she admired the child, telling the mother to keep it well; when it sickened the same day, to die a week later, the inference was obvious. Similar problems were attached to godparenting, for it was all too easy to give offence over this important sign of mutual friendship and respect. Jehennon Foelix had suggested that Claudatte Mengin might act as godmother to her first child then had to withdraw the offer because another promise had already been made else-where. The subsequent loss of a cow was blamed on her witchcraft, but when a second child was born Jehennon and her husband tried to make amends by asking George Mengin, Claudatte's husband, to be godfather. This too turned out badly because the suspect wanted her son to take the role instead and was annoyed when the midwife said he was too young; when the baby died a few months later, this was inevitably blamed on Claudatte. High infant mortality rates were general across Europe, with many babies languishing then dying for no obvious reason. These deaths inevitably formed one cause for suspicion; difficulties with breastfeeding, another very common problem, were often blamed on witchcraft too. Older women, who provided the normal source of advice in such cases, could easily find themselves in ambiguous positions. When Zabel Rémy lost her milk, her relative Dion Rémy (who was about seventy-five at the time) came to her aid; she made Zabel drink some wine, then damped some coarse cloth, warmed it by the fire and applied it to her breasts. Another witness remembered, however, that she had not been invited to the celebrations after the birth, was suspected by the parents, then invited to dinner in an attempt to secure relief.

Professional help in delivery was normally provided by midwives and it has been widely supposed that any misfortune might be blamed on their witchcraft, allegedly linked to their position as 'popular' healers in traditional folklore. Midwives have thus become a paradigmatic case of female medical specialists under attack from men who wanted to control them and destroy their autonomy. Whatever truth there may be in these wider claims, the putative association with witchcraft is illusory. No statistical evidence of any significance has been produced to support it; where figures have been established they show that midwives were rather under-represented among the accused.[8] The theme is present in demono-logical literature mainly because the *Malleus Maleficarum* went on about witch-midwives at some length and was copied by later writers. There seems to be a connection with the idea that witches ate the flesh of unbaptized children or used their remains to make poisons; midwives were supposed to be the main providers of the bodies of stillborn babies. There are odd cases where this idea surfaced, as with the one Lorraine witch who actually fits the stereotype, Jennon Petit; she admitted digging up the bodies of the infants she had killed on behalf of her master Persin, who then made powder with them. In general, however, it is easy to understand why midwives were rarely accused; they were selected precisely because they were regarded as trustworthy persons by the community so that it must have taken a catastrophic drop in their standing for them to become suspects. A rare instance of association between child-care and witchcraft tends to bear this out, for in the German city of Augsburg a number of lying-in servants found themselves on trial. These were women who specialized in helping out in households around the time of childbirth, but they lacked the skills or status of midwives and were much more vulnerable in consequence.[9]

Women who had difficulties bearing children, with frequent miscarriages or stillbirths, were liable to blame these on witchcraft, perhaps displacing their worries about their own failure to meet expectations. Mengeon Cohn and his wife Agathe had objected strongly when the local mayor's wife proposed Heuratte Chappouxat for election as midwife at le Vivier, drawing attention to the great misfortunes which might arise from having a witch in that position. She was naturally angry when they succeeded in getting someone else chosen, so now Agathe blamed her for three successive stillbirths. Motherhood is, of course, a long-term affair and as children grew their own behaviour often appeared as the original point of tension. They might taunt supposed witches directly or perhaps insult them through their own children. Mothers were always defending their children against others who attacked them; this could be thought the reason for a witch's resentment, or if threats of violence to a child were followed by sickness, the moment at which the bewitchment had actually occurred. Didier Goeury's mother went to tell Jean Pelisson off after he had beaten her son for no reason, saying she could beat her own children if it were necessary and meanwhile he should attend to his own, who badly needed discipline. Soon after, she fell fatally ill, while the surgeons and doctors declared her bewitched. When the sons of Claude Henry and Barbelline Antoine fought, the former was hurt, which led to a quarrel between the parents and relatives; the following Sunday the boy's grandmother, Marion Henry, was met with silence when she greeted Barbelline in church, then promptly fell ill and died. She would have sent for the suspect if one of her sons had not prevented this. When Marye Sotterel asked the eight-year-old son of Meline Hanry where he was going, he replied 'That's enough for you, great witch', after which she chased him and beat him; he fell ill next day and died a month later.

Animals and bewitchment

If there was one area in which people thought of bewitchment more readily than in connection with their own illnesses, it was over the misfortunes of their animals. Domestic animals are extremely vulnerable to infectious diseases and small accidents; even with modern techniques their ailments can be difficult to diagnose and treat. Furthermore, a substantial amount of the capital of early modern society, especially in the rural world, was tied up in these fragile creatures. If the medical profession was rudimentary, the veterinary one hardly existed at an official level. Every peasant needed some practical skills in treating animals; in difficult cases they turned to neighbours reputed skilful in healing, including herdsmen, shepherds and smiths. The usual range of practical and pious remedies was on offer; quite large numbers of magical prayers survive. This was probably because suspected witches saw them as perfectly normal and accepted forms of treatment, so were ready to repeat them before the judges. In other respects the bewitchment of animals followed the same pattern as that of humans. It usually followed quarrels and threats, was closely linked to these by its timing and frequently led to demands for the witch to effect a cure.

With animals even more than with humans, one is conscious of how flexible the diagnosis of illness might be. Strangeness and suddenness were taken as signs of witchcraft – the cow which ate normally but wasted away, the horse which dropped dead in the stable. Slaughtermen and others who cut up dead animals would sometimes claim that they were rotten inside, something which must proceed from witchcraft. Mayette Gaste was suspected of causing the death of a horse whose flesh was found to be blackened as if burned, so that the butcher said it had been given a drink by some evil persons. Commonest of all was the allegation that an animal had died 'as if rabid', a curious example of having it both ways, with the natural explanation being simultaneously advanced and rejected. Perhaps the symptoms of animals which lashed out at their masters and foamed at the mouth were thought similar to those of demonic possession. The various infections which resulted in the feet and legs rotting away were also cited as proof of bewitchment, although they seem all too plainly natural to a modern reader. The accused were obviously bewildered by some of the charges, protesting that the sickness had been natural, that animals were always dying and that they had lost as many themselves. On other occasions they alleged ill-treatment or various faults in handling the animals. Claudatte Ferry argued that the goats and cows she was accused of bewitching had suffered from a sickness which had affected many animals that winter, while some of them might also have been weak because their owner was feeding them on a poor substitute for hay.

Milking cows were very susceptible to infections (such as brucellosis and other disorders), which often coincided with minor disputes over requests for purchases or gifts of milk. A routine pattern saw these episodes interpreted as witchcraft. Demenge Saulnier claimed that Margueritte Liegey had asked his wife to sell her some wood and after several refusals went to the door of the stable, turned round and came back. This was repeated three times, then she asked to buy milk, responding to a further refusal with a threat that she would repent. Their only cow then sickened, only recovering within hours of a threat to beat her. A more elaborate belief occasionally surfaced that witches had the capacity to take milk away from their neighbours, using a kind of snare or other device. The child Mongeotte Pivert, whose confessions led to the deaths of several members of her family, alleged that her father set snares for neighbours' cattle to pass over, then took the threads home and warmed them by the fire before rubbing the backs of his own cattle to obtain more milk. Virtually all these beliefs seem to have been applied only to a minority of cases, so that yet again the identification of witchcraft must have depended as much on awareness of a suspect as it did on the nature of the misfortune.

This applied in the case of one specific nexus of beliefs, that in werewolves. The notion that witches could be transformed into the likeness of other animals, such as cats and hares, was particularly threatening when extended to these dangerous and much feared predators. The number of known cases across Europe is very small, despite the fairly widespread belief, so it is very hard to understand why it occasionally surfaced in a prosecution. Attacks by wolves might be interpreted in this way on the grounds that a particular animal had been singled out, a notably unconvincing attempt to give the normal behaviour of predators diabolical purposiveness. More plausible stories picked up on claims that the wolves had an abnormal appearance; according to Boguet, when Perrenette Gandillon turned herself into a wolf and killed a child, the creature had no tail and human hands in place of its front paws.[10] In 1573 rumours were circulating that the villages near Dole were 'infested with wolves the size of donkeys' that ate people and were impossible to capture; these were naturally supposed to be werewolves.[11] Alternatively they behaved unnaturally, like the wolf which strangled the foal of Claudon Jean Claudon, refusing to loosen its grip when burning sticks were put against its throat. Earlier the same day his son Curien (who was guarding the herd) had quarrelled with one of Claudon Marchal's sons, and this was not the only suspicion of the kind against him. The extreme and sensational cases were those of wolves which devoured children, bringing together the werewolf theme with the cannibalism sometimes found at the sabbat. When the children of Grattain were running after the wolf which had taken Claudon Didier Vagnier's child, Claudette Dabo was seen in the vicinity and a strong rumour spread that she had eaten it. The whole business of shapeshifting is a curious mixture of ancient folklore and practical everyday fears, which lurks around the fringes of witchcraft belief without ever becoming an integral part of it. Figures for later periods suggest that quite large numbers of children were attacked by wolves; apparently only a tiny minority of these events were openly attributed to werewolves.

Accidents and poverty

Another large area of bewitchment was that of damage from a range of physical causes. Work accidents – including injuries inflicted by sharp tools, falling objects and the like – made occasional appearances in the depositions. A variety of other accidents might be presented as life-threatening, as when millwheels disintegrated suddenly after a quarrel with the suspect. This happened to Colas Chretien at Moyenmoutler just as his wife was telling him of a quarrel with Mongeatte Joliet and warning him to be careful how he tried to clear the frozen millwheel which had only just been repaired. Newly built structures were known to collapse after visits by local witches.

Livelihoods could be put at risk in similar ways. The frequent disputes over milk might be followed by an inability to make butter churn; there were various folkloric remedies, including putting a heated horseshoe or other metal object in the cream, a move some thought would cause severe pain to the witch responsible. Ovens or forges would mysteriously refuse to reach the correct temperature, however much fuel was added. Francois Pelletier had a dispute over the price of some work he did for Hellenix le Reytre, then found the hides he had in store had rotted, causing him serious losses. He wisely reduced his price, then she advised him to use his own cellar for storage in future, which proved successful.

Serious damage to crops was most readily linked to witchcraft through the stories of hail, rain or frost being made at the sabbat. Individual witches were much less likely to be blamed here, although very selective damage or marked immunity might start tongues wagging. Jeanne Lienard was playing with fire when she told several people at Laveline that they ought to be generous with their alms to her, since she had preserved their crops from hail three years earlier when she had let the neighbouring parishes be laid waste because their inhabitants were so ungenerous to her. It was hardly surprising that one of the witnesses said that everyone feared her, and for himself 'he would as soon see a wolf as her when she came to his house begging'. Under interrogation she freely admitted these remarks, giving the obvious explanation that she wanted to persuade the villagers to be generous, while admitting that she knew no way to protect them in fact. This was an odd case in many respects; the accused told a series of fanciful stories, sounding very confused or even deranged, confessed under torture, then withdrew the confession, resisted a second round of torture and was finally released. Vines and fruit trees might suffer as well as grain crops, while gardens could prove strangely infertile. A run of bad luck was as threatening in these sectors of agricultural life as it was with animals. Behind local fluctuations there lurked the spectre of general economic failure, bringing personal ruin with it. In maritime communities, such as were found in Scotland, England, parts of Scandinavia or the Basque country, weather magic extended to the sinking of ships. Fishing villages which lost significant numbers of menfolk were extremely vulnerable, for this was one activity in which women could not replace them. Violent suspicions of this kind might lead to direct action, as with an incident in 1573 involving some sailors from Enkhuizen, anchored off the Dutch island of Ameland. At the request of the inhabitants, who believed a woman living on the island to be responsible for wrecking ships, they threw her into the sea, then beat her to death with an oar.[12]

Like every other aspect of bewitchment, this one reminds us just how precarious life must have felt to most ordinary people. Neither prosperity nor good health were to be counted on for the morrow. Those who stayed fit themselves might still be dragged down by the burden of a sick or crippled spouse or child. The unlucky could end up as vagrants and beggars, despite the very real degree of charity and mutual help offered by the community. Often the loss of status was felt as keenly as the more direct privations. The fears and tensions just below the surface occasionally surfaced in witchcraft accusations, with specific threats attributed to the suspects. Marguerite Carlier of Oisy-le-Verger, tried in 1612, allegedly told Antoinette Pannequin 'that she would see her husband die in poverty, as had happened, and that she herself would have to beg, as well as telling the children of the late Wattencourt to their shame that they too would go begging'.[13] Jean Diez seems to have made a speciality of such threats, for Zabel Gillat alleged that he told her and her husband 'he would bring them down so far that they needed a beggar's wallet', and having been rich they lost so many animals that they indeed became poor. Her husband Demenge added that every time he quarrelled with Jean some misfortune followed, and that he told the witness 'as for him and le grand Colas, he would cause them to die shamefully, in public view, because of the charges they made against him'. The other man intended was evidently George Colas Bergier, to whom he remarked on the road from St Die 'you see George, you are a rich man, comfortable and with much property, while I only have my bill-hook, but within three or four years at the most you will become so poor that you will have nothing left with which to beg your bread, while I will become prosperous'. George replied 'that this depended on the will of God, and it was for him to permit it or not', to be told 'that he knew for certain that it would turn out so, and that he knew many things'. According to his widow, although from that moment on they worked as hard as anyone else and were not extravagant, they were slowly reduced to desperate poverty. This will not have been an isolated experience around this time. The peak decades for persecution were ones in which communal and family bonds were being tested to the limit, for European society was passing through a phase of change accompanied by severe hardship for many.

Notes

1   S. Bradwell, 'Mary Glover's late woeful case', 5–6, 19 in M. MacDonald, ed., *Witchcraft and Hysteria in Elizabethan London* (London 1991).

2   W. B. Cannon, 'Voodoo death', *American Anthropologist,* new set 44, 1942, 169–81.

3   J. Favret-Saada, *Deadly Words: Witchcraft in the Bocage* (Cambridge 1980), 78–911.

4   For brevity, the archival sources used in this chapter have been omitted from this edition. Full references can be found in Robin Briggs, *Witches and Neighbours* (HarperCollins, London 1996), ch. 2.

5   *The most wonderfull and true storie, of a certaine witch named Alse Gooderidge of Stapenhill* (London 1597), 1–4. Summaries and extracts from the pamphlet in C. H. L. Ewen, *Witchcraft and Demonianism* (London 1933), 176–81, and G. B. Harrison, *Lancaster Witches* (London 1929), xxxiv–viii.

6   Pierre de Lancre, *Tableau de l'inconstance* (Paris 1613), 356.

7   Christina Larner, *Enemies of God: The Witch Hunt in Scotland* (London 1981), 141.

8   The absence of midwives among witchcraft suspects is confirmed by E. W. Monter in Chapter 5 of this volume. See also D. Harley, 'Historians as demonologists: the myth of the midwife-witch', *Social History of Medicine* 3, 1990, 1–26.

9   L. Roper, 'Witchcraft and fantasy in early modern Germany', in *Oedipus and the Devil* (London 1994), 199.

10   H. Boguet, *Discours des sorciers* (3rd edn, Lyon 1610), 361–28.

11   C. F. Oates, 'Trials of Werewolves in the Franche-Comté in the early modern period' (PhD thesis, London).

12   H. de Waardt, 'Prosecution or defense: procedural possibilities following a witchcraft accusation in the Province of Holland before 1800', in M. Gijswijt-Hofstra and W. Frijhoff, eds, *Witchcraft in the Netherlands from the Fourteenth to the Twentieth Century* (Rotterdam 1991), 83.

13   Robert Muchembled, *La Sorcière au village* (Paris 1979), 170.

Chapter 4

Wolfgang Behringer

WEATHER, HUNGER AND FEAR

Origins of the European witch-hunts in climate, society and mentality

I

THIS CHAPTER DOES NOT BEGIN by addressing the continental legal system, but a more fundamentally anthropological theme: the continental climate, changes in the ecological system and, as its indicator, the weather – at first glance a banal phenomenon. However, during the major witchcraft persecutions of Central Europe in the sixteenth century, accusations of weather-magic recurred with striking frequency. Midelfort has already shown how important the question of weather-magic was for the revival of witchcraft persecutions in Southwestern Germany in 1562–3.[1] The charge of weather-related magic was not new; it reflected a pattern of beliefs present in pagan antiquity and survived in popular culture into the Early Middle Ages. Virtually all Germanic law codes professed a belief in weather-magic, contained in proscriptions against it. In contrast, the church denied the possibility of weather-magic, threatening the belief therein with severe penalties, exemplified by prohibitions established by the Council of Brega in 563. However, examples from the High Middle Ages reveal that this campaign met with little success and, long before the rise of a cumulative concept of witchcraft, groups of individuals were collectively persecuted for alleged weather-magic: Agobard of Lyon implicated southern French peasants in repressions, while a chronicler from the Bavarian monastery at Weihenstephan accused peasants in the Bishophric of Freising of being instigators of a persecution of weather-magicians – against the will of their ecclesiastical and secular overlords.[2]

In the late fifteenth and early sixteenth centuries, the discussion of weather-magic accusations achieved new prominence. Although the belief was long considered theologically suspect, the *Malleus Maleficarum* unquestionably imputed to witches the ability to effect weather-magic, even as jurists and other theologians argued against this possibility. In his consideration of the *Malleus* in 1489, Ulrich Molitor placed the question of weather-magic before all others.[3] After witchcraft persecutions set in again in the 1560s, the issue of weather-magic returned to the centre of debate: an influential evangelical preacher, Thomas Naogeorgus of free-imperial Esslingen, blamed witches for hail damage to the harvest, calling for their persecution,[4] just as the representatives of Lutheran orthodoxy at Tübingen in the neighbouring Duchy of Württemberg energetically struggled against these beliefs with the traditional argument that only God was in a position to influence the weather.[5]

Why did theologians argue so vehemently about the role of weather-magic? That the charge played such a decisive role is not surprising when one considers the importance of climate in agrarian life. The exact time and location of this debate is even more conspicuous. Most participants were from the Upper German-French-Swiss border regions: Institoris, an Alsatian, came from Selestat, Molitor was the Episcopal Procurator of Constance and Brenz was a Tübingen reformer. Although the agrarian infrastructure of Central Europe lacked large urban areas on a par with Istanbul, Naples, and London, it suffered from chronic over-population with a population density greater than England, Scandinavia, or Eastern Europe, probably parts of Italy and the Iberian peninsula as well, all areas recently consigned to the 'periphery' of witchcraft persecutions. Central Europe suffered from a particularly sensitive infrastructure and backward agricultural practices when compared to England, Italy, and the Netherlands. Owing to its location, the agrarian economy of Central Europe, largely dependent on vineyards and wheat, was especially vulnerable to climatic disaster.

Nevertheless, the primary motivation behind the engagement of continental theologians with weather-magic derived more from its dramatically virulent manifestations. Whereas common *maleficium* involved individuals in conflict, charges of weather-magic were frequently raised by entire communities. These collective accusations directed against a fictive collective rather than individual culprits justified the employment of any means necessary to track down the conspiracy. In this sense, peasant perceptions corresponded with those of Christian demonology. That a crime as heinous as the destruction of crops by weather-magic could be committed by a single person seemed inconceivable, a preconception lending the crime an added dimension. If the authorities refused to bend to popular pressure, communities occasionally responded with open unrest.

A characteristic example is provided by the largest witchcraft persecution in German-speaking regions during the sixteenth century in Trier, which claimed some 300 victims and was previously written off to the personal persecution complex of the Prince-Elector. In an impressive dissertation on the witch trials in Trier and the County of Sponheim, Walter Rummel proves the inadequacy of this old interpretation. Actually, the persecuting impulse 'was fostered almost completely "from below", from communities and their representatives'.[6] The administration of the ecclesiastical territory was nearly paralysed as communal committees wrested judicial authority from its hands as a consequence of this campaign of extermination, while the administration fought in vain to win back the initiative. A local witchcraft ordinance of 1591 mentions that 'communities . . . have conspired and established a pact very nearly resembling a revolt'.[7]

And this was no mere apology, as confirmed by Eva Lahouvie's recent investigations into the social logic behind 'village inquisitions' conducted in the territories of today's Saarland, of the Teutonic Order, as well as Electoral Trier, the Duchy of Lorraine and their associated territories. With a dynamism shocking for the 'age of absolutism', subject populations imposed their will on politically weak administrations. Their methods of witch-finding reflected precious little of the refined techniques attendant on Roman law or inquisitorial theory. Committees formed by free primitive elections held within their respective communities acted without legitimation from the ruling elite and naturally beyond elite interests. Instead, they represented the 'self-initiative of comradeship toward witch-hunting'. The committees acted on behalf of village communities, following the interests of the peasant population alone. These circumstances unmistakably explain the laconic remarks of a contemporary chronicle from Trier on the causes of the great persecution: 'Because everyone generally believed that crop failures over many years had been brought on by witches and malefactors out of devilish hatred, the whole land rose up to exterminate them'.[8]

Obviously, rain, snow, and hail were not invented in the sixteenth century and illness and death are constant companions in humanity's path through history. However, just as people differentiate between 'natural' and 'unnatural' illnesses, so too have they differentiated between 'natural' and 'unnatural', i.e. magically conjured weather. One important cause of witchcraft persecutions in the second half of the sixteenth century appears to have rested in popular perceptions of 'unnatural' types of weather (e.g. cold winters, persistent snowfall, evening frosts late in the spring, wet summers, floods, severe hailstorms, etc.). In the eyes of contemporaries, 'unnatural' weather deviated from long-experienced norms.

Let us examine climatic history in the period identified by researchers as the high point of the European witchcraft persecutions, the decades between 1560 and 1630. Closer analysis reveals a striking correlation between this epoch and a period of general climatic deterioration after 1560, sometimes known as the 'Little Ice Age'. Although dates for the onset of the 'Little Ice Age' vary slightly, there is general consensus that a climatic deterioration occurred in early modern Europe, marked by falling annual temperatures, a curtailed growing season, pervasive meridional cold streams from the poles, extreme winters, a lowering of the snowline on mountains, and the advance of Alpine glaciers.

Statistics based on an interdisciplinary study by Christian Pfister regarding the history of Swiss climate permit precise conclusions for individual years in Central Europe. Pfister provides the following median climate fluctuations: after a 'warm-phase' (1530–64), comparable to the recent 'warm peak' for the years 1943–52, there followed a climatic deterioration between 1565 and 1629.[9] Both epochs correspond closely to the boundaries recognized by witchcraft researchers. A relative lull in witchcraft persecutions for about a generation after the Reformation ended after they began to revisit Europe in 1563, provoking Johann Weyer to utter his famous remark that one would have believed that the age of witch-hunts had long passed. Unfortunately, a period now unanimously recognized as the peak of persecutions followed, years which conceal hidden climatic surprises; Pfister identified 'cumulative cold-sequences' for the years 1560–74, 1583–9, and 1623–8.

Thanks to his conclusions, changes in the ecological system in the late sixteenth century can now be identified and placed in precise context. Apparently unrelated reports of catastrophes by contemporaries, such as constant flooding after 1560, were part of an overall pattern of increased rainfall, and damage to mountain forests and pastures was exacerbated by clearing and cattle grazing necessitated by increased grain cultivation in valleys. Erosion, soil exhaustion, and the tillage of marginal lands in continental Europe led to declining yields, both in agriculture and live-stock, the latter evidenced by falling milk production. Cold wet years resulted in meagre late harvests and the need to stall feed livestock for longer periods on reduced quantities of fodder. Low temperatures also increased demand for kindling and caloric intake. A monostructure of consumables enhanced human vulnerability to fluctuations in crop yields. The common people's fear of hail storms, regularly attributed to the activity of witches, derived primarily from the threat to subsistence agriculture rather than from religious reasons.

By 1562, a heavy increase in wet weather was already apparent. Extreme cases, such as the freezing of Lake Constance, the largest alpine lake, in 1563 and again in 1572–3 for a full sixty days impressed contemporaries as unusual climatic developments and were recorded for posterity by chroniclers as centennial events. The climax of the cooling off that began in 1560 was reached in 1573. 'At that time, nature seems to have left its usual course' was the sober conclusion of one glacial researcher on the years after 1570, a comment very close to the view of contemporaries.[10] In the early 1570s, Central Europe was visited by a major famine, which must have profoundly shocked this relatively affluent society.

After 1586, colder winters were intensified by a period of cold wet springs. In 1587, snow fell until the beginning of July and, by mid-September, the valleys were again covered with snow. In 1588, storms besetting the Spanish Armada coincided with the wettest year of the century. The years 1584–9, particularly cold and wet, provided climatic impetus to the witch-hunts in Trier, the largest up to that time in German-speaking lands. The Trier witchcraft persecution was no isolated incident; a simultaneous hunt occurred in the Duchy of Lorraine, reported in the *Daemonolatria* of the witch-hunting judge Nicolas Rémy. Potential witch-hunts also threatened other parts of France, Germany, Switzerland, and Scotland. Furthermore, increased interest in maleficient magic – though without major persecutions – is apparent in Austria, England, Hungary, Italy, Poland, Spain and the Baltic region. In light of interwoven ecological factors, we cannot dismiss the unusual accumulation of reports concerning ecological catastrophes by contemporary authors as mere tropes. For, as the anonymous author of a pamphlet appearing in southern Germany noted in 1590:

> So many kinds of magic and demonic apparitions are gaining the upper hand in our time that nearly every city, market and village in all Germany, not to mention other peoples amid nations, is filled with vermin and servants of the Devil who destroy the fruits of the fields, which the Lord allows to grow with his blessing, with unusual thunder, lightning, showers, hail, storm winds, frost, flooding, mice, worms and many other things . . . causing them to rot in the fields, and also increase the shortage of human subsistence by spoiling livestock, cows, calves, horses, sheep, and others, using all their power, not just against the fruit of the fields and livestock, but yes, not even sparing kinsfolk and close blood-relatives, who are killed in great numbers.[11]

The direct connection between weather-magic, witchcraft persecutions and harvest failures made by contemporaries is even more obvious when one reconstructs the circumstances of individual hunts, for example, in the county court of Schongau, where sixty-three women were legally executed as witches in the years 1589–91. These hunts were not initiated by denunciations arising from previous hunts nor from outside accusations. Nor did they commence at the instigation of the authorities, local judges, or the parish clergy. Instead, popular pressure obviously motivated the authorities to act. In so far as documentary reconstruction is possible, the prerequisite was a series of storms damaging crops and resultant crop failures, as chronicled for the regions near Kempten, Memmingen, and Augsburg, culminating in peasant unrest. On 26 June 1588, a severe hailstorm decimated crops in the community of Schwabsoien, a Bavarian border community partially under the jurisdiction of the Bishophric of Augsburg whose 100 households the protocols of the episcopal Court Council in Dillingen referred to as consisting mostly of poor cottagers. Although the Bishop expressed his willingness to provide new seed for the coming year, the inhabitants remained unsatisfied: the village elite, among them the village judge Hans Kerbl, and the committee of four appeared before the county judge of Schongau requesting the 'extermination' of the witches held responsible for the disaster. For the relatively poor community, all means to that end was justifiable. They were even prepared to sell the communal forest to pay for the services of the renowned executioner of Biberach. In a communal meeting with their pastor, the villagers explained that they would gladly sell the forest, if the proceeds would go toward the extermination of the witches. Bearing this connection in mind, let us examine a letter of Duke Ferdinand of Bavaria responding to the report from the county judge in Schongau, Hans Friedrich Herwarth of Hohenburg. This letter, which initiated the Schongau inquisition on 24 July 1589, contains the following remarks:

> My dear servant, we have seen with our own eyes and not from your report alone, how inclement weather, showers and hail spoiled these poor people's dear fruits of the field . . . but are even more concerned with their plight . . . as the Almighty has allowed them to be so sorely afflicted by the Devil and his damnable agents, and we order that you should secretly pay close attention to evil persons and witches and in case any should come under sufficient suspicion, you should stealthfully nab them and immediately search their lodgings, chests, bed and containers with all industry to discover if suspicious magical affects, such as salves, wicked powders, concoctions, wax images stuck with pins, human limbs or legs, charms, insignia or other equally wicked objects can be found.[12]

Explicit reference is made to a common characteristic of major witch-hunts, the public demand for persecutions from a community whose harvest, i.e. their source of livelihood, indeed of their very existence, had been destroyed by inclement weather. The letter also reveals that this was not Herwarth's first report of suspected witchcraft:

In particular, we recall that you recently mentioned the sighting of a woman by two woodmen in a wood not far from Peissenberg followed shortly thereafter by a storm. You should investigate this incident industriously and, if circumstantial evidence is present, make arrests and immediately thereafter inform the executioner from Biberach that he should examine the woman's entire body to determine whether signs, notes or marks of the type the evil enemy uses to mark his servants are present on her, and ask the executioner how to recognize the witches, and, according to your findings, to report back to us and, if necessary, to accompany the report personally.[13]

Suspicion of witchcraft was given top priority. As we can see from the background and the contents of the letter, the Duke was not a fanatical witch-hunter but simply paternalistic to the concerns of his subjects. Contrary to the situation in Trier, an example well known throughout Germany, he wanted to remain on top of the situation and master the investigation against the witches, whose existence he never questioned, rather than allow himself to be driven by the populace. This much is clear from his instructions to the county judge. Despite the large number of victims, no one in the county seemed displeased with the results of the persecution. In 1594, four years after the conclusion of this great persecution, the County Judge of Schongau requested that Duke Ferdinand erect an 'eternal pillar' to commemorate the witch-hunt, because the power of the witches had been broken and harvests had returned to normal. Tangentially, his request sought to underscore costs incurred during the hunt in the hope of reimbursement, but one assumes that the request for a monument would have been appropriate only if it fit the mood of the populace.

Similar correlation between climatic catastrophes and witch-hunts like that of the 1580s recurred thereafter. In particular, climatic conditions in the years 1621–30 resembled those between 1586 and 1599, marked by cold winters, late springs and cold wet weather in the summer and autumn. 1628, the year in which witchcraft persecutions in Germany, indeed Europe in general, reached their absolute peak, is referred to by Pfister as 'the year without a summer'.[14] These persecutions benefited from the experience of witch-hunts conducted since the 1580s. When crop failures beset the Saar region in 1627, communities gathered under the 'village linden trees' (a traditional meeting place) to discuss plans of action and elect representatives in order to organize witch-hunts.[15]

In summary, the age of the great persecutions corresponded generally to the 'Little Ice Age' and the individual hunts corresponded to specifically catastrophic years. The era of extremely poor weather was followed by a phase that was cool, but dry. In those lands which played a role in subsequent development, in England, Holland, and France, the witch-craze was overcome by ruling elites and the number of persecutions began to decline. One might find it historically ironic that the philosophy of western Europe corresponded to climatic conditions, for it was cool and dry as well. Empiricist and Cartesian philosophy in the subsequent epoch formed the bulwark against a major relapse into the witch-craze, even when global cooling in the last thirty years of the seventeenth century peaked in an 'Ice Age summer' in 1675. The years between 1688 and 1701 have gone down in the literature as a renewed highpoint of the 'Little Ice Age'. During this period, several great witch-craft persecutions did occur, although I shall not address them here. After a time of renewed warming (1702–30) there followed a period (1730–1811) in which cold winters and wet, but warm summers predominated. The rise of the sun at the beginning of the eighteenth century not only melted glaciers, but a change in mental climate set in as well. Demands for witchcraft persecutions declined as the sun of the intellectual Enlightenment ushered in the end of belief in witchcraft.

Naturally, parallels between great intellectual movements and the history of climate are nothing more than an intellectual game. However, the same cannot be said of the synchronicity of climatic epochs and persecutions, because the weather played a prominent role in the origins of the great witch-hunts. Both phenomena had something in common; their simultaneity, at least in Central Europe. A look at the social history gives further indication that this was no coincidence.

II

Adverse climatic anomalies of the late sixteenth century were Europe-wide rather than just local events, and the same holds true of social-historical events, such as crop failures and rising grain prices, changing structures of demand, market fail-ures for manufactured goods, indebtedness, broken contracts, the firing of employees, poor nutrition among the lower classes, increased susceptibility to disease, and famine.

Hunger was the mark of inflationary crisis – its dreadful symbol, so to speak. Changes in social relationships were already underway, but serious transformations of the conditions of reproduction directly threatened subsistence and often provided the conditions for witchcraft persecutions. We are familiar with the anthropolog-ically oriented research of Alan Macfarlane which cites the role of neighbourhood conflicts in witchcraft accusations. Rainer Walz has gone beyond Peter Burke's 'Macfarlane-Thomas model' in recent years to suggest that not just one specific constellation of conflict, in this case alms-giving, but nearly every human relation-ship which went wrong might lead to a charge of witchcraft, owing in part to an imaginary scale of honour attached to such interactions.[16] Conversely, one might suppose that situations which seemed to call for magical assistance actually increased in these crisis-years; magic for the recovery of lost objects, absconded spouses, love, and health or countermagic against witches – all revolved around the ques-tion of existential security.

Despite the multiplicity of factors, the individual experience of threatening situations can be integrated into social history. In a primarily agrarian society, providing sustenance was of paramount importance. Malnutrition during famines in the early modern period increased susceptibility to disease. Crop failures led to inflation, making it impossible for large parts of the population to feed themselves adequately. Bread provided the staple of the early modern diet. The pious wish, 'give us this day our daily bread', was fully justified. Naturally, the lower classes were immediately affected by price-inflation on consumables, and literally starved in the streets during subsistence crises in the heart of Europe. Early modern crisis-years found their expression in the inflation of prices for basic food-stuffs, and such inflation is measurable. The basic statistics of Moritz John Elsas (published during his exile in Holland) though dated, give precise details on several of the most important German cities between 1300 and 1820.[17] Price figures should be viewed in relation to wages and not taken at face value. Dietrich Saalfeld's study of the basket of consumables, made on the basis of data from the imperial city Augsburg, demonstrates that, from the 1580s, a long period of inflation brought on by crop failures made all previous experiences pale into insignificance and caused a decisive decline in the standard of living in Southern Germany. Although there was no repeat of the extreme famine of 1570, the period of inflation still lasted almost a full decade, from 1585 to 1594, with only two relatively stable years. Even wages for craftsmen fell below the existence-minimum in Augsburg and heads of middle class families could no longer feed their families on a single income. Similar studies for England reveal that the trend in real wages was not limited to Central Europe.[18]

These periods of inflation had more dramatic impact in southern Germany because the Swabian textile industry had lost its traditional market in Holland as a result of the Dutch Revolt. Malnutrition spread, thereby lowering immunity to diseases. Two major plague epidemics in 1585–8 and 1592–3 decimated the population. The situation of subsistence crisis accounts for widespread witchcraft persecutions around the year 1590. The aforementioned chronicle of Trier explicitly mentions the constant lack of grain caused by crop failures as the background to the persecution of 1585–92. 'Scarcely any archbishop has ruled the diocese under such great burden, trouble and emergency as Johann [Archbishop Johann VII of Schwarzenberg 1581–99]. For the whole of his administration, he had to suffer the constant lack of grain, the ills of poor weather and the failure of crops in the field with his subjects. For only two of nineteen years were fruitful, 1584 and 1590.'[19] One assumes that the greatest European witchcraft persecution of the sixteenth century, in the bordering Duchy of Lorraine, took place under the same conditions.

In order to understand the effects of crop failures, it should be made clear that the greater part of the population, in the country as well as in the city, did not participate directly in subsistence agriculture, purchasing necessities at local markets. The entire range of shortages was transmitted to the lower peasant and urban classes at the market in the form of higher prices for basic consumables. The existentially threatening connection of crop failure and inflation caused a knee-jerk reaction based on demonology, as the consecrated bishop of Trier, Peter Binsfeld, argued in a polemic for exceptional measures to fight witches in 1589: 'Witches are traitors to the Fatherland, because they secretly conspire, as experience shows, to destroy the wine harvest, rot the fruits and drive up prices of grain'.[20] Such inflationary crises often had a supraregional or even Europe-wide impact as a consequence of the deficient transportation infrastructure afflicting trade-routes during periods of regional hardship. The inflation mentioned by the demonologist Binsfeld is the same one that afflicted northwest Germany and Bavaria after 1589 at the onset of major persecutions.

A similar correlation of persecutions and crop failure/inflation can be observed in the major witch-hunts of the seventeenth century, the worst ever. Thousands fell prey to them in Franconia and the Rhineland during the late 1620s. Here as well, contemporary chroniclers suggested a direct connection between 'unnatural' storms and exorbitant inflation. The peasant population in these regions was doubly hit, since – insofar as they relied on the wine industry – their crop as well as their income declined measurably. According to a contemporary chronicler at the beginning of a mega-persecution:

> In the year 1626 on the 27th of May, the vineyards of the bishophrics of Bamberg and Würzburg in Franconia all froze over, as did the grain fields, which rotted in any case. Everything froze like never before remembered, causing a great inflation. There followed great lamentation and pleading among the common rabble, questioning why his princely Grace delayed so long in punishing the sorcerers and witches for spoiling crops since the beginning of the year.[21]

The Würzburg witch-hunt, one of the largest in European history, claimed some 900 victims between 1626 and 1630.

It is possible that persecutions in the territories of the Archbishop of Cologne, Ferdinand of Bavaria (1577–1650), managed to outstrip the Franconian hunts. Gerhard Schormann recently has argued that Ferdinand conducted a centrally directed campaign of extermination against witches and that the authorities initiated the hunt in these areas – the old argument in new clothing.[22] However, this point of view has been vehemently rebutted by the latest archival research. The ostensive 'programme' of the Archbishop published long after the persecution, was nothing more than a regurgitation of a four-decade-old discussion from the Bishop's home, the Electorate of Bavaria, that dealt with the possibility of 'purging' the territory in conjunction with new domestic legislation. This programme achieved new prominence in the Bishophric of Cologne in 1627. However, the political structure of the Electorate of Cologne was so complex that a centrally directed persecution without the co-operation of the general populace and the intermediary authorities (nobility, monasteries) was quite simply impossible. In 1620, the Prince Bishop was even unable to defend his subjects against Dutch incursions as they managed to erect a hostile fortress on a Rhine-island directly opposite his capital in Bonn. Political handicaps restricted any eventuality of conducting a policy of repression. Though we can ignore neither the potential influence of religiously motived proclivities toward persecution (Prince-Bishop Ferdinand and his uncle Franz Wilhelm of Wartenberg can be counted among the Bavarian Jesuit party, which supported witch-hunting at this time) nor a desire for control, major persecutions broke out years after Ferdinand's ascension in any case, after the effects of agrarian pressure set in among the populace. Thomas Becker confirms that supplications from local communities preceded the outbreak here as well, in this case a petition of autumn 1626.[23] This opinion is corroborated by a publication of Hermann Löher, an exile in Amsterdam, describing the simultaneous role of local committees in the Rhineland.[24] For that reason, we have to agree with Becker: the Prince-Bishop had no persecutory programme, but simply responded to the situation. The administration did not act; it reacted. And it reacted as a weak administration does: it yielded to the desire of the populace for persecution.

Thus this administration behaved no differently than other weak administrations at the time: the ecclesiastical territories of Würzburg, Bamberg, Eichstätt, Cologne, Mainz, and others persecuted witches simultaneously from 1626 to 1630.

These great persecutions deserve better research. Where we already possess in-depth analyses, such as for the Prince-Bishophric of Mainz, the evidence shows that a 'seismographic' connection between inflation and persecutions exists. Each of the four hunts there was directly connected to an inflationary crisis; in Franconia the long-term crisis which began in 1624 led to the most excessive witch-hunts under Prince-Bishop Georg Friedrich of Greiffenclau, who ruled briefly 1626–9 and had 900 victims burned as witches.[25]

As elsewhere, criticism in Mainz involved the accusation of weather-magic and its sociological consequences. As early as 1593, in conjunction with the first major persecutions, the local official Jeremias Lieb complained, 'the common man has become so mad from the consequences of crop failures, the death of livestock and similar things, that he no longer holds them for the just punishment of God for our sins, but blames witches and sorceresses'.[26] Precisely because of these pre-Christian peasant beliefs, there exists a fundamental social-historical connection between crises of the Ancien Régime and the proclivity to persecutions. Crop fail-ures, attributed to witches, led to inflated costs for consumables and consequently to malnutrition and disease. Hunger and disease struck all of Europe during partic-ularly unfavourable years simultaneously. Only this method allows us to comprehend the otherwise chance synchronicity of peak waves of persecutions in lands as distant as Scotland and Bavaria.

III

The link to broader social developments is an important step in historically locating conjunctures of persecution. However, the synchronicity of subsistence crises and witch-hunts should not, indeed cannot, be interpreted as mechanical determinism. Times of crisis and disaster are historical constants but external forces do not summon forth mechanical human responses, since they are constructed within modes of cultural perception. Before the construction of an early modern, cumu-lative concept of witchcraft, mass persecutions were unthinkable. The complex and only partially researced phenomenon of its reception was, not surprisingly, hesi-tant. Characteristically, the witchcraft persecution of 1563 began in southwest Germany, traditional home of the initial hunt conducted by the papal inquisitor Heinrich Kramer (Institoris). Interestingly, the torturers/executioners employed during the trials in southern Germany initially came from the region around the Ravensburger persecution.

The so-called 'history of mentalities' is another important aspect. Turning first to 'collective mentalities' (i.e. expectations and outlook not merely attributable to individual views), we should consider characteristics of social groups or even entire epochs. This is not the pervasive 'fear in the west' which Jean Delumeau and others believed could be identified for the whole of the early modern period, but rather a concretely dated and localized fear with concrete causes and results. Not wishing to explore the individual psychology of fear, I merely want to point out evidence of 'fear' in contemporary sources in connection with subsistence crises. The 'Fugger-Zeitungen', weekly, handwritten reports sent to the merchant Philip Eduard Fugger from the major cities of Europe, specifically mentioned the term 'angst' only in connection with extreme crisis-years; elsewhere it was not employed. In 1586, the hungry poor lost their work and begged from door to door fearing for their lives, while the rich feared to go out in public. Angst had many faces, but had a common cause.

Also of interest are contemporary comments pessimistically describing the condition of the world and its constant decay. These remarks have often been viewed as topical stereotypes, but when eyewitness accounts frequently recur in connection with concrete historical circumstances, suggesting that 'recent years have shown themselves ever harder and more severe as time goes on, and a reduction in living things, people and animals as well as fruits and crops', they ought to be taken more seriously.[27] Meteorological anomalies and subsequent inflationary crises, as previously noted, were attributed to the will and deeds of 'evil persons', transformed and personified as enemies according to popular beliefs in the occult. Magical explanations always enjoy the advantage of justifying direct action. Without reflecting on the esoteric game of magic and counter-magic, the populace struck an alliance with the authorities, using the latter's own demonological theories and judicial rituals to achieve a popular aim, to exterminate the evil persons and uproot the scourge. To their chagrin, many authorities, normally unable to encourage plaintiffs to bring charges of magic before the courts instead of settling them within the community, now suddenly found themselves besieged on all sides by massive pressure from peasant communities to intervene, threatening vigilante justice and open unrest if they failed to do so. In turn, collective action with ritualized character psychologically offset the fear of evil persons, a euphemism for witches.

The quality of life varied greatly between classes and groups in early modern society and dearth during subsistence crises increased want among the lower classes while others profited from shortages. In essence, the shortage of resources added to economic and social tensions. Social unease arose in the imperial city Augsburg in the wake of the famine years 1570–1 when inflation struck. Contemporary descriptions portray dramatic scenes of unexpected unemployment, the first appearances of disease and increased social tensions; the helpless anger of those whose savings proved insufficient to purchase their 'daily bread' was directed against speculators, who hoarded grain in the hope of driving up prices further. Sources describe animosity against the rich and 'unchristian utterings' against usurers leading to curses and, ultimately, to acts of maleficient magic.[28]

As this example demonstrates, existential crises and the fear of the lower classes held grave consequences for the ruling elite, who escaped inflation, indeed profited from it, either directly through speculation or indirectly by using the temporary material want of the lower and middle classes to their advantage. The primary consequence, social polarisation, was matched by secondary transformation of interpersonal relationships at these times. The use of specific terminology reveals a toughening of social relations, reflected in an accentuated hierarchical and hegemonic ideology characteristic of the early modern state, as well as other social organizations. These tendencies included limited access to guilds and the lower nobility, the construction of ideologically binding norms by religious confessions, the disenfranchisement of oppositional groups, an almost maniacal proliferation of laws, a trend toward absolutist rule and a criminal justice system that applied unprecedented brutality against crimes of violence, property damage and moral infractions, which accounted for over ninety percent of all executions, in addition to crimes involving magic. Never before or since have so many people been legally executed in such a grotesque manner as in the years 1560–1630.

This new social toughness corresponded to a radical transformation of mentality among the ruling elite independent of nominal confessional allegiance and only indirectly connected to subsistence crises. In crass terms, they departed from an open, vivacious, pleasure-seeking, this-worldly oriented, 'Renaissance' mentality, with contact with the popular world of the carnivalesque, to seek refuge in dogmatic, confessional, ascetic, other-worldly oriented, religious principles that offered solace in a situation perceived as precarious. Normally, much breath is spent on the elucidation of opposing confessional tendencies rather than noting just how much the competing religious ideologies had in common. However, clear signs of a mentality transformation are just as apparent in Catholic as in Protestant areas, as is the case in the Jesuit province of Upper Germany, where Peter Canisius excited the population through stern sermons and sensational exorcisms. Witchcraft was a recurrent theme in his sermons, which Canisius accepted along with the theologically problematic issue of weather-magic. After the first persecution of 1563, he wrote:

> Everywhere they are punishing witches, who are multiplying remarkably. Their outrages are terrible . . . Never before have people in Germany given themselves over to the Devil so completely . . . They send many out of this world with their devilish arts, excite storms and wreak terrible havoc among our countryfolk and other Christians. Nothing seems safe from their horrid wiles and power.[29]

The sermons of both Catholic and Protestant preachers called for witchcraft persecutions, thereby reinforcing the peasants in their demands for witchhunts. Götz von Pölnitz characterized the reaction of the Augsburg elite to the missionary activities of Canisius as follows:

> The remarkable increase in reports concerning a mood of penance and ecstatic excitement awakened in the elite testify to an atmosphere of transition. They lie somewhere between the princely exuberance of the near-decadent late-Renaissance and the ascetic rigour of certain Counter-Reformation saints.[30]

The radical transformation of mentality manifested itself in personal catharses, virtual 'bolt of lightning' conversion-experiences among the nobility and princely dynasties, such as those of Dukes Albert V and William V of Bavaria in the 1570s. Furthermore, the 'Marian state-programme' developed in Catholic regions, offered the image of the Virgin as a counter-pole to that of the witch. The Virgin Mary, immaculate symbol of fertility, stood in stark contrast to the female personification of infertility, the witch. Infertility is meant in the widest sense of the word, for witches were held responsible both for human and agricultural infertility. It is at least worth mentioning the coincidence of the first witch-burnings in the Bishophric of Augsburg and the Duchy of Bavaria with the founding of the princely Marian Congregation.

In the wake of the 'second Reformation' of Calvinism and Tridentine Catholic reform, a climate of gloom set in that accurately reflected deteriorating living conditions. The dramatic transformation of attitudes transcended confessional allegiance, replacing the optimistic mood of the first half-century with pessimism. Hard times hardened social structures, even reaching into iconographic representations after 1560. Preachers inculcated an accentuated consciousness of sin in the ruling elite and directed them to attribute the origins of decline to the wrath of God, providing fertile ground for social disciplining, as well as mystic and apocalyptic visions; free from the worries of the every-day struggle for limited resources, the elite was circumspectly dragged along with the tide of change. Indeed, it was the elite who first felt the screws of self-discipline, work-discipline, ascetic manners, constant spiritual exercises and moral rigidity at princely courts after 1560. The depressingly sober seriousness with which these changes of habit we enforced, a 'remodelling of affectation', reached into the most private personal affairs. Duke William V (1579–97), who conducted the first Bavarian witch-hunt, lived in strict accord with a daily schedule of prayer and spiritual exercises, wore a penitential hairshirt and engaged in self-flagellation. His successors, Maximilian (1598–1651) and Ferdinand Maria (1657–79) signed devotional blood pacts to the Virgin Mary at Altötting; they can be interpreted as the antithesis of the witch's Pact with the Devil.

Historians now generally assume that the radicalization of attitudes towards witches took place after 1560, as mirrored in criminal legislation against witchcraft in England, Scotland, and Germany, the synchronicity of renewed witch-hunting in France and Germany around 1570, or the simultaneous climax of persecutions in Scotland, the Rhineland and Bavaria around 1590. However, the complex interaction of social developments, times of crises, traditional modes of behaviour and opposing ideological interpretations make it impossible to define the activities of elites as a simple reaction to popular demand for persecution. Here we arrive at a juncture that seriously challenges theories regarding the existence of 'collective mentalities' in the early modern era. Records of criminal interrogations reveal an extraordinary range of perceptions even among the common people, one equalled in expressions recorded by literate members of society. This range of perceptions surrounding the issue of witchcraft comes more often to the fore than with other themes. The question of the existence of witches, the physical reality of their deeds, the judicial possibility and political desirability of their persecution was debated like hardly any other problem of the age. In Catholic Germany, an ideologically motivated group supported persecutions with the opinion that both people and rulers risked the wrath of God, if they failed to uproot the evil and 'radically' weed out witches. Justifying their policy of extermination with 'correct enthusiasm for the honour of God' for which no sacrifice was too great, the radically penitential and atoning spirit earned them and their followers the name 'zealots'. Pope Urban VIII (1623–44) condescendingly referred to this group as the Zelanti. The 'zealots' viewed witchcraft as no isolated occurence. For them, its elimination formed part of a domestic policy aimed at establishing a hierarchical, other-worldly, Catholic, model state, a political theory set out by Adam Coritzen in his *Methodus civilis doctrinae seu Abissini regis historia* (1628). Other aspects of his programme included an end to fornication, the replacement of frivolities like gambling and dancing with spiritual exercises (i.e. Corpus Christi processions, ten hour prayers, etc.), the repression of popular culture and its replacement with a literate 'high culture' based on biblical authority. The total programme of internal reform accompanied foreign policies of missionary conversion and the destruction of confessional opponents. Fear of heavenly retribution provided the explicit motivation behind the desire for rigid measures.

The rapid advance of a gloomy world view after 1560, intensified after the 1580s, depicts a transformation of mentality which indicates, at least partially, a break with the past. This factor ultimately explains the sudden decision of ruling elites in some areas to give in to popular demands for persecutions. The traditional rejection of popular belief in weather-magic, also widespread among theologians, was temporarily rolled back along a broad front. It was the correspondence of interests, though for different reasons, between the upper and lower echelons of society that temporarily enabled the great persecutions around 1600. Where interests corresponded, as in some ecclesiastical territories of the Holy Roman Empire, or where authorities were too weak to maintain a state monopoly over violence, as in some Swiss cantons, major persecutions became possible. Religious and political factors surely played a role in the question of whether or not a hunt took place, but the fundamental forces behind persecutions have to be sought elsewhere.

IV

As numerous discussions have demonstrated since the first article on the subject appeared, every account of the connections between social history and witchcraft persecutions has given rise to misconceptions because a variety of other factors contributed to their immediate outbreak. And the potential for misconception is actually enhanced rather than reduced by the addition of exogenous climatic factors to the discussion. One frequent critique holds that a mechanical connection between inflation and persecution cannot be substantiated. However, this critique addresses a thesis which has never been suggested. Eva Gillies demonstrates the bankruptcy of the determimistic connection between crises and witch-hunts in her introduction to the German edition of Evans-Pritchard's *Witchcraft, Oracles and Magic amongst the Azande* by posing the anachronistic question of why a major social transformation like industrialization did not lead to witchcraft persecutions.[31]

The European witchcraft persecutions are tied to a specific epoch, the early modern period, and characterized by elite abhorrence of magic and its diabolical origins. In a certain sense, to use Claudia Honegger's twist on Max Weber, they were 'the other side of western rationalization', inseparable from central components of European modernization, such as the 'civilizing process', state building, criminalization, and secularization. These general trends, to include the toughening of social relationships and a depressing world view, are nothing more than an outline for the geography and chronology of witchcraft persecutions. The same holds for the judicial framework, mentioned briefly. On the other hand, strict rejection of witch-burnings by the authorities clarifies some of the regional variations in the intensity of persecutions through prohibition. This explains the absence of executions in the reformed Palatine Electorate, the fact that larger imperial cities like Frankfurt, Nuremberg and Augsburg rejected executions, or that important territories like the Duchy of Württemberg and Bavaria decided after complex debate against any further persecutions. Elite refusal to authoritize legal executions of witches prevented them to a certain, though not absolute degree, as one interesting example connected to the question of the origins of witchcraft persecutions illustrates. In the Austrian Voralberg region, the population called for witch-hunts, especially in crisis-years. The administration in Innsbruck suppressed their demands. In the years 1649–50, the valley of Prattigau managed to purchase its independence from the Habsburgs and joined the Swiss canton Graubunden. The inhabitants took the judicial system into their own hands and judges were elected and controlled directly rather than by co-option. Terrible persecutions began immediately thereafter, venting peasant demands pent-up for decades. This period has gone down in the canton's history as 'the great witch-killing'. Finally the 'guilty' parties could be punished for threatening the crops and thereby the livelihood of the peasants. Demonological theory, Roman law, elite attempts at acculturation or base motives like greed played no decisive role in these persecutions. Specifically, what we are dealing with here is an archaic ritual to drive out evil.

It is important to recognize the social background to the major persecutions within a specific epoch. Authorities certainly bear political responsibility for witch-hunts but, as recent research indicates, hardly in the sense that they provided the impulse for initiating persecutions. This is true not only in individual cases, but for major persecutions as well, often preceded by massive pressure from the population bordering on open rebellion against the established order. The general explanatory potential of 'fear stemming from social transformation' offers a point of access to popular motivations, but requires more precise clarification. It is important to note that in areas with major persecutions, social want brought on by the structure of agrarian societies was a greater problem than social transformation. England and Holland no longer suffered from this problem by the end of the sixteenth century, but in Central Europe demographic development was pushed to the limit, as had previously occurred at the beginning of the fourteenth century. Shortages and attendant social differentiation marked this society and rendered it highly susceptible to climatic fluctuations in temperature and precipitation. Crop failures resulting from inclement weather led to inflation, malnutrition, and hunger. Increased susceptibility to disease or even major epidemics were the consequences. Such climatically induced crop failures occurred with greater frequency after 1560 during the period climatic historians refer to as the 'Little Ice Age', and periods of inflation dragged on. We can identify enough correspondence between cyclic agrarian crises and conjunctures of witchcraft persecutions that it is possible, without doubt, to speak of a fundamental social-historical correlation. The major persecutions were rooted in years marked by agrarian crises. The connection of persecution with agrarian crisis explains the synchronicity of witch-hunts in geographically distant regions. Furthermore, it explains the publication dates of demonological literature and territorial decrees against witchcraft. The nexus of causality between agrarian crisis and persecutions is based upon four supports. First, witches were held directly responsible for weather damage and crop failures, despite the official teachings of theologians. This explains the vehemence of discussion around the issue of weather-magic. Second, illness and death multiplied in the wake of crop failures, especially among children, who were also held accountable as witches. Third, latent conflicts emerged virulently because shortages of resources during agrarian crises increased social tensions, adding a psychological dimension that needed to be resolved. Fourth, witch-trials provided 'positive' feedback, leading to further accusations in the region. In an attempt to limit potential misunderstandings, let me again emphasize that the increased execution of witches after 1560, and especially after 1585, was not simply a result of agrarian crises in connection with the 'Little Ice Age'. A second decisive factor, the glum depressive world view shared by elites, also corresponded to the toughening of living conditions among the lower classes during the 'Little Ice Age'. Henry Kamen has characterized some of the conditions of this 'Iron Century' between 1560 and 1660 and Theodor Rabb has clearly demonstrated that the theme of re-establishing stable conditions dominated the seventeenth century after the unrest around the year 1600.[32] Hartmut Lehman has recently argued that the general phenomenon of witchcraft persecutions, and not just their limitation, should be viewed in the context of the struggle to re-establish order.[33] In the complete framework of interaction between communities and the authorities, witchcraft trials were an extraordinary mechanism for resolving crises. To that degree, despite the quickly recognized risk that they could become dysfunctional, the participants often initially viewed persecutions as functional rituals.

Now we need to ask why certain regions of Europe proved particularly susceptible to persecutions at certain times. The answer lies in a fundamental correlation to agrarian crises. These shortages varied in intensity according to regional distribution of wealth, as well as structures of trade and communication. Centres of international trade like Holland and England were apparently little affected. Similarly, lands on the thinly settled periphery (Scandanavia, Eastern Europe, the Iberian peninsula, European colonies) were also little affected, since the possibility of diffusion in open spaces served to decrease pressure. The semi-peripheral areas with their relatively high population density were especially hard hit by witchcraft persecutions because their agricultural products, like grain and wine, were highly susceptible to meteorological disasters. This is as true of Scotland as for parts of France, Switzerland, and Germany, while the agrarian economy of Southern Europe was spared climatic deterioration as a benefit of its latitude. Behind the major European witch-hunts, we can detect three archaic factors affecting every agrarian society, but particularly so in Central Europe during the early modern era. The exact conditions were quite specific, in effect, that rulers and subjects believed commonly in the existence of 'inner enemies' and sought their eradication, each for their own reasons. The authorities fought for religious salvation, while subjects harboured more material interests. And it was their interests that called the tune of persecution. The campaign against witches might be viewed as a metaphor. Its complex origins in climatic history, social history and the history of mentalities, today understood as its major causes, were, for contemporaries, reducible to three simple concepts: weather, hunger, and fear.

Translated by David Lederer

Notes

1 H. C. E. Midelfort, *Witch-hunting in Southwestern Germany, 1562–1684* (Stanford, Calif. 1972), 88–90.

2 Agobard of Lyon, 'Contra insulsam vulgi opinionem de grandine et tonitruis', in J. P. Migne (ed.), *Patrologiae cursus completus, Series Latina* (Paris 1844–64), vol. 104, 147–58.

3 Ulrich Molitor, *De laniis et phitonicis mulierbus* (1489); Martin Plantsch, *Opusculum de sagis maleficis* (Pforzheim 1507).

4 Günther Jerouschek, *Die Hexen und ihr Prozess* (Sigmaringen 1992).

5 Matheus Alber and Wilhelm Bidembach, *Em Summa etlicher Predigen vom Hagel und Unholden* (Tubingen 1562).

6 Walter Rummel, *Bauern, Herren und Hexen* (Göttingen 1991), 88 ff.

7 Behringer, *Hexen und Hexenprozesse in Deutschland* (Munich 1988), 267.

8 Emil Zenz (ed.) *Die Taten der Trier. Gesta Treverorum* (Trier 1964), vol. 7, 13.

9 Christian Pfister, *Klimageschichte der Schweiz 1525–1860* (Bern 1988), 118–27.

10 Bernhard Friedrich Kuhn, 'Versuch über den Mechanismus der Gletscher', *Hopfners Magazin* 1 (1787), 119–36, esp. 135.

11 Wolfgang Behringer, 'Hexenverfolgungen im Spiegel zeitgenossischer Publizistik', *Oberbayerisches Archiv*, 109 (1984), 346.

12 Behrenger, *Hexen und Hexenprozesse* (1988).

13 Ibid.

14 Pfister (1988), 40 f., 118 ff.

15 Eva Labouvie *Zauberei und Hexenwerk* (Frankfurt 1991), 86 f.

16 Guido Bader, *Die Hexenprozesse in der Schweiz* (Affoltern 1945), 116 ff.

17 Moritz J. Elsas, *Umrss einer Geschichte der Preise und Löline in Deutschland*, 3 vols (Leiden 1936–8).

18 Roger Schofield, 'Family structure, demographic behaviour and economic growth', in Walter and R. Schofield (eds) *Famine: Disease and the Social Order in Early Modern Society* (Cambridge 1989), 279–304, esp. 289.

19 Zenz (1964), vol. 7, 13.

20 Peter Binsfield, *Tractat von Bekanntnus der Zauberer und Hexen* (Munich 1592), 38–9

21 Ignaz Denzinger, 'Auszuge aus einer Chronik der Familie Langhans in Zeil', *Archiv des Historischen Vereins* 10 (1850), 143.

22 Heinrich Schultheis, *Ausfuhliche Instruktion* (Cologne 1634), 466.

23 Thomas Becker, 'Hexenverfolgung in Kurköln', *Annalen des Historischen Vereins für den Niederrhein* 195 (1992), 202–14.

24 Herrmann Löher, *Hochnotige Unterthanige Wemütige Klage Derfrommen Unschültigen* (Amsterdam 1676).

25 Horst-Heinrich Gebhardt, *Hexenprozesse in Kurfurstentum Mainz* (Aschaffenburg 1989), 349 f.

26 Herbert Pohl, *Hexenglaube und Hexenverfolgung* (Weisbaden 1988), 145.

27 Pfister (1988), vol. 2, 94.

28 Robin Briggs, *Communities of Belief: Cultural and Social Tensions in Early Modern France* (Oxford 1989), 91.

29 Bernhard Duhr, *Die Stellung der Jesuiten in den Deutschen Hexenprozessen* (Cologne 1900), 23.

30 Gotz Frhr. von Pölnitz, 'Petrus Canisius und das Bistum Augsburg', *Zeitschrift für Bayerische Landeskunde* 18 (1955), 352–94, quote 382.

31   Edgar Evan Evans-Pritchard, *Hexerei, Orakel und Magie bei den Zande* (Frankfurt 1978), 7–35.

32   Henry Kamen, *The Iron Century: Social Change in Europe* (London 1971); Theodore K. Rabb, *The Struggle for Stability in Early Modern Europe* (New York 1975).

33   Hartmut Lehmann, 'The Persecution of Witches as Restoration of Order', *Central European History* 21 (1988), 107–21.

Chapter 5

E. William Monter

THE SOCIOLOGY OF JURA WITCHCRAFT

WHAT SORT OF PERSON WAS ACCUSED of witchcraft? Recent scholarship has diligently concerned itself with this question and has reached some important but differing conclusions. From England, Keith Thomas observes that 'it is necessary to bear in mind that the judicial records reveal two essential facts about accused witches: they were poor, and they were usually women'.[1] From Germany, Erik Midelfort claims that the traditional stereotype of the old-woman witch tended to dissolve during the major panics, and that people accused of witchcraft during panics tended to be somewhat wealthier than the average citizen.[2] Since patterns of witch-hunting in the Jura region do not conform precisely to either the British or the German model, we should not be surprised if a sociological analysis of the Jura evidence yields some results that differ from both these pictures.

We propose to begin our inquiry into the nature of Jura witchcraft suspects first by examining the worst witchcraft panic anywhere in the region: the 1571–1572 crisis of plague-spreaders or *engraisseurs* at Geneva, when nearly a hundred people were either killed or banished within twelve months. This was the only occasion when more than two dozen people were arrested for witchcraft in one year in one legal jurisdiction – although in many important ways it was similar to the dozens of smaller panics in the other parts of this region. On the whole, these people closely resemble the British description of typical witches, 'poor and usually women'. Their poverty is suggested by what we know about their occupations. A half of all suspects for whom we have such information were unskilled laborers or their wives; the others came from families of artisans or fishermen, with a locksmith and an ironmonger at the top of the group. None of them belonged in an elite occupational or social category.[3]

Sex, however, seems to have been more important than wealth in determining panic suspects; perhaps we should reverse Thomas's order of priorities to read 'usually women, and poor'. Fewer than one in twelve of these accused *engraisseurs* were male. The question of why women predominated so heavily in witchcraft accusations has frequently been asked, ever since the days of the *Malleus Maleficarum*, but often in a curiously perfunctory manner, as if the answer really depended on some more important underlying mechanism (for example, the demonologists believed that a propensity for heresy was the root cause; today, Thomas believes that a refusal of charity or other traditional obligation was the basic cause). But it seems reasonable to me to examine the purely sexual side of witchcraft accusations as a primary line of investigation by itself.

It is not enough to learn how many women relative to men were accused of witchcraft in a particular place; we must also learn exactly what kinds of women were most likely to be accused. The Genevan panic of 1571 included forty-five widows and fourteen spinsters among its victims, as against thirty-two married women living with their husbands. Comparative data suggest that this exceeded the usual rate of widows, but not by much. Data from other parts of the Jura are less complete, but they too indicate an important percentage of widows among suspected witches; nowhere does their level drop below one-third. Overall, the rate of spinsters among suspected witches seems roughly analogous to their rate in the general female population, at least in the Jura: under one-tenth in rural districts, over one-fifth in the towns. (In seventeenth-century Sweden one adult woman in three was unmarried and one in six was widowed, thus confirming the general impression that only widows were heavily over-represented among accused witches.)[4] Of course, this superabundance of widows among accused witches might merely reflect their relatively old age, rather than being a primary clue: we know that the archetypical witch of sixteenth- and seventeenth-century Europe was an old woman – whether married or widowed or single made little difference.

Because sixteenth- and seventeenth-century records are always imprecise, we have little reliable data about the exact ages of the undistinguished and frequently illiterate people who were accused of witchcraft. In the Genevan panic of 1571, for instance, we know the ages of only thirteen of them. Age profiles must be constructed with extremely fragmentary information; the ages given have often been rounded off to the nearest five, or even ten, years; and the final samples are disappointingly small. But the results are interesting. In the 1571 Genevan panic, only three of the accused whose ages we know were under fifty, and the median age was sixty. Other Jura fragments corroborate these results. Only the meticulous Genevans kept track of the age of suspected witches with relative frequency, but their results – only one suspect in four under age fifty, and a median around sixty – seem typical of rural regions as well. Considering that in early modern Europe old age for women began soon after forty, when childbearing ended, these figures provide strong confirmation for the stereotype of the witch as an old woman.

The roots of the stereotype seem simple and obvious. The broad misogynistic streak in European letters, which flourished during the Renaissance, and the miso-gynistic elements embedded in some parts of the Christian tradition and re-empha-sized during the sixteenth-century Reformations, will suffice to explain why demonologists could agree on why women rather than men were 'naturally' prone to witchcraft. This point can be neatly illustrated by the most famous sixteenth-century demonologist, Jean Bodin: at the beginning of his *République,* when describing the order of a household (the prototype of all larger societies), he put the wife in the very last place, behind the father or *chef,* behind the children, the servants, and the apprentices.[5] Four years later, Bodin the patriarchal social theorist became Bodin the demonologist – and his sexual politics remained unchanged.

If we begin by emphasizing how often these accused witches were elderly widows or spinsters, we can argue that witchcraft accusations can best be understood as projections of patriarchal social fears onto atypical women, those who lived apart from the direct male control of husbands or fathers. These defenseless and very isolated women became the group most often exposed to charges of witchcraft.

Complementing this argument is another, which says that witchcraft must be seen as a magical means of revenge for real or imagined injuries. People who rely on magical means of revenge are primarily those who are incapable of using the more normal or socially approved means of revenge such as physical violence (very common in early modern European villages) or recourse to law courts. Older women who lived apart from direct patriarchal control were unable to revenge their numerous injuries in either of these ways. Thus they had only magical revenge – or at least society assumed they had magical means of revenge, which amounted to the same thing in terms of both popular fears and legal consequences.

Compared to sex, poverty and other factors appear to be secondary, but not insignificant. As we have seen, the data from the Genevan panic of 1571 suggests that most witches came from poorer families – unlike southwestern Germany, where rich people were frequently accused during panics. Although it is true that very rich or prominent people were never tried for witchcraft in Geneva, there are instances elsewhere in the Jura region of *notables,* rich and prominent people, being accused. For example, Leonarde Bregille, executed for witchcraft at Besancon in 1659, came from a prominent family who were fined the huge sum of 30,000 francs – ten to thirty times as much as the other witches condemned with her. Some accused witches came from the bourgeoisie of such towns as Neuchatel, Porrentruy, or Montbeliard (just as there were eleven victims in the Genevan panic of 1571 who held Genevan citizenship), but they generally represented the lower strata of municipal citizens. In the little town of La Neuveville, on the border between Neuchatel and the Bishopric of Basel, two sisters, one of them married to a magistrate, were accused of witchcraft and fled to avoid arrest in 1610. The municipality seized their property, 'in order to serve as an example to others and to squelch the sinister suspicion of supporting the rich and condemning the poor'. After three years of negotiations and protests by their relatives, one of the sisters apparently got the charges against her dropped by paying an enormous fine of 2500 ecus. And sometimes a member of the family of a rural *notable* went on trial as a witch: the wife of the chatelain at Boudry (Neuchatel); the wife of the lieutenant at Colombier (Neuchatel) or the wife of a village *voeble* in Ajoie (Bishopric of Basel). Such examples are not surprising., since we know that witchcraft cut across most social boundaries in the lands of the Holy Roman Empire; but in the Jura region they seem to have been comparatively rare, less frequent than in southwestern Germany or in Alsace, for example.[6]

It is important to realize that in the Jura region some kinds of people considered elsewhere to be common witchcraft suspects are almost completely absent – most notably, midwives and children. There were no midwives and no children among the Genevan *engraisseurs* of 1571, but one might easily argue that this was a special sort of panic. Among the thousand-plus witchcraft dossiers from the whole region, however, there are only a tiny handful where a practicing midwife or wetnurse was accused, or where the *maleficia* concerned the children the woman had delivered or nursed: in this mountainous, dairying region, dead cows figure more prominently among *maleficia* than dead children. The relative scarcity of children among persons convicted of witchcraft is even more unusual. In Geneva, children were never put on trial for witchcraft; elsewhere, they were sometimes tried but very rarely condemned to death, apart from a few instances in Franche-Comté during the 1628–1630 and 1657–1659 panics.[7] This does not mean that children were absent from the social drama of Jura witchcraft, but rather that their role was a special one: they often testified against adults, including their parents, sometimes by telling lurid tales about Sabbats which their parents had forced them to attend, and sometimes as the victims of demonic possession who ultimately identified the adults who had bewitched them. Boguet wrote a chapter about "How Midwives, if they are Witches, Kill the Children they Deliver"; but unlike the vast majority of his chapters, it offered no concrete examples from his own experience. The same chapter cited four children who accused their parents of taking them to Sabbats; all had been interrogated by Boguet, who felt obliged to note in his text that 'it is true that [the children] have not been convicted of any act of witchcraft'.[8] Bringing witchcraft accusations was partly a child's game in the Jura, as in many other places, but it was not often very dangerous for the child.

Now we must turn from static to dynamic analysis, moving from the 'whos' to the 'hows' of witchcraft accusations – from questions about what kinds of people were accused to considerations of the manner in which accusations were generated. We shall proceed first by examining how one small panic started in Franche-Comté and how it spread, and then by considering the motives behind a single, isolated example from a mountain village in the heart of the Jura.

The panic which lasted from autumn 1657 until late spring 1658 was the worst that ever afflicted the *bailliage* of Quingey. It began in September 1657, when the judge of the barony of Montfort (an important fief within the *bailliage*) arrested a forty-three-year-old peasant named Renobert Bardel, together with his mother and his two sons, aged thirteen and eleven. This took place during the larger panic which engulfed much of the province that year under the leadership of Inquisitor Symard (who, however, never visited Quingey). Renobert's mother, when liberally plied with wine, confessed everything asked of her, and his sons were also easily persuaded to confess (very little torture was used). Renobert himself was more stubborn and survived at least one round with the strappado before confessing in November 1657. He was executed shortly after his confession and apparently implicated no one else, but his mother and sons were far more loquacious: their lives were prolonged a bit so that they could implicate others and then confront the suspected witches they had named. These three were the direct source of several other arrests both inside and beyond the barony of Montfort in November and December.

The net of witchcraft suspects spread out from the Bardel family in two easily identifiable directions – one of them that of geographical proximity to the original accusers, the other ties of kinship. In the first category were some neighbors of the Bardels in the village of Montfort, above all Clauda Bernard, 'la Regnaude' – the first person outside Renobert Bardel's immediate family to be arrested and the first non-Bardel to be killed for witchcraft at Montfort (she died on December 23, 1657, with Renobert's mother and his sons). Clauda Bernard was another voluble confessor who implicated many others, including her kinswoman Anthonia Bernard of Montfort and another relative, Berthe Bernard, who lived with her husband in the village of Breres, far away from Montfort and the Baron's jurisdiction. Clauda Bernard and the Bardel children had also denounced several of their neighbors at Montfort and the neighboring hamlet of Ronchaux: five women, including Anthonia Bernard, were arrested by the Baron's officials in November; they all confessed in due time and were all executed together at the castle of Montfort in April 1658, thus making a total of ten witches killed at Montfort within five months.

What spread this panic beyond the boundaries of the Baron's jurisdiction was the intervention of the chief prosecutor of the *bailliage* of Quingey, Claude Buhon. He arrested both of Renobert Bardel's married sisters and Berthe Bernard on the strength of the Montfort denunciations. And in the early winter of 1657–1658 Buhon also arrested three other women who were neither Bardels nor Bernards: two were widows (one had been arrested before, in 1646, while the other had been suspected of witchcraft in her village for twenty years); the third woman was a magical healer who had been practicing in her village for twelve years. Their trials proceeded more slowly than those of the Bardel sisters or Berthe Bernard; however, between October 1658 and June 1659, five of these six women were executed at Quingey, while the other was condemned to death but eventually set free by the provincial parlement upon appeal.

A few other cases ensued from this second layer of arrests, mainly two young girls who confessed voluntarily to witchcraft: one was the daughter of a Ronchaux woman accused by the Bardels and Clauda Bernard, while the other lived in the same village as Françoise Bardel and one of the widows arrested by Buhon. The first girl was sentenced to death in August 1660 by the Baron of Montfort's judge, but the provincial parlement reduced her sentence to whipping plus banishment.

Thus, at least eighteen people were arrested in the *bailliage* of Quingey during this panic, and fifteen of them were eventually put to death for witchcraft (ten at Montfort and five at Quingey between January and June 1659). Of these eighteen, six belonged to the immediate family of the first suspect and three were Bernards, while another six were neighbors of theirs living in Montfort or Ronchaux. Three of the accused were children between the ages of eleven and thirteen. Only three cases were not directly tied to the original core of accusers (Clauda Bernard and Renobert Bardel's mother) by either kinship or geographical proximity – and these three were archetypical witchcraft suspects, old widows or magical healers. Seven out of approximately thirty villages in the *bailliage* of Quingey were eventually affected by this panic.

If the Quingey panic provides a clear-cut illustration of how witchcraft accusations spread out from an original nucleus, the case of Marie Joly in 1592 shows with equal clarity how an isolated accusation was generated. A middle-aged married woman, Marie lived in a small village in the mountains near Biel, in the Protestant part of the Bishopric of Basel. Her first accuser was the mayor of the neighboring hamlet of Plagne, who claimed that Marie had told him he would die by her hand. Then a woman testified that Marie once gave her a large white root to eat, which caused her to foam at the mouth and bite stones; when her family threatened to denounce Marie as a witch, she brought some soup which cured the other woman that very evening. Next, a man reported that when Marie was prevented from entering his bedroom for the traditional *poussenion* on his wedding night, she became furious and threw a stick onto his bed through a window; he fell ill, and his wife was afflicted with sleepwalking for three months: he was cured only after Marie tapped him on the shoulder with a stick. Another man discovered the day after a quarrel with Marie's husband, that his horses would only walk backwards; he threatened her and was told that his horses would be cured next morning – which duly happened. Another man was less lucky: he quarrelled with Marie and discovered that three of his horses were unable to do any work for a full year. Still another man who quarrelled with her was told, 'if you have oxen, you won't always have them'; that very evening one of his oxen died. Once, when some witches had been arrested in the nearby village of Boujean, local rumor had predicted that Marie would be arrested too; although bedridden, she had summoned her sister and tried to take sanctuary in the parish church. Four other hostile witnesses were heard. One man became sick at the village fountain after quarrelling with her. Another lost several animals within a year after his daughter-in-law refused to accept some herbs from Marie. Another man lost a horse two days after quarrelling with her. The last man 'had lost the power to drive animals and had even become deaf' after an argument with her.

This was enough to have her arrested and sent to the castle of the *bailli* of Erguel, where she was confined for six weeks and examined twice by magistrates from Biel. She was confronted by her accusers, but denied everything imputed to her. (These confrontations revealed that one of her accusers was dying and requested a reconciliation, which Marie had to be compelled to perform, and that Marie had given out a recipe for curing sick animals which she had learned from a woman of Boujean who was later burned as a witch.) Finally she was tortured for two days, 'according to Imperial law', but still confessed nothing. After the pastor of St Imier had written a long letter in her defense, she was released from prison and her village was compelled to pay the sizable costs arising from her trial.

This is an archetypical case of the village witch, capable of injuring man or beast after any argument, and of curing them sooner or later with a bowl of soup or a tap on the shoulder. Her accusers came from the immediate vicinity (Plagne, the other hamlet represented, is only a kilometer from her village) and mainly from a few clans: three of the four accusers from Plagne were Grosjeans, and three of the most important accusers from her own village were Voiblets. Marie Joly was fortunate insofar as she was never accused of killing people or of making hail – her *maleficia* were milder ones – and she had the raw courage to withstand two bouts with the strappado; so she became one of the lucky minority of accused witches who escaped the stake in her particular region. Perhaps what caused her village, which had tolerated her for so many years, to pass the legal threshold and arrest her was the threat (unaccompanied by any consequences) made against the mayor of Plagne, who probably summoned outside authorities as a preventive measure.

Recent scholarship, mostly in England, has created detailed explanations for the dynamics of isolated witchcraft accusations, while Germany has offered an important model for the dynamics of witchcraft panics. How far does each agree with the Jura evidence?

First, Jura panics do not seem to have been radically different from those in Germany, except (as we have seen) that they tended to remain relatively small and never led to a breakdown of the basic stereotype of the accused witch, an old woman. And the explanations offered here for the spread of these small panics, namely kinship and neighborhood, are certainly not novelties for the sociology of European witchcraft. The importance of kinship was stressed by the demonologists themselves, and has been repeated and refined by modern scholarship;[9] and neighborhood, while not so obvious a factor, has also been stressed by a few recent scholars.[10] The model proposed by Muchembled for the Cambresis region – in which isolated accusations were generated by the *sanior pars* of the village, older members of important families, during an age of increasing religious discipline and economic dislocation, and carried through *despite* their cost, in order to purge the village of undesirables fits fairly closely with the small-scale panics and isolated cases of the Jura region.

However, the social dynamics of Jura witchcraft do look significantly different from the well-known model which has been proposed from British evidence:

> Two essential features thus made up the background to most of the allegations of witchcraft levied in sixteenth- and seventeenth-century England. The first was the occurrence of a personal misfortune for which no natural explanation was immediately forthcoming. The second was an awareness on the victim's part of having given offence to a neighbour, usually by having failed to discharge some hitherto customary social obligation. As often as not, the link between the misfortune incurred and the obligation neglected was furnished by the frank expression of malignancy on the part of the suspected witch . . .
>
> The overwhelming majority of fully documented witch cases fall into this simple pattern. The witch is sent away empty-handed, perhaps mumbling a malediction; and in due course something goes wrong with the household, for which she is immediately held responsible. 'The requests made by the witch varied, but they conformed to the same general pattern.[11]

This clear and simple model does not work very well in the Jura region. Of course there are some cases, especially in Franche-Comté, where it is precisely repeated; but there are a few other instances, especially in Fribourg, where it is precisely reversed: where the spurned beggar later accused his uncharitable neighbor of witchcraft. Why could Jura beggars behave this way, instead of being mere victims, as in England? Sometimes they did so because they were already condemned themselves, and continental practice offered condemned witches a full opportunity to accuse anyone else of the same crime. But even more important is the fact that lack of charity could buttress a witchcraft accusation in the Jura because it was a negative personality trait, and Jura witches had a great many negative personality traits. Unlike the accused witches in England, who were in a position of moral superiority when they supposedly revenged themselves through black magic, Jura witches were likely to be in a morally inferior position. Delcambre's description of Lorraine witchcraft suspects will also fit the Jura region:

> If no individual . . . no matter how upright, was immune from prose-
> cution for witchcraft . . . immorality nevertheless constituted an
> unfavorable prejudice in this domain. A fairly large number of those
> accused of such crimes were people of ill repute and slight desirability:
> thieves, swindlers, sexual perverts, rapists, fornicators, the incestuous,
> people without religion and blasphemers, poisoners, and above all quar-
> relsome or bad-tempered persons, those 'inclined to an extreme anger',
> furnished an appreciable contingent to the tribe of witches.[12]

Thieves, sexual offenders, and above all habitual quarrellers (like Marie Joly) are easy to find among Jura witchcraft suspects. The sizable minority of men accused of witchcraft included many thieves and several with grave sexual crimes on their consciences. Only a handful of men were charged with witchcraft in the *bailliage* of Ajoie, but among them was one who had committed incest and another who was arrested in 1611 for 'theft, witchcraft, incest, and sodomy'; one of Neuchatel's male witches was Raoul du Plan, head of a gang of highway robbers and murderers operating for many years over much of French Switzerland; at Fribourg, eight of the fifty-nine men arrested for witchcraft were also accused (and convicted) of sodomy, while many more were thieves. Perhaps the most interesting example of all are the cases preserved at Lausanne: here among the fragments of approximately 115 trials, one finds 29 instances of confessed thefts, 19 instances (12 women and seven men) of such serious offenses as adultery, bearing illegitimate children, abor-tion, infanticide, incest and sodomy, and even four cases of confessed murderers, including one where the official sentence noted that 'the renunciation of God and deeds of witchcraft are greater than the other [crimes], deserving greater punish-ment'. The Lausanne evidence suggests that a sizable number of accused witches really did have some serious crime or crimes on their consciences; indeed, it some-times happened that the memory of his crimes led a person to fall into despair, during which the Devil persuaded him that he was already damned and should thus become a witch (this was relatively frequent among the men who had committed sodomy).

But of course most people accused of witchcraft were women, and in all prob-ability most Jura women accused of witchcraft were not habitual thieves or guilty of major sexual offenses. Certainly, many of them were habitual quarrellers: Merzine Clerc of Fribourg, a typical example, was arrested for bewitching a girl while refusing to give her alms, but her real fault seems to have been her reputa-tion as a bad neighbor *(mauvaise voisine)* in the village where she had lived for almost fifty years — a woman who had been reprimanded by her parish priest and who had openly rejoiced when her daughter-in-law had been arrested as a witch. Hundreds of Jura witch trials began with a cascade of 'informations' scrupulously recording the incessant quarrelling among village neighbors, often followed by an unexpected illness or accident. The important thing about these quarrels is that they were morally ambiguous: Marie Joly, for example, was neither more nor less at fault than her neighbors during most of her arguments. In other words, the magical punishment inflicted by Jura witches after a quarrel was not so much an act of justi-fied revenge, as the British model proposes, as a gratuitous display of the witch's malignant disposition — and a sign of her physical and legal powerlessness.

We must imagine the mental state of most Jura witchcraft suspects in the sixteenth and seventeenth centuries as dominated by an awareness of sin and guilt; they were unlikely to be innocent victims of others' guilt projections. 'Sin' is an even more basic concept than guilt. As Delcambre has emphasized, witchcraft trials took place in an atmosphere saturated with religious values, and these values are apparent at many different points in Jura region trials. There were instances when judges persuaded a suspect to confess by urging her that in no other way could she save her soul, often with an eloquence that the clergy could barely match. One Protestant witch was beaten by the Devil because he was 'careful to read the Holy Scriptures'; two more fortunate Catholic witches confessed their crimes to a priest and received absolution for them, so that the Devil ceased to trouble them for a time (in such cases, the secrecy of the confessional remained unviolated). There was even one instance where a Catholic witch insisted to his skeptical interrogators that the Devil who recruited him was named Martin Luther.[13]

Notes

1   Keith Thomas, *Religion and the Decline of Magic* (Penguin, Harmondsworth 1973), 520.

2   H. C. E. Midelfort, *Witch-hunting in Southwestern Germany, 1562–1684* (Stanford, Calif. 1972), 175. His remarks apply particularly to the two best documented panics from southwestern Germany.

3   The archival sources for this chapter can be found in the original version of the text: E. W. Monter, *Witchcraft in France and Switzerland: the Borderlands during the Reformation* (Cornell University Press, Ithaca, NY and London 1976), ch. 5.

4   See Midelfort, *Witch-hunting*, 184 and nn. 69–73 *passim*, for an intelligent discussion of this point, which stresses spinsterhood more than widowhood.

5   Bodin, *Les Six livres de la République* (Paris 1576), 8. Bodin published his *Demonomanie des sorciers* only four years later, with the same printer.

6   Compare Midelfort, *Witch-hunting*, 178: 'We can in fact conclude that [in southwestern Germany] a fairly even distribution of wealth emerges among those executed for witchcraft, with even some disproportion toward the wealthier'.

7   This seems to be one instance where a clear difference can be seen between Protestant and Catholic governments in the Jura, since recorded trials of children cannot be found in Protestant states, but are sometimes found at Fribourg or Porrentruy as well as in Franche-Comté. They were always a tiny minority of all witch trials, however.

8   Henri Boguet, *An Examen of Witches*, trans. Montagne Summers (John Rodker, London 1929), ch. 31.

9   Virtually all the important demonologists agreed with Boguet, who made kinship with a convicted witch grounds for suspicion: see article 36 of his 'Manner of Procedure'. See also Midelfort, *Witch-hunting*, 186–7.

10   See especially Alan Macfarlane, *Witchcraft in Tudor and Stuart England: A Regional and Comparative Study* (2nd edn, Routledge, London 1999), ch. 12, which is devoted to 'Kin and Neighbors'.

11   Thomas, *Religion*, 557, 554.

12   E. Delcambre, 'Psychologie des inculpes lorrains', as translated in E. W. Monter, ed., *European Witchcraft* (New York 1969), 105.

13   Luther was dressed in black, 'young and looking like a pastor'. His judges were obviously nonplussed by this answer: at Ducly's second interrogation, 'being seriously and straightaway examined' about the Devil's name, he again answered 'Luther', and they let the matter drop. The trial of his son Pierre a week later also revealed some signs of religious hypersensitivity: for example, a pilgrimage to Rome in a jubilee year, made in order to expiate a private thought, never spoken in public, that God did not exist.

Chapter 6

David Gentilcore

WITCHCRAFT NARRATIVES
AND FOLKLORE MOTIFS IN
SOUTHERN ITALY

Demonologists and inquisitors

ALTHOUGH ITALIAN INTELLECTUALS and the Papacy had done much to formulate the standard view of witchcraft during the Middle Ages, they afterwards did relatively little to encourage its development. A survey of Italian and Spanish witchcraft literature suggests that a stereotypical view of the phenomenon was never widespread in the Mediterranean.[1] In Italy early work on the subject may be characterised by Gianfrancesco Pico della Mirandola's *Strix* (1523), which, instead of being voluminous and encyclopedic, was a lively and elegant dialogue.[2] The character of Dicaste, resembling a lay or ecclesiastical judge, regarded witches as heretics who went to 'synagogues' or 'sabbaths' (like the Jews, we could add), insulted the cross (like the Albigensians) and performed their own perverse rituals (literally so, as they were upside-down versions of Catholic rituals). Peter Burke has described this conceptualisation of alien beliefs as the exact opposite of one's own in terms of the intellectual principle of 'least effort', because it is far less demanding than entering into the structure of those beliefs.[3] This approach may be of especial use in helping us to decipher the writings of later demonologists, who were more severe and condemning towards the witches. These works and their authors were part of a world-view which expressed evil as an inversion of good: to maintain its intellectual coherence, demonism was therefore linked with all privations of good.[4]

In accounting for the rise in accusations against suspected witches in much of Europe during the late sixteenth and early seventeenth centuries the importance of the courts themselves should not be underestimated. Although the essentially functionalist theories are quite helpful in accounting for reactions from below, we must also note 'the extension of public judicial systems and a greater willingness to bring to court disputes where witchcraft was suspected'.[5] The activity of preachers and confessors was also crucial in convincing people that the proper means of reacting to supposed acts of sorcery and witchcraft was through the episcopal tribunals.

Denunciations and confessions alike frequently began by citing the confessor's suggestion to bring the case to court; indeed absolution often depended on it. In explaining the character and content of the accusations and confessions we must account for these historical processes of mediation between the different cultural levels of the complex society that was early modern Europe.

It has been suggested that the change brought about by the 'judicial revolution' in England and elsewhere from restitutive to abstract justice allowed for the victimless crime of simply being a witch, a 'servant of Satan'.[6] This may help to explain the relative absence of witchcraft persecution in Mediterranean Europe. Here, traditional forms of justice held sway within the inquisitorial and episcopal courts, based on penance, and such concepts as the victimless crime and truth by self-accusation were foreign.[7] Although the Roman Inquisition was far more concerned with illicit magic – the crime which included witchcraft – than the Spanish, neither treated the matter with great severity. In the Otrantine diocese of Oria accusations of witchcraft numbered only eight, out of a total of forty-six for 'magic and superstition'; and of the eight, five did not reach a verdict (according to surviving records). Furthermore, most of the accusations were made during the episcopate of Bishop Labanchi (1720–46), in clear contrast with the neighbouring tribunal at Gallipoli, for which there are no surviving accusations of *maleficium* after 1620 (and none at all for diabolical witchcraft), and with the Inquisition at Naples, which was most active during the early decades of the seventeenth century.[8] This would seem to suggest an increased role of the bishop and his tribunal in the prosecution of *maleficium*, although his pastoral visitations give no indication of any extraordinary judicial zeal on his part. None the less the activity of his court against crimes of magic (in elite and popular varieties) and sorcery did not lead to the prosecution of suspected witchcraft offenses, of which the court was somewhat dubious and treated with leniency.

This relative lack of severity was due in part to the emphasis that the Roman Inquisition placed on judicial propriety, especially where witchcraft accusations were concerned. The common view that witchcraft was more pagan superstition and ignorance than diabolical apostasy – a view having its roots in the ninth-century *Canon episcopi* – was coupled with the rare use of torture, central control and assigning little weight to the denunciations made by accused witches. The 'Instructio pro formandis processibus in causis strigum, sortilegiorum, at maleficiorum' has been called the 'fullest and most eloquent expression' of this responsible attitude.[9] It was circulated first in manuscript form among the provincial tribunals of the Inquisition (in Italy and abroad) before appearing in print, first in the second edition of Eliseo Masini's *Sacro Arsenale* (1625) and later in appendix to Cesare Carena's *Tractatus de* Officio Sanctissimae Inquisitionis (the Cremona edition of 1655). When it was finally published in Rome as a thin pamphlet in 1657, it was without the references to the illegal meddling of secular magistrates. As Tedeschi suggests, this may have been done in order to avoid compounding the conflict with the secular courts, which were at this time accusing the Holy Office of being lax in the prosecution of witchcraft, contesting its jurisdiction and augmenting the severity of their own procedures.[10]

Yet the 'Instructio' reflected longstanding inquisitorial practice, preceding its first citation in a 1624 letter written by Cardinal Giovanni Garcia Millini, a senior

cardinal of the Holy Office, to the Bishop of Lodi in response to procedural questions. It seems to have been meant to check the severity and haste of the courts
caused in part by the *Malleus maleficarum,* counselling care in gathering evidence,
in particular before imprisoning, torturing or handing a suspect over to the Holy
Office. In 1626 the Cardinal wrote to the apostolic nuncio of Florence, advising
him that matters of witchcraft were 'most fallacious and, as daily experience shows,
much greater in men's apprehension than in the reality of occurrences – each
disease, the cause of which is not immediately discovered or an efficacious remedy
found, being much too facilely reduced to sorcery'. The letter-writing activity of
Cardinal Millini testifies to the centralising concern of the Holy Office in maintaining the judicial propriety of its provincial branches, especially where it operated
through the episcopal courts, as in the Kingdom of Naples.

The increasing activity of the ecclesiastical courts in the decades following the
Council of Trent does not alone suffice to account for the number of accusations
made before it. Most of the cases for 'magic and superstition' were initiated from
below. What led neighbours to accuse a woman (usually) of sorcery, as opposed
to merely accepting or tolerating her ambiguous role as village wise woman, realising that someone who could heal could also harm? It has been suggested that in
taking the *magare* to court, the accusers may have been dealing with illicit magic
in the way they thought would be most effective, especially as a last resort. But
what about the accusation of 'witchcraft'? How does this more specific accusation
fit into the general scenario, and how do accusations in the Terra d'Otranto compare
with findings for other parts of Europe?

Maleficium and accusations of diabolical witchcraft

Because the charge of diabolical witchcraft was based on a criminalisation of a set
of magical activities, suspects were not selected at random, but generally had a
prior reputation for *maleficium,* based on the recognition of a series of more or less
public 'performances': blessings, incantations, curses and manipulations. As a result,
various levels of labelling were employed by neighbours which, depending on other
factors, might or might not result in a formal accusation before the court.[11] This
seems to have been true throughout Europe, independently of whether the accusations culminated in a large-scale witch-hunt. Because witchcraft was essentially
an imagined crime, the initial stages of accusation and prosecution are thus the most
important in attempting to determine the contributing factors, with the result that
a qualitative study of the trial records is potentially more revealing than a quantitative one. Furthermore, the trial records do not always give us the information
we need (such as age, marital status, occupation, dealings with neighbours), so that
our interpretation of the social dynamics leading to accusations must be based on
a relatively small sample.[12]

Richard Kieckhefer has suggested that there are four different classes of trial
document which the historian of witchcraft must take into consideration.[13] They
vary in their level of 'reliability' as a source for determining actual belief and practice according to their origin. Thus the most valuable are those trials which begin
with the original 'spontaneous' depositions of witnesses or charges of defamation.

These are followed by trials which although initiated by a judge or prosecutor, seem to be free of learned influence. Less reliable still are those trials which show signs of judicial coercion and may contain information deriving from representatives of the intellectual elites. Finally, those trials containing charges of diabolism are the least reliable, because of obvious meddling from above. One trial can, of course, belong to several types. Frequently the first part of a trial will belong to the first type, only to be transformed into the fourth type toward the end. In this instance, the two sections should be studied separately, paying due attention to the dynamics of the case.

Although Donna Laura de Adamo of Francavilla Fontana was persuaded to make her 1678 denunciation of two *magare* by her confessor, the depositions seem to be free of learned influnce. The denunciation was used to introduce the subject of popular healing rituals. The witnesses in the case linked the practice of sorcery with other negative attributes like prostitution, singling out one of the women, Gratia Gallero, not only as a '*magara* e fattucchiara', but a 'public prostitute and loose woman', the object of 'public talk and rumour [which] for many, many years has circulated and circulates among the people of this town'.[14] As far as the Church was concerned, the possession of a bad reputation or 'fame' – the *malafama* of many Otrantine trial records – was a virtual crime in itself, so that it was almost always mentioned in conjunction with charges of illicit magic. Common too were links with moral shortcomings like 'filthy behaviour' or religious deviance, like blasphemy or absence from church. But in this trial both *magare* were careful to keep up appearances:

> Sometimes [Gallero testified] when I went to the Madonna di Finemundo I confessed myself and told the confessor that I had made and given salt, blood and enchanted herb; and at Easter I took communion, for fear of being excommunicated. Furthermore I heard mass almost every day, but when the high point of the mass was reached I didn't look at the Host or Chalice directly, but hid, turning my face the other way, because I knew that I was given to the Devil and damned. When I recited the rosary sometimes, I found myself regretting it. I went accompanying the Viaticum and to sermons and other devotions to show that I was a Christian like any other.[15]

It is with the confessions of the two suspects that the trial takes a quantum leap. From the charges *of maleficium* (principally love philtres and ligatures) made by the deponents against the women, we pass suddenly and directly to the satanic pact, night flight and the witches' sabbat. Their depositions both open with an expression of their desire to save their souls, confess all and be forgiven, after which they succinctly describe the pact, only commenting on the spells of which they were accused when specifically asked to do so by the court. Clearly there has been some sort of judicial prompting, perhaps in the form of counsel to the defence, but without the supporting documentation we can do no more than hypothesise. Our trial record has now shifted to a 'fourth-class' document! None the less Gallero's account is not bereft of originality. After being taken to the sabbat by the other *magara*, Cinzia Maietta, Gallero saw 'an ugly form of man' seated 'as at court', surrounded by others, 'who resembled the figures of demons painted in the picture and church of St Anthony Abbot in this town'. One wonders if this last parallel was hers. The place where the witches united was the walnut-tree of Sobrino (not the usual one at Benevento), and there she promised herself to the head Devil. She was then presented to her personal Devil, who went by the all-too-common name of Martiniello, a version of the name frequently applied to familiars in Italy and France.[16] This was followed by the usual dancing and songs blaspheming God and the heavenly host. Then came the feasting, each woman seated beside her own demon. They ate roast meat, without salt, and – according to the path of least resistance mentioned above – 'exactly as we Christians bless the table at the beginning and thank God at the end, so in reverse fashion we cursed and blasphemed God, the Trinity, Father, Son and Holy Spirit, the Madonna and the Saints.' Interestingly enough, the witches of Francavilla who attended 'li balli' were divided into various companies, of which Gallero said Nicodemo Salinaro – the learned magician – was the head. Certainly this was a curious mingling of different levels of society, learned magic and demonology with popular magic.

This connection is explained in part by the fact that Maietta's husband was a potter (she painting the vases he made), and Salinaro had asked him to make special 'magical' vases for his rituals.' Maietta's own account of the diabolical pact contains another topos, that of poverty. As the trial began she and her husband were living in a rented house, since the one they owned had been taken away from them because of debts. She recounts that several years before, while walking along the road bemoaning her own misery, she called out to the Devil for help and he appeared to her in the form of a shepherd, promising riches – promises which were never fulfilled. Despite the importance of the Devil in her confession, most of her spells have nothing to do with him, and the court seems primarily concerned with ascertaining if she knows any other maleficos. On one occasion, however, she was instructed by her demon to obey the wishes of Giovanni Guisa, who had Maietta, Gallero, Salinaro and a certain Caterina Ciminello assemble together at the Capuchin monastery one night. They were there to punish Fra Giovanni Battista, exorcist, who had allegedly been sent for (by the diocese?) because he was 'experienced in recognising those who have been bewitched', and who they were afraid was aware of Guisa's use of sorcery to cause a man's death. The beating they gave the friar was more on the conventional side, however:

> Together we tormented the said Fra Gio: Battista, who was here to exorcise the said D. Michelino; and we tormented him in this way, that is, the said Gio: Maria [Guisa] held the Capuchin father by his feet, upside down in the air, Nicodemo beat him from behind, la Tauricella [Gallero] pulled him by the sleeves, I by the ears, and the said Caterina beat him on the arms.

Not exactly the stuff of which demonological treatises were made, and yet we must still account for the various witchcraft motifs. The social tensions which resulted in the accusation and prosecution of suspected *magare* have been discussed elsewhere. The sorcery they were seen to perform was believed to bring about real results, whereas witchcraft existed totally in the mind. The role of the Church, as well as the 'monkish fantasies' of inquisitors and demonologists, is clear even in areas like the Terra d'Otranto where there were no witch-hunts. It was not for lack of effort. An ecclesiastic of Latiano unofficially examined several women who, he affirmed, had confessed to the satanic pact and numerous acts of sorcery, resulting in deaths. Convinced of their guilt, he wrote to the bishop of Oria, asking him to conduct an investigation and 'make them abjure publicly and express detestation of their errors'. The bishop should then decide whether to have a public confession and release them, or have the Holy Office pass them over to the secular arm which, he admits, might take a while because of the slow pace at which the Holy Office operates (suggesting that he thought it was overly careful in its procedures). Since the missive lacks both date and signatory, the Holy Office may have been right in regarding the activities of the local episcopal courts with some suspicion. None the less, it reveals the hatred which at least some ecclesiastics bore towards suspected witches, and the possibility that the greater severity of the secular courts better reflected the more widespread hatred of witches.

Spared the religious uncertainties of the northern European confessional conflicts and not as affected by the social and economic change which increased village tensions elsewhere, both of which have been identified as factors leading to the rise in witch trials, only three accusations in the diocese of Oria *began* with a charge of witchcraft. It is now a matter of accounting for these. What made the demonology of the judges acceptable both to those who made the accusations and those who 'spontaneously' confessed?

Witchcraft and popular culture

On the one hand, we should not ignore the possible contributions of traditional folk culture, elusive though it often is. Belief in night-flying witches existed in parts of Germany as far back as the eleventh century, and diabolical evidence emerges in trials before its codification by demonologists, theologians and lawyers. In this regard, anthropologists have found two sorts or levels of belief: first, a widespread belief in malefice, and second, a belief in the night 'witch', who flies through the air and assembles for cannibalistic feasts. The former belief is concerned with and present in daily life, while the latter, less commonly found, represents communal fears and fantasies. Research in modern-day Greece – where the diabolising of traditional beliefs typical of western Christianity did not take place – has explored narratives which deal with a whole host of spirits, demons and fairies, like the exotika and the nereids. The latter, for example, are beautiful female spirits who tempt, trick and harm men, and form 'a dancing, naked, ecstatic community of the night, musical and wild'.[17] Similar beliefs existed both in Graeco-Roman antiquity and among the pre-Christian Germanic and Celtic peoples, surviving into the Middle Ages, before being interpreted by mediaeval inquisitors in terms of Satan-worship.[18]

The mythical dimension of the sabbat stereotype was such a success, as Carlo Ginzburg has suggested, 'because it embodied in a perverted form the structure of an ancient myth, deeply rooted in the folklore of various parts of Europe'.[19] Beginning with fourteenth-century French trials against lepers and Jews, the satanic attributes were then transferred to those myths regarding communication with the dead or battle against evil spirits to ensure the fertility of the crops. The inquisitorial view could then be extended outside the original areas through the use of torture and other physical and psychological pressures, facilitated by periods of religious or socio-economic crisis.

In this respect, witchcraft accusations and confessions represent the interaction between the beliefs of judges and inquisitors on the one hand and popular beliefs in *maleficium* on the other, and their content may vary according to the integration of local belief systems – and their symbolic representations of the sacred – into the wider uniform system of the sabbat (and all its implications).[20] At the level of popular culture, people were concerned with the effects of a cunning woman's maleficent power – attempting to evade or neutralise it – rather than with its practical origins. But when accusing a suspect before the episcopal tribunal they came into contact with an institution which operated within a different framework. For this reason, the trials often consist of several different levels of discourse, as mentioned above. Of course, it is all but impossible to retrieve the local belief system in its pure state, but important elements can be recovered without the historian revealing too many of his own assumptions in the process.

In the footsteps of Ginzburg, Gustav Hermingsen has explored the Sicilian fairy cult of the *donni difuora* (literally, the 'women from outside', as in the Greek *exotika*) using a series of trial summaries sent between 1547 and 1701 by the Sicilian office of the Spanish Inquisition to the archives of la Suprema in Spain. Before being transformed into stereotypical witches by the inquisitors, the *donni* were believed to perform good deeds, healing people, assisting them in their spinning and other tasks and helping them find hidden treasure. Among those accused, Henningsen found no persons of wealth. Where financial status could be determined, they were poor women. This led him to describe the cult as a 'daydream religion that allowed poor people to experience in dreams and visions all the splendours denied them in real life'.[21] This suggestion is an important clue in understanding such beliefs, including the role of the pact with Satan in witchcraft accusations and confessions in the Terra d'Otranto and elsewhere, which we shall be discussing below.

The Devil

Of course, the standard explanation favoured by demonologists for women's attraction to the Devil was their insatiable lust. In a case of demonic obsession . . . Maria Salinaro described the Devil as a 'handsome young man' with whom she had often 'had sex for several hours, even through the posterior part'. In another confession three years later she stated that she had made her original pact with the Devil 'for the convenience of being able to give vent to my wild desires in the vice of dishonesty that had become my habit'. And in 1704 a forty-five-year-old widow, Antonia Donatino, confessed to making a pact with the Devil, who visited her while she was in bed, making love to her for more than half an hour, and 'he left me so tired, and almost dead'.

Why all this sex? G. R. Quaife has recently suggested that not only did such confessions reflect the misogynistic theories of demonologists, they also reflected the unsatisfied sexual needs of women. Noting that few male peasants seem to have engaged in fore- and after-play, Satan 'brought pleasure into the dull lives of disturbed, bored and frustrated women, even if only in the imagination'.[22] Such fantasies, he concludes, could result from an absence of sexual activity, severe depression (following a husband's death, for example) or advanced senility. Then again, it may also have been a case of the suspected women telling the inquisitors what they thought they wanted to hear, given their wish to escape punishment and given the lack of pleasure they seem to have derived from such relations. The rather uninhibited accounts of sexual relations may also reflect the strong physical component present in popular magic as well. In any case it would be wrong to make too much of it. As Mircea Eliade has remarked, rural populations are only moderately interested in sex, and the witches sought other goals than the simple gratification of lust.[23]

Taken in context, it would seem that the sexual fantasies express a desire on the part of the women to transmute their own condition. Significantly, the Devil offers all sorts of things, such as money and magical powders. The victims of these temptations were almost always poor, helpless women, and the Devil's promises were closely related to their plight, giving us little reason to doubt the reality of such fantasies. Antonia Donatino admitted to making her pact with the Devil because of his promise to take care of a meddling ex-lover of hers. More common was the hoped-for satisfaction of economic needs, not unusual considering that many accused witches were weak and helpless, with no other means of power or influence. Such was the case of the peasant Rosa Tardea who lamented 'that the more she toiled, the poorer she saw herself get'. She was one of Maria Salinaro's 'disciples', an indication that Salinaro really believed her obsession and counselled the Devil's help to others. Alternatively, she may have been so anxious to confess that she listed her 'disciples' to please the court. Another woman she claimed to have converted to the Devil was Francesca Antonia di Toripietto, married to a poor peasant. As the Devil had helped Salinaro, Salinaro advised di Toripietto that 'if she wanted to be well, and be supported and helped, it would be good to call the Devil for help'. She must have so advised the entire neighbourhood, for she listed twenty-one other 'disciples', none of whom were interrogated by the episcopal court. Perhaps her previous confessions had stretched the court's patience and credulity to the limit, for by 1741 the intellectual climate regarding witches was changing.

Temptations could also be induced by religious fear and despair, such as the lack of hope in salvation. It tells us something of the nature of religious instruction – and perhaps of the ability of oral culture to shift orthodox beliefs to suit its own psychological needs – that the Devil frequently promised to pay women's debts and lead them into heaven. Antonia Donatino confessed that the Devil appeared to her and said, 'I am your Angel and I've come here to grant you Paradise'. He returned often with the same promise, and told her (and this is the strange part) that she must recite the rosary, give alms to the poor and fast on Saturdays! When Leonarda Mingolla was asked by a somewhat doubting court what prayers her Devil had her recite, she replied: 'I worship you, oh lord and Devil, attend to my soul.' How can this confusion of divine and diabolical be explained?

In a 1519 case examined by Carlo Ginzburg, a suspected sorceress described two similar visions, one of the Virgin Mary and one of the Devil, both of which were coming to her aid. For the inquisitor the vision of Mary must therefore have been a result of the Devil's trickery, whereas for the suspect both were equally real. According to the popular conception of the sacred, both the Devil and the saints of heaven could give succour in time of need. In Ginzburg's words,

> divinity, as Chiara [the suspect] can understand and venerate it, is a divinity which intervenes to draw her from her misery, first casting a spell on her landlords who have put her out, then healing them so that she may return to her land: and it matters not whether a celestial or diabolical divinity is involved.[24]

As we have had occasion to observe with regard to lay visions, the Church – as part of its attempt to define and control the sacred – sought to impose a distinction between divine and diabolical visions, thereby acknowledging the similarity of forms they could take. A woman of Vicenza was returning home one evening in 1560, giving vent to her anguish and misery, and 'grieving over and lamenting with mournful voice the heavy burden of [her] children without any means of providing for their needs', when she heard a voice calling her. She turned about and 'saw a woman dressed in white like a nun's habit who tried to console her with comforting words, and she revealed herself to be the blessed Mary of God and Queen of heaven the Virgin Mary'. Perhaps because of its resemblance to many a devilish temptation, the Inquisitor-General in Rome, Cardinal Michele Ghisleri, declared the vision a 'diabolical illusion'.

Yet the whole historical period was fraught with ambiguity, for the years of diabolical temptation were also those of the great mystical ecstasies of the baroque saints. The language and experience of both was remarkably similar. According to Fulvio Salimbeni, 'if the witches lie prostrate and exhausted when the Devil has visited with them, the female mystics confess to an ineffable sweetness and a state of complete languor when Jesus visits them'. The seventeenth-century mystics sought *aneantissement* (loss of self before God), as a prelude to spiritual union: a kind of 'life in death' which left them physically drained. Compare this with Antonia Donatino's words describing her relations with the Devil [see p. 104]. The ambiguity is similar to that which existed between the recognised visions of canonised saints (or those about to be), and the visions – considered diabolical and heretical – of those not accepted into sainthood. Operating more often on a basis of shame than of violence, the authorities were determined to control the autonomous figures of sorceress and 'priestess' (the pseudo-saints examined by the Church). As far as the Inquisition was concerned both they and the witches were misled by the Devil, the 'Father of lies'.

This ambivalence may be explained by the fact that in popular culture the Devil, rather than being the personification of evil, had more the semblance of a demon. And in the confessions he appears 'more as a legendary figure of folklore than as the master of a demonic cult'.[25] Otherwise powerless women could boast to their neighbours of relations with 'their' Devil as a means of acquiring respect, as a forty-five-year-old *donna di fuora* who confessed 'that sometimes to please her listeners she had told them things that she had neither seen nor had any knowledge of'.[26]

Some of the narratives have a distinctly folktale-like quality. In 1745, on the advice of Abbot Filippo Coccioli, Giacomo Carrozzo denounced Antonia Macarella for relations with the Devil, based on what she had revealed to him (Carrozzo) in a conversation. Macarella told him that one day she was walking outside the town when someone called out to her. She immediately thought it was Vito Braccio, with whom she had had an affair, but who had since broken off relations, leaving her despondent. So she responded irately: 'What the Devil do you want?' The voice asked in reply: 'Don't you recognise me, since I'm the Devil, your friend?' After he had identified himself – appearing, as usual, in time of crisis – Macarella recounted that the Devil bade her to follow him, leading her to a 'certain place, where he made the earth open up' and they went inside.

The Devil (like some fairy-tale ogre) told her to wait there until he returned, adding that the treasure she saw about her was hers. Going deeper inside, Macarella found three mounds of gold and silver, and she put them in a sack, hoping to carry them off. But realising that she could not locate the way out of the cave, and looking about in dismay, she saw an image of the Virgin Mary, 'with such large eyes', and another one facing in, frightful in appearance, 'with such wretched hair, that is, dishevelled'. The latter image warned her that she would not be able to leave unless she took all of the treasure, a truly herculean task. At this point she grew afraid and, dropping the riches she was carrying, found the exit and quickly returned home and went to bed. That night the Devil visited her, and she explained her plight, but fearing the reaction of her husband sleeping in bed beside her, told the Devil to return another time.

Two features of this narrative are particularly striking. Firstly, the accuser's obvious belief in it, since it forms the principal evidence against Macarella – or at least the possibility that he thought the court might believe it. Secondly, its resemblance to a folktale is intriguing. Although the absence of sufficient data makes it difficult to historicise the various elements of such tales, the Devil is here portrayed more as a mischievous sprite, whom the hero always manages to outwit, than as the prince of darkness. Tales of the duped Devil were most likely derived from the folklore about stupid trolls and giants and, according to J. B. Russell, reflected the resentment that the humble felt for the powerful.[27]

Throughout the trial records the scholar can usually manage to separate popular from learned belief, sorcery from witchcraft, or account for transformations in the latter when taken on by the former. In the same way, it would seem that the Devil remained 'un-diabolised' in popular culture: a trickster capable of fulfilling fantasies and even bestowing Paradise to those who call upon him.[28]

Judicial reactions

How did the courts react to this? The answer must be, with scepticism, although the accusations themselves were taken seriously enough. Sorcery, more than witchcraft, seems to have been their primary concern. In 1742 Bishop Labanchi of Oria, writing in support of the episcopal court's jurisdiction over the case against the suspected witch Giustina Quaranta, made no mention of witchcraft. She was to be prosecuted 'for the many times she had blackmailed people, threatening them with evil if they did not give her the things and money she wanted from them, such that she had become infamous and kept people almost in dismay'. And if the episcopal prosecutors were still credulous, the representatives of the Holy Office were not, making certain that judicial standards were maintained. In the case against Caterina Patrimia, the court was inclined to believe Patrimia's confession until an inquisitor pointed out that it was impossible to stipulate a pact of ten years' duration with the Devil, as Patrimia claimed to have done, after which time she had withdrawn 'to look after the interests of her soul'. According to theologians, the inquisitor declared, the Devil always exacted a promise not to return to the Catholic faith. In the context of the inquisitorial 'Instructio' discussed above, the inquisitor's report charged that the trial records were full of legal invalidities: no formal charges had been laid, no statements had been taken other than those of the two suspects, which anyhow lacked their signatures or marks. Furthermore, Patrimia's sin could not have been apostasy since the formal pact with the Devil had to be finalised by eleven rites, including the Devil's baptism, of which there is no trace; and, he went on, no other documents supported Patrimia's confession that she was a witch. In fact, several priests had even testified as to her Christian behaviour. Because of these points, and the inadequate defence offered the two women by the promotor fiscal, they should be immediately liberated and absolved, the representative of the Holy Office concluded. At this point the trial came to an end.

The last surviving accusation of witchcraft laid before the episcopal court of Oria dates from three years later. As the court had made accusations of magic – beneficent and maleficent – and witchcraft possible, it now rendered them very unlikely. In part the attitudes of the educated levels of the clergy, which provided the judges and prosecutors, were slowly changing. Not that they now denied the possibility of witchcraft: it was more a case of the increasing impossibility of establishing certain proof in particular instances. At the popular level, belief in sorcery continued much as before. And if a belief in witches and the satanic pact managed to filter down and affect notions of malefice, it had no means of expression, for the courts were increasingly reluctant to regard such accusations seriously.

It would seem that in the Terra d'Otranto witchcraft accusations do not provide the enigma that they do in other European regions. The close relationship of witchcraft to *maleficium* is clear, as is the role of demonologists and inquisitors in gradually diabolising aspects of popular belief, though without the impact made elsewhere. When the Devil does make an appearance, it is not usually as the personification of evil, but as the trickster of folklore. Or he may appear in visions as the bestower of favours, in which guise the ambivalence between divine and diabolical sources of power is readily apparent. This ambivalent sense of the sacred is consistent with that manifested in other areas of the system, such as the pragmatic relationship between popular healing rituals and sacramental remedies. It was this ambiguity that the Church had sought to counter following the Council of Trent, as it attempted to define, regulate and reform access to and attitudes towards the sacred.

Notes

1   Brian Levack, *The Witch-Hunt in Early Modern Europe* (London 1987), 202.
2   See Peter Burke, 'Witchcraft and magic in Renaissance Italy: Gianfrancesco Pico and his Strix', in S. Anglo, ed., *The Damned Art: Essays in Literature and Witchcraft* (London 1977), 32–52.

3   Ibid., 40. This suggestion complements the argument of Stuart Clark in Chapter 11 of this collection.

4   Julio Caro Baroja, *The World of the Witches*, trans. N. Glendinning (London 1964), 104.

5   John Bossy, *Christianity in the West, 1400–1700* (Oxford 1985), 78.

6   See Chapter 15 in this book by Christina Larner.

7   Cf. Bossy, *Christianity*, 139.

8   William Monter and John Tedeschi, 'Toward a statistical profile of the Italian Inquisitions, sixteenth to eighteenth centuries', in G. Henningsen and J. Tedeschi, eds, *The Inquisition in Early Modern Europe: Studies on Sources and Methods* (Dekalb, Ill. 1986), 146.

9   John Tedeschi, 'The Roman Inquisition and witchcraft: an early seventeenth-century "Instruction" on correct trial procedure', *Revue de l'Histoire des Religions*, 200 (1983), 188.

10   Ibid., 176.

11   See Chapter 15 by Larner.

12   Cf. Levack, *Witch-Hunt*, 117.

13   Richard Kieckhefer, *European Witch Trials: Their Foundations in Popular and Learned Culture, 1300–1500* (London 1976), 45.

14   The phrase 'common whore and witch' was also used in the same way throughout England, according to Alan Macfarlane, *Witchcraft in Tudor and Stuart England* (2nd edn, London 1999), 277–9.

15   For full citations of the archival sources used in this work, see the original version in David Gentilcore, *From Bishop to Witch: The System of the Sacred in Early Modern Terra d'Otranto* (Manchester University Press 1992), 238–58.

16   According to Giuseppe Bonomo the name Martin was frequently applied to billy-goats (perhaps in reference to Martin of Tours, protector of cuckolds), which the devils closely resembled, according to demonological works.

17   Richard and Eva Blum, *The Dangerous Hour: The Lore of Crisis and Mystery in Rural Greece* (London 1970), 218–19. The authors suggest that women narrate accounts of the nereids as a way of keeping men in line; it also offers a harmless means of expressing the dream-like 'antithesis of the marital state'.

18   Norman Cohn, 'The myth of Satan and his human servants', in M. Douglas, ed., *Witchcraft Confessions and Accusations* (London 1970: ASA Monograph 9), 11.

19   Carlo Ginzburg, 'The witches' sabbat: popular cult or inquisitorial stereotype?', in S. Kaplan, ed., *Understanding Popular Culture* (Berlin 1984), 45–6.

20   Cf. Robert Rowland, '"Fantasticall and devilishe, persons": European witch-beliefs in comparative perspective', in Ankarloo and Henningsen, eds, *Early Modern European Witchcraft*, esp. 178–89.

21   Gustav Henningsen, '"The Ladies from Outside": an archaic pattern of the witches' sabbath', in Ibid., 200.

22   G. R. Quaife, *Godly Zeal and Furious Rage: The Witch in Early Modern Europe* (London 1987), 99–102.

23   Mircea Eliade, 'Some observations on European witchcraft', in his *Occultism, Witchcraft and Cultural Fashions* (Chicago 1976), 91.

24   Carlo Ginzburg, 'Stregoneria e, pieta popolare', in *Miti, emblemi, spie: Morfologia e storia* (Turin 1986), 17.

25   Kieckhefer, *Witch Trials*, 36.

26   This incident is described in Henningsen, 'Ladies from Outside', 198.

27   Jeffrey Burton Russell, *Lucifer: The Devil in the Middle Ages* (Ithaca, NY 1984), 76.

28   The difference between popular and learned ideas about the Devil is also described in Chapters 17, 18 and 23 of this book.

PART THREE

The Idea of a Witch Cult

EARLY MODERN ACCOUNTS OF the collective activities of witches — and particularly the rites associated with the sabbat — were often as repulsive as they were bizarre. The ritual slaughter of infants, the feasting on excrement and human flesh, and the act of copulation with the Devil all appeared frequently in depictions of the satanic mass. Such activities were, as Jean Bodin noted in 1580, 'the most detestable crimes of which the human mind can conceive'.[1] In the absence of any credible evidence that such practices ever took place, modern readers might find it hard to imagine how such allegations emerged. To put it bluntly, why should any culture create such sickening myths? The emergence of the idea of collective satanism is not only an intriguing psychological puzzle: the myth played an important role in the whole history of European witchcraft. As Erik Midelfort points out in Chapter 7, the notion that witches acted together was one of the prerequisites for the large-scale persecutions which blighted Germany in the late sixteenth and early seventeenth centuries. By encouraging the courts to pursue the associates of alleged witches, the fantasy of communal Devil worship could spark an explosion of accusations that transformed isolated cases of *maleficium* into panics involving dozens of individuals. In the most extreme instances, like the panic in Trier between 1587 and 1593, hundreds were executed and whole villages decimated. Though the horrors of the German persecutions were not repeated throughout Europe, the idea of a witch cult was significant elsewhere. In the Franche-Comté region between France and Switzerland, William Monter has shown that an initial accusation of witchcraft could fan out into a serious panic, fuelled by the denuciations by witches of their alleged accomplices (see Chapter 5). Even in areas where the idea of the sabbat was not fully developed, and played only a minor role in the confessions of the accused, the notion of collective witchcraft could give impetus to persecutions. The panic in Essex in 1645 was encouraged by the conviction of local authorities that they were dealing with a 'horrible sect of witches'.[2] When the first suspect named her supposed confederates, this set in train a series of accusations based on local suspicions of *maleficium*. It is significant, perhaps, that the idea of collective witchcraft was usually absent in English trials before this date, and the Essex persecutions claimed far more victims than any previous prosecutions for the crime.

For Midelfort, the lethal idea of a witch cult derived from the 'panic-striken demonology' of learned theologians and lawyers. He suggests that the fantasy of the sabbat was largely unknown in peasant communities, but was imposed by scholars as a by-product of the extension of imperial law in the sixteenth century. This emphasis on the role of elites can be challenged, however. Wolfgang Behringer argues in Chapter 4 that fears of collective witchcraft reflected the widely held belief that large-scale *maleficium* like weather magic was normally the work of groups of witches. In Chapters 8 and 9, two other historians, Carlo Ginzburg and Éva Pócs, take this idea a step further: they argue that key elements in the theory of the sabbat originated in traditional beliefs that were not confined to an educated minority. Ginzburg challenges the claim made by Norman Cohn (see Chapter 2) that allegations against witches were essentially a continuation of the accusations levelled at mediaeval Jews and heretics. He suggests that this cannot account for important features of the sabbat, notably the idea that witches travelled through the air to attend their secret gatherings. Moreover, he cites beliefs recorded in trial records that appear to be alien to demonological stereotypes, and were therefore unlikely to have been imposed by legal authorities. For Ginzburg, such evidence suggests that the concept of the sabbat originated in a common set of popular traditions, centred on 'spirit travel' to the land of the dead, which were reinterpreted as satanic witchcraft by the courts in the early modern period.

While Ginzburg's chapter raises fascinating possibilities, it relies largely on fragmentary evidence scattered over western and central Europe. It does not demonstrate that traditional beliefs about spirit travel were integrated into a coherent, living belief-system which was misrepresented as satanism during the period of persecutions. This is a major weakness of the argument, at least when it is applied to Europe as a whole. There is, however, strong evidence that fully developed beliefsystems based on spirit travel did exist in certain areas. Ginzburg's major work on the Fruili region of Italy, and Gustav Henningsen's study of fairy cults in Sicily, have shown that peasant belief-systems could provide the raw material for theories of satanic witchcraft.[3] In Chapter 9, Éva Pócs provides similar evidence from seventeenth- and eighteenth-century Hungary. She demonstrates that a popular concept of witches' meetings was reported to the courts throughout this period, and received only relatively minor modifications from the authorities. In these extraordinary depositions, witches and their victims were transported to an 'alternative world' that existed in parallel to reality, where they engaged in feasting, magical feats, battles and punishments. Like Behringer, Pócs suggests that fears of collective witchcraft were as common among ordinary people as they were among elites, though she traces these fears to folkloric concepts of the sabbat instead of the belief in large-scale *maleficium*.

The evidence from central Europe and Italy shows that folk beliefs could provide the basis for ideas about the witches' sabbat. But did such beliefs influence demonological thinking in the heartlands of Europe's witch trials – Germany and Central Europe – and other regions like France and the British Isles? This idea is challenged robustly by Robert Muchembled in Chapter 10. Muchembled maintains that the sabbat was 'simply and solely a figment created by theologians, whose ideas governed the imagination of the elite classes of Europe in the late Middle Ages'. It had no strong roots in popular culture, though its exponents were sometimes prepared to incorporate aspects of folklore into the doctrine. In this interpretation, the success or failure of witch persecutions depended on the willingness of local communities to accept the alien concept of collective witchcraft. Where this took place, it was part of a much wider process of 'acculturation', by which leading figures in the localities acquiesced with central governments to impose order in their communities. Muchembled's work provides a useful critique of Ginzburg's interpretation of the origin of the sabbat, and suggests an alternative source for the myth of a witch cult. His position can be criticised, however. Robin Briggs has argued that Muchembled places too much emphasis on socio-political trends, to the exclusion of other factors relevent to the development of witch beliefs.[4] In this respect, his work reflects the general tendency of historians to seek single-cause explanations for witchcraft phenomena. It can also be objected that Muchembled assumes the existence of a sharp distinction between elite and popular culture. While there were undoubtedly differences between the beliefs of ordinary people and the educated minority, there is a danger in his interpretation of overlooking the many common features between the two.

The final chapter in this section is less vulnerable to this criticism. Like Muchembled, Stuart Clark argues that the concept of collective witchcraft could have emerged without the existence of folk beliefs resembling the sabbat. But instead of political factors, he stresses the role of 'inversion' in the development of an imaginary witch cult. Clark points out that early modern people tended to think in terms of absolute opposites, so that most social, religious and political conventions were defined in terms of their negative mirror images. This inclination was apparent in festivals like the 'feast of fools', which turned conventional social hierarchies temporarily upside down, and in a wide range of artistic and academic practices. In this context, it was possible for demonologists to construct the major features of the witch cult by simply reversing the positive aspects of their own view of society. Indeed, it was even necessary for them to do so, since the existence of a good society presupposed the possibility of its wicked opposite. To Clark, the business of describing in detail the frightful events of a witches' sabbat was a 'necessary way of validating each corresponding, contrary aspect of the orthodox world'. Thus the principle of inversion goes some way to explaining the psychological riddle posed at the start of this introduction: it made sense for scholars to emphasise the most repellent aspects of satanic witchcraft because each feature of the demonic anti-society affirmed the goodness of the normal world. The idea of inversion also provides an alternative explanation for some features of the sabbat that might otherwise be attributed to folklore. Clarke suggests, for example, that the idea of witches turning themselves into animals was an inversion of contemporary ethics: it replaced reason with animal instinct and morality with bestial desire.

Taken together, the five chapters in this section suggest at least two possible origins for the myth of a witch cult. They provide potential ammunition for two very different historical arguments. It would be possible, if one wished, to combine the ideas of Muchembled and Clark to explain fears of collective witchcraft without any reference to popular traditions of spirit travel or the 'alternative world'. Equally, Pócs' study of the Hungarian trials could be used to support Ginzburg's thesis that the sabbat originated in folklore. But neither approach would produce a complete or wholly convincing interpretation. It is best to accept that the complexity of the surviving evidence means that different explanations must be advanced for different regions, and often more than one source was involved in the development of the myth. With this in mind, it is worth noting that the fantasy of the sabbat varied from place to place, and was often coloured strongly by local legends. In Sweden, for instance, the witch panic of 1668–76 was fuelled by stories of the sabbat linked to the legend of the 'blue mountain' Blakulla, a traditional haunt of witches and demons.[5] Such examples show that sabbat beliefs could entwine learned demonology with folklore in creative and unpredictable ways, thus making the search for an original source rather pointless. Like many other aspects of the witch persecutions, the fantasy of the sabbat can be best understood when one resists the lure of a simple, single-cause explanation.

Notes

1   Alan Kors and Edward Peters, eds, *Witchcraft in Europe, 1100–1700: A Documentary History* (University of Pennsylvania Press, Philadelphia 1972), 215.
2   Matthew Hopkins, *The Discovery of Witches* (1647), 2.
3   Carlo Ginzburg, *The Night Battles: Witchcraft and Agrarian Cults in the Sixteenth and Seventeenth Centuries* (Johns Hopkins University Press, Baltimore, Md 1992); Gustav Henningsen, 'The Ladies from Outside: An Archaic Pattern of the Witches' Sabbath', in Bengt Ankarloo and Gustav Henningsen, eds, *Early Modern European Witchcraft: Centres and Peripheries* (Clarendon, Oxford 1990).
4   Robin Briggs, 'Many Reasons Why: Witchcraft and the Problem of Multiple Explanation', in Jonathan Barry, Marianne Hester and Gareth Roberts, eds, *Witchcraft in Early Modern Europe* (Cambridge University Press 1996), 52–3.
5   Robin Briggs, *Witches and Neighbours* (HarperCollins, London 1996), 52.

Chapter 7

H. C. Erik Midelfort

HEARTLAND OF THE WITCHCRAZE

MAXIMILIAN I, HOLY ROMAN EMPEROR and the 'last knight of the Middle Ages' kept a magician, Johannes Trithemius, Abbot of Sponheim, at his court. On one occasion, the Emperor asked him to settle empirically the rival claims of the pagan and biblical worthies by bringing them back to earth. We do not know what the famous humanist abbot made of this imperial request; nor can we tell what spectacles and illusions he produced to entertain the court at Innsbruck. What we do know is that Trithemius had a reputation as a learned necromancer.

But was his art witchcraft, a demonic gift made possible only by a pact with the Devil? No one in the early sixteenth century seems to have thought so. Indeed, Germany was alive with learned magicians in those years, men whose neo-Platonic convictions led them to harness the magical forces of the cosmos. Henry Cornelius Agrippa of Nettesheim and Theophrastus Bombastus von Hohenheim, known more simply as Paracelsus, flourished in the early sixteenth century and tried to bring magic to the aid of philosophy and medicine. Dr Faust may even have given himself to the Devil before his death in 1540, thereby engendering a myth that has firmly linked Germany and the Devil together ever since. And yet it is worth noting that none of these magicians was ever even prosecuted for witchcraft. Theologically they all deviated from Christian orthodoxy, but even dabbling with demons did not endanger their lives. Later in the century, David Leipzig might actually sign a pact with the Devil and receive a punishment no more severe than expulsion from his university.

In a court of law all of these men might have been convicted of witchcraft, but the interesting point is that no-one thought of bringing charges against them. In 1563, in his famous *De Praestigiis Daemonum,* Johann Weyer complained bitterly that these *magi infiames* got off scot free while deluded old women were convicted and executed by the hundreds. Weyer's sense of outrage illustrates the important point that, regardless of what the theologians and jurists might say, witchcraft in Germany was not simply a crime of mental or spiritual deviation; it was not primarily heresy or apostasy or learned diabolism. Rather, witchcraft was mainly a social offence: the use of harmful magic by a secret conspiracy of women. The German prosecutors who assumed the task of rooting out the godless witches knew whom they were looking for. And they were so successful that they made the German-speaking territories the classic land of the witch-hunt. It is certain that the Holy Roman Empire and Switzerland executed far more witches than any other parts of Europe. How can we account for this?

Recent studies have illuminated the important extent to which witchcraft trials remained popular in inspiration or became subject to learned influence and inter-ference. It has become clear that down to 1550, and probably much later, the common folk of the village feared witchcraft not as a demonic conspiracy but as a practical threat to the fertility of their fields, flocks and families. Witches were popularly imagined as solitary sorcerers, practicing their malefic magic through the manipulation of cursing tablets, ointments, charms, and all the mysterious rubbish that could be combined in a *Hexentopf*. Their baneful poisons could cause hailstorms and untimely frosts; sickness in man and beast; impotence, miscarriage and death. These were everyday threats to country life, and it is not surprising that common people accused the local crone of enviously casting evil spells. Indeed it is probable enough that some of the locally accused were guilty as charged of at least *trying* to harm a neighbour or secure his affection with love magic. Through-out the centuries of the witch-hunt these locally inspired and locally controlled sorcery trials continued to be common. They usually ended as abruptly as they had begun, with the execution or banishment of one or two witches. There was nothing peculiarly German in this procedure and nothing to cause the panic that the great witch-hunt inspired. But the true panic did not remain rooted in these rural concerns and did not rest content with the extermination of one or two geriatric outcasts.

To have some understanding of the difference, we may look with profit at some of the frightful trials that became characteristic of Germany, especially in the prince-bishoprics and ecclesiastical states of central Germany. Between 1587 and 1593 the Archbishop Elector of Trier sponsored a witch-hunt that burned 368 witches from just twenty-two villages. So horrible was this hunt that two villages in 1585 were left with only one female inhabitant apiece. In the lands of the Convent of Quedlinburg, some 133 witches were executed on just one day in 1589. At the Abbey of Fulda, Prince Abbot Balthasar von Dernbach conducted a reign of terror in the first decade of the seventeenth century: his minister Balthasar Ross boasted of having sent over 700 witches to the stake, no less than 205 of them in the years 1603–05 alone. At the *Furstprobstei* of Ellwangen, ecclesiastical officials saw to the burning of some 390 persons between 1611 and 1618, while the Teutonic Order at Mergentheim executed some 124 in the years 1628–30. The Prince Bishopric of Würzburg endured a frightful panic during the 1620s: in just eight years Bishop Philipp Adolf von Ehrenberg executed some 900 persons including his own nephew, nineteen Catholic priests, and several small children. In the Prince Bishopric of Eichstatt some 274 witches were executed in 1629. At Bonn, the Archbishop Elector of Cologne supervised the execution of his own Chancellor, his wife and his secretary's wife. The worst ecclesiastical excesses may well have occurred in the Bishopric of Bamberg, where Bishop Johann Georg II Fuchs von Dornheim is said to have eliminated 600 witches during his reign of ten years (1623–33), including his own Chancellor and one of the burgermeisters of Bamberg, Johann Junius.

Although these ecclesiastical territories were the most ferocious exterminators of witches, secular territories were not always far behind them in their zeal to purge the commonwealth. The tiny county of Helfenstein killed sixty-three witches in 1562–63. The Duchy of Brauschweig-Wolfenbuttel executed fifty-three between 1590 and 1620, while Duke August of Braunschweig-Luneberg eliminated seventy between 1610 and 1615 in the tiny district of Hitzacker. The County of Lippe tried 221 witches between 1550 and 1686 and another 209 in the town of Lemgo. All told, the Duchy of Bavaria probably executed close to 2,000 witches, and the secular territories of south-western Germany very likely accounted for another 1,000. Even the imperial cities hunted witches in sizeable numbers, both among their own burghers and among the peasants of their outlying hinterlands.

When we ask who these witches were, the German evidence agrees closely with that from most of the rest of Europe: they were women, usually old and poor, often widows. Overall, some 80 to 90 per cent of the accused were female, and one cannot begin to understand the European witch-hunt without recognising that it displayed a burst of misogyny without parallel in Western history. Scholars are still far from agreement as to the sources of this hatred and fear of women, but it is clear that the major trials sprang from fears that were no longer rooted merely in the vagaries of peasant misfortune. The thousands executed in these chain-reaction trials may have had to confess to harmful magic, but their chief crime was one of which peasants were generally unaware: the obscene worship of the Devil. Where and how had this idea penetrated the German-speaking lands?

The first massive persecutions in Germany are inseparably connected to the author of the famous *Malleus Maleficarum,* the Hammer of Witches, published in 1486: Heinrich Institoris, OP. In 1484 Institoris obtained from Pope Innocent VIII a bull *(Summi desiderantes)* urging German secular and ecclesiastical officials to co-operate with Institoris and his associate, Jacob Sprenger, OP, in the hunting of witches. Theologically, this bull contained nothing that previous popes had not said; but the bull had considerable importance because it seemed to sanction the subsequent activities of these two Dominican inquisitors. Reprinted with every edition of their *Malleus,* the bull seemed to bestow papal approval on their inquisitorial theories as well. So successful was this stroke of advertising strategy that the authors hardly even needed the approval of the Cologne University theologians, but just for good measure Institoris forged a document granting their apparently unanimous approbation. Armed with the bull, Institoris began a campaign in the diocese of Constance and executed forty-eight witches between 1481 and 1486. Although these efforts finally ran into the effective opposition of the bishop of Bressanone, Institoris assembled enough practical experience to enliven the manual he and Sprenger composed in 1486.

The *Malleus Maleficarum* is a remarkable treatise that actually reveals how far Germany still was from a full-fledged witch-hunting panic. True enough, the two Dominicans injected so much misogynist venom into their pages as to construe witchcraft almost exclusively as a crime of female lust. True, too, the *Malleus* recommends a degree of judicial terror and deception that helps us understand why those

accused of witchcraft often found that they had no real chance to defend themselves. But it is also true that the *Malleus* repeatedly mentions popular incredulity.
In the late fifteenth century Germans were still far from unanimous in their acceptance of the fine points of demonology. In fact, the *Malleus* itself is innocent of the
most important detail of late mediaeval witchcraft theory: the witches' dance or
sabbat. Institoris and Sprenger spent so much time working out the way that
witches co-operated with the Devil that they neglected to spend any attention on
the single feature that made massive, chain-reaction trials possible. Indeed it was
another 75 to 100 years before the orgiastic ritual of the sabbat had worked its
way into the obsessions of the learned and the imagery of the artists. It is noteworthy that German artistic representations of witchcraft in the late fifteenth
century agree with the *Malleus* in portraying a basically solitary crime. The famous
prints of Hans Baldung Grien and Albrecht Mer enliven the theme with visual jokes,
playing changes on the theme of the classical muses, but their figures are still far
from the lusting, turbulent, populous scenes of the late sixteenth and seventeenth
centuries.

The *Malleus,* for all its wealth of corrupt and confused argument, cannot be
viewed as the final synthesis of witchcraft theory. In its own day it was never
accorded the unquestioned authority that modern scholars have sometimes given
it. Theologians and jurists respected it as one among many informative books; its
peculiarly savage misogyny and its obsession with impotence were never fully
accepted. Emperor Charles V promulgated a criminal code for the Empire in 1532
(the *Carolina*) with a witchcraft clause that was still far from reflecting the spirit of
the *Malleus*. Article 109 read simply:

> When someone harms people or brings them trouble by witchcraft, one
> should punish him with death, and one should use the punishment of
> death by fire. When, however, someone uses witchcraft and yet does
> no one any harm with it, he should be punished other-wise, according
> to the custom of the case; and the judges should take counsel as is
> described later regarding legal consultations.

This article preserved intact the Roman legal distinction between harmful and harmless magic, a distinction that appeared impious to the authors of the *Malleus*. As
long as courts insisted that witchcraft prosecutions be closely tied to actual cases
of harm and loss, there was little chance of a chain-reaction trial breaking out.

Unfortunately, the witchcraft article of the *Carolina* did not make full theological sense, for it seemed to permit a more lenient treatment of the most diabolical
magic so long as it harmed no one. Through the middle and late decades of the
sixteenth century in Germany, one can mark the advance of two notions, both
fateful for the development of the German panic trial; gradually, the witches' sabbat
became a common obsession among the ruling elite; and, just as gradually, territorial laws were altered to allow for the execution of witches whose only crime
was association with the Devil, regardless of harm (*maleficium*) to anyone. In 1572
the Criminal Constitutions of Electoral Saxony declared, for example, that 'if
anyone, forgetting his Christian faith, sets up a pact with the Devil or has anything
to do with him, regardless of whether he has harmed anyone by magic, he should

be condemned to death by fire'. With a law such as this, one could proceed to torture a suspect until one had not only an admission of guilt but a list of the names of others seen at the witches' dance. These persons could then in turn be examined and tortured if necessary. A panic might be under way.

To return to our earlier question, it seems clear that the German holocaust of witches depended both on torture and on the learned obsession with the sabbat. But where had local courts and the petty princes of Germany obtained their notions of the sabbat? And let us make no mistake that it was an illusion: no careful researcher has discovered even a trace of a true witch-cult with sabbaths, orgies, black masses and Devil worship. So how did this inquisitor's nightmare become part of the secular law of hundreds of German jurisdictions? Here the notion of the peculiarly German reception of Roman Law is useful again. For as Roman procedures replaced traditional ones in the sixteenth century, local judges were frequently at a loss as to how to proceed. Roman procedure dictated the rational device of seeking learned counsel, as we have seen in the witchcraft article of the *Carolina*; and, beginning in the mid-sixteenth century and with regularity in the seventeenth century, local districts turned to the juridical faculties of the German universities. In this way local procedures all across the Holy Roman Empire were tied to the Roman legal theories of the professors – but, just as fatefully, local witchcraft theory was now dependent as never before on the demonological illusions of learned jurists. In requiring ignorant petty judges to take counsel, the *Carolina* in effect undercut its own prudent Roman witchcraft doctrine, and opened the door to the possibility that the panic about the witches' sabbat could spread beyond the learned studies where it had first taken root.

The Holy Roman Empire thus became the classic land of the witch-hunt, not so much because of the 'German temperament' as because of the German legal system, a system that allowed bishops and other ecclesiastics an unparalleled degree of influence in their territories, and permitted university professors to become full members of the judicial mechanism. Episcopal and professorial fantasies still need close investigation, but at least it seems clear now where we need to look in order to understand how popular and peasant notions of merely harmful magic were perverted into the witchcraft delusion. We may find that the full panoply of demonology never became deeply rooted in the villages, that local accusations almost always stemmed from some local misfortune. At any rate it appears that small-scale witch-trials could survive long after the chain reaction panics had disappeared. Across the Empire the mass trials proliferated between c. 1570 and c. 1630. Some regions had flare-ups again in the 1670s, but by 1630 in most places the worst was over.

How shall we understand this decline? A common answer has been that the magistrates and learned elites of Europe finally gave up their belief in witchcraft. Without their support, trials were no longer possible. This may help explain why even the small, local trials withered away in the eighteenth century; but by then the large, chain-reaction trials had been dead for a generation or more.

One reason for the disappearance of large trials is that during the seventeenth century they came increasingly to involve children. Most of the huge trials after 1625 featured children as accusers and even as the accused. In several cases it was finally recognised, if not by learned university jurists then at least by local officials, that the testimony of minors was simply not credible. Critics of witchcraft trials, from Johann Weyer in the sixteenth century to Friedrich von Spee in the seventeenth, had long maintained that tortured evidence was equally unreliable. Slowly but surely the territories of the Holy Roman Empire put on the brakes, becoming much more cautious in the use of torture than they had been. Already in 1603 the Protestant Archbishop of Bremen, Johann Friedrich, published an *Edict Concerning Witchcraft* that made continuation of the trials almost impossible. In 1649 Queen Christina of Sweden put an end to witchcraft trials in Verden, which was controlled by her country after the end of the Thirty Years War. Bishop Johann Philipp von Schonborn ordered the end to trials in Würzburg in 1642 and carried this caution to Mainz when he became Elector and Archbishop there in 1647. Similarly Prince Bishop Christoph Bernhard von Galen put a stop to trials in Munster. By the 1670s the legal faculties of Tubingen and Helmstedt were urging extraordinary caution in the application of torture. Although the enlightened Professor Christian Thomasius of Halle won renown for his dissertation *De Crimine Magiae* (1701) and for his other attacks on the witchcraft theory and demonology of the learned, by then the true age of witchcraft trials was over.

A glance at witchcraft in Denmark can serve as a comparative check on the picture presented here of the Holy Roman Empire. The Lutheran Bishop of Sealand, Peder Palladius, urged vigorous prosecution of witches in 1544 and reported that successful trials were uncovering 'swarms' of witches in Malmo, Koge, and Jutland, and that at Als and in the nearby islands a chain-reaction trial had sent fifty-two witches to the stake as 'one of them betrays another'. But all of these trials dealt with specific cases of *maleficium,* and in general the Danish trials never developed the fascination with the Devil and the sabbat that one finds just to the south. The main reason for this surprisingly 'backward' condition (one much like that of England) was the promulgation of two laws in 1547. The first forbade the use of testimony from those convicted of infamous crimes, such as theft, treason, and sorcery, against others. The second held that 'no person shall be interrogated under torture before he is sentenced'. These two rules effectively cut off the spread of massive chain-reaction trials like those of 1544. It was no longer possible to torture suspects into confessing their horrible misdeeds or into naming those whom they had seen at the witches' dance. From beginnings that seem similar to those in Germany, Danish trials were thus steered into an English path. Even without ideas of the sabbat, the best recent estimate suggests that the Danes tried some 2,000 persons and executed something less than 1,000. A further reason for the Danish 'mildness' is that after 1576 all death sentences had to be appealed to the high court *(Landsting),* which often proved more cautious than the local courts. After 1650 cases dropped off dramatically to just a few per annum. As in the Holy Roman Empire, however, the popular fear of *maleficium* survived long after the elite had put an end to actual witchcraft trials.

In the rest of Scandinavia, however, the picture was somewhat different. In Norway, where the records of about 750 trials survive between 1560 and 1710, torture was seldom used and only one quarter of those accused (mostly those convicted of causing the death of a person or an animal) were executed. But in Sweden, although the use of torture was infrequent in the sixteenth century, church leaders convinced the government that all found guilty of making a pact with the

Devil should be sentenced to death. From 1668 until 1676 a major witch panic gripped northern Sweden (with repercussions in Finland until 1684): thousands were accused, interrogated and tortured; over 200 were executed. After 1672, persons accused by several witnesses were executed even if they did not confess. The panic abated only in 1676 where several child-witnesses involved in a major Stockholm trial admitted that their stories of Sabbaths and Covens were entirely false.

These Scandinavian trials all serve to point up the extremely pernicious effects of legalised torture and the idea of the sabbat. Wherever the testimony of witches and the possessed could be excluded, trials remained small and manageable; but whenever these restraints were relaxed, the Scandinavians rapidly imitated the legal excesses of the prince bishops of central Germany. Local suspicions of *maleficium* seem to have flourished throughout northern Europe for centuries, certainly surviving long into the nineteenth century, and even into our own. By themselves, however, these suspicions never led to more than a few trials or lynchings. It was the fateful intervention of learned and thoughtful lawyers and theologians with their panic-stricken demonology that sent thousands of women to their deaths. It is a legacy for the learned to ponder.

Chapter 8

Carlo Ginzburg

DECIPHERING THE WITCHES' SABBAT

THE THEME OF WITCHCRAFT in Europe, formerly considered marginal and even frivolous, has since the early 1970s become a subject of international discussion among historians. However, few of the numerous studies have devoted much attention to the sabbat – the nocturnal meeting of witches and sorcerers – although it is clearly of decisive importance in the history of witchcraft and witch-hunting.

The principal exception is Norman Cohn's work *Europe's Inner Demons* (1975), which makes two main points: (1) The picture of the sabbat which took shape in the first decades of the fifteenth century was a modern elaboration, by lay and ecclesiastical judges and demonologists, of an aggressive stereotype that had been applied in former times to Jews, the early Christians, and mediaeval heretical sects; (2) There was no ritual reality corresponding to this image.[1] The nocturnal assemblies described with so much macabre and picturesque detail in the trials and treatises of demonology were like the sect of witches and wizards who supposedly took part in them – a projection of the fears and obsessions of judges and inquisitors.

The first point of Cohn's argument seems to me to be unacceptable, since it postulates the continuity and homogeneity of a stereotype, which in fact underwent radical modification at a particular time owing to the introduction of different elements belonging either to the world of scholarship or to that of folklore. All this suggests that the sabbat is to be regarded as a culturally mixed phenomenon rather than a mere projection of the dominant culture.

The main components of the stereotype as described by Cohn are sexual orgies, cannibalism, and the worship of a bestial divinity. But apart from the chronological hiatus between the beginning of the eighth century and the end of the eleventh the documentary evidence on which this interpretation is founded presents a still more glaring discontinuity as regards content. The anthropophagy attributed to mediaeval heretical sects was a sort of endo-cannibalistic ritual wherein the children of incestuous unions were devoured at nocturnal meetings. The image of the witch pursuing the children or adults of a community in order to eat them or make them fall sick is very different and much more directly aggressive. To discover how it can have come into being, I propose to analyse a body of evidence differing from that presented by Cohn.

We may begin with the rumour which spread in France during the summer of 1321, that lepers had conspired to poison wells and rivers. This charge was almost immediately extended to the Jews, who were accused of having instigated the lepers, sometimes at the behest of the Muslim rulers of Granada and Tunis. In this way the pre-existing notion of an enemy within, the accomplice and instrument of an external enemy, led to a ferocious persecution which was the first of its kind in European history. An examination of chronicles, confessions extracted by torture, and deliberately fabricated evidence leads to the certain conclusion that two plots were brewed in France at that time by the lay and ecclesiastical authorities: one against the lepers, and the other, immediately afterwards, against the Jews. After burnings at the stake and other massacres, lepers were segregated and Jews expelled. Both measures were advocated, some months before the discovery of the alleged plot, in a letter addressed to Philip V of France by the consuls of the seneschalsy of Carcassonne.[2]

In 1347, at a time when the Black Death was raging in Europe, an accusation similar to that of 1321 again emanated from Carcassonne. This time, according to the authorities, it was only the Jews who had poisoned the waters to spread the plague. Once again, the conspiracy was discovered by torture and as a result of persecuting the Jewish communities of the Dauphiné and regions around Lake Geneva. But in the same area some decades later, in 1409, the inquisition accused Jewish and Christian groups of jointly practising rites that were 'contrary to Christian faith'. This enigmatic description probably referred to the notion of the diabolical sabbat that begins to take shape in the Formicarius, a treatise by the Dominican Johannes Nider, written in 1437 during the Council of Basle, and based on facts concerning witch-trials that he had been informed of by the inquisitor at Evian and a judge from Berne. Nider stated that in the past sixty years or so a new form of sorcery had arisen: a sect in the full sense, with a ritual involving Devil-worship and profanation of the Cross and the sacraments. This chronological evidence is corroborated from the other side of the Alps: at the beginning of the sixteenth century, the Dominican inquisitor Bernardo da Como writes that it appears from the record of trials in the archives of the local Inquisition that the sect of witches had originated some 150 years earlier.[3]

Thus the picture of the sabbat took shape in the Western Alps about the middle of the fourteenth century, half a century earlier than the date traditionally accepted by scholars. More important than the earlier dating, however, is the 'lepers–Jews–witches' graduation that emerges from our reconstruction. The creation of the image of a sect of witchcraft, additional to that of isolated witches and warlocks, must be regarded as a separate chapter – destined to be a most important one – of the segregation or expulsion of marginal groups which characterised European society from the fourteenth century onwards. It is also an instructive event from the theoretical point of view. Initially it stemmed from a deliberate political inten-tion, or even a plot, which was assured of success by a prompt popular response. But the successive links in this chain make it impossible to speak of a plot. The scheme of a hostile group conspiring against society was progressively renewed at all levels, but directed against targets that could not have been foreseen. The prodigious trauma of the great pestilences intensified the search for a scapegoat on which fears, hatred, and tension of all kinds could be discharged; the supposed nocturnal meetings of witches and wizards, who came flying from far away to brew their diabolical schemes, embodied the image of an organized, omnipresent enemy with superhuman powers.

As we know, witches and wizards flew to the sabbat, sometimes in animal form or riding on animals. These two elements of flight and metamorphosis were not part of the aggressive stereotype concerning the sect of well-poisoners. They are first heard of in 1428, in certain witch-trials at Sion in the Valais and at Todi (we shall come back to this synchronism later). That these themes originated in folklore has long been known, but scholars have never gone beyond this evident fact. Certain popular beliefs, antedating the sabbat proper but linked to it in many respects, provide us with a clue.

The best-documented case is that of the Friulian *benandanti*. These persons, denounced by their fellow-villagers in about 1570, told the inquisitors that during the year, when the Ember Days came round, they fell into a sort of trance. Some of them, mostly men, said that they then went fighting in far-off places, 'in the spirit' or in a dream, armed with stalks of fennel; their adversaries were witches and wizards, armed with sorghum stalks, and they were fighting for the fertility of the fields. Others, mostly women, said that, either 'in the spirit' or in a dream, they witnessed processions of the dead. All those questioned attributed their extraordinary powers to the fact that they were born within a caul. The inquisitors, having overcome their first astonishment, tried to make the *benandanti* confess that they were sorcerers and had taken part in a witches' sabbat. Under this pressure the *benandanti* altered their story by degrees so that eventually – but more than fifty years later – it conformed to the stereotype of the sabbat, which had not previously figured in the proceedings of the Friulian Inquisition.

The inquisitors' reaction is very understandable. The nocturnal excursions of the *benandanti* were preceded by a kind of trance which left the body as if dead, after which the spirit left it in the form of an animal (a mouse or butterfly) or riding on an animal (a hare, dog, pig, or the like). This clearly suggested the animal metamorphoses attributed to witches on their way to the sabbat. The evident analogy can be interpreted from a different point of view than the inquisitors'. In *I benandanti* (1966) I pointed out that in the case of witches as well as of *benandanti,* 'that state of lethargy – provoked by the use of sleep-inducing ointments or by a catalepsis of an unkown nature – was sought after as the ideal way to reach the mysterious and otherwise unattainable world of the dead, of those spirits that wandered over the face of the earth without hope of peace'. In my opinion it is here that we should seek the underlying unity of the myth of the *benandanti,* looking beyond the agrarian and the funeral versions. The sorcerers who are enemies of the fertility of the fields reflect the ancient notion of the unappeased dead; the processions of the dead are already a partially Christian image, similar to that of the souls in Purgatory. In either case the *benandanti,* men or women, appear as professional intermediaries between the community and the realm of the dead. My conclusion was that:

> Such phenomena as trances, journeys into the beyond astride animals
> or in the form of animals . . . to recover seed grain or to assure the
> fertility of the land, and . . . participation in processions of the dead
> (which procured prophetic and visionary powers for the *benandanti*) form
> a coherent pattern which immediately evokes the rites of the shamans.[4]

When writing the above words I confined myself to suggesting, without elabo-
rating, the analogy between *benandanti* and shamans: the distance between Friuli
and Siberia seemed altogether too great. But I now believe that the disconcerting
heterogeneity of culture, space and time between these realities can be offset, by
morphological research, the results of which may in the future serve as a guide to
historical reconstruction.

Wittgenstein, when proposing the idea of 'perspicious presentation' as an alternative to Frazer's genetic explanations, emphasized the need to find 'intermediate
links'.[5] In our case this implies the adoption of a firmly comparativist point of view.
As regards the 'funeral' *benandanti* who, in a dream, witness the processions of the
dead, two similarities or connections immediately suggest themselves. Firstly, with
evidence concerning the myth of the 'furious horde' or 'wild hunt', or the spirits
of the dead, usually conducted by a male deity such as Herlechinus, Odin, Herod,
or Arthur. Secondly, with stories (especially the famous *Canon episcopia*) of women
dreaming of flying by night, mounted on animals, in the train of Diana, or other
female divinities (Holda, Perchta, Herodias, etc.). All this adds up to a fairly substantial dossier, essentially Franco-German, but with an important extension to the Po
valley. Originally the material I was able to collect on the theme of battles for
fertility was meagre and more dispersed. As a parallel to the *benandanti* I was able
to find only the Dalmatian *kersniki* and the case, which appears to be exceptional,
of an old werewolf brought to justice in Livonia at the end of the seventeenth
century. But the second dossier expands in its turn to include a number of characters well-rooted in European folklore: the Balkan *zduhaéi*, the Hungarian *táltos*,
the Corsican *mazzeri*, the Ossetian *burkudzàutà*, Baltic werewolves, shamans of
Lapland *(noai'di)* and of Siberia.[6] What is the common feature of these beings (who
are deliberately mentioned here in no particular order)?

To begin with, they are certainly intermediaries between the world of the
living and that of the dead, to which they are given access in an ecstatic trance.
But an answer of this kind may be misleading, especially in view of the inclusion
of shamans in this variegated list. It might be thought that the connecting link
between all these figures is purely (and generically) a typological one: after all,
mediators between this world and the next, or 'shamans' in the vague sense, have
been found in the most various cultures. The resemblance that I have pointed out,
on the other hand, is a specific one, as is the reference to the shamans of Eurasia
– which, it may be remarked, has already been proposed for several of these figures,
in particular the *táltos*.[7] It is a resemblance which does not even exclude real and
precise superpositions, but it is not based on them. For instance, the fact that in
Friuli individuals born with a caul were regarded as future *benandanti,* and that
among the Yurak Samoyeds of Siberia they are regarded as future shamans, might
be interpreted as a superficial coincidence. But it takes on its full value within a
profound isomorphism embracing phenomena scattered over a huge geographical

area, of which we have information dating from remote antiquity (Herodotus already mentions belief in werewolves among the Neuri).

We cannot here go into the detail of this isomorphism, but it will suffice for the moment to point out that the existence of a deep-seated connection makes it possible to consider variants that are apparently diverse. Thus persons who are destined to undertake the ecstatic voyage are those born with some physical peculiarity (with a caul, like the *benandanti,* or with teeth, like the *táltos*), or at a particular time of year (the twelve days during which the dead were thought most likely to roam); or again, persons who have passed certain initiatory tests. They usually make the journey riding on animals or in animal form, but also sometimes on broomsticks (of course), or other modes of conveyance such as ears of corn, benches, or stools (among the Ossetes, or at Mirandola near Modena). During their ecstasy they fight against beings with diverse names (nearly always sorcerers or spirits of the dead) for various purposes: to ensure a good harvest, to conquer disease, or to scan the future. Their powers are known to their fellow humans, but except in the case of the shamans the ecstatic journey is made in private rather than in public.

These distinctive traits form a mythic combination that is clearly recognizable. We can discern fragments of it in trials for witchcraft, even at a late date, when we encounter what appear to be extravagant details alien to the demonological stereotypes – as when a Scottish witch in 1662 speaks of flying to the sabbat mounted on a straw or a beanstalk.[8] Conversely, even in fairly early evidence, we can perceive, grafted on to the substratum of popular belief, elements belonging to the stereotype of the sabbat: the presence of the Devil, the profanation of the Sacraments, or the negative transformation of beneficent or neutral figures such as werewolves. It is indeed clear that in this field the absolute dating of the sources (penitentials, annals, trials, etc.) is not necessarily identical with the relative dating of the phenomena they mention or describe. The consequences for research are evident. Chronology (one of the eyes of history, to use an antique metaphor) proves to be more or less unusable; so we must have recourse to the other eye, geography, reinforced by morphology. In other words, as far as this mythical, pre-sabbat level is concerned, historical research must endeavour to place in a temporal sequence the spatial dispersion of data, having first collated them according to morphological affinity.

Given a mythical complex that has left traces from Scotland to the Caucasus and from the Mediterranean to Siberia, any attempt at interpretation seems extremely hazardous. We may begin by citing the alternatives that are theoretically possible. The analogies that exist may be attributed (1) to chance; (2) to the necessity imposed by mental structures common to the human species; (3) to diffusion; or (4) to a common genetic source. Hypothesis (1) can be ruled out: the convergences are too many and too complex to be put down to chance. I would also firmly exclude hypothesis (2), in all its possible formulations. 'Mental structures' may be taken as meaning either psychological archetypes or dispositions of a formal character. But the mythical complex we are speaking of presents too many variants to be identified with supposed but unprovable archetypes, and too many specific coincidences to be identified in terms of a formal disposition. We are thus left with the third and fourth possibilities: diffusion or a common genetic source.

We may say at once that neither can be summarily dismissed. The theory of diffusion no doubt rests on linguistic parallelism, that is to say the fact of borrowings, in both directions, between Indo-European and non Indo-European languages. Such borrowing, either in the historical or the proto-historical period, might well have been accompanied by the transmission of mythical complexes such as that we are concerned with. The very close resemblance between Friulian *benandanti* and Ossetian *burkudzauta* is surprising in view of the geographical and cultural distance, even though both belong to the Indo-European language area. But the existence of Ossetian loan-words in Hungarian may suggest a chain extending from the Caucasus to Friuli and comprising similar morphology phenomena such as the Frulian *benandanti*, the Balkan *zduhaci,* the Hungarian *táltos,* and the Ossetian *burkudzauta.* On the basis of such reasoning and the valuable evidence provided by linguistic borrowings we might seek to link, one after the other, all the points on the globe that we have briefly mentioned, beginning with culturally contiguous areas such as Lapland and Siberia, Friuli and Dalmatian, and so on. It is not, of course, necessary to postulate a unique source of diffusion.

From all that is said above, it is clear that the diffusion hypothesis is based on numerous facts but an equally large number of conjectures. The alternative hypothesis of a common genetic source is certainly more economical, but involves a linguistic base that is evidently more conjectural. Linguists have long argued as to the possibility of proving, by a comparison between Indo-European and Uralian languages, the prior existence of an Indo-Uralian linguistic community, but this hypothesis has aroused much criticism and is far from being generally accepted. Even if it were proved, this would not be proof of the origin of the myths of shamanist inspiration, with regard to which we spoke of a cultural stratum antedating the differentiation of the languages of Eurasia, though such origin would then at least be historically plausible. Like all simple hypotheses this one is extremely attractive, but it is at present a hypothesis and no more.

The divergence between the two hypotheses relates only to the manner and time of the process of transmission, which, on the diffusion hypothesis, might have continued until relatively recent times. But whether we opt for diffusion or a common source, the origin of these myths must in all probability be referred to a very distant, proto-historic period. This antiquity seems to be confirmed by the fact that they coincide with the central core of the fairy-tale genre.

Vladimir Propp, at the end of his *Morphology of the Folktale* (1928), posed the question whether the unexpected discovery of an underlying structure common to all fairy-tales would imply that they derived from a single source. He commented that: 'The morphologist is not entitled to reply to this question. He must pass on his conclusions to the historian, or else become a historian himself.' Propp was to adopt the second course. But in the last pages of the *Morphology* he already anticipated the direction his research would take: the 'single source' of fairy-tales was not to he sought in a geographical or psychological domain, but in a central core of religious representations. He added a 'small example' of a parallel between fairy-tale and belief:

In the stories, Ivan [i.e., the hero] is transported through the air by three fundamental types of mount or vehicle: a flying horse, a bird, or a flying ship. But these are precisely the same as those which carry the souls of the dead – the horse being the usual with herdsmen and farmers, the eagle with hunters, and the ship with dwellers of the sea-coasts.

This in fact was neither a small example nor a random one, for, very soon afterwards, Propp was to formulate – though still necessarily in a conjectural manner – the central thesis of his work on *The Historical Roots of the Fairy-Tale* (1946): 'It may thus be accepted that one of the primary elements in fairy-tales, that of a miraculous voyage, is a reflection of the religious concept of souls travelling to the next world'.[9]

The fundamental historical nucleus of the structure found in fairy-tales is to be sought here. But in the *Morphology* Propp discovers that this structure implies the presence of two functions that are almost always mutually exclusive: (1) the fight with an antagonist and the victory over him; (2) the difficult task and its accomplishment. In the few cases where both are present, (1) always precedes (2). Hence a further hypothesis: 'It is very possible that historically both types existed, that each had its own history, and that in a distant past two traditions met and fused together'.[10] In *Roots*, however, Propp dwells almost exclusively on the relation between fairy-tales and initiation rites (function (2)). The research on the sabbat, the conclusions of which are summarized here, also throws light on the mythic-religious core of the past (battles fought in a state of trance against the souls of the dead) elaborated in function (1). More generally, this research illustrates the decisive importance, traceable over a very large cultural area, of the image of the traveller, male or female, in a trance in the world of the dead, in relation to the genesis and transmission of the narrative structure – perhaps more ancient and certainly more durable – elaborated by the human species. All this makes it possible to supplement with strictly historical data the too rigorously evolutionist typology indicated by Propp in *Roots*. But the tribute paid by Propp to the then dominant Stalinist orthodoxy does not detract from the genius of his luminous work, indissolubly linked with the *Morphology* written twenty years earlier in the atmosphere of formalist research. The link between morphology and history that Propp specifically proposes in these two works is an example of incalculable fruitfulness.

Thus the stereotype of the sabbat represents a fusion of two distinct images. The first, a product of the learned culture (judges, inquisitors, demonologists), centred on the supposed existence of a hostile sect, inspired by the Devil, members of which had to renounce their faith and profane the Cross and sacraments. The second image, rooted in folk-culture, was based on belief in the extraordinary powers of particular men and women who – in a state of trance, and often in animal form or riding upon animals – travelled to the realm of the dead in order to bring prosperity to the community. As we have seen, this second image was much older than the first, and infinitely more widespread. Both took shape in the Western Alps shortly after 1350. It is very possible that the convergence between these widely different cultural complexes was facilitated by the presence of heretical Vaudois (Waldensian) groups in the same area at the same time. The original doctrines of these groups had long been mingled with local folk traditions and dualistic beliefs of the Catharist type from East Central Europe, which lent themselves to being interpreted as Devil-worship. The intervention of inquisitors brought all these scattered elements to the point of fusion, and so the sabbat myth was born.

After fusion, diffusion. Besides inquisitors, judges, and demonologists, the process was aided by preachers, especially S. Bernardino da Siena. The latter's sermons on 'enchantment, witches and spells' at first met with incredulity in Rome: as he said later on, 'my words made them think I was dreaming'. But trials and burnings of witches were to follow without delay. The records of the Roman trials have not survived; but the trial of Matteuccia di Francesco at Todi in 1428, two years after S. Bernardino's sermons in that town, shows clearly how the idea of the sabbat, which had already crystallized despite its novelty, had merged with an old system of magic beliefs. After a long enumeration of curative and amatory spells, Matteuccia confessed that she had turned herself into a fly by means of an ointment made from the blood of newborn infants, and had been carried to the walnut-tree at Benevento by a demon in the form of a he-goat.

Probably the Todi magistrates had obtained, by violence and pressure, a full confirmation of what S. Bernardino's preaching led them to expect. He himself, as he tells us, gained his information from other Franciscans who had been at work in Piedmont: this explains how the idea of the sabbat developed simultaneously in the Western Alps and at Todi.

For the next two and a half centuries the trails for sorcery that took place all over Europe were full of confessions similar to that of Matteuccia and basically stereotyped, though often embellished with details from local tradition. But it must not be thought that the sabbat idea developed with the same rapidity everywhere. At the end of the fifteenth century, the author of the famous *Malleus Maleficarum* had no more to relate on the subject of diabolical assemblies than what Nider had learnt from his informants at Evian and Berne: they were, that is to say, unable to add anything to a dossier already fifty years old. At the end of the sixteenth century, resistance to the inquisitors' pressure by the *benandanti* shows that the image of the sabbat which had come into existence about two centuries earlier at the other extremity of the Alpine chain has still not made its mark on Friulian folklore. In general the European geography of the diffusion of the sabbat idea is extremely variable, with many gaps and time-differences: among the former we may notice (save for a few exceptions) the case of England.

We have seen that the stereotype of the sabbat included elements, such as flight through the air and the assumption of animal form, which, although re-elaborated in a symbolic context different from the original one, clearly originate from a stratum of folk-culture. In some cases the modification to which they are subjected is very slight or completely absent, so that we may discern more or less extensive fragments of this stratum, otherwise totally covered.

The conclusions summarized here relate only to the composite mythical structure which can be discerned in descriptions of the sabbat. I am of course well aware that my capacity, linguistic and otherwise, is inadequate to the extent and complexity of the subject-matter. But the chronological and geographical diffusion of accounts of the sabbat, and their stereotypical character, poses questions which one can only attempt to answer by means of global interpretation. One must sometimes take one's eyes off the trees in order to view the forest.

Notes

1   See Chapter 2 in this collection for Cohn's argument.
2   Malcolm Barber, 'The Plot to Overthrow Christendom in 1321', *History* 66 (1981), 1–17.
3   Norman Cohn rejects the statement by Bernado da Como, overlooking the fact that it agrees with Nider's indications. Cohn, *Europe's Inner Demons* (London 1975), 145.
4   Carlo Ginzburg, *The Night Battles: Witchcraft and Agrarian Cults in the Sixteenth and Seventeenth Centuries* (London 1983), 59 and 32.
5   Ludwig Wittgenstein, *Remarks on Frazer's Golden Bough* (London 1979), 9.
6   On *zduhaci* and *táltoso*, see Gábor Klaniczay, *The Uses of Supernatural Power*, trans. Susan Singerman (Princeton, NJ 1990), ch. 8. On werewolves, see Maia Madar, 'Estonia: Werewolves and Poisoners', in Bengt Ankarloo and Gustav Henningsen, eds, *Early Modern European Witchcraft: Centres and Peripheries* (Clarendon, Oxford 1990), ch. 9.
7   The author's hypothesis on the relation between *benandanti* and shamans was subsequently supported by Mircea Ehiade, 'Some Observations on European Witchcraft', *History of Religions,* 14 (1975), 149–72, esp. 153–8.
8   Robert Pitcairn, *Ancient Criminal Trials in Scotland* (Edinburgh 1833), vol. 3, II, 603–4 ('Confessions of Issobell Gowdie').
9   Vladimir Propp, *Morphologie du conte* (Paris 1970), 178 ff.
10   Ibid., 173.

Chapter 9

Éva Pócs

THE ALTERNATIVE WORLD OF
THE WITCHES' SABBAT

Journeys

IN THE HUNGARIAN WITCH TRIAL NARRATIVES that concern
visions, the terms 'enchantment' and 'abduction' have a range of meanings. In
their primary senses they refer to an altered state of consciousness in which the
supernatural is perceived, apparitions are experienced, and occasionally a journey
is made to the alternative world. Bewitched individuals lived through experiences
such as demonic witches entering houses and holding their merriments there,
injuring their victims, or taking them to the witches' sabbat.

The enchanted person lying in trance may be observed by others, at the same
time that both the injured party and the witches can travel on soul journeys. In the
account of a 1747 witch trial in Kiskunhalas, Anna Hos reported seeing her husband
in bed,

> lying there stiff, barely drawing breath, and she called to her husband
> 'what happened to you, are you asleep?' For a long while she and her
> stepdaughter tried to awaken him . . . and after a long time he awoke
> and cried out, 'My Lord Jesus help me! Fiery witches took me to
> Maramaros, and they put six hundredweight of salt on me'.[1]

The narratives of witches' confessions were strongly influenced by the expectations
of the court: witches had to confess to 'witches' companies' or even to a pact with
the Devil, which obviously meant that their testimonies included the traditional
demonological witches' sabbat doctrines along with any relevant personal experiences.

We can presume that, through the medium of sermons, the literature of visions
substantially influenced local traditions concerning witnesses and the accused, and
the visual experience of church frescoes also probably played a role. It is possible
to trace Christian visionary imagery of heaven and hell in several themes in the

terrestrial otherworlds of witches. While visionary literature lent Christian motifs of the otherworld to narratives on the witches' sabbat, witch-hunting demonology gained its place and influence over the participants in the trials through the court's questions to the accused. This mainly had the effect of making experiences tangible, rational, and 'terrestrial'. All this is because the alternative of experience, a 'real' adventure in the otherworld or a narrative, was always present for the people at the trial, whereas looking at it through the eyes of the court, one form of witches' sabbat alone was what certainly existed: an authentic terrestrial gathering of heretic God deniers who actually and physically participated. If they flew, it was accomplished with the help of the Devil, but they flew in a physical sense. The other demonological alternative was that the adventure of the witches' sabbat was nothing other than devilish illusion.

Scenes

According to hundreds of Hungarian witness accounts, one of the common scenes of witches' sabbats and merriments was in the house or yard of the injured party, where the bewitched was compelled to take part in the merriments of the witches. On other occasions the victims were transported farther away – they were dragged or carried – but only in a few instances were they taken beyond the borders of the village. 'Carrying' is a particular form of abduction and a term that appears frequently in the trials. It refers to a rapid horizontal flight by the abducted to actual terrestrial sites, such as 'Laposdomb' (Flat Hill), 'the stove of Janos Vas', 'Antal's pear tree' and so on. This flight in pairs does not constitute the real witches' sabbat, but its essence is the same. The abducted party arrives in an alternative world with the witches; the narratives also refer to a parallel world existing in terrestrial scenes. References to breaking away from earth are often attached to narratives about more 'realistic' carrying; for example (from Otomany, Bihar County 1735), 'her feet could not touch the ground'; and 'she walked on the tree tops'. Another example, from Kisvarda, Szabolcs County, speaks of rapid horizontal flight: 'with a speed like the winds she was rushing down the road . . . Mrs Mihaly Sandor passed her at speed on a brownish horse'.

The scenes of group witches' sabbats, if not in or around the house of the injured party, mostly occurred on a hillock, a hill, or a mountain top. Presumably this is no accident, given that these are the symbols of the universal 'sacred center of the earth'. Specified hills, such as Gellért and Tokaj, as well as unnamed surrounding hillocks were commonly mentioned examples. Going to Gellért Hill would probably have been a legendary topos in those days; even in Hungary's Modern Age legends, it is the most frequent scene of the witches' merriments. Every kind of landscape surrounding the village was represented: vineyards, meadows, gardens, forests, fields, valleys, and waters. References to cities and palaces are striking among village scenes. It is not out of the question that the 'vast, monstrous cities and vaulting arches', the 'palaces and churches' relate to the heavenly city of Christian visions through a series of linked stages of transmission.[2]

In the eyes of the interrogator, who knew nothing about 'soul trips', witches could not possibly fly except with the help of the Devil. Therefore, admitting to flying constituted an admission of witchcraft and indirectly indicated participation in the witches' sabbat. So it was not accidental that, in Hungarian trial minutes as elsewhere, a question about flying followed an accusation of witchcraft: 'Did you fly about the rooftops?' was the question to a witch from Feketeardo in 1732.

Transformations

Those who were abducted became demons themselves, like their abductors. This is true of Hungarian demonic night witches too. In one descriptive example, Mrs Marton Viragos, a witch from Bihar County, spoke to the women of the village about 'whether [her illness] was caused by a human' – that is, whether or not it was *maleficium*. One of the women told her, 'You bumped your head into the roof beams when you were a fairy', meaning that she had become ill when she was a fairy, and she was a fairy when the fairies visiting her house had enchanted her to dance (and caused her to bump her head against the roof beams).

The record of the 1747 trial of Mrs Andras Gulyas, in Kassa, contains unique elements that suggest a probable visionary experience. Appearing in the text are spirit horses, victims who are turned into horses, and witches that saddled them, as well as a rather ghoulish company of riding witches. The other world is signi-fied by the symbolism of encircling or losing one's way, and on another level there is a reference to the abducted victim's trance state. Mrs Gulyas enters the house in the night, the witch from Göncz

> saying 'Do you know what I asked from you? You dog! Come here, dog!' With this she threw the bridle over her head and turned her into a horse there and then. Leaving the place with a mighty noise, she tied her to the door post . . . then she mounted the horse, and by which time there were three waiting outside in front of the gate on black horses . . . thus they went to Szina. A black horse in fancy decoration preceded them everywhere, [and] it was glittering with light.

Then later the witch

> just threw the bridle over her neck, [and] sat on the back of the fatens [the victim]. Going toward the fields of Rosál the fatens saw a powerful steed and with grand preparations it glittered with light. Following this steed while they were going to the fields of Rosál, the fatens still had her senses, but after that where the fatens was carried she did not know. Only as she finally came home to town did she come round once more, [as] Mrs. Gulyas made the fatens circle her own house three times.

A totally different way of traveling to the witches' sabbat was to fly on magical objects. The basis for this motif of legends was the demonological idea of 'satanic help'. The topoi of the literature of magic, as well as motifs from tales that referred to magical objects, magical spells, and magical transformations, constituted a rich source of ideas for such help. Flying on objects created through illusion was a recurring motif of court narratives. Witches claimed (although mostly in confessions following torture) to have traveled on carpets with the help of the wind, a cannonball, or carts that rose into the air through magic, as in Erzsébet Hampa's 1737 trial in Sumeg:

> The six horses mentioned previously were naught but cats in truth, two black cats belonging to Ilona . . . the carriage was only a sieve and a bolter sieve thrown to the air, which were put together like wheels and were started with a whiplash . . . they traveled like the wind.

Societies

The figure of the Devil, particularly in the making of pacts, appeared only occasionally in narratives about witches' merriments or witches' sabbats. What was an indispensable part of the narratives was being together as a group, the actual society of witches. We can read about the society of witches in contexts at different levels, from narratives on experiences of death troops to confessions following torture where guilty partners were enumerated. We know that participation in the sabbat was a key focus of interrogation, in order to expose the assumed conspiracy. The company of witches, like other features of the witches' sabbat, was not invented by demonologists to serve the aims of interrogation. This society, just like the Devil making a pact, had a popular basis. In the first century of the hunts there was no mention of the Devil at all in the narratives about the witches' sabbat. Apparently, the conspiring society of witches organized by devils did not exist then, not even in the minds of Hungarian judges. It seems probable that the peasant witnesses conceptualized only one type of company: the gathering of the dead with supernatural witches and their demonic relatives, fairies, and werewolves.

The ghoulish nature of these troops can often be traced to witches' sabbats: these witches are 'the evils', 'the evil souls', or children with fiery eyes in 'the troop'. What was really connected to the dead was the troop's black or white flag, which grew to extraordinary supernatural proportions at night. That was a repetitive motif: witches came to the house at night carrying a flag, and as the 'troop of the dead' they called their victims to them with flags. The troop flags disappeared upon the dispersal of the group, but they were of great size and are described as 'very beautiful and shiny' or 'scarlet silk with golden dots', and as being made of silk, gold, copper, or embroidery.

Like other accessories of the witches' sabbat, the flag may be understood through the eyes of the interrogators and the words of the tortured confessors as magical objects created through illusion. One, for example, 'reached from the Hill of Tokaj as far as the River Tisza when it was unraveled'. The flag is an emphatic object rich in meaning, the positive symbol of the alternative world with its simultaneous connotation of death and heaven. The latter examples suggest that it had some connection with the fairylike 'heavenly' joys of the otherworld. Its parallels were the flags of southeastern European fairy troops, or the heavenly flags of religious visions.

Fairy merriments

Witches with fairy attributes are mentioned several times in the trial records. They brought glittering beauty to the houses in which they appeared, and they abducted their victims into their companies and their fairylike witches' sabbats by making music and dancing. Negative witch characteristics are totally absent from some of these source narratives, which depict an alternative world full of beauty and joy that contrasts with the miseries of the terrestrial world. So, fairylike witches' sabbats also belong in the world of desire. One account from Hodmezövasarhely in 1739 reports, 'in the group they all seemed of beautiful and gentle colors, and even if they are in rags at home, there their clothes are all of straight beauty'.

The most important motif of the fairy sabbats was the merriment with dance. Around sixty narratives concerning fairy merriments emerged from Hungarian trials across the country (excluding Transylvania), where, as in Romania, it was the witches with a werewolf or unbaptized demonic character who attended sabbats. The heart of fairy merriments was the feast, and the stories about it refer to cooking and baking, food and beverages, cooks and servants. At times we are witness to a wonderful range of dishes and drinks: from ten seeds of millet they feed 'the entire company' as guests, or three thousand of them drink from a single drilled vine root. The mythological topos of magic food from antiquity and the Middle Ages was often broadened with the motif of the magically timed harvest (for example, wheat harvested before Pentecost or grapes harvested at Christmas time). These themes are known from the elite literature of magic, as well as from village crop magic. The accessories of a fairylike witch feast were golden and decorative, as in southeast European or Celtic fairy heavens. According to confessions made in a 1728 trial in Komarom, the company of Mrs Mihaly Olah enjoyed themselves with silver and golden glasses while they traveled over water on a bolter sieve. On another occasion, 'they comforted [the injured party] with an extraordinarily sumptuous feast'.

This fairy world of desire realized in dreams and apparitions was characteristic of the fairy beliefs of the central southeastern Europeans – it also has close parallels in the Celtic, Italian, and Scandinavian regions – and it lent particular fairy attributes to the witches' sabbat in many areas. Something fairylike is always closely linked with the archaic and demonic witches' world of the dead – so much so that at times the shiny, heavenly features are missing from the image of the feast, and a 'black' fairy world of the dead appears before us. The following example concerns a 'black' troop of fairies with whom, however, it was possible to have a good time. From Mrs Gyorgy Gemes's 1739 trial in Hodmezövasarhely, we learn that her husband, when she fell ill, asked that she 'take me in that black troop, how long is it since I was there? . . . my dear dove, it is an age since I drank from that good old wine of Tokaj, that we drank in the black troop, give me a glass of that'.

The underworld and hell

Demonologists imagined the feast of the desired world to be a dinner in hell with lizards, snakes, and frogs, as the French demonologist Pierre De Lancre described the end of an illusory feast. In narratives about witches' sabbats, the glittering table became 'a tussock in the meadows', the golden glass turned into a shinbone, and the girl who had been taken to dance was transformed into a boat. These are motifs from legends about witches and fairies known throughout the region. They are presumed to have been very popular in the early modern age, and have had their enduring formulation in legends dated as early as the trial documents.

Hell appeared in narratives about witches' sabbats as a consequence of these processes – for example, in the demonological context of the illusory feasts of plenty, if the fairy banquet had an infernal ending. On the other hand, there was also a 'popular' hell present in the texts, which was on earth (as were all the other worlds of the witches), and only certain symbols of hell referred to its connection to the underworld or the Devil. From these symbols the most frequently occurring were the scenes of the feasts: mill, cellar, wine cellar, pub, stable, pigpen, oven, or cauldron. These symbolic terrestrial hells are known mainly from the narratives that refer to the hellish merriment of the Balkan and central European underworld demons. Presumably they entered the narratives about witches' sabbats through those demons. Chimneys and chimney flues also represent hell; witches of the underworld used them as a passageway to reach the sabbat.

Certain food types could also signal the satanic, infernal nature of the feasts. Examples are the stone bread and stone pears that witches ate at their merriment in wine cellars. Animal bones, stones, and animal or human excrement, which appeared as the transformed food and trappings of illusory feasts, are the antithesis of the appetizing dishes of golden banquets. Repugnant actions occurring in the context of witches' sabbats could also denote the underworld or the Devil: for example, the serving of slurry or manure dinners, defecating into dishes, or urinating or vomiting into barrels at the end of feasts. A great number of the dishes possessed the character of the underworld, consisting of such things as water animals or creatures that slither and slide – that is, hellish animals and concoctions from visions and demonological literature. Examples include references to a 'sliding animal' and the 'inside of a snail' and to frogs and turtles.

The origins of the witches' sabbat

Tracing the origins of the witches' sabbat in all their complexity would be an impossible task. The few connections between the texts mentioned only hint at the linkages that interwove around Europe in the Middle Ages and the early modern age. However, the search for the foundations of the witches' sabbat in popular belief is more promising ground since these elementary images are astonishingly homogeneous throughout Europe. The sabbat was in essence a visionary experience, an 'alternative adventure'. Carlo Ginzburg, in tracing the origins of images of European witches' sabbats, came to the conclusion that the ancient European basis of these was the journey to the realm of the dead.[3] His findings were confirmed by our detailed research in central and eastern Europe, as well as by Gustav Henningsen with his research on fairy cults in Sicily (1990), and later by Wolfgang Behringer in his book about the Stoeckhlin fairy magicians (1994). Visions of the dead and witches (Ginzburg did not emphasize the latter, since he focused on the precursors) offered the common European fundaments of images of the witches' sabbat. The most important basis for these was European belief in doubles, *mora*, and werewolves. All of this of course refers to the undemonologized popular witches' sabbat. That can be much more clearly understood from the eastern and central European documentation than elsewhere in Europe because in this region theological doctrines did not overshadow that sabbat to such a great extent, and consequently the doctrines are easier to peel away from the 'original' images, as mentioned earlier. I think that the references here constitute enough evidence to assert that the following phenomena, among the general European elements of the sabbat, had a strong 'predemonologic' foundation in this region: flying, turning into an animal, gathering of the dead and demons, and the sabbat itself as a trance and dream experience.

Notes

1   For full citations of the sources used in this Chapter, see the original version in Éva Pócs, *Between the Living and the Dead* (Central European University Press, Budapest 1999), ch 5.
2   See Colleen McDannell and Bernhard Lang, *Heaven: A History* (New Haven, Conn. and London 1988), 69, 89.
3   For Carlo Ginzburg's argument, see Chapter 8 in this collection.

Chapter 10

Robert Muchembled

SATANIC MYTHS AND CULTURAL REALITIES

WITCH-HUNTING IS A LITURGY OF FEAR. It spreads obses-
sions that are essentially those of the learned, but which inspire real dread
and anxiety among the peasant masses. Holding up to the latter a mirror of satanism
and sorcery, magistrates and demonologists exacerbate the social rifts innate in rural
society by conferring on them a cultural, moral, and religious justification. Every
villager can recognize his own beliefs and practices, real enough to him, but diabolical in the eyes of his betters; each man must then decide in what fashion to present
his own image. The intensity and continuity of persecutions depend on the good
pleasure of those in authority, but also on the receptivity of some peasants to the
message offered them. It is thus possible to define communities that are 'open' or
'closed' to persecution, and more generally to propose an overall explanatory
model, valid for several European countries in the sixteenth and seventeenth
centuries. Is not witch-hunting, despite its spectacular appearance, simply an
episode in the conquest of the West European countryside by the forces of law and
order? In other words, is it not the universal story of the advance of public authority
against particularism, against the rural custom of settling disputes between man and
man with the least possible recourse to outside tribunals? In this way the myth of
diabolism opens the way to a sociology of authority.

Satanic myths and genuine fears

In my opinion the sabbat – a nocturnal, demoniac meeting of witches and warlocks
– is simply and solely a figment created by theologians, whose ideas governed the
imagination of the elite classes of Europe in the late Middle Ages. Drawing on the
composite tradition of persecutions of the Jews, the early Christians, and various
heretical sects – as Norman Cohn has brilliantly described[1] – the theologians revived
stereotypes that had no popular basis, in order to demonstrate the existence and
progress of a huge satanic plot designed to make the powers of evil triumph upon

earth. Such ideas unquestionably reflected the disarray of authority and especially of churchmen, confronted with the fissures that portended the disruption of Christian unity in the sixteenth century. Persecutors and heirs of the Inquisition, the new fraternity of demonologists imagined that they were themselves persecuted, that the world was given up to diabolism, and that secret Devil-worshippers were plotting to frustrate their purposes. Their imaginary sabbat was a reversal of the Christian liturgy, a copy of the Mass in which each separate feature was given a negative coefficient – a dark, morbid parody of the original.[2]

However, this construction of the mind did not become fully effective until later, more especially in states strongly influenced by the Tridentine Counter-Reformation such as the Spanish Netherlands. There, witch-hunting became most intense and widespread between 1590 and 1620 as a result of princely edicts issued in 1592 and 1606, which let loose a fearsome campaign of repression by courts composed of laymen.

It does not seem necessary in this chapter to repeat the arguments that I have developed at length elsewhere.[3] The main point to bear in mind is that the sabbat is an alien notion to the peasant actors in these dramas. The witnesses who depose against women accused of witchcraft never mention it. The accused themselves do so only in confessions extracted by torture and generally dictated by very precise questions from their judges, who supply the necessary demonological details as the basis for a verdict on the standard model. As we know, these include a record of initiation, symbolized by a bodily mark insensible to pain and confirmed by copulation with the demon; then comes a description of the Sabbat and a list of the wrongs and wicked actions committed by the accused in everyday life with the aid of the powders and unguents furnished during the nocturnal ceremony.

The fact that satanism is a direct product of demonology and of the judicial practice based upon it is confirmed by the experience of certain countries where, exceptionally, the procedure in trials for witchcraft does not centre on proof of dealings with the Devil. This applies to England, or to Denmark as described by J. C. V. Johansen.[4]

This being so, few authors at the present day maintain that the sabbat was a reality in any shape or form. Some indeed, like Pierre Chaunu in France, still believe in the Devil and in diabolic agency, and consequently still defend a hypothesis that has never been proved by concrete evidence. Others see the sabbat as containing an element of folk culture. But lest they be charged with seeking to revive Margaret Murray's unacceptable theory of the cult practised by European witches, these authors are either obliged, like Mircea Eliade, to speak of imaginary orgiastic practices reflecting the longed-for return to an ancient phase of culture, or else, like Carlo Ginzburg they postulate the existence of a ritual based on a highly composite mythical structure inferred from various descriptions of the sabbath.[5] This latter procedure is the most subtle, but is methodologically flawed, depending as it does on arbitrary associations, with no reference to chronology or, above all, to the social structure of the groups who are supposed to preserve this ritual in the myths of which they inform the judges. When the history of ideas is studied in this completely abstract fashion there is a grave risk that the investigator will describe his own mental processes rather than the subject of his research, by imposing an arbitrary significance on his collection of brief, out-of-context citations, thus in effect applying the structuralist method to his own unconscious. Taking into account, moreover, the number of exceptions, from Holland to Denmark and England, would it not be much better to fasten on a genuine stratum of folklore – the procession of the dead, for instance – in the two latter countries, where the culture of the learned has not succeeded in complicating the problem for us by imposing the concept of the demonic sabbat? In Denmark it is easy to identify popular beliefs, or such as represent a recombining of learned culture and that of the masses, for example, the belief in wizards entering a church by the keyhole. It is all the more striking that there is no mention whatever of a ritual form comparable to the Sabbat. But, basically, Carlo Ginzburg's reduction of the nocturnal assembly to certain structures leads him to describe universal human practices, including the cult of the dead, without regard to their essential feature, the cultural forms specific to a particular group at a particular time.

Any myth, in fact, is subject to precise sociological forms and does not exist as a mere category of the mind. This is true of the sabbat myth, which creates realities and chains of events which may affect its own consequences. Being a liturgy of fear it leads, domino fashion, to a multiplicity of trials: a witch denounces her fellow-participants in the alleged sabbat, and one after another is burnt at the stake.[6] But more important than this, a wave of fear spreads throughout the countryside, arousing feelings of dread and even panic, with consequences of two kinds: an exterminating fury against witches, expressed within the bounds of law, and an upsurge of social antagonism, brutality, and private vengeance, directed especially against supposed witches, but also against other persons.

The repressive mania can in this way take hold of an entire region. On 7 July 1612 the lieutenant of the castellany of Bouchain in Hainaut wrote to the Privy Council of the Archduke and Archduchess of the Netherlands that

> this district is strangely infected by persons abandoned and enthralled
> to the Devil, of all ages and of either sex, so that in the past two years
> I have convicted more than eighty in this town and in six villages, besides
> many suspect and banished and fourteen others now prisoners.

One suspect, a woman, had entered a plea for pardon: the castellan advised the Privy Council, the supreme court in such matters, not to grant it, 'to prevent indignation and disturbances among the populace, which is much incensed against persons of this kind'.[7]

The lieutenant's statement is borne out by the financial accounts of the viceregal domain. Trials for witchcraft were rare in the castellany of Bouchain before the end of the sixteenth century, when they were instituted under a royal ordinance of 1592. There was a lull from 1601 to 1608, despite a second edict against sorcery in 1606. A suspect was tried in 1608, and a married couple in 1609. Then came a dramatic increase: 22 cases in 1610, 59 in 1611, 22 in 1612, 21 in 1613, 12 in 1614, and 15 in 1615. A return to moderation followed: 12 trials between 1616 and 1619 (8 of which were in 1617), only 1 between 1620 and 1647, and 8 more between 1648 and 1652. The 175 who stood trial between 1608 and 1652 consisted of 123 women, 18 men, and 34 children.

Thus the castellan's figures of 1612 were correct. He was himself responsible for the wave of persecutions, having applied the edict of 1606 in all its rigour, which ensured that those denounced by the first culprits were brought to book in their turn. But such epidemics of persecution only reach their full extent thanks to a veritable phobia taking hold of the population of a region thought to be contaminated, so that the inhabitants come forward in huge numbers to testify against local sorcerers. The trials in the castellany were confined to two towns, Bouchain and Denain, and six villages. We have a record of their sequence: Rieuz and Lieu-Saint-Armand began in 1610 with 15 accused; then Bouchain with 43 cases in 1611, and Lieu-Saint-Amand with 20 more in 1612. Neuville-sur-Escaut had 6 cases in 1613, Fechain 15 in 1615, and Villers-en-Cauchie 8 in 1617.

The sentences were as severe as was commonly the case for witchcraft: 45 per cent of the accused were executed, one acquitted, the rest banished for refusing to confess or because they had no fixed abode, or put 'in care' if they were too young to he executed. Out of thirty-four children tried between 1611 and 1619, thirteen were put to death regardless of age: this was before the edict of 30 July 1612, which laid down that boys under 14 and girls under 12 should be imprisoned until puberty. This was done in the case of twelve children, three of whom were subsequently executed. Thus Anne Hauldecoeur was kept in confinement from 1 September 1614 to 11 July 1619, on which day she was put to death, having been barely 7 years old when first imprisoned!

Like their elders, the child sorcerers and sorceresses of Bouchain fell victim to the convergence of three phenomena. Firstly, anti-sabbat legislation; secondly, the zeal of a minor functionary of the Crown – the castellany being the lowest in the hierarchy of princely courts; thirdly, the demand for purification expressed by the communities themselves and directed even against children of tender age, who were merely sons and daughters of those accused of witchcraft.

A comparison with Artois, the province bordering on Bouchaimi and Hainaut, shows even more clearly how this conjunction of forces accounted for the witch-hunting frenzy. In the very large governorship of Arras, which comprised hundreds of villages and belonged to the same state as Bouchiain, the same edicts at the same period produced only a few dozen prosecutions. Only one example of a spread of the epidemic type can be discerned: this was in the castellany of Oisy-le-Verger, at the eastern extremity of the governorship and in the immediate vicinity of Bouchain. This conspicuous variation is clearly due to a certain moderation on the part of the Artois judges, and also to a slate of mind amongst the population such that the sabbat bogy failed to arouse reactions of panic fear and widespread denunciations of witches. We do not find in Artois the equivalent of documents signed by 'the sounder part of the people' of certain villages in Cambrésis and Hainaut, calling for local witches to be prosecuted, and even offering to help pay the legal costs.[8]

In my opinion, the acceptance or rejection by local communities of the myth of satanism put about by the authorities was the decisive factor accounting for the success or failure of repressive measures. The Danish ordinance of 1617 directed that accomplices of the Devil should be put to death and that ordinary practitioners of witchcraft should be exiled. Over 300 trials took place in Jutland from 1617 to 1625, but the bulk of them fell under the second heading, as though the first related to a foreign ideology. On the other hand, the Norwegian decree of 1593 was applied in a manner reminiscent of the Netherlands and other Continental states.[9] In Sweden, the repression in the late 1660s is to be explained by the propagation of the Continental model among the educated middle class and by 'immense pressure on the part of the lower class, an almost unanimous demand for extensive legal action against witches'.[10]

This attitude, however, of appealing to the law for protection against the dangers it has itself conjured up, is not the only possible reaction. Many sought other remedies, more brutal and more traditional, against the witchcraft in their midst. The incessant burnings of witches and the propagation of rumours created an atmosphere of intense anxiety. There were even localised outbreaks of panic, such that children, at Bouchain or in Sweden, would inform against anyone at all; relatives would suspect one another, and neighbours still more so. The era of suspicion was born: it was aggravated, in the Spanish Netherlands for instance, by the authorities' willingness to reward those who denounced the perpetrators of grave crimes. As early as the reign of Charles V, those who informed against Protestants were promised a portion of their confiscated goods. Such practices continued on an increasing scale: police forces were thin on the ground, and rewards to informers were a means of giving some degree of efficacy to the judicial system.

Thus the siege mentality of the time was reinforced by the horrific deeds attributed to witches and warlocks. The official persecution that took place in several provinces of the Spanish Netherlands after 1606 was matched by a wave of private vengeance against the supposed votaries of Satan. A princely pardon, granted by a letter of remission, was a sign that the authorities were not over-scandalized by such behaviour. In 1607 the gatekeeper of a town in Luxembourg beat to death a woman who had been accused of witchcraft in a civil suit, but who had been acquitted. His act of violence was accounted for on the ground that he had spent all his money on the court case. On 15 October 1607 two brothers at Wissegem, a village in the Franc de Binges, murdered an innkeeper who had come to their house to demand the settlement of a debt. They pleaded that they had acted from desperation: they had lost three horses shortly before, and were firmly convinced that sorcery was at work. A fortune-teller in Bruges had told them that this was so, and that the guilty man (whom he did not name) lived near their village church and had a 'young, slender wife': the victim answered this description.

Both these incidents are indirectly related to the ordinance of 1606 against witchcraft, and also stem from deep-seated rural beliefs. The connection is still clearer in the case of Claude Ausseau, a farmer in a Hainaut village who was ruined in about 1607 by the mysterious death of all his cattle. Word had got about that a certain widow had been accused of witchcraft and imprisoned at the instance of her own son. On the patronal feast-day of the village, Claude went to visit her with two men who undertook to make her confess, but who beat her to death. Claude, while claiming to be a mere accomplice, went into voluntary banishment and was pardoned seven years later. There is no evidence that he blamed the dead woman for his misfortunes, but his behaviour illustrates the effect of the official witch-hunt on the peasantry.

The other side of the coin: living popular culture

The demonological construction is an intimate blend of certain obsessions of the elite classes of Europe, with which Norman Cohn has dealt as they deserve, and elements of the social reality and popular culture of the time. It is only the latter that I shall be concerned with here.

These elements have nothing to do with any organized non-Christian cult, even of a residual or mythic kind. At all events it is impossible, in my opinion, to formulate such delicate questions concerning the origin of the practices and beliefs involved: the problem is manifestly a false one, after a thousand years of Christianity and syncretism, at the very least, between ancient pagan traditions and those of Catholicism. The important thing is to consider the vision of the world and the attitudes current at the time of the witch-hunts; this may help us to understand, through the conflict of cultures and the crisis, what was vital to one part of the community and rejected by others.

The sabbat-myth enables us to list conveniently the various elements in question: the human body (with the Devil's mark); the nocturnal ritual; the role of women; wealth, reputation, and human relationships, all of which the spell casters sought to destroy. Each of these phenomena has a normal aspect of its own, which the demonologists and those who inspired them refused to acknowledge.

Magistrates saw the Devil's mark as a presumption of guilt, a tangible sign that Satan had taken possession of a human body. This idea struck a chord in the peasant mind, reflecting as it does a 'magic' conception of the body's powers, which, however, need have nothing to do with demonology. Artois villagers, for instance, regarded the body as a kind of microcosm, directly related to the outside world and equally capable of acting upon it or being acted upon by it. Thus there is a symmetry or interrelation, for example, between rain or mist and a person's tears. Consequently a witch can call up a storm by using a stick to ruffle the waters of a pond, while uttering mysterious words – she is, in fact, extending into the macrocosm her power over her own body. Belief in the efficacy of the forces inherent in every human being was so widespread that people would avoid contact with a stranger, lowering their eyes so as not to meet his; they would even defend themselves, weapon in hand, if such a person tried to touch them or come close enough to be reached by the sword held in the outstretched arm. As we have seen, the evil eye or 'Vaudois eye' of which the Rumegies peasant spoke was supposed to be capable of killing dogs and causing diseases. The myth of satanism transposes these beliefs – which are far from being extinct in the twentieth century – into the realm of diabolism: that is to say, it invites superstitious rustics to cease believing in the power of human beings and concentrate all of their fears on the Devil, whose counterpart is the no less unique figure of a God able to save mankind. In other words, a monotheistic explanation is offered to people who are in reality both Christian and polytheistic, since they are disposed to believe themselves surrounded by a plurality of forces.

By a still clearer process, the notion of the sabbat is used to diabolize the hours of night. Darkness is the Devil's domain for theologians, but for them only; in the countryside, at our period, it was full of folk and animation. It was at night-time that bands of armed young men roamed about after the day's work, seeking ritual but very real combat with other groups of youths, generally from neighbouring parishes. Unmarried lads would serenade their girls with the aid of musicians, sometimes at a very late hour; sometimes they would enter the house with the father's tacit consent – this was especially the case in Artois and Flanders. On the way home, drunkenness and passion led to many nocturnal brawls that were by no means trifling, as we see from hundreds of letters of remission granted to perpetrators of homicide on such occasions. On Sundays and great feasts such as St John's day there was dancing in the villages, as well as in the surrounding country, after nightfall. Processions and pilgrimages likewise offered an excuse for jollity. Pieter Aertsen's *Returning Pilgrims*, painted before the last quarter of the sixteenth century, depicts a scene of dancing, music, games, and love-making. True, it is by daylight, but in all probability the merriment will continue after dark. This is confirmed by other sources, even at the height of the Counter-Reformation. We read of a party in the Beaunne region, returning home from a wedding on 2 October 1622. They halt at a mill, an arquebus-shot away from a certain village, and start dancing at 2 in the morning. Would not a demonologist have been certain to regard this as a witches' sabbat, instead of an ordinary peasant diversion?

Trials for witchcraft include charges that reveal a clear desire to put a stop to such amusements by night, and even by day. The more obstinately the peasants defended their customs, the more diabolic they seemed to the authorities. In 1613 a young man of Recourt in the castellany of Oisy in Artois was accused of frequenting a sabbat 'with a yellow pipe, whereon he whistled'. Need we see in this anything more than a frolicsome band of youths and musicians? Far more so as an archducal ordinance forbidding young people to dance in villages was in force from 1609 to 1610 in that region, as in other Netherlands provinces; heavy fines for infringing it were inflicted in the governorship of Arras, to which Recourt belonged. Here we have trials for sorcery buttressing legislation that was much disobeyed, populating the night-time with demons so as to deter young folk and others from what had been their accustomed pleasures.

The link between women and sorcery – an enormous theme, on which I shall only touch in outline – is connected with the same fierce determination to stamp out the 'errors' and 'superstitions' of rural communities. I have described elsewhere the importance of the peasant woman in transmitting and preserving popular culture.[11] In the 'satanic' version of the sabbath she similarly occupies a central place. For women are the exact equivalent, in their own culture, of demonologists and judges in theirs. They bring up children, but in a very different way from that in which theologians and magistrates seek to educate the people. Certainly the elite culture was capable of taking children in hand and exterminating those guilty of evil thoughts: around 1610, this horrible task was performed by the lieutenant of the castellany of Bouchain. But such actions were scarcely acceptable in themselves, and compromised the future of the entire community; accordingly, in 1612, the official's zeal was curbed by archducal order. The rule thus laid down was intended to prevent the depopulation of a region, and was imitated by the authorities in several other states. One effect was to increase the importance of the school system in educating the younger age groups and above all limiting the pernicious influence of mothers. Thus the ferocity of magistrates towards women was not only a matter of virulent anti-feminism: it was also a way of casting the main responsibility for diabolism on the weaker sex, and avoiding the disastrous results of applying too strictly the terrible notion of hereditary witchcraft. With relatively few exceptions, the *Malleus Maleficarum* – the witch hammer – fell on witches but spared their children. Better still, the persecutors relied on children to inform against their mothers, sometimes on a massive scale: thousands of children did so in the epidemic persecution of 1670 around Lake Siljan in Sweden.[12] In such cases the demonologists succeeded in inducing the young generation to reject their unworthy mothers, guilty of witchcraft. Those mothers who were spared received a severe warning not to behave like the rest: in other words, they had henceforth to regard as devilish the unlawful beliefs and customs that they had shared with other peasant women and were imparting to their children.

Among the various 'superstitions' or 'spells' that are described at length in the trial records we find innumerable magic formulae designed to affect the course of events in regard to property, reputation, or social relations. With much variation among different countries and regions, these ideas are the staple of popular witchcraft in the true sense and can be found everywhere, including countries like England and Denmark where the name of the Devil is almost absent from the trials and the witches' sabbat plays a minor part. Here we can really point to structures valid throughout Europe, derived from pre-Christian religions and gradually modified by more than a thousand years of Christianity: a syncretism in a state of permanent evolution, in which it is hard to isolate the constituent elements, but which is different in character from the purified monotheism which supplies a model to the demonologists. One of the main characteristics of this system is that it enables men and women to believe that they can affect their own destiny by means of rites, by the aid of diviners and sorcerers of all kinds, or again by praying to statues, saints' relics, and so on.

For those who have recourse to such intervention, Christian signs and symbols are often simply a reinforcement, so that, as a twentieth-century historian puts it, the sacred and the profane overlap without difficulty. Do not Danish wizards show a preference for casting spells in churches?[13] Similarly, Bénigne Morand, a villager of the district of Gray in Burgundy, is described as knowing the use of

> signs and charms, so that on Good Friday of the past year 1634, being in the church of Seey (his village) he did write signs on a laurel leaf during the divine service of the Passion, whereof many were witnesses; and did confess and say that if a hen were to eat of the said leaf she could not be killed even by an arquebus-shot.

Bénigne Morand's method of protection against bodily harm is paralleled, in the Tournaisis region, by the use of 'mighty names' on the part of young men who wished to be proof against wounds incurred in fighting. Long lists of such beliefs could be drawn up, but they were more and more frowned on by the religious reformers of the sixteenth and seventeenth centuries. The authorities had previously tolerated them, but did so no longer: they were an integral part of the sabbat myth, tarred with the brush of diabolism. Those, such as Bénigne Morand, who practised them were an occasion of scandal. A sharp distinction was henceforth drawn between what was sacred in the orthodox sense, supervised by the clergy, and what was profane and secular, belonging to everyday life. The latter, never-theless, was also subject to moralization, and, for instance, to the eradication of 'superstitions' that were defined in the synodal statutes of French dioceses.

Both in the demonological mirror and in the peasants' mind, the features of the popular culture fade into a blur behind the single figure of Satan. This more or less coincides with the acme of the witch-hunting process, in all those countries where the sabbat myth falls on fertile ground as far as the peasantry is concerned; and it portends the establishment of a new overall relationship between the law and the rural population, between authority and its subjects.

From private vengence to public order: a European pattern?

The persecution of witches is an effect of the acculturation of rural areas by the religious and political elite. However, it only reaches a high degree of intensity when the judicial system is reinforced by agents within the rural community. It is a fundamental error to see witch-burning as a purely religious phenomenon; it was in fact part of a much wider movement, whose object was to make country folk respect law and order and discontinue the practice of private vengeance. From this point of view one can compare the different European countries so as to establish a pattern of the sociology of authority which will take account even of those coun-tries where witchcraft was not severely persecuted.

The myth of satanism, conceived by theologians but applied by lay judges, produced condemnations on a massive scale. It is too often forgotten that the actual burnings were the work of the civil power. The Church furnished ideological weapons and continued in the modern era, in the Spanish Netherlands for instance, to counsel rulers in their fight against devilry. But the persecutions were carried out by royal officers, like the lieutenant of Bouchain already mentioned, or by magistrates who found themselves peasants appointed by the local lord. All these were cogs in a judicial system in which demonology played a specific part. Certainly, village aldermen and the lord's lieges had only an imperfect knowledge of the prin-ciples they were applying: some could neither read nor write, as was the case in about 1679 with the lieutenant of the barony of Bouvignies in Flanders. But all were agents of the law and were imbued with its ideas of penal repression: and in several European states these ideas were taking on a different form. Royal justice no longer endeavoured merely to keep the peace, as in the Middle Ages, but estab-lished a whole scale of crimes and punishments culminating in the notion of high-treason (lèse-majesté) this occurred in the Spanish Netherlands with the ordi-nances of 1570, and in France in 1670.

Sorcery, of course, headed the catalogue of crimes; being lèse-majesté against the Almighty, it was the most frightful misdeed imaginable. But we must remember, witch-hunters were not solely engaged in persecuting witches. Much more frequently they had to deal with all sorts of other crimes: to these they were either traditionally indulgent, as with crimes of violence, or progressively more severe, as, for instance, towards thieves, vagabonds, and offenders against morals and reli-gion. In absolutist countries, in particular, as a direct result of the evolution of the sovereign power, there was an attempt through the legal machinery to concentrate and watch over the population and to establish a uniform system of penalties, if not of courts.

This political and institutional change is one of the factors which led to the persecution of witches. The criminal law which emanated from the new political structures created a framework for persecution; and the use of torture, which was in no way confined to witch-trials, naturally multiplied convictions. Few witches were burnt in countries that did not use torture, or used it to a limited extent, such as England, Scotland, Denmark, and Sweden: this is a sign of a different evolution of the penal system, a mutation of political structures in a different direction from the absolutist kingdoms. This is no doubt one explanation of the unique situation in the United Provinces, where witches ceased to be persecuted at the beginning of the seventeenth century. Legal particularism was strong in Dutch territory; the notion of *lèse-majesté* commanded little sympathy after the revolt against the king of Spain, and the ordinances of 1570 were certainly not applied in the independent Netherlands.

Political and legal forms are not the whole story. The absolutist countries did not all persecute witches to an equal extent; on the other hand, persecution was strong in Protestant countries, though here in my opinion two opposite types are to be discerned. Those states, such as Geneva or Scotland, where political and religious power was concentrated in a hierarchical form, persecuted more ruthlessly than those in which authority was more diffused.[14] Exceptions can be found, but I believe there is a link between the incidence of executions for witchcraft and the strength of the process whereby the population was brought under political and administrative control. Emulation among the states of different religious persuasions also played a part, for instance in south-west Germany.

Persecuting zeal could be more thorough still. Well-known officials such as Pierre de Lancre, or obscure ones like Charles Van der Camere, lieutenant of Bouchain castellany around 1610, were personally responsible for dozens or hundreds of executions. Their actions had, of course, to appear within the law to be encouraged by higher authority and sanctioned by the judicial system. This brings us back to our previous theme, as bloodthirsty judges could not last long unless their acts conformed to the needs and standards of the society they lived in. Such was the case in England during the 1640s, when witch burnings increased in number but reflected a period of crisis. Conversely, it was not easy for sceptics to impose their way of thinking except in areas where witch-hunting had no deep roots in society such as the United Provinces in the seventeenth century.

All this does no more than account for the existence of the phenomenon. Its intensity and duration depended in part on the efforts of the magistrates but still more on the reactions of the peasantry itself. I have described the effects of the wave of fear that swept the countryside when the myth inculcated by the upper orders of society was given tangible form by incessant executions. Some peasants reacted in a traditional manner by identifying those of their neighbours who practised witchcraft and driving them out of the village or exacting summary justice. Others denounced the supposed malefactors to the courts or, more often, assembled in crowds to bear witness against the objects of popular suspicion.

The key question is: why did peasants in the second category act as they did? How and why was it that one section of rural society preferred to get rid of sorcerers and witches by invoking the law instead of by private vengeance?

The picture painted by the demonologists was by no means accepted every-where as a matter of course. In the Netherlands, the satanic myth was very clearly defined by time ordinances of 1592 and 1606, but the ensuing witch-hunt differed greatly in intensity from one province to another. In the county of Artois, at the opposite extreme to Flanders and Hainaut, the persecution was moderate and short-lived: by and large, it ceased in 1620. Artois was three-quarters rural, and very few of the population were avowed Protestants; it was loyal to the Spanish monarchy, and its lawyers upheld the same values as their colleagues in Flanders and Hainaut. Yet its record as regards witch-hunting is similar to that of the United Provinces, with which it had nothing else in common from 1579 onwards.

The only possible explanation in this case is that the peasant communities in Artois were for the most part averse to legal proceedings: they remained firmly attached to the principle of private revenge, which led to innumerable acts of violence. They apparently detected as many witches in their midst as did the peas-antry of neighbouring regions, but preferred to deal with them extra-legally. Their deep mistrust of the courts is shown by (1) the absence of epidemics of persecu-tion, except for a few cases in the castellany of Oisy, situated in the eastern part of Artois and in the vicinity of Bouchain; (2) the rarity of denunciations by those accused; and (3) the absence of any request by the village communities for the prosecution of witches by the courts.

Artois, in short, appears to have been 'closed' to the extension of official justice to rural areas, whereas Flanders and Hainaut were much more open. It should be noted here that the local custom in Artois generally allowed parents, if they chose, to leave their property to their male children only, whereas in Flanders all the heirs, male and female, had to be treated equally. At the beginning of the seven-teenth century, with the cessation of hostilities, a demographic upsurge took place in both regions; its effect was to increase tension within families and to widen the gap between well-to-do peasants and the rural masses. We may suppose that the impact of this phenomenon varied according to the firmness of family structures and the ability of parishes to close ranks against the outside world. In both respects the consensus appears to have been much more fragile in Flanders than in Artois. Faced with change, the Flemish peasants were, it seems, unable to preserve the equilibrium of their society except by appealing increasingly to the law against witches and also, still more frequently, against any of their number who might constitute a threat.

In my opinion, witch-hunts were not the outcome of war and grave civil distur-bance, but were associated with periods of rapid demographic expansion and economic change. These produced a ferment of social differentiation in the villages, especially if mass pauperization was increased by local customs on inheritance, as was the case in Normandy or Flanders with its egalitarian system. The changes were often favourable to the better off, but the resulting fissure exacerbated social tension and envy. Those at the bottom reacted by seeking a 'magic' revenge, uttering explicit threats, and probably believing in their efficacy. This state of things gave full weight to accusations that wizards and witches were ruining their neighbours, causing beasts to die and crops to fail. The example of Cambrésis shows that the alleged sorcerers, while not paupers or vagabonds, belonged to the most numerous and least well-off class of peasants, while those who brought charges or informed against them were often somewhat more prosperous and even rich, or else they were clients of local notables.

Some suspects, it is clear, were obsessively determined to bring down their more powerful neighbours. Marguerite Carhier of Oisy-le-Verger in Artois uttered threats against those who appeared too 'high and mighty', such as a woman who, she thought, behaved slightingly to her at mass. She predicted to another family that the husband would die in poverty and the children would have to beg for their bread.

Fears such as these – together with a process whereby the superior class of peasants differentiated themselves from a popular culture that was more and more confined to the poor – brought about a fundamental rift in those villages that were most affected by demographic and economic change. There emerged a dominant, property-owning minority which sought the aid of law and authority in countering the real or magic threats of which it was the object, thus breaching the united front of the local community *vis-à-vis* the outside world.

In cases where the demonological doctrine, imparted from above, was not applied by zealous officers or welcomed by peasant 'notables' as a legal remedy against the customs and practices of their own society, witch-hunts might occur, but were no more than a straw fire. In some regions, where magical beliefs were no less common than elsewhere, executions might be few because the harmony of the countryside was little disturbed by demographic or economic changes. Right into the nineteenth century the Gevaudan district, as studied by Elisabeth Claverie and Pierre Lamaison, was still a peasant society based on violence. Breaches of equilibrium were corrected by private revenge; secret arrangements were preferred to lawsuits; the community distrusted the outside world and protected itself against it. Artois in the seventeenth century was similarly shut in on itself and that is why it and other such regions were spared hundreds of witch-burnings.

These witches were the victims of the demonological obsession of the Western elite classes, and also of the fact that some of their fellow citizens abandoned the principles of private vengeance, choosing instead to take their place in a world of law and order. The 'treason' of these rural notables, which took different forms elsewhere, consisted in their case of abandoning an archaic and magic culture disseminated by women. Attracted by the 'modern' forces in operation in towns and at the centre of the realm, they sought help from the law in casting off the restrictions that were still upon them, using the fear of penal sanctions to keep the masses in subjection and to thwart the sorcerers who planned their ruin. In a word, they turned to new methods to ensure their social domination.

In this sense the witch-hunt was a sign of twofold crisis. A crisis, firstly, of the mediaeval state and the unity of Christendom, giving birth painfully to new solutions: absolutism, the Counter-Reformation, the Protestant Dutch republic, the Calvinist theocracy, and so on. A crisis, secondly, of the rural world, coming to terms willy-nilly with modernity; obliged to submit to powers more instant and imperious than before; called on abruptly to give up its 'superstitions', its violent ways, the whole structure of a delicate internal balance framed over the centuries.

After a process of adaptation requiring several generations, the root-causes of witch-hunting disappear and so do the executions. Magistrates cease to believe in the satanic myth, and the elite cease to regard Christianity in its various forms as a citadel besieged by evil. New types of social equilibrium prevail in 'open' communities, while 'closed' parishes and regions, like Gevaudan, continue for a long time to exhibit forms, inherited from the Middle Ages, of internal consensus and mistrust of what lies outside.

Europe as a whole stands ready at this time to confront a tremendous future of economic and colonial development. Its vital force, the peasantry, produces more and better in a situation of demographic expansion. In the eighteenth century a new sociology of authority, varying in form, is associated with the relative docility of the peasant masses, itself an indispensable prelude to the rise of capitalism. We must not mistake the part for the whole: witch-hunting is fundamentally not a religious but a political phenomenon, and it is only one aspect of the penetration and opening-up of the countryside.

The witch gives way to the priest, and private vengeance to public order; the authorities invade the heart of the village.

Notes

1   See Chapter 2 in this collection.
2   For the principle of inversion in early modern witchcraft, see Chapter 11 by Stuart Clark.
3   Robert Muchembled, *Sorcières, justice et société aux 16 et 17 siècles* (Paris 1987), esp. 89–205; Muchembled, *Les Derniers buchers: une village de Flandre et ses sorcières sous Louis XIV* (Paris 1981).
4   Alan Macfarlane, *Witchcraft in Tudor and Stuart England* (2nd edn, London 1999); Jens Christian Johansen, in Bengt Ankarloo and Gustav Henningsen, eds, *Early Modern European Witchcraft* (Oxford 1990), ch. 13.
5   Pierre Chaunu, 'Sur la fin des sorciers an xvii siecle', *Annales* ESC 24, 4 (1969), 895–911; Mircea Eliade, 'Some Observations on European Witchcraft', *History of Religions* 14 (1974), 49–72; Margaret Alice Murray, *The Witch-Cult in Western Europe* (London 1921). For Carlo Ginzburg, see Chapter 8 in this book.
6   H. C. Erik Midelfort, *Witch-Hunting in Southwestern Germany, 1562–1684* (Stanford, Calif. 1972).
7   For full citations of the archival sources used in this chapter, see the original version in Ankarloo and Henningsen, *Early Modern European Witchcraft*, ch. 5.
8   Muchembled, *Sorcières*, 144–9.
9   Hans Eyvind Naess, in Ankarloo and Henningsen, *Early Modern European Witchcraft*, ch. 14.
10 Bengt Ankarloo, in Ankarloo and Henningsen, *Early Modern European Witchcraft*, ch. 11.
11 Robert Muchembled, *Popular Culture and Elite Culture in France, 1400–1750* (Baton Rouge, La 1985), esp. 66–71.
12 Ankarloo, in Ankarloo and Henningsen, *Early Modern European Witchcraft*, ch. 11.
13 Johansen, in Ankarloo and Henningsen, *Early Modern European Witchcraft*, ch. 13.
14 For an alternative view of the role of central authorities in witch persecutions, see Chapter 16 in this collection by Brian Levack.

Chapter 11

Stuart Clark

INVERSION, MISRULE AND THE
MEANING OF WITCHCRAFT

I

WE NO LONGER READILY UNDERSTAND the language of early modern witchcraft beliefs. Demonological classics like *Malleus Maleficarum* (1486–7) or Jean Bodin's *De la dimonomanie des sorciers* (1580) seem to reveal only an arcane wisdom. It is not apparent what criteria of rationality are involved, nor how the exegesis of authorities or use of evidence support the required burden of proof. Since individual steps in the argument are difficult to construe, its overall configuration often remains impenetrable. And the accounts given by other authorities like Nicolas Rémy and Pierre De Lancre of the ritual practices of witches and demons, notably those associated with the sabbat, appear sensational and absurd. Faced with such refractory meanings, some past commentators have tried to put Renaissance demonology to the test of empirical verification by asking if it described, albeit in exaggerated or symbolic form, the actual activities of real agents. Agreed (largely) that it did not, that there were no witches in fact, they turned with relief to sceptics like Johann Weyer who, even at the height of prosecutions, cast doubt on the reality of witchcraft phenomena by offering non-magical theories of causation. And with intimations of rationalism of this sort historians have continued to feel an intellectual affinity. A second popular approach has been the explanation of learned witchcraft beliefs in terms of social and socio-psychological determinants, especially those thought to be at work in the designation of criminal actions or the persecution of demonized 'out-groups'.[1] This too has had the advantage of bypassing the problem of their meaning by reducing them to epiphenomena; tracing them, for instance, to the periodic social need to relocate moral and cultural boundaries by means of accusations of deviance, or, again, to the neuroses which are said to accompany the repression of erotic or irreligious impulses in devout minds.[2]

Yet there is surely *prima facie* reluctance to dismiss Bodin as a victim of obscurantism or delusion, let alone regard a whole tradition of discursive argument, successfully sustained for nearly two hundred years, as essentially irrational. What is at stake are the criteria for interpreting a past world of thought without recourse to anachronism or reductionism, an issue recently debated by historians of ideas in a number of analogous inquiries. In the case of the history of political theory Quentin Skinner has persuasively defended a model of explanation in which the claim (stemming from Collingwood) that meaningful action can be sufficiently accounted for in terms of agents' intentions is complemented by J. L. Austin's stress on the performative quality of utterances. Since its explanatory force depends on seeing the point of a specific textual speech act for the author, Skinner also emphasizes the Wittgensteinian principle that what it makes sense for anyone to say is relative to a linguistic context or 'language game'. In political theorizing the intention to persuade presupposes such a framework of shared meanings in which certain concepts and rules for applying them in argument have a conventional life. It is these changing conventions of discussion which pre-empt anachronistic readings by limiting the range of possible meanings which a textual utterance can be said to have. Likewise it is the criteria of sense and nonsense which they embody to which appeal must first be made before cases of apparently bizarre rationality are rejected on the grounds of incoherence.[3]

Such a methodology has already rescued Hobbes's *Leviathan* from a series of critical mythologies; others like it have established the internal cogency of styles of thought like those associated with divine right monarchy or millenarian politics where little sense could previously be discerned.[4] The implication is that if the rationale which originally informed the literature of witchcraft is ever to be recovered, we must begin not by assuming some sort of mistake on the part of the authors but by locating individual texts in the linguistic framework, possibly extending far beyond demonology itself, in which they were expected to make sense as utterances of a certain kind. This would involve establishing what Skinner calls the 'range of descriptions' available to writers in a demonological tradition. It might lead us into a world where the criteria for saying that something was possible or impossible or made sense or nonsense were highly idiosyncratic. But Wittgenstein's point is not that these rules may not vary between language games but that their existence is the minimum formal condition for any linguistic engagement. Thus, if it could be shown that it did in fact make sense within such a world for scholars like Bodin and De Lancre both to accept the reality of witchcraft phenomena and attribute witches with certain ritual practices, then initial doubt about the felicity of demonological arguments would simply disappear. There would be no cause to look for an explanation of them other than that they followed recognized linguistic conventions, that they were part of what Peter Winch has called 'a coherent universe of discourse'.[5]

Doubtless the task of decoding the meaning of witchcraft texts in this way would be an enormous undertaking. In what follows I have chosen only one, albeit characteristic idiom, the stress on contrariness and inverse behaviour in demonism. Part at least of our puzzlement over this particular way of thinking and writing about witchcraft can be successfully removed by filling out the prevailing conventions of discourse, particularly political discourse, in the sixteenth and seventeenth centuries. Of central significance are those arguments considered appropriate for identifying and contrasting the key conditions of order and disorder. I want to argue that Renaissance descriptions of the nature of Satan, the character of hell and, above all, the ritual activities of witches shared a vocabulary of misrule, that they were in effect part of a language conventionally employed to establish and condemn the properties of a disorderly world.

II

That witches did everything backwards was as much a commonplace of scholarly demonology as it has been of romantic fiction since. But in this respect they were not alone. Throughout the late mediaeval and Renaissance period ritual inversion was a characteristic element of village folk-rites, religious and educational *ludi,* urban carnivals and court entertainments. Such festive occasions shared a calendrical licence to disorderly behaviour or 'misrule' based on the temporary but complete reversal of customary priorities of status and value. One typical recurring idea was the elevation of wise folly over foolish wisdom. Another was the exchange of sex roles involved in the image of the 'woman on top' or in transvestism. Clerical parodies of divine service substituted the profane for the sacred, and low for high office. Most pervasive of all were mock political authorities, the *princes des sots* or 'abbeys' or 'lords of misrule' who presided over ephemeral commonwealths complete with the paraphernalia of serious kingship but dedicated to satire and clowning.[6] Often these various modes of topsy-turvydom were invoked simultaneously, as in the ecclesiastical, Feast of Fools or the activities of the French urban confraternities, the *societes joyeuses.* Sometimes one relationship was explored; the street *charivari* in which partners in unequal or violent marriages were ridiculed by the symbolic ride backwards focused on the dangerous social and moral inversions implied when familial disorder threatened patriarchal rule. Similarly 'barring out' the master in English grammar schools has been shown to depend on assumptions about the limits of pedagogic government over pupils, especially with the onset of the vacation.[7] Whatever the case, however, seasonal misrule involved not simply riot or confusion but conventional styles of ritual and symbol associated with inversion – recognized forms of 'uncivil rule'.

It would be remarkable if no links could be established between these forms of inverted behaviour and descriptions of demonic practices, flourishing and declining as they did in the same period. Certainly there were borrowings from accounts of sabbat rituals where the world upside-down was an important theme of festival occasions at court. Conversely the demonologist Pierre Crespet located the witches' dance in a tradition including the bacchanalian revel, early Christian transvestism and the masquerades of the *Maschecroutte* of contemporary Lyon.[8] The inferior clergy of late mediaeval France celebrated Christmas and the New Year with burlesques which were readily attributable to God's ape – singing in dissonances, braying like asses, making indecent grimaces and contortions, repeating prayers in gibberish, censing with puddings or smelly shoes and, above all, mocking the sermon and the mass with fatuous imitations. As late as 1645 the lay brothers of Antibes marked Innocents' Day by wearing vestments inside out, holding liturgical books upside-down and using spectacles with orange-peel in them instead of glass.[9] According to the social reformer Philip Stubbes, English rural practitioners of misrule encouraged in their soliciting for bread and ale what was in effect a propitiatory sacrifice to Satan as well as a profanation of the sabbath.[10] In France attempts were made by Jean Savaron and Claude Noirot to link the history and etymology of popular entertainment with those of witchcraft; Savaron thought that masquerading was a form of demonic sabbat (*la feste de Satan*).[11] Moreover carnival Devil figures could be seen taking an important part in processions and even organizing festivities.[12]

But even if they shared no specific types of inversion, both festive behaviour and learned demonology were dependent on inversion itself as a formal principle. And this allows us to apply to witchcraft studies some of the questions currently being asked by historians and anthropologists about the meaning of misrule. To some extent attention has concentrated on the practical benefits accruing to a community from what is actually done at times of ritual licence. For instance it is argued that traditional institutions and values are reaffirmed by the mockery of offenders against social codes, the deflation of pretentious wisdom and overweening authority or simply the open expression of grudges borne against neighbours. In this fashion, misrule strengthens the community by symbolic or open criticism and its moderating influence. Alternatively the same carnivalesque practices have been associated with innovation and protest because they offer freedom to explore relationships potentially corrosive of existing structures and, therefore, not normally tolerated. Neither of these readings is particularly helpful when applied to demonology. For although the differing social functions are largely seen as latent in the behaviour, some attribution of intentions to agents is required in each case. In the first, we would therefore be committed to something like Margaret Murray's theory that Renaissance witchcraft consisted of rites of inversion actually performed by folk worshippers of a surviving Dianic fertility cult. And the second would involve accepting the connections which Le Roy Ladurie has claimed existed between conceptions of revolt based on a 'fantasy of inversion' shared by rural peasant insurrectionists, festival fools *and witches* in southern France at the end of the sixteenth century.[13] Yet the accredited historical evidence for maleficent witchcraft comes very largely from allegations or from stereotyped confessions; we therefore have few grounds for attributing witches with intentions of any kind, whether re-integrative or innovatory in character.

This forces us back to a second set of issues relating to misrule, concerning the conditions which must obtain if inverted behaviour is to be seen as having not only various social-functional uses but any meaning at all as an act of inversion. The starting-point here must be the fact, emphasized many years ago by Enid Welsford and recently reiterated by Natalie Davis and Keith Thomas, that misrule necessarily presupposes the rule that it parodies.[14] Thus the fool could only flourish, in fact or in literary imaginations, in societies where the taboos surrounding divine kingship and sacramental worship were especially rigid. The street theatre and cacophonous, 'rough' music of the *charivari* were effective precisely because all other ceremonial occasions were solemn; while turning social or sexual status upside-down, and the laughter it provoked, only began to make sense in a world of simply polarized hierarchies. The degree of meaningfulness of carnival misrule therefore depended on the extent of familiarity with such orthodoxies. And the performance of ritual inversion was only successful if accompanied by possibly complex acts of recognition. An example from modern anthropology is McKim

Marriott's failure to comprehend the Indian village festival of Holi as an actor but his subsequent understanding that its apparent disorder was 'an order precisely inverse to the social and ritual principles of routine life'.[15] Reverting to the language of use, there is the further suggestion that, simply in obliging the spectator to see the conventional world in the guise of its opposite, misrule embodies a cognitive function that, in part at least, must be essentially conservative – a restatement of the normal from a 'ritual viewpoint'. Stronger still is the claim that only by exploring this contrary perspective can men make themselves conceptually at home in a world of unchanging polarities.[16]

III

It was in a world accustomed to think in these ways about contrariety and disorder that the arguments of the demonologists made sense. In the face of Sadducism or qualms merely about publicizing witchcraft their whole intellectual engagement could be defended as an example, perhaps the paradigm case, of the principle that the appreciation of good consisted in the recognition and exploration of its opposite. In his *Daemonologie* (1597) King James claimed that:

> since the Devill is the verie contrarie opposite to God, there can be no
> better way to know God, then by the contrarie; . . . by the falshood of
> the one to considder the trueth of the other, by the injustice of the one,
> to considder the justice of the other: And by the cruelty of the one, to
> considder the mercifulnesse of the other: And so foorth in all the rest
> of the essence of God, and qualities of the Devill.

This applied to all specific offices and ordinances of divine origin, indeed to all features of a world imbued with an invertible morality. Thus James's own attempt in 1590–1 to write into the confessions of the North Berwick witches a special antipathy between demonic magic and godly magistracy had been a way of authenticating his own, as yet rather tentative initiatives as ruler of Scotland.[17] Similarly in Pierre De Lancre's *Du sortilège* (1627) it was the very fact that the Devil chose to mimic the Catholic liturgy which was said to be incontrovertible proof of its divinity.[18] The rationale of all such institutions would accordingly be seriously undermined without demonological science. Establishing in exact detail what occurred at a witches' sabbat was not arid pedantry or intellectual voyeurism but a (logically) necessary way of validating each corresponding contrary aspect of the orthodox world. And the full intelligibility of demonological literature was, in the end, dependent on success in reading into each individual facet of demonism an actual or symbolic inversion of a traditional form of life.

In this respect the most appropriate context of meanings was that of conceptions of disorder as a world turned upside-down by disobedience and tyranny. For demonic inversion was inseparable, in the first instance, from notions of archetypal rebellion and pseudo-monarchy. The Devil's original presumption prefigured every subsequent act of resistance, while the style of his rule in hell was, as Erasmus explained, a model for all those whose political and moral intentions were most unlike God's.[19] Although some sort of order could be discerned there, it was therefore fitting that it should comprise the opposite of perfect princely and paterfamilial government. Aquinas had established that demons only co-operated out of common hatred for mankind, not from mutual love or respect for magistracy. Though there were ranks among the fallen angels the criteria involved were those of greatness in malice and, consequently, anguish rather than worth and felicity.[20] These principles became essential to all formal demonology. Their relation to the wider context can be seen in a discussion such as D'Acuto's. Here the fact that demons had inverted the angelic nature is offered as one example, albeit historically prior, of a universal overturning wrought by the rebellion which constitutes sin. The contrarieties involved in the fall of Lucifer (for instance, from prince of heaven to tyrant of hell) and the qualities both of his subject devils and the corresponding moral faction of mankind are expressed in a series of the usual linguistic antitheses.[21] In effect, then, the Devil's regimen was a compendium of the paradoxes of misrule: a hierarchy governed from the lowest point of excellence, a society in which dishonour was the badge of status and a *speculum* imitable only by the politically vicious. This was worse than simple anarchy.[22]

Moreover there was a specific sense in which demonic allegiance was necessarily associated with disobedience and its consequences. The voluntary contract with the Devil which was thought to be the essence of malevolent witchcraft could be seen, primarily, as spiritual apostasy, symbolized by rebaptism at the sabbat. But the non-sacramental significance of baptism and the insistence on both the physical corporeality of devils and their political organization inevitably brought it as close to an act of literal, if indirect, resistance. English puritan demonologists argued that the proper spiritual response to the tribulations of Satan was that of Job, while using the language of politics to convey the essential rebelliousness of his agents the witches. William Perkins, for instance, recommended that the natural law enjoining the death penalty for all enemies of the state be extended to 'the most notorious traytor and rebell that can be . . . For [the witch] renounceth God himselfe, the King of Kings, she leaves the societie of his Church and people, she bindeth herself in league with the Devil'.[23] The text occasioning this argument, 'For rebellion is as the sin of witchcraft' (I Samuel 15. 23), could be used to demonstrate the identity in substance as well as in seriousness of the two sins. Hence the sensitivity of French and English writers to the double meaning involved in the word 'conjuration'; hence too the overtones in the claim made in the English *Homily against Disobedience* that rebels 'most horribly prophane, and pollute the Sabbath day, serving Sathan, and by doing of his work, making it the devils day, instead of the Lords day'.[24] While witchcraft was constituted by an act of revolt, rebels effectively promulgated the sabbat. Even the many commonplaces to the effect that civil rebellions could only result from bewitching or sorcery or from 'the mixing of heaven and hell' take on an added meaning.

These associations of ideas must have influenced the understanding of *maleficium*. For it was to be expected that witches should intend not only outright confrontation with the godly prince (as Lambert Daneau warned in theory and as was actually alleged in Scotland in 1590–1)[25] but the promotion of those other inversionary phenomena which were thought to be, or to symbolize, disorder. Thus it was widely accepted that they could destroy the marital hierarchy by using ligature to prevent consummation, by sowing dissension or by incitements to promiscuity. Pierre De Lancre and Sebastien Michaelis claimed specifically that witchcraft subverted familial authority by destroying filial love in its devotees and victims.[26] This echoed the earliest charges made against the alleged *maleficium* of the Vaudois by Johann Tinctor: 'Friends and neighbours will become evil, children will rise up against the old and the wise, and villeins will engage against the nobles'.[27] In the Richard Brome and Thomas Heywood comedy *The Late Lancashire Witches* (1634) a well-ordered household is attacked (in a 'retrograde and preposterous way') by such sorcery – the father kneels to the son, the wife obeys the daughter, and the children are overawed by the servants. The demonological point is hardly obscure but it is nevertheless underlined; a nephew comments that it is as if the house itself had been turned on its roof, while a neighbour protests that he might as well 'stand upon my head, and kick my heels at the skies'. Ligature and the symbolism of a *charivari* reinforce the same theme.[28]

The idea that witches could change themselves and others into animals is another instance of inversion. Although it became usual to argue that the transformations were illusory, the concept of metamorphosis itself, if it was entertained at all, suggested that instinct might replace reason and brutishness virtue. The further example of the natural disorders supposedly wrought by *maleficium* is perhaps the most explicit. Witches, with demonic aid, were assumed to interfere with elements and climate to achieve especially hurtful or unseasonable reversals. Their most powerful magic hardly knew these limits. Henry Holland thought that the notion 'that witches have power to turne the world upside down at their pleasure' was mistaken, but only because it suggested that this was not, indirectly, God's work.[29] Nicolas Rémy listed the detailed wonders:

> there is nothing to hinder a Demon from raising up mountains to an enormous height in a moment, and then casting them down into the deepest abysses; from stopping the flow of rivers, or even causing them to go backwards; from drying up the very sea (if we may believe Apuleius); from bringing down the skies, holding the earth in suspension, raising fountains solid, raising the shades of the dead, putting out the stars, lighting up the very darkness of hell, and turning upside down the whole scheme of this universe.[30]

These were extravagant claims, inspired by Ovid's *Medea* and *Circe* as well as Apuleius's *Meroe* and as popular with poets and dramatists as with demonologists like Rémy. Nevertheless we recognize, with him, the familiar lineaments of the *mundus inversus*. Indeed an important part of the meaning of all these various types of *maleficium*, whether in the family, society, the body or the world, was that they were conventional manifestations of disorder.

Once descriptions of the diabolical polity and the alleged intentions of witches are seen in this context, it becomes possible to read related meanings into the symbolic actions of the sabbat itself. Here many contemporaries were forcibly struck by the systematic and detailed inversions of liturgical forms, by what they recognized as a specious religious observance. Yet since religiosity was not confined to church worship, elaborate ceremonies of homage, however perverted, did not preclude other interpretations. In fact they facilitated an understanding of sabbat rituals in terms of the forms of the Renaissance court festival. Thomas Heywood's own account of the induction of witches is couched in part in the language of formal patronage and clientage and tries to evoke a mood suitable to 'the pompe of regalitie and state'. The rubric is minutely observed, but the (unstated) intentions are there to remind us of the irony of the situation.[31] The most sustained of such descriptions is, however, in Pierre De Lancre's influential demonology *Le Tableau de l'inconstance des mauvais anges et demons* (1612), where it is illustrated by an engraving by Jan Ziarnko. In form at least the occasion is unmistakably that of a court spectacle, organized by a 'master of ceremonies and governor of the sabbat' before the thrones of Satan and a designated 'queen of the sabbat'. A new client is presented, courtiers engage in a feast and various *ballets,* and there is instrumental music. An audience of aristocratic figures includes a group of women 'with masks for remaining always covered and disguised'. There is the same emblematic quality here as in other court festivals of the period, the same attention to detail in the performance, the same use of symbol and imagery, and the purpose is equally didactic. 'For an instant', it has been said, 'one catches a glimpse of the magnificences at the late Valois Court'.[32]

This impression of a festive hell is, of course, confirmed and not weakened by an absolute antithesis of content. In place of godlike monarchy and perfect Platonic love, the sabbat celebrated the most extreme tyranny and the foulest sexual debasement, and its aim was not to bring moral order and civil peace through the acting out of ideal roles but to ensure chaos by dehumanization and atrocities. If Ziarnko's engraving shows a court, it is, then, an anti-court and De Lancre's impresario is not, as it were, a master of revels but a demonic lord of misrule. Certainly the symbolic inversions are not merely those of the world upside-down but specifically those of so many anti-masque *mises en scène,* albeit in more horrendous forms – the elevation of the passions over reason by ritual depravities, physical reversals involving the priority of left-handedness and backwardness and even complete bodily inversions, vertiginous dancing, discordant music and nauseating food.

IV

Given the enormity of their sins and a world in which all phenomena were subject to inversion there was in fact no limit to the disorder of which (with the Devil's aid and God's permission) witches were capable. Nevertheless it is clear that audiences and readers were able and expected to make sense of their activities in a number of conventional ways, anchoring the meaning of witchcraft in terms of styles of thinking and writing about the world upside-down. Each detailed manifestation of demonism presupposed the orderliness and legitimacy of its direct opposite, just as, conversely, the effectiveness of exorcism, judicial process and even a royal presence in actually nullifying magical powers confirmed the grounds of authority of the priest, judge or prince as well as the felicity of his ritual performance. But it also had indirect meaning in terms of the many relations, both of causal interdependence and of 'correspondence', which interlaced the Christian and neo-Platonist universe. The Devil's tyranny was an affront to all well-governed commonwealths but also to every state of moral equipoise. The wider implications of attacks on the family, and of the fact that they were promoted largely by women, could hardly have been missed in a culture which accepted the patriarchal household as both the actual source and analogical representation of good government. The reversing of the human bodily hierarchies or of priorities in natural things had effects which could literally be felt throughout a world thought to be an organic unity of sentients. Especially resonant were references to the dance; for dancing not only had its own powers to confer (or destroy) order and virtue but figured the harmonic relations to which every phenomenon was subject. A single ritual act such as the anal kiss perverted religious worship and secular fealty, dethroned reason from a sovereign position on which individual wellbeing and social relations (including political obligation) were thought to depend and symbolized in the most obvious manner the defiant character of demonic politics as well as its preposterousness.

In these ways demonology superimposed image upon image of disorder. This profusion of levels of meaning made witchcraft beliefs ideal material for the literary imagination; but that they should have been integrated in performances as carefully structured as the court *ballet* and masque, shows how naturally they cohered with men's general conception of things. The best example of a dramatic fusion of this sort is, of course, in Shakespeare's *Macbeth*. It is a critical commonplace that the pervasive disorder in the play is expressed in a series of multiple inversions of contraries in the personal, political and natural planes.[33] Especially striking in the present context are the substitution of tyranny for true magistracy, both in fact and in Malcolm's self-accusation to Macduff, and the reiterated consequences of disobedience to anointed kings and fathers. Even without the explicit witchcraft it would have seemed quite appropriate that *Macbeth* should be prepared to turn the world upside-down, that his castle and kingdom should become a hell and that his actions should be inspired by ultimately deceitful incantations. Nevertheless the witches' presence is vital, for it establishes the two crucial features of the play's atmosphere. One is the sense of obscurity, uncertainty and dissimulation which clouds the subsequent action and its physical location with the effect of claustrophobia. The other is the repeated expression in linguistic antitheses of the inversions which this action embodies and provokes. Both are fixed at the very outset, not only by the famous ritual utterance, 'Fair is foul, and foul is fair', but also by the reference to a 'hurly-burly' with its suggestion of misrule and topsyturvydom.[34] We must suppose that the dramatic effectiveness of this opening scene presupposed the wider context in which demonism was traditionally understood.

V

A contextual reading of Renaissance demonology may not help us to answer the major questions about the genesis or decline of the European 'witch-craze', though it surely confirms the view that these were related to the fortunes of an entire world-view. My aim has been rather to sketch some of the conventions of discourse which governed the successful persuasion of audiences at the height of the persecutions say, between 1580 and 1630. In fact these turn out to be so important that it becomes difficult to explain, not how men accepted the rationality of the arguments, but how, occasionally, sceptics doubted it. What it made sense for demonologists to say depended partly on traditional metaphysical notions about the logical shape and moral economy of the world and partly on shared linguistic patterns for describing its most disturbing aspects. The first entailed a conception of evil for the sake of structural coherence, linking demonism with all privations of good; the second required inversion (both in forms of thought and forms of words) to ensure linguistic felicity, linking demonology with the articulation of key political concepts. The idea of witchcraft was not then a bizarre incongruity in an otherwise normal world; like all manifestations of misrule it *was* that world mirrored in reverse, and the practices of the alleged witches were no less (and no more) meaningful than those of ordinary men and women. It may be true that the demonologists, like other late sixteenth-century writers, were preoccupied with a disorder which appeared to characterize all their affairs. Grounds for such apprehension have been found by historians in an acute instability wrought by inflation, social mobility, sectarian violence and warfare. But to attribute the belief in demonic witchcraft to some determining 'social dysfunction' would not only beg philosophical questions about the way language gives such traumas the meaning they have but ignore the extent to which contemporaries found reassurance in demonological (and millenarian) explanations, even of chaos. In the same way the discovery of instances among believers of what we would today recognize as clinical insanity could never warrant the view that Europe was in the grip of a 'collective psychosis'. This would be to explain away what in effect was a constitutive assumption of its culture, whereas part of what we mean when we speak of a 'world-view' at all is surely that its constituents need no other explanation than their coherence one with another. The primary characteristic of demonological texts as historical evidence is not their supposed unverifiability but their relationship to what J. L. Austin called a 'total speech situation'; their meaning for the historian may be thought of as exactly symmetrical with their original meaning as linguistic performances.[35]

Notes

1   Applications of labelling theory to early modern witchcraft include K. Erikson, *Wayward Puritans: A Study in the Sociology of Deviance* (New York, 1966); E. P. Currie, 'The Control of Witchcraft in Renaissance Europe', in D. Black and M. Mileski (eds), *The Social Organization of Law* (London, 1973), 344–67.

2   N. Cohn, *Europe's Inner Demons: An Enquiry Inspired by the Great Witch-Hunt* (London, 1975).

3   Q. Skinner, 'Meaning and Understanding in the History of Ideas', *History and Theory*, 8 (1969), *Past and Present*, 3–53; Q. Skinner, 'Motives, Intentions and the Interpretation of Texts', *New Literary History*, 3 (1971), 393–408; Q. Skinner, 'Some Problems in the Analysis of Political Thought and Action', *Political Theory*, 2 (1974), 277–303.

4   Q. Skinner, 'The Context of Hobbes's Theory of Political Obligation', in M. Cranston and R. Peters (eds), *Hobbes and Rousseau* (London, 1972), 109–42; Q. Skinner, 'Conquest and Consent: Thomas Hobbes and the Engagement Controversy', in G. E. Aylmer (ed.), *The Interregnum: The Quest for Settlement, 1646–1660* (London, 1972), 79–98.

5   P. Winch, 'Understanding a Primitive Society', *American Philosophical Quarterly* 1 (1964), 309. Contrast Cohn, *Europe's Inner Demons*, where it is a reluctance to accept the 'manifestly impossible' elements in evidence for the reality of witch-craft events that sustains a view of demonology as an intellectual fantasy and leads to a search for an alternative socio-psychological causation.

6   E. Welsford, *The Fool: His Social and Literary History* (London, 1935), 197–217; N. Z. Davis, *Society and Culture in Early Modern France* (London, 1975), 97–123, 'The Reasons of Misrule', and 124–51, 'Women on Top'; P. Burke, *Popular Culture in Early Modern Europe* (London, 1978), 182–91.

7   K. V. Thomas, *Rule and Misrule in the Schools of Early Modern England* (Reading, 1976).

8   Pierre Crespet, *Deux livres de la hayne de Sathan et malins esprits contre l'homme et de l'homme contre eux* (Paris, 1590), 246–55.

9   E. K. Chambers, *The Mediaeval Stage*, 2 vols (Oxford, 1903), i, 317–18, cf. 294, 305, 321, 325–6; Welsford, *The Fool*, 200–1.

10   Philip Stubbes, *The Anatomie of Abuses* (London, 1583, STC 23376), Sigs. Miv–Mivr.

11   Jean Savaron, *Traitte contre les masques* (Paris, 1608), 3–4, 15–16; Claude Noirot, *L'Origine des masques, mommerie, bernez, et revennez es jours gras, de caresme prenant, menez sur l'asne a rebours et charivary* (1609), in *Collection des meilleurs dissertations, notices et traites particuliers relatifs a l'histoire de France*, ed. C. Leber, 20 vols (Paris, 1826–38), ix, 35–8.

12   See Chapter 17 in this collection by David Nicholls.

13   E. Le Roy Ladurie, *Les Paysans du Languedoc*, 2 vols (Paris, 1966), i, 407–14.

14   Welsford, *The Fool*, 193; Davis, *Society and Culture in Early Modern France*, 100; Thomas, *Rule and Misrule in the Schools of Early Modern England*, 34.

15   Cited by Turner, *The Ritual Process*, 185–6.

16   Ibid., 176, 200–1.

17   James I, *Daemonologie, in Forme of a Dialogue* (Edinburgh, 1597, 55; S. Clark, 'King James's *Daemonologie*: Witchcraft and Kingship', in S. Anglo (ed.), *The Damned Art: Essays in the Literature of Witchcraft* (London, 1977), 156–81.

18   Pierre De Lancre, *Du sortilege* (1627), 6–7.

19   Erasmus, *Christiani principis institutio*, trans. Born, 174

20   Aquinas, *Summa theologica*, i, q. 109, ed. Pegis, i, 1012–16.

21   Affinati D'Acuto, *Il mondo al roversica e sossopra*, 447–92.

22   A tract which brings together many of the features of the mentality of contrariety in an attack on the Devil's mockery is Artus Desire, *La Singerie des Huguenots* (Paris, 1574). The Huguenots, inspired by the Devil's desire to turn all things upside-down, have substituted for every true form of worship its exact opposite. This is said to bear witness to the 'advancement of Antichrist' and is expressed in a series of linguistic antitheses; it is also called 'witchcraft'. Ibid., 7–8, 22–4, 40v.

23   William Perkins, *Discourse of the Damned Art of Witchcraft*, in his *Works*, 3 vols (London, 1616), iii, 651; cf. Henry Holland, *A Treatise against Witchcraft* (Cambridge, 1590), Sig. Aiir.

24   Anon., *The Seconde Tome of Homelyes* (London, 1563), 292–3.

25   Lambert Daneau, *Les Sorciers*, trans. R.W. as *A Dialogue of Witches* (London, 1575), Sigs. Bii r–v; *Newes from Scotland* (1591).

26   Pierre De Lancre, *Le Tableau de l'inconstance des mauvais anges et demons* (Paris, 1612), 4; Sebastian Michaelis, *Histoire admirable*, trans. W.B. as *The Admirable Historie* (London, 1613), 254.

27 Johann Tinctor, *Tractatus de secta Vaudensium*, trans. as *De la secte qui s'appelle des Vaudois*, in J. Hansen (ed.), *Quellen und Untersuchungen zur Geschichte des Hexenwahns und der Hexenverfolgung im Mittelalter* (Bonn, 1901), 186–7.

28 *The Dramatic Works of Thomas Heywood*, ed. R. H. Shepherd, 6 vols (London, 1874), iv, 178 (Act i, scene I).

29 Holland, A *Treatise against Witchcraft*, Sig. Giii r.

30 Nicolas Rémy, *Daemonolatreiae* (1595), iii. I, in *Demonolatry of Nicolas Rémy*, ed. M. Summers (London, 1948), 141.

31 Heywood, *The Hierarchie of the Blessed Angells*, 472.

32 M. M. McGowan, 'Pierre De Lancre's *Tableau de l'inconstance des mauvais anges et demons:* The Sabbat Sensationalised', in Anglo (ed.), *The Damned Art*, 192–3.

33 L. C. Knights, 'How Many Children Had Lady Macbeth?', in his *Explorations* (London, 1946, repr. Harmondsworth, 1964), 28–48; Shakespeare, *Macbeth*, ed. K. Muir (Arden edn, London, 1951) 'Introduction'.

34 *Macbeth*, I. i. 3–11.

35 J. L. Austin, *How to do Things with Words*, ed. J. O. Urmson (London, 1962), 52.

PART FOUR

Witchcraft and the Reformation

WHEN THE ENGLISH PROTESTANT John Bale contemplated the horrors of the Roman mass in 1547, he declared that 'it serveth all witches in their witchery'. Expanding on his theme, he claimed that 'all sorcerers, enchanters, dreamers, sothsayers, necromancers, conjurers, cross-diggers, [and] Devil-raisers' owed their powers to the sacrilegious magic of the Catholic church.[1] Bale was entirely typical among his Protestant contemporaries in regarding 'popery' as the source of witchcraft; and this accusation was thown back with enthusiasm by polemical writers on the other side of the religious divide, who associated the reformed faith with satanic delusions and identified Luther as the Devil's spawn.[2] In the same period, both Catholic and Protestant authorities viewed the more radical elements within the Reformation movement as a threat akin to witchcraft. As Luther himself noted in his Commentary on St Paul's letter to the Galatians, Anabaptists were 'sorcerers and authors of witchery', whose false teachings were 'a manifest sign that they are bewitched of the Devil'.[3]

Witchcraft continued to figure in denominational conflicts in a rather different way after the end of witch persecutions in the eighteenth century. As Stuart Clark notes in Chapter 12, Protestant and Catholic historians tried to attach blame for the 'witch craze' to their religious opponents. In a less adversarial fashion, Clark himself has provoked recent discussion among historians about the differences between Protestant and Catholic demonology in the 1990s. While accepting that both sides developed essentially similar views on the crime, he identifies differences 'of scope and accent' in the ways in which they dealt with it. In Clark's view, one notable difference concerned the options available to counter *maleficium*. While Catholics retained sanctified objects and practices to ward off the power of evil spirits, their Protestant counterparts were prevented by their theological views from employing such methods: there were no Protestant equivalents to holy water or the mass. On the contrary, such ritualism was regarded as positively harmful by the reformers, who viewed it as evidence of Satan's dominion in the Roman church. As a consequence, Protestant demonologists tended to emphasise divine providence and utterly reject the power of sacraments to overcome the Devil. Clark also suggests that the religious preoccupations of the two sides encouraged them to focus on different aspects of witchcraft. For Protestant writers, who were particularly concerned with the 'covenant' between the individual and God, the pact between witches and the Devil was paramount. On the other side, the Catholic respect for ritual encouraged a greater emphasis on the ceremonial desecrations associated with the sabbat.

As well as exploring the variations between Catholic and Protestant demonology, Clark considers the relationship between witch persecutions and the Reformation as a whole. He suggests that the eagerness of both parties to associate their opponents with witchcraft was an essential aspect of religious identification in early modern Europe: the charge of witchcraft 'identified what it was that was so offensive about enemy faiths, as well as evoking the sense of an unbridgeable distance between them. To *be* a Protestant or a Catholic was thus, in part, to have precisely this view of one's foes'. Since both sides identified witchcraft so closely with their opponents, their desire to eradicate the crime can be viewed as part of their wider religious agenda. The efforts to suppress popular magic in some Protestant states, for example, were an expression of the anti-Catholic zeal that motivated their ruling elites, since magic was intimately connected with the 'superstition' of the Roman church. At a deeper level, Clark argues that witchcraft made sense in the ideological context of the kind of 'state churches' that emerged in the Reformation era. The religious uniformity that these institutions demanded was challenged by the 'counter-institution' of the witch cult, with its own demonic priesthood and practices organised under the leadership of Satan. The idea of witchcraft was also an essential element in the moral system of a confessional state, since it offered a mirror-image to the positive values that it sought to enforce. For these reasons, Clark suggests that the fear of witchcraft was confined to the advocates of 'church-type' religious organisations: witchcraft lost its meaning in the context of 'sect-type' groups like the Anabaptists, since they had no desire to impose their beliefs on the whole community, and no need for a satanic anti-church to mirror their own endeavours.

Clark's work offers an exceptionally rich and nuanced interpretation of the relationship between witchcraft and the Reformation. Its implications are taken up, directly and indirectly, by the other two contributors to this section. In Chapter 13, Edmund Kern examines the career of Jacob Bithner, a Protestant witch finder in the Austrian province of Styria, where the Habsburg dukes were imposing a Catholic Reformation in the face of resistance from local Lutheran magnates. In his capacity as *Landprofos*, the official reponsible for keeping public order within the duchy, the Lutheran Jacob Bither was accountable to both the Catholic dukes and the Protestant estates. His career as a zealous prosecutor of witches, therefore, provides an illuminating case study of the difference between Protestant and Catholic perceptions of the crime in the region, and the relationship between witchcraft and the emergence of a 'state church'.

In many respects, Kern's study confirms the view of Protestant demonology set out by Clark. It appears that Bithner accepted the existence of the sabbat – and sometimes included it in charges against alleged witches – but he was much more concerned with the role of the Devil in the practice of magic. Like the English demonologist William Perkins, he made no distinction between supposedly demonic and non-demonic magic, and held the practitioners of both to be equally culpable. In his dealings with the Habsburg court, however, Bithner's career indicates that the prosecution of witchcraft did not always go hand in hand with the imposition of religious orthodoxy. Kern argues that the dukes and their agents were content to allow a Protestant *Landprofos* pursue a campaign against witchcraft in their territory, but they regarded the prosecution of witches as a lesser priority than the restoration of Catholicism. Where the two campaigns came into conflict, the authority of local officials was overruled. In one particularly striking example from 1599, the bishop of Seckau intervened to stop the prosecution of a Lutheran student at the University of Graz so that he could make a public conversion to Catholicism, despite the fact that he had apparently confessed to signing a demonic pact. As Kern concludes, such episodes imply that 'overcoming Protestantism merited more support' from the Habsburg authorities than the persecution of witches.

While Kern focuses on a 'church-type' Reformation, Chapter 14 by Gary K. Waite considers the relationship between witchcraft and the Anabaptists, the most successful of the 'sect-type' groups to emerge in the sixteenth century. Throughout Europe as a whole, some 3,000 Anabaptists were executed between 1520 and 1565 for actions that, Waite contends, resembled those attributed to witches. Both Anabaptists and witches were sent to the flames for renouncing their original baptism and pledging themselves to an alternative religious community; and in the eyes of their persecutors at least, both groups came under the leadership of the Devil. As Waite reminds us, 'it was often the same court officials who tried both sets of victims, sometimes conducting such seemingly distinct trials during the same week'. This parallel has some fascinating implications for witchcraft research. For a start, it suggests that witch trials were an aspect of the more general impulse to persecute unorthodox religious groups that arose during the Reformation. The chronology of the persecutions also raises important questions, since the most intense attacks on Anabaptism occurred *before* the second wave of European witch trials, during a relative lull in the prosecution of witches. It appears, therefore, that magistrates turned their attention away from the activity of religious sects to concentrate on the far greater threat of satanic witchcraft in the late sixteenth century. Viewed in this way, the attempt to eradicate witchcraft was an alternative to the persecution of heretics. Since witches were more numerous than groups like the Anabaptists, and their activities provoked popular hostility as well as official concern, it was also easier to sustain the attack on this new and more terrible strain of heresy.

The link between Anabaptism and witchcraft also relates to Clark's observations about 'church-type' religious organisations in early modern Europe. For Protestant and Catholic churches of this kind, the threat posed by witchcraft and religious sects was essentially the same: both challenged the 'universal dominion' claimed by the official faith, and served as a frightful but necessary mirror image of the values of orthodoxy. The fact that such groups were clandestine, and appeared to exist at the very heart of the God-fearing community, could only add to the horror that they aroused. The fear of an 'anti-church' is not hard to detect in the proceedings against Anabaptists in the early sixteenth century. In 1528, for example, the interrogators of Augustin Wurzlburger, a Regensburg schoolteacher, accused of belonging to the sect, asked him about 'the secret assemblies attended by him and his fellows', and wanted to know 'what signs they used to recognise one another'.[4] Similarly, Gary Waite notes that the threat of heresy in 1540s Netherlands was 'heightened to the level of a secret and dangerous conspiracy' with the ultimate aim of overthrowing Christianity. The parallels with witchcraft are obvious. Moreover, the fear of Anabaptism and witchcraft was perfectly understandable in a culture that equated Christianity with a church-type model of religious organisation.

What of the Anabaptists themselves? Clark suggests that the threat of witchcraft was largely irrelevant to members of such 'sect-type' religious groups, since they made no attempt to impose conformity on the population at large. As Waite's chapter shows, however, this did not mean that sectarians rejected the idea of a demonic conspiracy. On the contrary, they attributed their persecution and the false beliefs of their Catholic and Protestant adversaries to the inspiration of Satan. For Anabaptists and other separatist groups, the Devil's servants were not a secretive cult but the rulers of their own society. It was this conviction that underpinned the doctrine of social separation adopted by Swiss and German Anabaptists in the 1520s, and later expressed by separatist preachers like the Englishman John Canne, who declared in 1634 that Christians were 'a faithful people called and separated from the world and the false worship and the ways thereof'.[5] In this respect, the beliefs of sectarians can be viewed as a curious inversion of the demonology of their religious opponents: they held that the Devil-worshippers had already overthrown the public institutions of Christianity, and their best option was to isolate themselves from the witch-like practices that dominated the world.

Notes

1   John Bale, *The Lattre Examinacyon of Anne Askew, Lately Martyred in Smythfielde* (London 1547), 60r.

2   One early English example, entitled 'A little Treatise Confownding the Great Hereses that Rayge', presented Luther as a 'poisonous dragon' and Protestant doctrines as filth 'from the Devil'. Frederick J. Furnivall, ed., *Ballads From Manuscripts* (London 1868–72), vol. I, 282.

3   Alan Kors and Edward Peters, eds, *Witchcraft in Europe: A Documentary History* (University of Pennsylvania Press, Philadelphia 1972), 199.

4   The proceedings of Wurzlburger's trial are reproduced in Hans Hillerbrand, ed., *The Protestant Reformation* (Harper & Row, London 1968), 137–42.

5   John Canne, *A Necessitie of Separation From the Church of England* (Amsterdam 1634), 165.

Chapter 12

Stuart Clark

PROTESTANT WITCHCRAFT, CATHOLIC WITCHCRAFT

I N 1584 REGINALD SCOT CLAIMED that only the Catholic Church took the subject of witchcraft seriously; it was, he said, 'incomprehensible to the wise, learned or faithfull; a probable matter to children, fooles, melancholike persons and papists'. In effect, 'witchmongers' and 'massmongers' were one and the same thing, whereas the religion of the gospel could stand 'without such peevish trumperie'.[1] All the same, he was obliged to acknowledge the demonologies of leading Protestant theologians like Daneau and Hemmingsen, and he deplored the way in which the ordinary English clergy lent credibility to popular witchcraft beliefs by recognizing the existence of healers and conjurors in their parishes and making allegations against local witches. In 1653, after nearly seventy more years of active Protestant publishing on the subject, another English sceptic, Sir Robert Filmer, was in no doubt about the essential consensus across denominational lines.[2] This shift of emphasis has been mirrored in modern times. Like Scot, Georg Langin and Wilhelm Gottlieb Soldan (anti-Catholic) and Johann Diefenbach and Nikolaus Paulus (anti-Protestant) blamed the witch trials on their religious opponents.[3] In the more recent past, historians have tended to concur with Filmer. Trevor-Roper argued that the evangelists of all the major churches were equally involved, both at the level of actual prosecutions and in the elaboration of theory, a view in which he has been followed by Jean Delumeau.[4]

What difference, then, did confessional disagreements make to witchcraft beliefs? Was early modern demonology, whatever the faiths of its authors, simply the uniform expression of a new form of social control – what Christina Larner called 'Christian political ideology'? If we look at the fundamental ingredients of demonology, there does seem to be little to distinguish the Protestant from the Catholic formulations. The thought patterns and linguistic habits that governed representations of witchcraft stemmed from cosmological traditions, communication theories, and evaluative strategies that transcended religious difference. That difference, with all its bitter irreconcilability, vastly exaggerated the tendency to polarize and dichotomize, but this tendency was not in itself peculiar to any of the major religions. Concerning the causal mechanics of demonism – the limitations on the powers of devils to effect changes in the natural world and their consequent resort to illusion – there was total agreement between the faiths, grounded on a shared intellectual indebtedness to Augustine and Aquinas. On the general causation of witchcraft phenomena, Zanchy, Casmann, and Pettus Martyr spoke with the same voice as Torreblanca, Binsfeld, or Del Rio. The eschatological view that witchcraft flourished because the world was in a state of terminal decline was, likewise, as common among French Catholic authors such as Michaelis, Nodé, and Le Normant, as among the writers of Lutheran Germany and Calvinist England – in this case reflecting the popularity of apocalyptic history in both major Reformations.

Even when we arrive at religion itself there seems paradoxically little evidence of strong theological or pastoral preferences. The tendencies in 'Augustinian Europe' that turned *maleficium* into a case of conscience, made 'witches' of the churches' competitors, and cast 'superstition' as religion's greatest obstacle worked their intellectual effects irrespective of clerical allegiance. There were, however, differences of scope and accent. Historians have long recognized that it is not a 'Protestant' judgement to say that Catholic reformers could not deritualize conduct to the same extent as their rivals. Lorichius was as anxious as any to say that no time, place, person, number, gesture (or whatever) was intrinsically more significant than any other. Yet, like any Catholic, he invested more in extrinsic significance than Lutherans and, especially, Calvinists did. The Roman Church had to spend more time making distinctions between the use and abuse of its practices than others did, as the pages dedicated by Lorichius to Catholic superstitions testify.[5]

For their part, Protestants simply did not have some of the doctrinal commitments that, like the belief in purgatory and the invocation of saints, gave ancillary encouragement to spirit activity. While allowing that there was no essentially Protestant doctrine of witchcraft, William Monter has also suggested that nearly all Protestant writers on the subject 'insisted on a few common elements', above all, the extent of divine power and providence.[6] Larner, too, while arguing that the different types of theological position prevalent in seventeenth-century Scotland are less important than the introduction of Christianity itself, provides for a theological emphasis on God's rewarding of sin with earthly punishments.[7] If it is not the case that Protestant authors dealt with themes that found no place in the Catholic literature, they nevertheless seem to have dealt with them to the neglect or exclusion of other elements in witchcraft beliefs, notably those concerning the sabbat and the other sensational aspects of demonism like metamorphosis and sexuality. As Teall again remarked, without either canon law or scholastic theology, Protestants' views about witchcraft 'rested on narrower foundations' than did those of the Catholics.[8] This preoccupation may be traced partly to the characteristic stresses in Protestant theology, particularly 'theocentricity' and anthropological pessimism. Covenant theory, likewise, gave extra inversionary meaning to the demonic pact, especially in its implicit form. Protestant biblicism provided little or no help on the subject of sabbats, but its influence over interpretations of witchcraft as a spiritual and moral problem could be total. Besides, the sabbat, with its pronounced anti-ritualism, was of much greater significance to Catholics. But probably the most important reason was that the typical Protestant author was more likely to be involved first-hand in clerical practice – indeed, he was usually a pastor with a flock, rather than an academic theologian with a student audience – and, therefore, more interested in the evangelical and homiletic aspects of witchcraft, than the theoretical and intellectual.

These qualifications apart, it remains difficult – with one important exception – to trace in demonology any serious repercussions of the doctrinally most divisive issues of the reform era – *sola scriptura, sola fide,* and so on. That the things that defined witchcraft for clerics were the things they largely agreed on is borne out by its universal placement in the Decalogue as a sin against the first Commandment. How to relate Old Testament and gospel, works and faith, sinning and salvation, could not have been more controversial; but that the Law was an indispensable element in such calculations was presupposed by all. However theology coped with it, and wherever it was placed in the catechism, it provided the essential benchmarks of human depravity. Although, too, the circumstances in which the individual sin of idolatry occurred might be hotly contested – above all, in connection with images – idolatry itself was a transgression that no Christian could do without. The aspects of doctrine and worship that underpinned it, notably the stress on a providential divinity who required total and undivided loyalty, were incontestable and, thus, shared. Elaborations of the first Commandment in Protestant and Catholic catechisms dealt, accordingly, with the same arguments, while those matters that did divide catechists on denominational lines did not – if the case of the Trent catechism and the evidence from France are typical – impinge on their understanding of witchcraft.

It therefore looks very much as though the history of demonology conforms to what reinterpreters of early modern religious change have, in the wake of Delumeau, been telling us – that the two major Reformations had so much in common that their similarities are more significant than their differences. Delumeau's own celebrated proposal was that, despite their doctrinal and liturgical rivalries, Protestants and Catholics were jointly attempting to 'Christianize' the average westerner.[9] In his own judgements about the state of the average westerner's religion before the reformers got hold of it, as well as their success or failure when they did, Delumeau was vulnerable to criticism. But there is scarcely any doubt that 'Christianizing' was what reformers of all the major churches *thought* they were doing, and that what they meant by this was, in part, the spiritualization of misfortune, the abolition of magic, and the discrediting and eradication of a wide range of popular cultural forms as superstitions. Seen in this light, demonology comes to have a crucial bearing on the impetus to reform, while evangelism makes better sense of clerical hostility to witchcraft. What was reflected in many witchcraft prosecutions, it has been claimed, was not so much the differences between the religions involved (or any inter-sectarian strife) as their common missionary determination to impose the fundamentals of Christian belief and practice on ordinary people. This is a principle that has been put to work in the cases of Calvinist Scotland, the Catholic Netherlands and north-east of France, the duchy of Luxembourg, Hungary, and the areas covered by the Mediterranean Inquisitions. It also applies well to the circumstances of the witch trials in the Catholic ecclesiastical territories of Bamberg and Würzburg.

The one exception to this all-party consensus lay in the area of remedies against witchcraft and against demonism in general. If ordinary people, fearing bewitchment, were not to counteract it by resorting to 'magic' and 'superstition', or rely solely on the lawcourts, how should they respond? Writers of all denominations agreed that they should appeal to the spiritual and moral protections of the Church (as well as to allowable medicine) and often concluded their discussions by listing the permissible alternatives and giving advice. But there could be little agreement across the churches about what specific remedies to list, given that Lutherans and Calvinists had removed entire areas of the traditional therapeutic repertoire. A Jesuit like Maldonado could offer these typical 'ecclesiastical' protections: exorcism, the name of Christ, the sign of the cross, saints' relics, reciting the Creed, fasting and prayer, the eucharist, holy water, and the word of God.[10] But by then, patently, no Protestant could possibly expect to ward off *maleficium* with relics or holy water, and Catholics too had to pay attention to their correct significance when using them. The remedies against demons and witchcraft were the same as the responses to any spiritual threat or physical misfortune, but these changed in nature and number according to which church was recommending them. This would seem too obvious a point to make, if it were not for the great importance of what was on offer to the central debates of Reformation history. This was so highly contentious an area because it lay at the very heart of what divided the faiths. Any witchcraft writer who prescribed an 'ecclesiastical' remedy involved himself necessarily in this wider polemic at least tacitly, and many took the opportunity to make a vigorous contribution to it. Thus discussions of the purely spiritual remedies offered by Protestantism not only defended the efficacy of faith, the Word, prayer, fasting, and vigils; they very often turned into denunciations of Catholic 'idolatry' and 'superstition'.

From 1564 onwards pronouncements in this area were naturally influenced by the canons and decrees of the Council of Trent. Benoist's advice for avoiding the effects of sorcery and demonism was clearly inspired by its measures for parochial discipline; he said one should attend mass on Sundays and feast days in the local church, not elsewhere, and hear the full version, not the low mass or one heard privately. A typical post-Trent specialist was Bishop Forner of Bamberg, who devoted twenty-two of his thirty-five witchcraft sermons to the pieces of spiritual armour that would protect Catholics from the Devil's assaults. All seven sacraments are there, plus some of the Church's sacramentals – benedictions (of holy water, salt, wine, oil, bells, etc.), exorcisms, and so on. Excluding those that Protestants too would have accepted, such as faith, trust in God, fasting and prayer, and renunciation of the Devil, Forner also offered devout invocation of the names of Christ and the Virgin, the protection of a guardian angel, saints and their relics, the sign of the cross, and the use of *Agnes Dei* and amulets made of the scriptures. The items were virtually the same (but there were only five of the sacraments) in the second of Crespet's *Deux Livres*, where he considered ways to resist the Devil's 'interior' assaults. Both authors were, in effect, writing essays in orthodox Counter-Reformation spirituality. For the most part they cite supporting testimonies and episodes from the history of each vehicle of grace or aid to piety. But they were also fashioning propaganda against the Church's enemies – heretics who denied the validity of its rites but whose own versions were powerless against devils. The evidence regarding the sign of the cross, for example, was sufficient, in Forner's eyes, 'to refute the unbelieving Calvinists, enemies of the truth'; the power of the eucharist in cases of demonic possession had already won over many of them.[11] According to the highly partisan demonology of Crespet, 'all the heresies, atheisms, enchantments, scandals, and vices that reign in France arise from nowhere else than the scorn that is shown for the Holy Sacrament and for the victorious Cross'.[12]

The case of remedies apart, the dominance of demonology by Decalogue theology meant that serious confessional divergence was only able to arise when idolatry – in the form of witchcraft, magic, or superstition – was detected in the beliefs or observances of a religious competitor. Agreeing, for the most part, on what witchcraft was, Protestants and Catholics were still free to identify it in each other's church – indeed, not only free but desperately eager. This is another feature of early modern religious life that might seem almost too obvious to deserve record. Without doubt, much of what was said was sloganizing and name-calling, but it was so widespread, so endemic in the discourse of religious difference, that it must be seen as constitutive of what opponents thought of each other, and not merely a decorative addition. However unthinking and repetitive, the surface of polemical invective usually reveals deeper meanings. Calling each other 'witches' helped religious enemies just to vent their anger and hatred but it also identified what it was that was so offensive about enemy faiths, as well as evoking the sense of an unbridgeable distance between them. To *be* a Protestant or a Catholic was thus, in part, to have precisely this view of one's foes.

In this sense, the greater currency given to conceptions of witchcraft by contemporary prosecutions for the crime undoubtedly influenced both the character and the intensity of confessionalization. Influences in the other direction are more elusive. Historians of the witch trials have found it difficult to substantiate Trevor-Roper's assertion that they resulted directly from mutual accusations of witchcraft between Protestant and Catholic communities, usually in situations of conflict and crusade. To the extent that accusations and prosecutions reflected reforming zeal, this may well have been the zeal to eradicate what was seen as laypeople's irreligion, rather than the errors of other Christians. It will be clear from what has gone before that the texts, at least, paid a great deal of attention to this sort of reformation, and less to straightforward interconfessional denunciation. On the other hand, acculturation also appealed precisely because true churches naturally wanted all the recruits they could win over. The obstacles to the godly society – the very need for it – could be blamed on false churches and the demons they served. Recalcitrant individuals who failed to respond could thus be demonized as 'witches' not because of any strict confessional allegiance but through a looser association of errors.[13]

Even so, there were countless depictions by adherents of each major faith of the 'witchcraft' inherent in the other, and these were reflected in demonological writings. Protestant propaganda to this effect in England is familiar from Keith Thomas's *Religion and the Decline of Magic* and the historian of its continental equivalents need only extrapolate from his findings. Religious reformers from the Lollards onwards asserted that Catholicism was inherently magical since many of its rituals relied on securing material effects from non-material causes – blessings, exorcisms, hallowings, and the like. These were attempts to endow physical things with powers beyond their natural capacities and, since they were spurious in this way, they fell into the category of tacitly demonic operations. All the church's *sacramentalia* were obviously vulnerable to such an attack, but so too was transubstantiation itself, which in many denunciations became a 'conjuration' and an 'enchantment'. Catholic priests were no better than magicians, sorcerers, and witches, it was repeatedly said. In this spirit, the liturgy of the reformed church in England was purged of its 'superstitious' and 'magical' elements, though never with sufficient rigour to prevent further attacks from ever more radical critics. 'By the end of the sixteenth century,' writes Thomas, 'there was substantial acceptance for the extreme Protestant view that no mere ceremony could have any material efficacy, and that divine grace could not be conjured or coerced by any human formula'.[14]

English witchcraft authors plainly shared these views and, since many of them were of 'puritan' persuasion they tended to express them forthrightly. Henry Holland (citing Hemmingsen) compared Catholic to 'heathen' magic, saint-worship to Devil-worship, and the sign of the cross to witchcraft by 'characters'.[15] For him, the 'witches' of Rome were 'more wicked then the Heathen Witches, for these abuse the Worde and Sacramentes of God'. Thomas Pickering introduced the 1610 edition of Perkins's *Discourse* by pointing out that the miracles associated with saints and their relics were 'but meere Satanicall wonders', while Perkins himself said they were 'Satanicall impostures' wrought by sensory delusion, that Catholic exorcisms were 'meere inchantements', and that the sign of the cross 'carrieth the very nature of a Charme, and the use of it in this manner, a practise of Inchantment'.[16] For Bernard, it was natural that among people most likely to blame witches for misfortune were the 'popishly affected' and among those most likely to become witches were the 'superstitious and idolatrous, as all Papists be'; after all, sorcery was 'the practice of that Whore, the Romish Synagogue', and devils could be relied on to teach popery during exorcisms.[17] Later, John Gaule repeated again the view that witches were more common in societies with 'superstitious' religions, notably Catholicism.[18] This was one of the refrains of English witchcraft theory, underlined by the universal association of Catholicism with the Antichrist, and by the conviction that the strengths of the true religion and of magic varied in inverse proportion. All would have agreed with the Welshman Charles Edwards, who remarked that since the faith was repaired even the fairies (which he took to be familiar demons) were not so bold as they had been in the time of the Papacy: 'It is a sign of the dawn of evangelical day', he wrote, 'when the insects of darkness went into hiding'.[19]

Continental parallels (indeed, sources) for these Protestant attributions of witchcraft to Catholicism are likewise abundant. The Tübingen theologian Heerbrand, for example, called Catholic rituals 'nothing but truly diabolical, ungodly, and magical blasphemies'.[20] Ellinger likened Catholic baptism to demonic magic, both of them relying spuriously on an intrinsic power in words, and the same objection could obviously be brought against the text of the mass.[21] In Denmark, Hemmingsen wrote of the supplanting of the 'diabolical impostures' of Rome by the true faith and of the Devil transfering his attention to countryside magicians instead.[22] It was widely alleged that several mediaeval Popes had practised magic and that the Jesuits were likewise magicians and witches. The assumption that the Pope was the Antichrist also cemented Catholicism's connection with the black arts. That it was the quintessence of superstition was a view so general to Protestant cultures that it ranks as the merest of commonplaces in the history of early modern religion. But it helped witchcraft authors too to explain away the centuries of darkness and error and to defend the need for radical change. Equally prevalent, of course, was the association of superstition with demonism.

In essence, therefore, the Protestant accusation that Catholicism was a religion based on witchcraft arose from questioning the sense in which specific religious rituals could be said to be efficacious. Catholics returned the accusation but not by raising the same questions about the rituals of their enemies. Instead, they took a long view of the church militant and argued that, from the example of Simon Magus onwards, heresy had always been intimately associated with magic. Theirs was an argument based on a simple dualism between God's true church and the Devil's false versions, backed up by a reading of history. That the mediaeval Church did indeed link heresy with demonism, that heretics were accused of crimes with close similarities to witchcraft, and that the first 'new' witches of the fourteenth century were assimilated to the 'old' heretics of the twelfth and thirteenth, are all commonplaces of modern scholarship and there is no need to rehearse them again here. The main point is that, for the Catholic controversialists of the post-Lutheran era, Protestant 'witches' were only the latest in a long series of demonic threats to the faith. It seemed, moreover, that the things that Protestants denied in Catholicism were precisely the things that were rejected, parodied, ridiculed, or otherwise subverted by witches – the Virgin, the saints, the sign of the cross, and so on. This was yet further evidence of the closeness of their alliance and not, as we might read it, of the working out of a particular representational and symbolic pattern.

A classic example of this polemic was the oration 'Cur magia pariter cum haeresi hodie creverit' given at a graduation ceremony at Louvain on 30 August 1594 by the English professor of theology, Thomas Stapleton. Deploring the practice of witchcraft in every part of Europe, Stapleton argued that this was a natural accompaniment to the equal spread of heresy, given the intimate links between the two. They had the same demonic origins, of course, but were also inspired by the same motives, notably 'carnal desire', hatred of authority, and curiosity, and they appealed to the same kinds of dissidents and waverers. The true faith was denied in both cases, at first in small matters, but eventually in essentials, leading to the systematic flouting of all the Church's laws and ceremonies. Moreover, heresy and magic were intrinsically connected:

> just as the wonderful effects of the magic art cannot themselves be attributed either to the magicians' own intelligence or to the artefacts they use, such as figures, images, and incantations, but are produced by a different intelligence, by the Devil himself, and only he does everything . . . so today the leading astray of the people by heretics does not happen because of the learning, eloquence, cunning, or wickedness of the heretics themselves, but through that same Satan whose servants they are and who works through them.

Magicians and witches, like heretics, were deceptive and difficult to discern, their threat to orthodoxy not always being acknowledged. They were betrayed by their use of superfluous, 'ceremonial' efficacies (magic) or by superfluous and novel doctrines (heretics).[23]

Five years after Stapleton, Del Rio opened the first Louvain edition of his massive demonology with an equally trenchant version, borrowed from another Jesuit, whose lectures he had attended in Paris, Juan Maldonado. Magic and heresy had been inseparable since Simon Magus, and the Hussite, Waldensian, and Lutheran movements had each seen an increase in witchcraft. According to Del Rio, most of those who had recently confessed to the crime in Trier had admitted to being 'infected' by demonism as a result of the spread of Lutheranism. England, Scotland, France, and Flanders had been poisoned with the same venoms by Calvinism, but magic would always follow heretics because demons 'inhabited' them, just as they had worked the pagan idols, and used them like courtesans to deceive men, because heresy aped the magic arts and led to 'curiosity' in knowledge, and because of the negligence of churchmen.[24]

The French Counter-Reformation witchcraft authors Nodé, Crespet, Massé, Michaelis, and Boucher were especially vocal in their denunciations of the 'witches' who had overrun the Protestant territories in Germany and the British Isles and were threatening France. Their whole view of witchcraft was premised on a historiography of heresy seen as the continuous expression of demonism.[25] Nodé, for example, traced it to the later mediaeval heresies, in particular to Hus, Wyclif, and Luther, and feared a future alliance between witches and Huguenots.[26] All the mediaeval heresies, said Massé, had had links with the magic arts, and the Anabaptists' resort to prophecy by divination was only a further example (this did not stop him calculating numerologically that Luther, Karlstadt, Zwingli, Oecolampadius, and Calvin were all part of the Antichrist).[27] Michaelis complained that the Genevan authorities neglected the laws against witchcraft but added that he was not surprised by this: 'for besides their rage in depressing as much as in them lies the honour of God and his Saints . . . they have the property that all Hereticks naturally have, to love Magicians and Sorcerers'.[28]

Throughout Europe, indeed, Catholics could link the flourishing of witchcraft to the prevalence of the new heresies. In this way, witch-*hating* was certainly influenced and exacerbated by confession-hating, even if (so-called) witch-*hunting* resulted from additional, more complex, and, indeed, earlier circumstances. To the extent that counter-reforming was seen as a sectarian as well as an evangelical process – entailing the obliteration of the enemy faiths as well as the improving of lay piety – anti-witchcraft legislation could be presented as one of its key ingredients. This was the argument of one of the most influential proclamations, the Ordinance of 1592 issued by the Viceroys of the Spanish Netherlands in the name of Philip II. In this sense, it is not the case that the disputes of the Reformation era had no major impact on the history of witchcraft. Actual prosecutions, in reflecting, say, Protestant zeal, were reflecting what that zeal meant, and it meant anti-Catholicism; thus, witch-hunting could have been directed against things that were defined in terms of their anti-Catholicism, even if it was not necessarily directed against Catholic individuals. The same was true, presumably, for Catholic zeal. Stapleton demanded equal detestation of magic and heresy from his audience; for him, an age of religious reform must, of necessity, be an age of anti-magic and vice versa:

> For such is the affinity between them, being related in so many different
> ways . . . that there is not a Christian who does not fight against the

outrages of heresy and magic with the same hatred, and dread them with equal detestation. Just as to have dealings with magicians and witches, and to make peace with them, is abhorrent to all Christians, so the same commerce with heretics is to be rejected. Just as we imprison magicians by public authority, expel them from the community, and inflict terrible punishments on them, so we must take the same pains and use the same force against heretics. Just as the arts of magic, and their professors and books, cannot be suffered among Christians and are destroyed by sword and fire, so the same is decreed for heretics.[29]

In some respects, it has proved fruitful to look for the interesting differences concerning witchcraft within, rather than between, the major faiths – matching the suggestion that both were divided internally by similar doctrinal disputes. It was Erik Midelfort's argument, for example, that during the sixteenth century all three confessional groups in south-western Germany were split internally between those who took a strongly 'providential' and, thus, moderating view of the crime, and those who adopted a more 'fearful' and punitive perspective in the manner of the *Malleus Maleficarum*. This was not a question of confessional commitment but of how far men of religion were prepared to spiritualize human experience by raising its significance beyond the plane where physical harms by witches and devils and physical punishments and remedies against them mattered most.

Ultimately, however, the religious reasons for taking witchcraft seriously or not can be related to differences between what (following Ernst Troeltsch) we might call the 'church-type' and the 'sect-type' churches of early modern Europe. Atheists, libertines, and other 'unbelievers' who (when they existed at all) recognized no religion and no church were, presumably, not touched by any demonology either. But church members had very divergent social doctrines, moralities, and even theologies, depending on the type of organization to which they belonged, and these were reflected in their views about religious deviance. For Troeltsch (writing in 1912) a 'Church' was, in principle, universal, because its aim was 'to cover the whole life of humanity'; compulsory, because it tried to impose its values and institutions on all the members of a society; and conservative, because it embraced and became integral to the secular order and reinforced that order's social and political hierarchies. He spoke of it utilizing and interweaving with the state and its ruling classes and becoming dependent on them. 'Sects', on the other hand, were highly selective, always voluntary, and usually radical. They:

aspire after personal inward perfection, and they aim at a direct personal fellowship between the members of each group. From the very beginning, therefore, they are forced to organize themselves in small groups, and to renounce the idea of dominating the world. Their attitude towards the world, the State, and Society may be indifferent, tolerant, or hostile, since they have no desire to control and incorporate these forms of social life; on the contrary, they tend to avoid them; their aim is usually either to tolerate their presence alongside of their own body, or even to replace these social institutions by their own society.[30]

The Church, moreover, controls access to the supernatural by associating it with ecclesiastical conformity, channelling asceticism into the achievements of a heroic class of monastics, and monopolizing the means to salvation; for the Sects, on the other hand, the supernatural is directly available to the individual through the personal asceticism of detaching from the world and (for example) refusing 'to use the law, to swear in a court of justice, to own property, to exercise dominion over others, or to take part in war'. The Church is sacerdotal and sacramental, claiming a monopoly of truth and power and the right to supervise faith and punish heresy. The typical characteristics of the Sect, in contrast, are:

> lay Christianity, personal achievement in ethics and in religion, the radical fellowship of love, religious equality and brotherly love, indifference towards the authority of the State and the ruling classes, dislike of technical law and of the oath, the separation of the religious life from the economic struggle by means of the ideal of poverty and frugality, or occasionally in a charity which becomes communism, the directness of the personal religious relationship, criticism of official spiritual guides and theologians, the appeal to the New Testament and to the Primitive Church.[31]

This is an ideal-typical distinction, of course, but its relevance to the history of witchcraft is that it suggests a further important differential in the very meaning of the crime. In the context of church-type religious organizations – in effect, 'state churches' – witchcraft was a serious counter-institutional competitor for the allegiance of potentially all Christians. Its significance lay precisely in the challenge it posed to universal domination, and the magistrate must play a part in stamping it out. The powers of the Devil threatened directly the miraculous basis of church-type authority and had to be carefully downgraded to the status of mere wonders. The witch was the apparent rival of the official priesthood, whether professionally as purveyor of alternative therapies, or sacramentally as perverter of the vehicles and signs of grace. The ceremonies of the sabbat were invariably the inverse of required liturgical norms, and its entire mood was in direct contravention of a church-type asceticism based on what Troeltsch called 'the repression of the senses'. Superstition was always tied to conceptions of true religion as a public and official cult. At the same time, the Devil, hell with its terrors, and witchcraft itself were all contributors to the moral systems of the state churches and, in some respects, indispensable to their functioning. They provided the mirror-images of their positive equivalents, and they were sanctions against sinning. Punishing demonism and witchcraft made a valuable statement about collective orthodoxy and its enforcement. In every way, then, the witchcraft found in traditional demonology was an ecclesiastical crime, and the fact that it allegedly flourished among the laity was an affront to religious evangelism. Its very significance was relative to the expectations of church-type Christians.

Transferred into the realm of the sects, witchcraft presumably lost all these terrors. Detached from claims to monopoly and inclusivity, religious deviance takes on altogether different connotations. Sects that turned their backs on the world and its institutions could not have treated religious apostasy either as a threat to ecclesiastical unity or as a token of social and political disorder. Since secular magistracy had no relevance to church affairs whatsoever, there was no transfer to be made from the spiritual to the political meanings of witchcraft. In eschewing worldly values and morality, they were necessarily emptying many of witchcraft's perversions of their meaning, as well as abandoning the punitive legalism that fuelled witch trials. Alienation from the world entailed the irrelevance of that world's perceived foes. If the orthodox state church was degenerate, then its claim to be environed with demonic enemies lost its force. To reject the sacramental channels of grace and their priestly administrators was simultaneously to redefine things like blasphemy and profanity and remove competition altogether from religious service. To give up evangelism and 'magisterial' dogma was, likewise, to abandon official correctness as a test of faith. 'The individualism of the sect', wrote Troeltsch, 'urges it towards the direct intercourse of the individual with God'; at the same time, an ideal of religious fellowship holds the group together in brotherly association. Its ethic is that of the gospel rather than the Law – the Sermon on the Mount rather than the Decalogue – and its spirituality is highly personal and subjective. None of this, it seems, would have accommodated traditional fears of witchcraft. One can imagine the Devil acting as instigator of malice between sect-type Christians, in which case the 'witches' among them would have been disciplined, eventually by exclusion from the elect group, like any other evildoers. But with their ideals of fellowship and their programmes of mutual support, sectarian communities were less prone to the interpersonal disputes that lay behind traditional witchcraft accusations. And in any case, the Devil was much more likely to be seen as a spiritual opponent, making 'witchcraft' no more than an inward obstacle to personal achievement and 'hell' a name for its whereabouts in the soul.

The views of the early modern sectaries concerning witchcraft are a neglected subject. The history of radical religious groups in Germany, Switzerland, and the Netherlands certainly bears out much of Troeltsch's typology of sect-type churches, and makes it clear that they often took up doctrinal and moral positions that were, in principle, inimical to traditional demonology.[32] These included the abandonment of the idea of territorial reform, the rejection of magistracy and capital punishment in religious affairs, pacifism, confessional toleration, perfectionism and mysticism, and psychopannychism or mortalism (the doctrine of the sleep or death of the soul prior to the resurrection). Sectaries and mystics were much more likely than orthodox witchcraft theorists to prefer figurative to literal readings of biblical texts. One historian of the Anabaptists speaks of their indifference to theology.[33] It is also difficult to see how they could have equated witchcraft with heresy. Advocates of witchcraft prosecution did sometimes say that reluctance to invoke a secular punishment for the crime was an 'anabaptist' error. Only their intense eschatology linked the sect-type churches to their magisterial competitors, and, even here, spiritualized readings of the last times tended to predominate over the literal ones required for serious witch-hating. It is somehow indicative that Thomas Müntzer should have preached that Exodus 22:18 was to be rendered as 'Thou shall not suffer evildoers to live', and that Giacomo Aconcio's *Stratagematum Satanae* (1555) treated the Devil in entirely symbolic terms as the motivator of religious discord.[34] No doubt accused of witchcraft (amongst other crimes) by their many enemies, the radicals may well prove to be the least 'demonological' of all the religious groups of the age.

This seems to have been the case with the Netherlands Anabaptists and spiritualists of the sixteenth century, of whom the most renowned, David Joris of Delft, taught that original sin was an inner (and thus reversible) process, that the Devil was merely the fallen nature of each individual, and that witchcraft was 'nothing'.[35] Among the Dutch witchcraft writers of the next century, it was the Mennonites Jan Jansz Deutel, Antonius van Dale, and Abraham Palingh who initiated the most sceptical arguments, adopting a strict spiritualism and providentialism that eclipsed demonic physical activity altogether and made the idea of the witches' pact untenable. Mennonites were also active among the Collegiants, a radical religious movement that drew on Dutch Arminianism and Cartesian philosophy, and, after decades of exploring spiritualism, free prophecy, and other undogmatic and nonexclusive forms of piety, took Bekker's arguments further than even he had taken them by arguing against the activities of good as well as evil spirits.[36] It is known that Johann Weyer corresponded with his youngest brother, Matthias, a spiritualist and mystic, concerning the ideas of Menno Simons's associate, Dirck Philips, and those of the founder of the Family of Love, Hendrick Niclaes, both of whose works Johann had evidently been reading. Whether their radical theologies were consistent with his own heavy reliance on the Devil as a physical agent must, however, be doubted.

In England, too, it was the sectaries of the 1640s and 1650s, together with their clandestine predecessors, who were associated with the kind of radical anti-Calvinism that rejected a physical hell and physical devils. The symbolic location of hell in the hearts of men and women was suggested by, or attributed to, the Familists, John Everard, the 'ranter' pamphleteers Jacob Bauthumley and Lawrence Clarkson, and the 'digger' prophet Gerrard Winstanley.[37] Much of the mystical recategorization that went on in 'ranter' literature was directed specifically against those traditional religious polarities that sustained orthodox witchcraft beliefs, but which 'ranters' wanted to transcend. Robert Norwood, for example, explicitly rejected the notion of *concordia discors* in favour of the view that the creation was composed of 'Severalls, or Divers'. Dualisms may still have been prevalent in radical religious writing but the urge to resolve them spiritually turned them into aspects of the unregenerate world.[38] It was in order to spiritualize the Devil and witchcraft, and to defend mortalism, that Lodowick Muggleton published a 'true interpretation' of the witch of Endor story in 1669. 'There is no other Devil', he wrote, 'or spirit, or familiar spirit for witches to deal withal, or to work any enchantments by, but their own imagination'.[39] In giving the Devil only a symbolic existence, the religious sects encouraged the view that was also central to witchcraft scepticism, that his role in human affairs could never take a material form.

Of great significance, in this respect, is the evidence linking the two most effective witchcraft sceptics in England with religious radicalism. In the case of Reginald Scot, this takes the form of an association with Abraham Fleming, whose theology was similar to Scot's but whose *Diamond of Devotion* has suggested to David Wootton contacts with Elizabethan Familism. Among alleged Familist beliefs was the usual view of the spiritualists, but also the view of Scot, that the witches and devils in scripture should be treated metaphorically. Moreover, in the 1665 edition of *The discoverie of witchcraft* a further anonymous treatise was added as 'book 2' to Scot's own supplementary 'Discourse of divels and spirits', containing arguments presumably felt to complement those in the original text but derived from the radical theology of the 1650s. Amongst them was the reduction of demonic activity to mental operations internal to the 'hell' that was the state of mind of evil persons.[40]

John Webster was a Grindletonian in the 1630s and later an anabaptist and seeker. There were important elements of Behmenism, perfectionism, and antino-mianism in his sermons and writings, and his eschatology was non-literal. In 1653 he preached that 'in the Day that the Soul turns to the Lord, then . . . that hell men so much talk of, he sees to be really in himself, and that himself is the very Image of the Devil'. 'Antichrist' and 'witches' were also thought to be external deceivers, he said on another occasion, but 'however man is carried out to look for all these things without him, yet be sure these Sorcerers, these Wizzards, these Necromancers . . . Devils, Antichrists, all are in thine own bosome. Here is the true Necromancy and Witchcraft, the true Antichrist'. By 1677, when Webster published *The displaying of supposed witchcraft,* he was conforming and had given up active radicalism. But he was still deploying this earlier theology, and nowhere more so than in his insistence that the only way to talk about a demonic pact was in purely 'mental' and 'spiritual', not 'visible' or 'corporeal' terms.[41]

As in Continental Europe, the religious radicals of mid-seventeenth-century England were accused of weakening witchcraft belief – in this case, by Restoration Anglicans. There were even occasions when the labelling processes at work in tradi-tional witchcraft beliefs were thrown into reverse. When Winstanley called the clergy 'witches' and said that their interests were demonic, was he not turning round a field of force that, for half a century, had led zealots like George Gifford and Arthur Dent to reject popular culture as implicit, if not explicit, sorcery? One of the most extraordinary things about Winstanley's extraordinary book, *The law of freedom in a platform* (1652), is that he *retains* the death penalty for witchcraft but defines a witch as 'He who professes the service of a righteous God by preaching and prayer'.[42] This is not to escape completely from the mentality of witch-hunting, but it does demonstrate vividly the rejection by the unorthodox of the church-type religiosity of those who usually promoted it. One of the reasons, we may suppose, for the decline of witchcraft prosecutions and of witchcraft beliefs in general was the coming of a religious pluralism that permitted the members of all types of churches to coexist and spelt the end of the confessional state.

Notes

1   Reginald Scot, *The Discoverie of Witchcraft* (London 1584), quotations at 472 and sig. Biv, see also sig. Biiv and 4–6.

2   [Robert Filmer], *An Advertisement to the Jury-Men of England* (London 1653), 3.

3   Georg Langin, *Religion und Hexenprozess* (Leipzig 1888); Wilhelm Gottlieb Soldan, *Geschichte der Hexenprozesse,* ed. Max Bauer, 2 vols (Munich 1912); Johann Diefenbach, *Der Hexenwahn vor und nach der Glaubensspaltung in Deutschland* (Mainz 1886).

4   H. R. Trevor-Roper, *The European Witch-Craze* (Harmondsworth 1969), 64–7, 72–3; J. Delumeau, *La Peur en Occident* (Paris 1978), 359–60.

5   Jodocus Lorichius, *Aberglaub* (Freiburg 1593), 30–2, 43–93.

6   E. W. Monter, *Ritual, Myth and Magic in Early Modern Europe* (Brighton 1983), 31.

7   For Christina Larner's argument on this point, see Chapter 15 in this book.

8   J. L. Teall, 'Witchcraft and Calvinism in Elizabethan England', *Journal of the History of Ideas*, 23 (1962), 28–9.

9   J. Delumeau, *Catholicism between Luther and Voltaire*, trans. J. Mosiser (London 1977), 161.

10   Juan Maldonado, *Traicte des Anges et Demons* (Paris 1605), fos 232v-42v.

11   Friedrich Forner, *Panoplia Armaturae Dei* (Ingolstadt 1625), 254, 172–3.

12   Pierre Crespet, *Deux Livres* (Paris 1590), fo. 408v, see also 390v, 396–7r, 403v-4v.

13   For valuable cautions regarding the complex interrelationship between religious change and witchcraft prosecutions, see Robin Briggs, *Communities of Belief: Cultural and Social Tensions in Early Modern France* (Oxford 1989), 395–7. The possible impact of the Reformation on witch-hunting is discussed by Levack, *The Witch-Hunt in Early Modern Europe* (London 1987), 93–115.

14   Keith Thomas, *Religion and the Decline of Magic* (London 1971), 51–77, gives many illustrations.

15   Henry Holland, *A Treatise Against Witchcraft* (Cambridge 1590), sig. E1 r; see also B1 r-v.

16   William Perkins, *A Discourse of the Damned Art of Witchcraft* (Cambridge 1610), 'Epistle Dedicatorie', 25–6, 150, 152.

17   Richard Bernard, *A Guide to Grand-Jury men* (London 1630), 73–4, 95–7.

18   John Gaule, *Select Cases of Conscience* (London 1646), 16–17.

19   Charles Edwards, *Hanes y Ffydd Ddiffuant* (*History of the Unfeigned Faith*), facs of 3rd edn of 1677, ed. G. Williams (Cardiff 1936), 238 (trans. kindly provided by Prys Morgan).

20   Jacob Heerbrand, *De Magia* (Tubingen 1570), 13–15, quotation at 15; other examples from the German south-west in H. C. E. Middlefort, *Witch Hunting in Southwestern Germany* (Stanford, Calif. 1972), 63.

21   Johann Ellinger, *Hexen Coppel* (Frankfurt 1629), 6–11.

22   Niels Hemmingsen, *Admonitio* (Wittenberg 1564), sigs F1v-F3r.

23   Thomas Stapleton, 'Cur magia pariter cum haeresi hodie creverit', in *Orationes Academicae Miscellaneae Triginta Quatuor* (4 vols; Paris 1620), ii, 502–7 (quotation at 505).

24   M. Del Rio, *Disquisitionum Magicarum* (Lyons 1608), 'Proloquium'.

25   J. Pearl, 'French Catholic Demonologists', *Church History*, 52 (1983), 457–67. For the conflation, in French Catholicism, of Protestant heresy with witchcraft, see A. N. Galpern, *The Religions of the People* (Cambridge, Mass. 1976), 157–8; P. Benedict, 'The Catholic Response to Protestantism', in J. Obelkevich, ed., *Religion and the People* (Chapel Hill, NC 1979), 174, n. 22 (p. 307) on the pronouncements of the provincial council of the dioceses of Normandy at Rouen in 1581.

26   Pierre Nodé, *Declamation* (Paris 1578), 58–66, see also 8–10.

27   Pierre Massé, *De L'Imposture* (Paris 1579), fos 111r-20v.

28   Sebastien Michaelis, *Pneumology, or Discourse of Spirits* (London 1613), 71.

29   Stapleton, *Orationes*, 507.

30   Ernst Troeltsch, *The Social Teaching of the Christian Churches*, trans. Olive Wyon, 2 vols (London 1931), i, 331.

31   Ibid., i, 336.

32   See especially the classic study, much influenced by the Troeltschian typology, by G. H. Williams, *The Radical Reformation* (3rd edn, Kirksville, Mo. 1992).

33 Michael Mullett, *Radical Religious Movements in Early Modern Europe* (London 1980), 65, 103.

34 G. H. Williams, ed., *Spiritual and Anabaptist Writers: Documents Illustrative of the Radical Reformation* (London 1957), 66; *Radical Reformation,* 154.

35 For the attitudes of Dutch Anabaptists towards witchcraft, see Chapter 14 in this collection by Gary K. Waite.

36 Deutel's *Een kort tractaetje tegen de toovery* was written in 1638 and first published in 1670.

37 For these and many other examples, Christopher Hill, *The World Turned Upside Down* (London 1972), 23, 149, 172, 176–7 and esp. 136–45; Thomas, *Religion and the Decline of Magic*, 170–1.

38 N. Smith, *Perfection Proclaimed* (Oxford 1989), 230–44, esp. 235. On Norwood's Ranter associations, see Hill, *World Turned Upside Down*, 18 1.

39 Lodowick Muggleton, *A True Interpretation of the Witch of Endor,* 5th edn (London 1856), 1; Christopher Hill, Barry Reay and William Lamont, *The World of the Muggletonians* (London 1983), 122–4.

40 Scot, *Discovery*, 39–72.

41 See Peter Elmer, 'The Library of Dr John Webster: The Making of a Seventeenth-Century Radical', *Medical History Supplement*, 6 (1986), 2–12 (quotations from Webster's 1650s sermons cited p. 3 and n. 7).

42 Gerrard Winstanley, *The Law of Freedom in a Platform*, in George H. Sabine, ed., *The Works of Gerrard Winstanley* (Ithaca, NY 1941), 597. Immanuel Bourne, *A Defence of the Scriptures* (London 1656), dedication, complained that the Quakers too called the clergy witches.

Chapter 13

Edmund Kern

CONFESSIONAL IDENTITY AND MAGIC IN THE LATE SIXTEENTH CENTURY

Jakob Bithner and witchcraft in Styria

IN THE FINAL DECADES of the sixteenth century, the duchy of Styria (loosely comprising the province of the same name in the Republic of Austria and a portion of Slovenia) experienced the initial effects of an emerging Catholic Reformation, sponsored by the ruling house of Habsburg. In an ultimately successful effort, ducal authorities, following the policies established by Archduke Charles of Styria (1564–1590) and his son Archduke (later Emperor) Ferdinand (1590–1638), began to attack Lutheran religious practices by co-opting the religious cause of Catholic orthodoxy as a political goal, pressuring first the common people of rural villages and towns, and then advancing gradually against the local nobility. During this early phase of Catholic Reform, secular courts also began to prosecute numerous persons under charges of magic and witchcraft, and to initiate a series of trials that would continue simultaneously with the consolidation of Catholicism throughout the seventeenth century.

Yet, paradoxically it would seem, one of the most vociferous witch-hunters in Styria during this early period of Catholic ascendancy was an avowed Lutheran from Saxony, the *Landprofos* Jakob Bithner. In a series of reports to the Styrian estates dating from 1580, he outlined his interests in eradicating all manifestations of magic and superstition, and described his involvement in no fewer than twenty-three of the thirty-nine known cases of witchcraft between 1578 and 1600.[1] (Only three other cases occurred in Styria during the sixteenth century.) Because of the ambiguous and indeterminate religious complexion of Styria during this period (an avowedly Catholic duke pursuing his religious prerogatives on the one hand, and a strong Lutheran nobility securing their own liberties on the other), the example of Jakob Bithner seems strikingly appropriate for further examination of the issues of witch-hunting and confessional identity.

The steps taken by the Habsburg dukes in the late sixteenth century can be best understood with reference to the paradigm of confessionalization, which has emerged as a useful conceptual tool in the recent literature on early modern Central Europe.[2] Heinz Schilling's 'The Reformation and the Rise of the Early Modern State' describes the process of confessionalization within the developing states of Central Europe in the early modern period. For Schilling, confessionalization implies the 'fragmentation of the unitary Christendom' that had existed in the Middle Ages into at least three distinct confessional churches: Lutheran, Calvinist or Reformed, and Roman Catholic. He further asserts that the development of these confessional churches was inextricably linked with the 'grand process of state building between the fifteenth and seventeenth centuries' that gave rise to unified territorial states typified by an emerging bureaucratic administration, an enlarged sphere of state prerogatives, and an enhanced role for ruling dynasties and courts. In short, the process of state-building led to a concentration of power within an increasingly sophisticated political apparatus that adopted confessional orthodoxy as one of its goals. Thus, 'confessional church and confessional state combined to regulate religious and church life', with widespread social and cultural repercussions.[3] In this process, confessional identity became an important measure of one's allegiance to the state, regardless of how authorities defined orthodoxy within a large variety of specific political circumstances.

As a Lutheran estates' official experiencing directly the Habsburg effort to reinstitute Catholic orthodoxy, Jakob Bithner found himself caught up in the antagonisms between crown and estates in what has been conceptualized as the political 'dualism' inherent in the late mediaeval/early modern corporative state, or 'Standestaat'. Within the charged religious atmosphere of Styrian confessionalization, these antagonisms centered on the question of who held the political authority to determine the religious identity and allegiances of Styria: the Catholic dukes or the largely Lutheran estates? Although the ultimate success of confessionalization in Styria was never assured, by 1600 the Catholic archduke Ferdinand, building on the slow advances made by his father, Charles of Styria, between 1578 and 1590, enjoyed the relatively successful reintroduction of Catholic clergy in the villages and towns of his duchy, despite the fact that the nobility maintained their personal liberties. At the level of estates administration and within the ducal court in Styria, little institutional change had taken place since efforts for religious reform had proceeded without numerous specific attacks against the estates' institution itself, which continued to deliberate and make decisions as it had done before. The crown did, however, continue to exert personal pressure against confessional holdouts among the nobility. Thus, by 1628, when the Styrian duke, Emperor Ferdinand II, compelled the nobility to convert or be forced into exile, major personnel changes in both the diet itself and its administrative organs had already taken place. The process of confessionalization in Styria had produced major successes, and alongside them Habsburg claims to sovereignty in religious matters had been greatly enhanced.

But it is easy to overstate the case for political dualism within the Styrian *Standestaat,* since it grants priority to only one political issue, namely princely authority (or sovereignty) and estates' resistance to it, to the exclusion of many others in which the crown and estates had significantly overlapping interests. A concern for social order within the duchy is one such area of overlapping interests, and the Styrian *Landprofos* represented the sovereign just as much as he did the estates in the continuing effort to maintain order throughout the land. The office of *Landprofos* was established by the predominantly Lutheran estates of the duchy in 1578 to help ensure public security and order, in line with a developing sense of *güte policey*, common to both estates and ducal officials.[4] Although the official was appointed and paid by the estates, he also had to take an oath of loyalty to the Catholic archduke, making the question of his political allegiance an issue for potential dispute. At face value, this situation in itself did not necessarily present a problem, since the office of *Landprofos* did not have competency for the specifically religious issues over which the estates and crown contended.

The official's duties entailed primarily control of the many wandering and marauding *Knechte* or *Kriegsleuth* (mercenaries), who were about in the land, but also included control over the increasingly worrisome number of 'roaming', 'idle' [masterless] persons, 'the poor about in the land', 'dangerous' [lawless] people, and 'wicked, roaming riffraff'. In practice this included apprehension of those traveling throughout the land without the appropriate passes and transferring them to the nearest regional courts for detention, investigation, and punishment. The *Landprofos* sent regular reports to the estates and to the duke's court, including general assessments of the safety and conditions of the duchy's roads, footpaths, bridges, and postal routes. Appointed *Landprofos* in March 1580, Bithner immediately expanded his duties to include actions against sorcerers and witches, whom he believed to be particularly active among the vagabond groups under his charge, contending that 'not only did the marauding mercenaries wander from time to time in the land, but so did other dangerous persons, who caused profanation with robbery, sorcery and similar vices, and who gave themselves entirely over to indolence.' Given Bithner's continued activities, the estates apparently approved Bithner's expanded role, sanctioning an official link between sorcery and vagabondage in the process. For Bithner and the estates, the threat to *güte policey* from such persons was self-evident.

Prohibitions against sorcery were also apparently self-evident, since such practices were outlawed in the judicial regulations promulgated by Charles of Styria in 1574. Sections of at least six articles contained in the *Ordnung* outline what grounds were required to interrogate a suspect, what activities were outlawed, and how such trespasses were to be punished. In practice, however, these regulations allowed individual officials and magistrates tremendous personal discretion, since none of the articles mentions the specific types of sorcery and divination that they were intended to regulate. Similarly, the *Ordnung* is mute on such topics as the Devil and witches' sabbaths – demonological themes paramount in the European-wide phenomenon and essential for an understanding of the Styrian witch-hunts. According to his own understandings of sorcery and *güte policey*, Bithner filled such details into the silences left by the regulations.

The thirty-nine Styrian cases of witchcraft between 1578 and 1600 represented in court documents and Bithner's reports do not depict a series of large-scale panics, or witch-hunts, but suggest rather a pattern of various individual cases. According to the documents, at least seventy-four individuals found themselves accused or under suspicion of magical activities, but many other unnamed persons are mentioned as well. Of the sixty-seven persons whose sex is known, forty-four were women (66 percent) and twenty-three were men (34 percent). When the cases involved individual persons and did not lead to further accusations, men and women appear in roughly even numbers. In the relatively few cases evolving into larger trials (four or more defendants), women are listed among the accused in much greater numbers than men (twenty-six of thirty, or 87 percent).

At least some form of judicial proceedings was begun in twenty-nine of the thirty-nine cases. Twenty-three cases concerned accusations against only one person, who was suspected or formally accused of witchcraft; three cases implicated two persons; two cases implicated three persons; and four cases eventually included charges against four persons in each. Only two cases of the thirty-nine can be described as truly large-scale, relative to these other cases: a 1580 trial in Maribor with nine accused and a 1584–1585 trial also in Maribor with thirteen named accused and numerous others implicated. The remaining five of the thirty-nine Styrian cases did not involve any formal charges and are depicted only in Bithner's reports, in which he claims numerous persons or groups active in witchcraft fled when word of his approach reached them.

The reports of Jakob Bithner must be understood within the larger context of Styrian witchcraft cases between 1578 and 1600, which include examples of both demonic and nondemonic magic: accusations of simple *maleficia* (harmful magic that was demonic in some cases and non-demonic in others), references to organized witches' societies, and elements of diabolical sabbaths (both suggestive of fully fledged Devil worship).[5] It should first be noted that a few trials for *maleficia* occurred in or near the Austrian territories in the decades preceding the witch-hunts of the early modern period, and some of the cases even included diabolical elements, such as a case from around 1400 when a woman was fined for sorcery and for associating with the Devil. What was missing, however, was a consistent pattern of diabolical magic or continuing references to the sabbat stereotype associated with learned discourse on the topic. The first seventeenth-century case dates from 1513, and was non-demonic in form. Two additional trials took place in 1546 and 1548. The first, a rather large trial in which six women were tried and likely executed, included charges of participation in the diabolical sabbat (including nocturnal flight and intercourse with the Devil), and represents the first time that sabbat stereotype appears in Styrian documents. On the other hand, the second trial, which occurred in Seckau, corresponded to the earlier, non-demonic pattern, and included charges against an individual woman who was fined for causing sickness among her neighbors' animals. Within the larger Austrian context, these early Styrian trials contribute to a highly fragmentary series of relatively infrequent trials dating from the fifteenth century which sometimes included diabolical aspects, but mostly involved only *maleficia*.

Given this larger context, it would be difficult to contend that Bithner introduced many new elements into the Styrian situation, since the sabbat stereotype had appeared well before his arrival there. Nonetheless, his letters to the estates emphasize (often savagely) the demonic origins of *maleficia* and the prevalence of this diabolical influence throughout the land. Ten of the twenty-three cases of magic, in which Bithner played a role, resulted in some form of judicial proceedings with allegations of diabolical elements: of these ten, one case concerned a self-described *Planetenleser* or astrologer, who possessed books and instruments interpreted as demonic by Bithner; two cases included descriptions of pacts with the Devil – to bring great wealth to a man in one case, and for assistance in overtly malevolent purposes in the other; the seven remaining cases referenced membership in witches' 'societies' or included elements associated with diabolical sabbaths.

Bithner's emphasis upon demonic magic is most evident in his accounts of the pacts made with the Devil and his reports of alleged witches' sabbaths. The most common elements in Bithner's own narrative commentaries on these events are the suspects' associations with the Devil and the existence of organized societies to which the suspects belonged. In one of Bithner's reports from 1581, he recounted events from 1579, concerning the 'sorcery' trial of four women in Cilli who confessed to belonging to a society with many other members. Emphasizing the continuing threat to order from such persons, Bithner included an extract from the confession of one of the accused: 'The society was so large, that she did not know everyone whom the Devil had brought together'. Although there is no way of knowing Bithner's full meaning when he spoke of groups of 'sorcerers' throughout Styria, he always applies the term 'sorcery' to the crimes of those confessing to participation in witches' societies, and he never uses the term 'witchcraft', which is found in some other German-language sources from the time. Too much should not be made of this fact, since many words related to magic had ambiguous or synonymous meanings. But it is important to note that like many, or perhaps most, of his contemporaries, Bithner made no distinction between what some theorists understood as separate categories of non-demonic and demonic magic; his words implied instead the diabolical nature of all such practices.[6]

Less common, but still found among the reports, are accounts of witches' sexual relations with the Devil – occurring, not surprisingly, in cases involving female suspects. Two related cases dating from 1580, one in Arnfels, the other in Maribor, contain accounts of sexual activity. In Arnfels the accused, Barbara Striglin, was said to have borne a demon, ostensibly after intercourse with the Devil. Not a single aspect of this birth, reported to Bithner secondhand, can be understood as resulting from human sexual relations, since according to the report, Striglin's pregnancy ended when the demon flew from her body in the form of a large raven, leaving a gaping wound in her side. Both of these cases, as well as the other five cases that suggest the existence of organized societies, include other elements, such as night flying, frenzied dancing, animal metamorphosis, and child murder often associated with the sabbat stereotype. But it is important to note that most of the cases which occurred in Styria in the late sixteenth century involved accusation of general sorcery (*maleficia* such as animal magic, weather magic, divination, the retrieval of lost objects, harm of human beings), and did not evolve into large-scale trials which featured the highly elaborate imagery of the sabbat stereotype. Despite Bithner's familiarity with sabbat imagery and his willingness to accept the existence of witches' societies, such themes do not always appear in his representations of magical activities. Far more important was the fact that the Devil inspired all magical activities, regardless of how they manifested themselves and not necessarily always in the same way.

There is little within Bithner's writings to suggest that his representations of diabolical magic came particularly from his professed Lutheran beliefs. Rather, his activities against witchcraft and superstition can be attributed to ideas about the diabolical nature of magic common to both Catholics and Lutherans at the time.[7] How his religious faith influenced his witch-hunting activities must be understood within the religious-political context of Catholic confessionalization in Styria. It may seem that his witch-hunting contributed to the Catholic cause, as the process of Habsburg-sponsored religious reform proceeded in the duchy, but to see his reports to the estates exclusively in this light would be a misunderstanding of his activities and the role of his confessional identity within them. Although Styria was fast becoming what can be termed a Catholic cultural area, since Tridentine orthodoxy had been adopted by the princely court as a political policy, the late sixteenth century was experiencing only the earliest phases of this process. I would even contend, with reservations, that this was true for other ostensibly Catholic or Protestant areas of the empire at the time. It is important to situate matters of confessional identity within local practice, rather than in the religious–political statements of orthodoxy promulgated by the various faiths (e.g. Canons and Decrees of the Council of Trent in 1563, Heidelberg Catechism in 1563, Formula of Concord in 1577), for despite the apparently comprehensive nature of these prescriptive documents, confessional identity remained a controversial and fragmentary construct, created as much by reaction to the prescriptive statements as by the statements themselves. The clear, disjunctive categories of Catholic, Lutheran, and Calvinist conform more to modern notions of denominational churches than to the contested definitions of religious orthodoxy in the late sixteenth century, and as such, they lack explanatory power without reference to specific situations.

The example of the Lutheran Bithner prosecuting witches in a state increasingly subject to the forces of Catholic confessionalization illustrates how both Catholics and Lutherans in Styria often acted in like ways to root out magical practices in accordance with a shared notion of *güte policey* unrelated to confessional differences or the political dualism present in the antagonisms between crown and estates. Nonetheless, a difference of emphasis can be seen in a number of cases when issues of religious orthodoxy were involved.[8]

The first case concerns charges of witchcraft against the newly installed Catholic pastor of Oberwölz in 1590. The villagers, who disliked the priest's Catholic zeal, accused him of weather magic after he threatened them with divine retribution, if they did not change their ways. After a series of terrible storms convinced them that the harvest would be especially bad, they beat the priest, forced him to leave the village, and began a lawsuit against him in the ducal court at Graz.[9] The Catholic court immediately dismissed the charges against the priest, and brought a finding against the villagers, holding them responsible for false accusation and impious behavior. As *Landprofos,* Bithner was called upon to arrest those responsible and make them available for punishment, although he made clear that he did not like it, and emphasized his dismay by stressing the steps taken by the pastor to foster 'his religion' among the parishioners 'against their conscience'. Likewise, he reported that the storms had indeed taken place in the area, with the attendant destruction of grain, and that not only were such activities possible but likely. To punctuate his dismay, Bithner continues his report with an account of a beggar he had apprehended, who – among other things – could practice weather magic. For the Catholic court, issues of orthodoxy clearly superseded suspicions of magical activities, since it installed the pastor specifically to institute the religious reforms to which the parishioners objected.

A second telling example is represented in the accounts of several exorcisms that occurred in Graz in 1599 and 1600, the final years of Bithner's activities as

Landprofos. Although he was not directly involved in these cases, they serve to illustrate once again a difference of emphasis within the Styrian court – overcoming Protestantism merited more support than did stamping out illicit magic. During this two-year period, two women and one man were exorcised by a religious commission consisting of the Habsburg court chaplain, Jesuits at the University of Graz, and local Franciscans. The three cases were unrelated except in the way in which they were conducted. Each became a lengthy public display, used in a propagandistic way by the Habsburgs and their clerical allies, and the reports based on these exorcisms had indisputably anti-Protestant tones.

As would be expected, the Devil or individual demons were paramount in each of the three exorcisms, but it is interesting to note that according to the accounts, the demons reported of their interactions with the local Lutheran community, in one case going so far as to travel in the belly of the Lutheran preacher from Eisenerz. In the case of one of the women, a local physician who had treated her came under suspicion of sorcery, of compact with the Devil, and ultimately of causing her condition with three demons he kept in a bottle.[10] After these formal accusations had been made, a witchcraft investigation was begun, but through the intercession of the bishop of Seckau, Martin Brenner, the witchcraft charges were dismissed. The man who was exorcised was a noble Lutheran student at University of Graz, who was allowed to convert publicly to Catholicism, despite having sold his soul to the Devil in a written document. In none of the cases was anyone tried and punished for what appeared to witnesses as either willful compacts with the Devil or premeditated attempts to inflict demons on others. We can see in these cases that issues of religious orthodoxy took precedence over attacks against magic, despite the clearly diabolical nature of the cases.

Witch-hunting *per se* was not against Habsburg interests at the time, but it was not a priority of the court either. In these circumstances, Bithner carried out his duties as he saw fit, including active suppression of magical practices among the populace, by diabolizing those practices. The ducal court in Graz had no reservations, since witchcraft was something to be despised by Catholics as well, but when persecution of magic interfered with the dynasty's religious prerogatives, it did not receive full backing, was suppressed outright, or was simply ignored. In the exorcisms themselves we can see another theme played out within the specific religious-political context of Styria – namely, an attempt to link the Devil and, by extension, diabolical sorcery with the Lutheran cause. The Antwerp-born Spanish Jesuit, Martin Del Rio (theology professor at the University of Graz, 1600–1603), explicitly made this connection in a later edition of his witchcraft treatise, *Disquisitionum Magicarum Libri Sex,* using the possession of the Lutheran noble in Graz as an example. He thus equated the impulse towards Protestant heresy with the impulse towards demonic magic.

Bithner's reports to the Styrian estates apparently lend credence to the claim that the early modern attack on magic and its attendant linkage of such beliefs with diabolism was not exclusively a manifestation of either Catholic or Protestant doctrines, but rather a shared tactic in an overall missionary effort to reform the common people of Europe. In particular, Jean Delumeau, in *Catholicism between Luther and Voltaire,* argues that reformers of all confessional identities sought to 'Christianize' a populace deemed ignorant of the basic tenets of religious faith.[11] Although Delumeau's claim might be a bit overstated, current scholarship treating the religious changes of the sixteenth and seventeenth centuries continues to develop this theme, and tends to emphasize similarities among confessions over differences between them.[12] Although Stuart Clark's point about 'differences of accent' in Lutheran theoretical literature is well taken, he also contends that it is particularly worthwhile to situate such issues within the specific contexts of clerical practice.[13] Since historians cannot escape the continuous play of similarity and difference among the religious confessions that emerged in the late sixteenth century, they must avoid using the disjunctive categories of Catholic, Lutheran, and Calvinist as universal explanations for complex historical events. Nevertheless, conceptions of confessional identity and sectarianism certainly have utility within historical scholarship if applied to specific examples of religious and political practice.

Thus, Jakob Bithner is not a simple example of a Protestant working for a Catholic cause, though he may have indirectly contributed to one. The specific religious-political context of Habsburg state aggrandizement and Catholic confessionalization situated Bithner's witch-hunting practices within local circumstances, which the disjunctive categories of Lutheran and Catholic doctrines on witchcraft cannot explain. Bithner's own confessional identity, nonetheless, had meanings we can interpret in other ways – meanings that illuminate the complexities of witch-hunting in Styria. While Bithner carried out the duties of his office, he also actively worked to maintain Lutheran religious liberties in the duchy. Despite his efforts, Catholic interests within the archduke's court (and increasingly complex state apparatus) forced the appointment of a Catholic *Landprofos* and sent Bithner himself – unprotected by noble prerogative – into exile in 1600. He had become a victim of the changing conception of *güte policey* that began to define religious deviants as threats to the social and political order. After his exile, Bithner no longer had a role to play in the Styrian witch trials, but the phenomenon whose early phases he had helped to shape continued in his absence. The last trial for witchcraft in Styria ended in 1746.

Notes

1   All archival materials referred to in this chapter are located in the Steiermarkisches Landesarchiv, Graz, Austria. For full references, see the original version of this chapter in *Sixteenth Century Journal*, 25(2) (1994), 323–40.

2   For confessionalism in general, see J. Delumeau, *Catholicism between Luther and Voltaire*, trans. J. Mosiser (London 1977); for Central Europe, see R. Po-Chia Hsai, *Social Discipline in the Reformation* (London 1989).

3   Heinz Schilling, 'The Reformation and the Rise of the Early Modern State', trans. Heinz Schilling and Thomas A. Brady, Jr, in *Luther and the Modern State in Germany*, ed. James Tracy (Sixteenth Century Journal Publishers, Kirksville, Mo. 1986), 21–30.

4   For a general survey of the development of policing in the region, see Marc Raeff, *The Well-Ordered Police State: Social and Institutional Change through Law in the Germanies and Russia, 1600–1800* (Yale University Press, New Haven, Conn. 1983), esp. 1–10, 43–179.

5   The categories of non-demonic and demonic magic were hardly clear to contemporaries since some writers argued that magic which was not explicitly demonic could in fact be implicitly so. See Richard Kieckhefer, *Magic in the Middle Ages* (Cambridge University Press 1990), esp. 8–17, 56–94, 151–201.

6   This is not surprising, since the intricacies of sixteenth-century debates over the nature of magic may not have been known to an estates' official such as Bithner; he may not even have been aware or the existence of such an esoteric discourse.

7   This argument can also be found in Erik Midelfort's book, *Witch Hunting in Southwestern Germany, 1562–1684* (Stanford, Calif. 1972).

8   See Chapter 12 by Stuart Clark for the similarities and 'differences of accent' between Protestant and Catholic demonology.

9   This is a nice example of popular demand for action against witches believed to be harming the weather, and relates to Chapter 4 by Wolfgang Behringer.

10 These grossly physical ideas about the Devil differ from the more abstract conception of Satan developed by Protestant and Catholic theologians. See Chapters 17, 18 and 23 in this collection for other differences between learned and popular opinions of the Devil.

11 Delumeau, *Catholicism between Luther and Voltaire*, 175–202.

12 See, for example, Hsia, *Social Discipline in the Reformation*.

13 See Chapter 12 by Stuart Clark.

Chapter 14

Gary K. Waite

BETWEEN THE DEVIL AND THE INQUISITOR

Anabaptists, diabolical conspiracies and magical beliefs

THIS CHAPTER EXPLORES THE INTERSECTIONS between the heresy of Anabaptism and the supposedly even greater apostasy of demonic witchcraft. Anabaptism challenged the institutional churches because of its rejection of the official social structure and hierarchical understanding of the cosmos. The early Anabaptists, moreover, depicted the ecclesiastical authorities in apocalyptical terms as the antichrist (the son of the Devil), thereby turning the accusation of a diabolical conspiracy on its head.[1] However, once a relative truce had been declared with Lutherans, and Anabaptists had been persecuted into an underground and largely sectarian existence, it seems many authorities turned around 1566 to the suppression of magical deviance with increased fury and near unanimity. This chronological development leads to several related questions: first, did the perceived threat of Anabaptism have anything to do with this revival of diabolical conspiracies? Second, did the popular or official image of Anabaptists change in any way after the rise of witch-hunting? Third, was there any overlap in official perception of Anabaptists and witches during the critical decades of the 1540s to 1560s?

This much is agreed upon: the flare-up of the persecution of witches followed close upon the heels of the waning of large-scale heresy prosecution by 1565, although there were a number of individual cases of prosecution for witchcraft that took place coterminously with the trials against religious dissidents. However, it was not the isolated witch who brought periodic bouts of terror to the hearts of Europeans through the later sixteenth and seventeenth centuries, but the belief that witchcraft was a diabolical conspiracy between Satan and groups of women and men meeting secretly at night who performed perverse inversions of Christian rites, worshipped the Devil, kidnapped and roasted unbaptized infants, and plotted the overthrow of Christian society. Certainly belief in magic and witchcraft was endemic to European society, but it was not until the fifteenth century that this stereotype of the diabolical and conspiratorial witch was fully developed. Even so, persecutions of these supposed diabolical agents seem to have died down by the end of the century, and soon the inquisitorial and secular courts were preoccupied with religious dissidents. Brian Levack's suggestion of a chronological intersection between heresy persecution and witchcraft trials has been recently pursued by William Monter, who has calculated that there were some 3000 legally sanctioned executions for heresy from 1520 to *c.* 1565, and about two-thirds of these victims were Anabaptists.[2] He argues that the apparent rise of Anabaptism from the ashes of the German Peasants' War of 1525 and the fear of further sedition provoked by these religious dissenters led to the secularization of heresy trials in the German Empire, the Low Countries and eventually elsewhere in Europe.[3] Monter asks why this momentous attack on heresy by secular states has not seriously been seen as contributing to the even more horrific assault on accused witches. The reason is perhaps quite simple: historians of the Reformation and historians of witchcraft, in Monter's words, 'rarely read each other's works', a conclusion that is perhaps unfair in some cases, but is too often corroborated when reading the secondary literature in both fields.[4] It is this major gap in our understanding of the persecution of both heretics and witches that this chapter broaches, seeking to communicate to scholars of both the Reformation and the witch-hunts.

Given what we now know about early modern popular culture, it seems likely that ordinary people who witnessed the fiery executions of both Anabaptists and accused witches would have confused the two sets of victims, especially since contemporary polemicists condemned Anabaptists as a demonic sect threatening the Christian religion. Perhaps ordinary people also misconstrued some Anabaptist ideas or practices as somehow magical and demonic. Lutheran and Reformed polemicists showed little caution in demonizing their more radical opponents, and in some cases, associating them with sorcery. In his *Lectures on Galatians* Luther wrote the following in a passage about witchcraft:

> Thus in our day we, too, must labour with the Word of God against the fanatical opinions of the Anabaptists and the Sacramentarians . . . For we have recalled many whom they had bewitched, and we have set them free from their bewitchment, from which they could never have been untangled by their own powers if they had not been admonished by us and recalled through the Word of God . . . So great is the efficacy of this satanic illusion in those who have been deluded this way that they would boast and swear that they have the most certain truth.[5]

Of course Luther distinguished between physical and 'spiritual' witchcraft. However, not all of his readers, or those who heard Luther's ideas second hand, made such careful distinctions.[6] That Menno Simons (*c.* 1496–1561) found it necessary to respond to charges that he and his fellow Mennonites were demon-possessed illustrates the potential ramifications of such polemical characterization.[7] Instead, Menno argued, infant baptism was a 'ceremony of Antichrist, a public blasphemy, a bewitching sin'. While this position may have led some opponents to believe that Anabaptists were demon possessed, Menno responded that,

> We consider those possessed of the Devil who speak the Devil's words, who teach the Devil's falsehood instead of truth, steal God's glory from Him, and sadly deceive souls . . . we hate the word of the Devil from

our inmost souls . . . This is an evident sign that we are not possessed
of the spirit of the Devil but of that of the Lord. If we were of the
Devil as we are reviled, we would walk upon a broader road and be
befriended by the world and not so resignedly offer our property and
blood for the cause of the Word of the Lord.[8]

In other words, the true agents of the Devil are the religious and civic authorities
that vigorously pursue the Anabaptists.

A start to examining the implications of Anabaptist rejection of infant baptism
can be found in the published court records relating to Dutch Anabaptists.[9] These
are the records of the court officials, reflecting the interrogations as understood
and recorded by the prosecutors. We can then turn to a source that presents the
perspective of the arrested Anabaptists themselves as they underwent their interrogations and reflected on their final days. This is the martyr book *Het Offer des
Heeren* (1570), and while the documents in this work too have undergone a complicated process of transmission and editing, they reflect the authentic voice of the
persecuted. Both of these types of sources provide important information on the
relationship between accused heretics on the one side and their official interrogators on the other.

Before tackling the persecution of Anabaptists, it might be useful to survey
briefly how Lutherans and other early Evangelicals were treated and regarded in
the courts prior to the arrival of Anabaptism in the Netherlands *c.* 1530. Examination of these published sources, which are admittedly incomplete, reveals that the
authorities in the vast majority of cases regarded the early Lutheran movement as
a form of academic heresy, as almost an 'in-house' conflict among clerical factions.
This is especially the case between 1519 and 1521, for it was Luther's learned
supporters within the Augustinian monasteries who won the greatest attention on
the part of the authorities, leading them to become the first martyrs of the
Reformation in the Netherlands. Unlike the case with the later Anabaptists, the
Lutherans' theological positions were taken seriously and rebutted in a learned
manner by their orthodox opponents. In only one of the published sources is there
any serious attempt to link Luther's heresy with diabolical notions, and that was a
response to Luther's own characterization of the Pope as antichrist. This reference
occurred in Charles V's second placard against Lutheranism, issued 8 May 1521
(his first placard of 20 March 1521, made no such reference). In it Charles V's
theologians note that Luther had scandalized the entire church, especially when he
called the fifteenth-century Council of Constance, which had burned Jan Hus at
the stake, the 'synagogue of Satan'. In response, and with intended irony, the writer
concludes that 'the person of the aforesaid Martin is not a man, but a Devil under
the species of a man, bedecked in the habit of a religious, in order better and more
easily to bring the human race into eternal death and damnation'.[10] Even this bit
of scholastic gamesmanship, based as it was on Aristotelian logic and modelled after
the very doctrine of transubstantiation rejected by Luther, was not taken up in later
placards or, apparently, even by interrogators of early Lutherans to implicate the
Lutheran Reformation seriously in a diabolical plot. Instead, Charles V's public
commission to inquisitor Frans vander Hulst and accompanying placard of 23 April
1522 toned down the diabolical rhetoric, so that Luther and his ideas are listed as

schismatic, heretical and leading to eternal damnation, but his person is no longer described is a demon.[11] As the evangelical movement became more popular and lost its learned leadership under the pressure of persecution, there may have been a tendency to characterize it as a greater diabolical threat, but the available published sources do not reveal this as a significant development. Despite the authorities' opposition to Luther's reform movement and heretical ideas, Lutherans could prove useful in opposing even more radical forms of heresy, such as that of the infamous slater Loy Pruystinck (de Schaliedecker), whose quite unorthodox opinions, including his rejection of hell, eternal punishment and the physical resurrection, as well as his affirmation that the Holy Spirit was none other than human reason resident in each individual, won many followers in Antwerp. In 1525 Pruystinck travelled to Wittenberg to convince Luther of his pantheistic notions but Luther's response was hardly positive, hastily dashing off a missive to his followers in Antwerp warning them of this mischievous spirit and his dangerous ideas. Ironically, when in January of the following year Pruystinck and nine of his supporters were arrested for heresy, his crime was identified as 'Lutheranism', undoubtedly to Luther's chagrin. In spite of his public recantation in February, Pruystinck continued to spread his ideas throughout the city, attracting not only an adoring crowd of poor sympathizers who bowed down when he passed by adorned in his bejewelled rags, but also a number from the middle and upper social strata. In 1539, reform-minded dramatists in the city wrote a Lutheran play that opposed the more radical notions of Pruystinck, thus maintaining the support of the local authorities for their dramatic activities. Finally in 1544 Pruystinck and several of his prominent supporters were arrested and executed. This one example does help reveal why Luther's reform, however distasteful it may have seemed to orthodox theologians, did not elicit the same level of panic on the part of the authorities.

Anabaptists in the authorities' perspective

As with most secular court materials, the Anabaptist court records present very skimpy summaries of the proceedings; however, a few things can be gleaned from them. First, it appears that what most concerned court officials was the extraction of confessions about the principal beliefs of heretical Anabaptism, most notably its rejection of infant baptism and transubstantiation and the adoption of adult baptism. The records describe this latter act as a renunciation of one's original baptism, and hence of the church and Christian society. In most cases, the accused had come to regard infant baptism as ineffectual and the priestly consecrated Host as ordinary bread. Furthermore, some Anabaptist parents were discovered because they had not had their infants baptized, in itself a criminal act.[12] Given the physical obviousness of pregnancy, it must have been difficult to hide a pregnancy and birth from the authorities. This may have been the reason why a rumour appeared during the height of Anabaptist activity in Amsterdam in 1534, suggesting midwives were smuggling newborn infants out of the city. Count Hoogstraten expressed considerable concern over this news, although Amsterdam's magistracy denied any knowledge of such occurrences, doubting that such was even possible. The ability of many Anabaptists to hide their unbaptized infants from the authorities, however, may have led to increased suspicion regarding midwives, who, perhaps not surprisingly, figured largely in witchcraft beliefs.[13] As with the case of midwives suspected of witchcraft, the presumed collusion between midwives and Anabaptist parents finally led the Groningen authorities in 1569 to issue a decree ordering all midwives to be examined by the States General to see 'if they are Catholic and of good reputation' before being allowed to perform their work in the region.

Increasingly, especially after Anabaptists had successfully taken over Münster in 1534, authorities sought to uncover the conspiracy of Anabaptism, to extract from the accused the names of all others who had attended the secret meetings and who were also supposedly plotting insurrection.[14] Thus descriptions of the sect included the appellative 'seditious' as well as the more typical 'heretical'. The imperial placard against Menno Simons of 7 December 1542, described him as deceiving the simple people with his false teaching during secret, night-time meetings. Like diabolical witchcraft, the crime of rebaptism, because of its inherent social danger, was treated as an exceptional crime of *lese majestatis,* of treason against both divine and human authority. The concern over heresy had therefore been heightened to the level of a secret and dangerous conspiracy. Mandate after mandate ordered local officials and clergy to uncover people hiding in attics or cellars, 'to keep their eyes on any who did not attend yearly confession or mass and to report on the kind of lives they led, those with whom they associated, any secret meetings at their homes, as well as to relate the presence of any strangers in their midst.' Furthermore, on 6 January 1536, Karl van Egmond, Duke of Guelders, ordered all the clergy of his domain to conduct a visitation in Drenthe and the region of Groningen to discover any heretical beliefs. To underscore the authorities' seriousness regarding the presumed Anabaptist threat, in most areas of the Low Countries those convicted of such heresy were, like convicted witches, burned at the stake, although under certain conditions the accused might be accorded the mercy of a drowning or beheading.

Fears of an Anabaptist conspiracy to overthrow Christendom did not dissipate quickly. Two decades after the Münster debacle the court of Friesland issued a placard denouncing the increase in dangerous heretics hiding in their midst who reject all the sacraments, steal from people and churches, and secretly plot a godless revolt to expel and exterminate Christians. To accentuate the danger of this threat, the president of the court, Hippolitus Persijn, calls these Anabaptist heretics 'an evil race of men and monstrous creatures'. Of course, part of Persijn's concern was to counteract the Batenburgers, a small group of militant Anabaptists who commited acts of robbery and violence as a means of visiting divine vengeance upon their persecutors.[15] Yet Persijn makes no distinction between militant and peaceful Anabaptists, such as the Mennonites, presumably wishing to keep the size of the fearful conspiracy as large as possible. Three years later the stadholder of King Philip II attempted much the same thing in his attempts to force the city of Groningen to fall in with the king's policy of harsh suppression of Anabaptism, telling the city fathers that the Anabaptists and related sects were gaining the upper hand in the city and would soon overthrow it. The city council responded in a very interesting fashion: its members knew of some women who refused to baptize their children, but they did not consider these to be dangerous, nor were they aware of any portentous buildup in militant Anabaptist forces. In other words, in this case the local civic authorities had become acquainted with their Mennonite residents and knew them to be no threat to law and order, whereas the more distant royal government continued to propagate a conspiratorial vision of these heretics. Interestingly enough, one of the worst outbreaks of executions in the Netherlands for witchcraft occurred in the Groningen Ommelanden, the rural area outside of the city, where twenty executions took place in 1547 and another five in 1562.[16] Unlike Friesland, where the Court of Friesland kept a firm hand over local courts and controlled heresy hunting, completely suppressing potential witch-hunts, the Ommelanden courts had a relatively free hand and were more easily manipulated by 'foreign' pressures to prosecute, such as the royal government or advocates of witch-hunting from East Frisia. At the same time it seems both Groningen's and the Ommelanden's officials strongly resisted royal pressure to prosecute Mennonites, forcing the stadholder in 1567 to hire, without the approval of the local authorities, a band of mercenaries to 'rob, disturb and hunt down' Mennonites in the Ommelanden. Evidently, in this region of the Netherlands, witchcraft was perceived as a much more serious threat to social order than was Anabaptism, royal propaganda notwithstanding. In neighbouring Friesland, however, it appears that judicial officials were content to limit their efforts in counteracting heresy to Anabaptism.

Such broad-ranging conspiracies usually had at their centre the leadership of the Devil. Yet the Devil figures hardly at all in the published court records. Of course, this could simply mean that his presence and activity were assumed. It could also mean, as it did in many witchcraft cases, that the accused themselves did not mention the Devil, even though the interrogators constantly attempted to put a demonological slant on the accused's confessions. Before examining the applicability of this theory for Anabaptist trials, it will be illuminating first to examine the few cases where the Devil is mentioned. Then we can turn to the *Het Offer,* where the Devil figures more prominently.

In the four volumes examined, the name of the Devil, or the adjective diabolical, appears only seven times, and in two volumes, not at all. Of all of these, only in one case was the name used by an accused Anabaptist. One of the reasons for the apparent neglect of the Devil (at least in the official court records) has to do with the attitude of the accused themselves toward the magical and diabolical beliefs of their day. The Anabaptist rejection of all Catholic ritual led them to regard all sacraments as priestly magic. Anabaptists rejected the doctrine that Christ was corporeally present in the consecrated host, because they could not understand how Christ could be physically present both in heaven and in the bread. Most revealing is the confession of the Anabaptist leader Adriaen 'the one eyed' Pieterszoon, who, on 12 May 1534, admitted to the Amsterdam magistrates that he had told some people walking to the 'Holy Place' [*Heilige Stede*], the shrine memorializing the city's miracle of the Host, that the bread and cheese in his hands were as good as the bread (Host) sitting in the shrine's monstrance. He also remarked to some others that if the body of Christ was indeed in the Host, then it should bleed when broken and he challenged these people to bring 'fifty gods' (Hosts) which he would stab with a knife and if they bled, he would believe in the sacrament. Even more brazenly, he had stated in the city hall that the Host is merely baked bread and priests cannot make gods, for God is in heaven. Apparently the city's bailiff [schout] had responded to Adriaen's disbelief by referring Adriaen to the miracles which took place on a daily basis at the Holy Place shrine. To this Adriaen replied, 'the Devil can perform these miracles as well as God'. This, the only reference to the Devil recorded from the lips of in accused Anabaptist in these sources, reveals quite clearly the anti-miraculous (at least in the Catholic sense) perspective of many Anabaptists, perhaps even a commonsense scepticism which contrasts with both the miraculous and learned demonological theory. At the same time, Adriaen's threat to desecrate the Host is not totally removed from the realm of magical beliefs; judging from accusations made against Jews in the later fifteenth and sixteenth centuries, it seems to have been widely believed that desecrated Hosts did bleed, confirming the reality of transubstantiation in the face of doubters.[17] Adriaen most assuredly knew of these beliefs, and his comments must therefore be seen as a direct challenge not to official theology, but to popular religion, to magical thinking.

The Anabaptists' perspective

The accounts of Mennonite trials composed by the victims and collected by an anonymous editor as Het Offer des Heeren [The Offering of the Lord], fill in the picture of the official accounts of interrogations. Unfortunately, only a handful of Het Offer's martyrs appear in the published sources surveyed above and merely one of these, the trial of Lysbet Dircxdochter in Leeuwaarden, Friesland, in 1549, adds considerable new detail. In this account of the interrogation of Lysbet, a former nun executed for her rejection of the sacraments of the church, the authorities ask her what she believed about the 'most worthy, holy sacrament'. In her own account, she responds that she had read nothing of a holy sacrament in the Scriptures, only of a Lord's Supper. To this the gentlemen of the court respond, 'Silence, for the Devil speaks from your mouth.' Preparing her for torture, they strip her against her pleas to force her to confess the names of her associates. She holds firm and is drowned as a heretic. Lysbet's experience in the interrogation room was not far removed from that of accused witches; she was questioned according to a set script, stripped and tortured to uncover her cohorts, and accused of diabolical inspiration. We must not forget, in spite of our proclivity to make sharp distinctions between different fields of study such as heresy and witchcraft – reflected in the practice of pulling Anabaptist records out of their juridical contexts and publishing them separately – that it was often the same court officials who tried both sets of victims, sometimes conducting such seemingly distinct trials during the same week. One would therefore expect the interrogators to carry over techniques and ideas from one interrogation to another, although in most cases the Dutch authorities were able to distinguish clearly between those accused of Anabaptist heresy and those charged with diabolical witchcraft. As seen in the case of Lysbet, and a few of the other cases from Het Offer which we will examine now, accusations of diabolical guidance provided one common thread between the two sets of judicial victims.

Another case is that of Claesken Gaeledochter, executed by the Court of Friesland on 14 March 1559. Claesken records that she was asked the standard questions, what she believed about baptism, who had baptized her, why she had not baptized her children. Then she adds, 'these are the questions which he [the inquisitor] asked me. But he had many more words, and when I did not answer him well, then he said that I had the mute Devil in me, for the Devil places himself as an angel of light in us, which was true of all heretics' (p. 324). (This would have been a reference to a specific demon whose job it was to cause its servants to remain mute when questioned by the authorities.)[18] When two monks were brought in to convince her of her errors, Claesken notes that because of her stubbornness, they too insisted she was controlled by the Devil: 'The beginning and end was that I had the Devil in me, and that I was deceived' (p. 328). After the inquisitor compared her rebaptism with the baptism of a Jew — which by this time was believed to be of little effect — Claesken writes that 'all that he kept saying was that we had it all from the Devil, and that we had the proud Devil in us'. Faced with Claesken's intransigence, the inquisitor concluded that the Devil had called her. She refuted this conclusion by asking, 'is the Devil now of such a nature that he rejects the evil and does the good?', for that is what she and her colleagues have done in their baptism (p. 336).

If the accounts presumably composed by the victims themselves can be trusted (and there seems little reason to doubt their veracity on this point), it appears that the Devil was a more prominent figure in interrogations than the brief trial summaries provided by the authorities would lead us to believe. Anabaptists were apparently accused of being under the lordship of the Devil, even to the degree of possession.[19] Their response was that their godly lives gave the lie to this allegation. Those in league with or possessed by the Devil hardly committed acts of charity toward their fellow humans.

In several instances, Anabaptists charged their interrogators with being those truly in league with the Devil. Hans van Onerdamme, tried in Ghent in 1550, apparently answered the monks who demanded he swear on his baptism and faith to tell the truth: 'What, will you swear much? I regard not your swearing, for it is a craft of the sorcerers [toouenaers], who swear against the truth.' He notes that three of his co-religionists had been returned to the Catholic fold in the course of their trials, something that Hans blamed on the monks' 'bewitched swearing, that they did not keep themselves from the Devil's deception', for they did not have the gift of disputation (p. 110). He compares his opponents to the Egyptian sorcerers who opposed Moses, and concludes his remarks to the gentlemen of the court, 'now understand, you noble sirs, the misuse and abuses of your state or ministry, for we confess it not to be of God, but of the Devil, and that the antichrist has so bewitched and blinded your eyes, through the deceit of the Devil, that you do not perceive yourselves to be what you are' (p. 114). Similarly after his interrogation in the prison of Antwerp in August 1551, Jeronimus Segersz wrote to his wife that 'we must oppose the princes and mighty of this world, yes the spirits that work in the air, which is the old serpent and Satan' (p. 134). He warns her of the Devil which seeks to damn their souls and of the false prophets which have only the teaching of the demons (pp. 145–6). Peter van Weruick, imprisoned in Ghent in 1552, writes to his sisters and brothers that they must distinguish between what is the worship of God and that which is really the worship of the Devil and idolatry. Those who perform righteousness are the children of God, he continues, while those who sin are from the Devil (p. 188). Peter was not reticent to make his opinion known to his interrogators; he reports that he told them 'perhaps your teaching is the teaching of the Devil, for it is against the truth' (p. 190). Another Anabaptist, Claes de Praet, who was eventually executed in Ghent in 1556, was told by Pieter Titelmans, the infamous inquisitor of Flanders, that he had been deceived by the Devil and misled by artisans and that he should now be instructed by the learned. Claes responded, 'why then do they [the learned] lead the life of a Devil?' (p. 244).

The Anabaptist belief that Catholic practices were witchcraft (or sorcery) seems to have been widespread. The lengths that Anabaptists would go to avoid baptizing their infants suggests that they viewed the Catholic rite as one that would, at the very least, taint their children with the diabolical. (On the other hand, spiritualists like David Joris depreciated the importance of externals such as water baptism while at the same time denying the physical existence of the Devil.)[20] In 1553 in Kortrijk Joos Kint was interrogated by inquisitor Titelmans. She confronted him bravely, responding to his demand she renounce her rebaptism by stating 'my faith and baptism I know, but I have nothing to do with your swearing, I would then confess to you sorcerers'. She then warns him not to tell others that she had recanted or that she had a Devil in her, not to mention that she was damned among the simple folk. Several times, in fact, she told her accusers to 'get behind me Satan' (pp. 224–6). For these courageous souls facing their own destruction, it was quite clear who were truly in league with the Devil.

Were there any incidents wherein the authorities conflated beliefs about witches and those about Anabaptists? Joke Spaans has recently discovered some intriguing evidence from Amsterdam witchcraft trials of the 1550s and 1560s where under torture two accused witches appear to have changed their accounts of a meeting with a Mennonite or other sectarian leader in order to conform to their interrogators' views of the Devil. One of the accused, Volckgen Harmansdr of Blokzijl, was executed in 1564 because 'before the enemy she had denied her baptism and christendom [*doopsel ende chrisdom*]'. In her first testimony, Volckgen describes this 'enemy' as a weaver from the Waterland. Spaans plausibly suggests that this could have been a Mennonite, for a relatively high proportion of both Waterlanders and weavers were attracted to this branch of radical reform. In the Amsterdam court records there were also numerous reports during this period of Waterland Mennonites proselytizing in the port city. In any event, in her later confession Volckgen changes the character of the 'enemy' to fit the accepted appearance of the Devil. Spaans also rightly points out that those who underwent sectarian 'rebaptism' were like witches charged with having denied their original baptism and Christian faith. In other words, both Anabaptists and supposed witches were accused of renouncing their original baptism and hence opening themselves to demonic control. The difference is that Anabaptists were not, as far as I have been able to determine, charged explicitly with making a pact with the Devil, the key charge against witches.

Conclusions

It is much easier to describe what this investigation into one form of sixteenth-century religious heresy and witchcraft belief has not shown rather than what it has proven. Certainly I do not wish to revive the old 'witchcraft as heresy' school – that witchcraft was a Christian heresy which developed out of French Catharism – so well demolished by Norman Cohn and Richard Kieckhefer, who discovered that the fourteenth-century documents providing the link between heretical Cathars and the earliest witchcraft trials were forgeries.[21] As far as I have been able to determine, of all the major religious traditions of the sixteenth century, Anabaptists were the least caught up in magical beliefs or practices (apart from those, I suppose, who emphasized immediate revelation).[22] On the other hand, I think it fair to suggest that scholars have been too reluctant to return to the question of the relationship between heresy and supposed demonic sects, especially in the sixteenth century. At least at the level of officialdom, and perhaps too of popular perception, the prosecution of sixteenth-century Anabaptism and of magical deviance had much in common. For one thing, rejection of infant baptism carried with it, in the minds of sixteenth-century people, several diabolical ramifications, not the least of which was the increase in the number of unbaptized and 'unexorcised' individuals who were presumed to be much more susceptible to diabolical influence. Perhaps too the supposed collusion of midwives in assisting Anabaptist parents avoid baptizing their newborn infants helped rekindle suspicions that midwives were in league with the Devil to supply him with unbaptized infants. These and many other parallels between persecution of Anabaptists and witches appeared during the decades of the 1540s to 1560s, precisely the moment when authorities across Europe were becoming less concerned with Anabaptism but even more worried about the menace of witchcraft.

Notes

1   For an early example of this apocalyptical ideology from Holland Anabaptists, see Gary K. Waite and Samme Zijlstra, 'Antiochus Revisited: An Anonymous Anabaptist Letter to the Court at the Hague', *Mennonite Quarterly Review*, 66 (1992), 26–46.

2   Brian P. Levack, *The Witch-Hunt in Early Modern Europe* (2nd edn, London and New York, 1995), 120; William Monter, 'Heresy Executions in Reformation Europe, 1520–1565', in Ole Peter Grell and Bob Scribner, eds, *Tolerance and Intolerance in the European Reformation* (Cambridge, 1996), 48–64, esp. 49.

3   Monter, 'Heresy Executions', 50.

4   Ibid., 62.

5   Martin Luther, *Works*, vol. 26, *Lectures on Galatians*, 194–5.

6   Martin Luther certainly believed that his phrase 'Freedom of the Christian Man' had been badly misused by the German peasants as a slogan of rebellion in 1525. Notwithstanding Luther's protest, the rebellious peasants 'thought of the enterprise as their contribution to the Reformation'. J. M. Stayer, *The German Peasants' War* (Montreal and Kingston, Ont. 1991), 35.

7   For Menno's defence, see his comments in 'Brief Defense to All Theologians' (1552), in John C. Wenger, ed. and Leonard Verduin, trans., *The Complete Writings* (Scottdale, Pa, 1956), 535, and in 'Reply to False Accusations' (1552), Ibid., 571–2.

8   Menno, *The Complete Writings*, 133, 140.

9   For full citations of the Dutch sources used in this chapter, see the original version in Werner O. Packull and Geoffrey L. Dipple, eds, *Radical Reformation Studies* (Ashgate, Aldershot 1999), ch. 8.

10 Paul Frédéricq, ed., *Corpus Documentorum Haereticae Pravitatis Neerlandicae* (Ghent 1892–1906), vol. 4, docs 47, 67.

11 Ibid., docs 72 and 79.

12 In May 1538 Uulbe Claeszoon was executed for refusing to baptize his infant, who had died 17 weeks after birth. Pieter Pieterszoon was condemned in January 1569 for abducting his newborn daughter from her mother so that she could not be baptized.

13 Robin Briggs argues in Chapter 3 of this book that there is no statistical evidence to support the argument that midwives were especially targeted as witches, and his research from the Lorraine trials shows that they were instead under-represented. For an alternative view, see Anne Llewellyn Barstow, *Witchcraze: A New History of the European Witch Hunts* (San Francisco, 1994), 113. The *Malleus Maleficarum* (1487) argued that midwives frequently offered up unbaptized infants to the Devil.

14 This is seen, for example, in the case of Andries Clacszoon of Doonrijp, tried on 16 March 1535 by the Court of Friesland, who freely confessed to rebaptism, to holding conventicles in his house, and who was convicted for being a member of the 'rebellious' sect of Anabaptists in Münster.

15 For the Batenburgers, see Gary K. Waite, 'From Apocalyptic Crusaders to Anabaptist Terrorists: Anabaptist Radicalism after Münster, 1535–1544', *Archiv für Reformationsgeschichte*, 80 (1989), 173–93.

16 Marijke Gijswijt-Hofstra, 'Six Centuries of Witchcraft in the Netherlands: Themes, Outlines, and Interpretations', in Marijke Gijswijt-Hofstra and Willem Frijhoff, eds, *Witchcraft in the Netherlands from the Fourteenth to the Twentieth Century* (Rotterdam, 1991), 1–36, esp. 26. See also Marijke Gijswijt-Hofstra, 'The European Witchcraft Debate and the Dutch Variant', *Social History*, 15 (1990), 181–94.

17 R. Po-Chia Hsia, 'Jewish Magic in Early Modern Germany', in R. Po-Chia Hsia, ed., *Religion and Culture in the Renaissance and Reformation* (London, 1987), 81–97; see also his *The Myth of Ritual Murder: Jews and Magic in Reformation Germany* (New Haven, Conn., and London, 1988). At the same time, Adriaen and his cohorts were able to tap into a rising tide of scepticism regarding the Catholic miraculous tradition; in the same year as Adriaen's boast, city fathers heard several complaints about Amsterdamers who closed their doors and windows when the processional priests carrying the blessed Host in a monstrance to the 'Holy Place' passed by.

18 There were dozens of such demons noted in the various 'Devil's books' of the sixteenth century. For the *genre* as a whole, see Chapter 18 by Erik Midelfort.

19 See Chapter 17 in this book for the classic signs of possession. They included convulsive movements or seizures, speaking in a voice different from one's own, expressing horrible blasphemies, and exhibiting eyes that bug out, a grossly extended tongue, and a head wrenched nearly backward facing.

20 Gary K. Waite, '"Man is a Devil to Himself": David Joris and the Rise of a Sceptical Tradition towards the Devil in the Early Modern Netherlands, 1540–1600', *Dutch Review of Church History*, 75 (1995), 1–30.

21 For the exposure of these documents as fakes, see Chapter 1 in this collection by Richard Kieckhefer.

22 On this point, see Chapter 12 by Stuart Clark.

PART FIVE

Witchcraft, the State and Social Control

WHY DOES MODERN HISTORY begin in 1500? The division of the past into mediaeval and modern epochs has long been a source of dispute between historians. The Protestant Reformation, for example, can be understood only in the context of the Middle Ages – indeed, one historian has argued convincingly that it was 'a mediaeval event' – but the conventions of academic history insist on placing it in the 'modern' era.[1] Outside the academic world, the blurred distinction between the mediaeval and the modern age is reflected in the tendency of people to locate any event before 1800 'in the Middle Ages'.

There is, however, one phenomenon associated with the sixteenth and seventeenth centuries that appears to be unmistakably 'modern'. This is the emergence of the 'nation state': the independent, centrally governed territory with its own political institutions, bureaucracy and laws. The extent to which the countries of early modern Europe conformed to this ideal will always provoke disagreement among historians; but it appears that several factors combined after 1500 to increase the authority of secular rulers across Europe. The Reformation undermined the power of the papacy in both Protestant and Catholic regions, and placed the clergy more firmly under the control of lay magistrates; the new technology of printing encouraged the development of administrative systems, and allowed central authorities to communicate more effectively with outlying areas; and changes in legal practices tended to place more power in the hands of government institutions, while limiting the independence of alternative jurisdictions like the church courts. It has been argued that the combination of these factors produced the 'confessional state', typified in the late sixteenth century by Bavaria, Scotland and Spain: political entities identified with one religious denomination, and possessing the means to impose standards of belief and behaviour on their populations.[2] Understandably, the coincidence of this period of 'state-building' with the major European witch-hunts has encouraged historians to seek links between the two phenomena.

The relationship between the confessional state and witchcraft is considered in this section.

In Chapter 15, Christina Larner presents a thoughtful and influential discussion of the status of satanic witchcraft as a *crimen exceptum* – that is, an exceptional crime for which extraordinary procedures were thought to be necessary. In many respects, she argues that witchcraft was indeed a crime like no other: it was committed in secret, and involved a transgression of social norms more extreme than any other imaginable act. Nonetheless, she suggests that the prosecution of witches should be viewed as part of a more general pattern in early modern society. Witchcraft was one of a number of crimes removed from the jurisdiction of church courts and prosecuted with increased severity by secular authorities; other offences of this kind included sexual misconduct, infanticide and religious dissent. These were 'abstract crimes' against a model of correct behaviour embraced by governing elites. The ultimate purpose of their suppression was to enforce social control, a term which for Larner includes 'all the norms, ideologies, and sanctions by which certain types of social behaviour are encouraged and others discouraged'. It is against this background that the persecution of witches should be properly understood:

> The punitive treatment of deviance not only demonstrates the control
> of rulers but also asserts the values of conformists. The advantage of
> witchcraft over other crimes in this context is that it sums up all forms
> of non-conformity. Witches are evil. The prosecution of witches is a
> peculiarly economical way of attacking deviance.

For Larner, the rise of witchcraft prosecutions was greatly encouraged by the emergence of the confessional state, and its decline began when religious ideology was no longer needed to sustain the authority of ruling groups and their supporters.

Larner's approach has considerable merits. By focusing on the rise of confessionalism, she avoids the mistake of attributing witch persecutions to either Protestant or Catholic doctrine: rather, she suggests that the 'politicisation of religion' on both sides of the divide encouraged the persecution of real and imagined 'enemies of God'. On this point her argument complements the work of Stuart Clark, who suggests in Chapter 12 that the existence of 'state churches' in Protestant and Catholic regions was a prerequisite for witch persecutions. Larner's thesis also goes some way towards explaining the high incidence of women among witchcraft suspects: like adultery and infanticide, witchcraft was a hidden crime against the ideal of the pious, well-ordered household that confessional regimes were determined to uphold; and deviant women represented the most obvious threat to this ideal. Larner's work has been complemented by the findings of historians in other fields: Lyndal Roper has shown that elite groups in sixteenth-century Germany used the Reformation to police sexual deviance and impose new regulations on marriage;[3] and Anthony Fletcher has drawn attention to the brutal suppression of the 'secret crime' of infanticide in early Stuart England.[4]

These qualities have not, however, protected Larner's work from serious criticism. Robin Briggs has argued that she places excessive emphasis on the role of elite groups, and suggests that the claim that 'ideological crimes' legitimized new regimes is 'hardly less wrong' than Margaret Murray's fanciful notion of a pagan witch cult.[5] Some of the weaknesses of Larner's thesis are illustrated in Chapter 16 by Brian Levack. Levack contends that central authorities, far from initiating witch persecutions, were often responsible for restraining the excesses of local officials who wished to eradicate witchcraft in their neighbour-hoods. Taking the example of Scotland – where Larner's primary research was also based – he shows that only a minority of witch trials directly involved the central government, and these trials resulted in an unusually high level of acquittals. The bulk of prosecutions were initiated from below, though they took place under warrants issued from Edinburgh. The use of torture, which was instrumental in securing many convictions, appears to have been largely illegal: local groups exploited the lawful practice of 'pricking' for the Devil's mark to extort confessions from alleged witches, though such forced confessions were regarded as unacceptable by the higher courts. In Levack's view, it was the *failure* of the central administration to control events in the localities that allowed most persecutions to occur; and he argues that a similar state of affairs applied in many of the other emerging nation states of early modern Europe. This conclusion is consistent with some recent reseach from other areas, notably Behringer's study of Germany in Chapter 4.

Can these conflicting interpretations be resolved? The evidence presented by Levack makes it hard to argue that central governments normally initiated witch trials; but this does not mean that Larner was completely mistaken to attribute persecutions to the need of elite groups to legimise their authority. The key issue is the *level* at which this process took place. As Levack notes, those responsible for the bulk of the witch trials in Scotland were not 'private individuals' or 'vigi-lantes': they were members of local elites who went to some length to obtain permission from central government to investigate witchcraft in their own commu-nities. They 'were acting as the rulers of their towns and villages', and used 'the judicial authority of the state' for their own ends. In a period of increased concern about social order, sexual conduct and religious conformity, it is understandable that local leaders sometimes sought to eliminate the percieved threat of witchcraft; and this process might well have increased their standing among their neighbours, particularly if they were acting with the delegated authority of the state. The exer-cise of social control was probably one component of the witch persecutions in sixteenth- and seventeenth-century Europe, though it was not necessarily the product of the centralised, confessional state.

Notes

1   Heiko Oberman, *Luther: Man Between God and the Devil*, trans. E. Walliser-Schwarzbart (Yale University Press, New Haven, Conn. 1989), ch. 2.

2   For the emergence of confessional states in Germany, see R. Po-Chia Hsia, *Social Discipline in the Reformation* (Routledge, London 1989); for a similar argument, see Richard Muchembled, Chapter 10 in this collection.

3   Lyndal Roper, *The Holy Household: Women and Morals in Reformation Augsburg* (Clarendon, Oxford 1989).

4   Anthony Fletcher, *Gender, Sex and Subordination in England, 1500–1800* (Yale University Press, New Haven, Conn. 1995), 277–9.

5   Robin Briggs, 'Many Reasons Why: Witchcraft and the Problem of Multiple Explanation', in Jonathan Barry, Mariane Hester and Gareth Roberts, eds, *Witchcraft in Early Modern Europe* (Cambridge University Press 1996), 52–3.

Chapter 15

Christina Larner

THE CRIME OF WITCHCRAFT IN
EARLY MODERN EUROPE

I

WITCHCRAFT WAS KNOWN AMONG lawyers during the time when it was a capital offence as *crimen exceptum*. They meant quite simply that since it was not amenable to the normal principles of proof, normal standards of interrogation and court procedure would not meet the situation. It was necessary to use torture to extract a confession. It was necessary to admit the evidence of those not normally allowed to bear testimony in courts of law: women, children, interested parties, and convicted felons. The crime of witchcraft went on the statute books, or became otherwise the responsibility of secular powers, at a time when jurisdictions were becoming more centralized and more rationalized and when standards of proof were becoming rather closer to those of our own day. Ideas such as those that juries should not have an interest in the conviction of the accused, confessions should not be extorted by threat or force, witnesses should have seen the crime committed, witnesses should not be intimidated or bribed, were, if not operational, at least current. The management of trials for witchcraft apparently ran counter to much of this emerging rationalization and depersonalization of criminal law and practice.

Nor was it merely among lawyers that witchcraft was regarded as a special case. Commentators in general and the populace at large regarded the trial of a single witch as particularly worthy of note compared, for example, with a trial for theft, slaughter, cattle raiding, or a sexual offence. Large-scale trials evoked widespread horror, titillation and anxiety. This anxiety was not, of course, normally about the innocent being accused, though such anxiety did occur, even among those who fully accepted official legal demonology. James VI of Scotland, for example, withdrew his general commission against witchcraft in 1597, partly on the grounds that people were raising accusations of witchcraft simply to pay off old scores.[1] The burghers of Bavaria realized that the innocent were being involved when accusations were levelled at those at the top of the social scale.[2] All felt anxious when those of previously good character were drawn into the net, for no-one then felt secure. But the basic anxiety was about the prevalence of witchcraft. There was really no period in the whole of the witch-hunting era when the indictment, trial and execution of a witch was regarded by either authorities or populace as completely routine. A witch was, by definition, an abnormal person. The execution of a witch was a demonstration of group solidarity. It removed the provocative deviant and redefined the boundaries of normality to secure the safety of the virtuous community. For witch trials to have been made a routine procedure would have robbed them of their principal social meaning. The legal understanding of *crimen exceptum,* therefore, had echoes in the popular image of it. Witchcraft was more than crime for the practitioner was an enemy and the witch process was directed against the eradication of public enemies.

Yet, at the same time, it is only as a crime that we have detailed knowledge of it and as a crime it undergoes a sea change with regard to the meaning attached to it by the populace. In times and places where the social control of witchcraft was unofficial and not reinforced by state or tribal sanction, our knowledge of this control is through the very limited access of participant observation in present-day societies or the chance of literary survival or anecdote. Even if more lavish material were available about unofficial activities designed to control witchcraft in times and places where witchcraft was not a crime, it seems likely that this would suggest that the interest of church and state made it a qualitatively different phenomenon. Partial evidence for this lies in the fact that unofficial torturing, lynching and illegal execution is almost unknown except during the running down of official prosecutions and just after the removal of the death penalty. The sole known instance of lynching in Scotland occurred in 1704 when the High Court at Edinburgh refused to convict Janet Cornfoot and sent her back to her native Pittenweem where her neighbours strung her up between a boat and the pier and stoned her to death. France, Poland, and Germany likewise had some very dubious executions in the eighteenth century, but none thereafter. The implication of this is that the labelled witch, in a community in which the control of witchcraft is not reinforced by state authority, is found to be less fearful. She fulfils the function of defining the normal standards and boundaries of the local society by being placed on its margins. She explains evil events, but she does not threaten the community's well-being to the extent of needing to be eliminated. The local purpose of defining certain types of human behaviour as criminal is to give clear boundaries to the prevailing norms and customs. Crime, is, therefore, something to live with. For the state, crime was in theory something to be eliminated but, through the redefinition of crime, crimes were and are continually created. The crime of witchcraft was abolished through the formal repeal of witchcraft acts but it had already been abolished *de facto* by the repeated refusal of the late seventeenth- and early eighteenth-century courts to provide enough examples.

For scholars of the twentieth century, witchcraft is also *crimen exceptum* in a different sense. Witchcraft is widely regarded as being unique because it is 'impossible' and special, in that we not longer regard it as a crime. The putting of witchcraft on the statute books and the widespread prosecutions and executions for witchcraft are therefore deemed to require 'explanation' in the sense that the eighteenth-century habit of executing small boys for the theft of objects of small value does not require explanation. The development of an educated demonology is deemed to require 'explanation' in the sense that the development of an educated theology does not. We still inflict a variety of punishments for theft. We still encounter educated persons who believe in the resurrection of the body and the life everlasting. Historians, like sociologists, ought to regard all aspects of remote systems of thought as requiring explanation. In practice, variants of beliefs and practices with which we are culturally at ease do not require it, or at least not at the same level as the culturally alien. The manner in which commentators today view the criminalization of witchcraft in Europe as *crimen exceptum* is an example of this selective process. It bears little relation to the reasons why the lawyers and commentators of the period so regarded it, other than that both are agreed that there is a special problem about evidence.

II

The suggestion that witchcraft should be put back into the criminal context from which it has been extracted does not mean that it is not reasonable to regard it as *crimen exceptum*. Rather, it is hoped that a consideration of the general criminal context will indicate factors which affected a wider range of crimes than witchcraft and which, incidentally, throw more light on witch-hunting. What follows can only be suggestive, since the detailed study of early modern criminal archives has barely begun.

Three possible areas for exploration are the relationship of the crime of witchcraft to the 'judicial revolution', the criminalization of women, and the role of moral panics in social control. It has been suggested by Parker and Lenman[3] that the judicial revolution involved over a considerable period of time (but coinciding with a process which in a Marxist frame of reference is known as the transition from feudalism to capitalism) a change from restorative, interpersonal justice, to abstract, rational, bureaucratic justice with repressive sanctions[4] – the reverse, in effect, of Durkheim's ideal types of legal authority in pre-industrial societies. There was also an increase in the proportion of the sometimes elusive category of victimless crimes. False coining had long been known, but newly grown in status were adultery, blasphemy, bestiality and the Scottish crime of mass-mongering. Indeed, a noticeable feature of sixteenth-century Europe was the secularization of crimes formerly dealt with in ecclesiastical courts. Both England and Scotland passed Acts formally incorporating in statute law a number of such misdemeanours, witchcraft merely being one item among them. On mainland Europe the secular courts steadily encroached in Catholic as well as Protestant areas. The *Constitutio Criminalis Carolina* promulgated by Charles V in 1532 imposed the death penalty for witchcraft.[5] There was also a shift in responsibility from the accuser to the court official, which had the effect of making frivolous or vindictive accusation possible. It also meant that there were those who were responsible, without personal interest, for pursuing the perpetrators of crimes, thus allowing witch-hunting to flourish. Those whom previously the *lex talionis* would have deterred were able to make accusations with impunity.[6] So far as witchcraft was concerned, a system of restitutive justice encouraged anxiety about sorcery and *maleficium*: these crimes had 'victims' alleged to have suffered in their persons, the persons of their kin, and their property from the *maleficia* of the accused. *Maleficium* bridged both the old type of crime against the person and the new type of crime against property, though witchcraft was a rather limited form of crime against property since it ususally involved damage or injury rather than theft. A system of abstract justice, however, made possible the victimless crime of simply being a witch, of being the servant of the Devil. A rationalized theology demanded that the kingdom of Satan possess a social structure of devils and witches to balance that of God with his angels and his saints. These demonic and heavenly hierarchies were pitted against each other in a struggle of variable inequality depending on the orthodoxy of the exponent. This particular rationalization, made possible by the move to a system in which abstract triumphed over restitutive justice, helps to account for the paradox of witch prosecutions coming to the fore at a time when the rules of evidence were becoming more rigorous.

The list of other activities which became prominent as crimes at the same time as witchcraft consists largely of religious and sexual offences. Soman, a pioneer in the treatment of witchcraft as a category of crime among others, has studied the appeals to the parlement of Paris from 1565 to 1640. He found that witchcraft cases were most commonly found alongside cases of incest, adultery, sodomy, and infanticide, and that by and large the figures for all of them rose and fell together.[7] Before turning to the theme of general moral panics suggested by these findings, it is worth looking at an issue contained within the wider one of social control: that of the criminalization of women at this time. Previously kept out of the courts on the grounds that their fathers or husbands were legally responsible for their actions and that crimes committed by them must have been through coercion by their men folk, women suddenly appeared in the courts in large numbers, the old women as witches, the young as infanticides. Soman has suggested that as many women were executed for infanticide in France as for witchcraft. This raises questions which cannot yet be answered about possible changes in the status of women at this time and about the role of women in the moral order. Certainly one factor in the witch-hunt as a whole which has not really been sufficiently examined, despite its obviousness and despite the fact that it was asked continually by commentators and authors of demonological handbooks at the time of the hunt, was that of why witches were women. Most commentators, if they deal directly with the question at all, answer it tautologically by saying that the witch stereotype was always that of a woman, or that women were accused because they, and particularly poor women, were the most socially defenceless category and therefore likely to be accused, or that since men were sometimes accused, and since women accused other women of witchcraft, sexual prejudice was not at issue.[8]

Monter has pointed out that male witches tended either to be related to a female suspect or to have committed some additional crime,[9] and Scottish findings support this. Midelfort notes that the proportion of males rose in major hunts and, as already mentioned, suggests that in these extreme panics the stereotype broke down. The question of to what extent and under what circumstances males got involved in witch-trials, however, is a diversion which distracts attention from the wider issue of female criminalization. The questions which ought to be asked about the witch-hunt are why the stereotype of a witch is that of a woman, and why women were criminalized for the first time on any scale in this period. If women were to be put in the courts as suspected criminals it had to be for new crimes which were either virtually sex-specific, like infanticide, or sex-related. Where existing standard crimes like theft, short-changing or arson were concerned, the behaviour of women was still widely regarded as being the responsiblity of their husbands or fathers, although occasional prosecutions of women did occur.

Witch beliefs represent the inverse of the positive values of any given society. In a patriarchal society the characteristics of the ideal women will be delineated by men: 'her voice was ever soft, gentle, and low, an excellent thing in woman' – and women will identify with this male-delineated ideal. Individual women who deviate too far from it will be identified as witches. The fact that other women will also so identify them does not mean that there is, therefore, no hostility to women in witchcraft accusations. There is hostility to women who exhibit characteristics normally appropriated to men by men, such as independence and aggression, and who fail to fulfil functions thought appropriate to women, such as the nurture of men and children. The stereotype of witch is set by males as a negative standard for women. Female security lies in conforming to the positive standard and therefore women, who for this very reason rarely engage in bonding (the term used by sociologists to describe the male habit of forming sexually exclusive groups and communities for work, relaxation, emotional security, and selfhelp), reinforce their own individual positions by joining in attacks on deviant women. The role of Queen Christina of Sweden, herself a deviant but a powerful one, in suppressing witch-hunting may, therefore, have a different significance than that given it by Trevor Roper.

The anthropological literature has been under-used on this issue. We note only two examples. Nadel in *Nupe Religion* describes Nupe witch-hunting as historically specific rather than endemic in that it related to a period when women had taken over the roles of money lenders and traders in a developing economy. The male craftsmen were very often in debt to these women and were dependent on them. The women, on the other hand, led independent lives, travelled, took lovers and rarely had children. They violated the norm of the caring, submissive female and they, in particular, were frequently accused of witchcraft.[10]

A different angle is stressed in Goody's account of discussions with African women as to why women were more often accused of witchcraft than men. She received the reply, familiar in a sixteenth-century context, that they were more evil. Goody goes on to argue that, unlike men, women have no legitimate outlets for aggression and that, with actual violence either forbidden or impractical, sorcery is their only weapon.[11]

Work on the status of women in Europe in the sixteenth and seventeenth centuries is still in its infancy.[12] There is not yet enough evidence to determine whether there was a significant change at this time of which the embryonic change in legal status was only a part. There is some indication that an increasing complexity in the division of the labour of men may have played some part. It has been suggested that the development of the medical profession may have been a contributory factor to the witch-hunt, in that wise women healers came under the jealous scrutiny of chirurgeons and physicians. While this does not seem to have been of major importance it was certainly a factor in a minority of cases, and it indicates further the variety of ways in which social change could exploit and buttress the new secular capital crime of witchcraft. The third suggested expansion of interpretations of the witch-hunt related to the role of moral panics in social control. The term 'social control' indicates more than merely a radical view of 'law and order'; it includes all the norms, ideologies, and sanctions by which certain types of social behaviour are encouraged and others discouraged. The interest here is in the position of the crime of witchcraft as an item in a list of previously ecclesiastically controlled crimes dominated by sexual behaviour. The work of Soman suggests that in France the rate for witchcraft and for sexual offences (in which infanticide can be included since this crime is closely identified with a penal attitude to pre-marital sexual inter-course) rose and fell together. It has also been noted that in Scotland in 1649, a year of civil war and witch-hunting, the landlord class were for the first time accused of sexual offences by the dominant covenanting clergy.[13] Whether or not such correlations are frequent has yet to be established, but they are suggestive. It has been pointed out that new regimes tend to be repressive, not only in that the new leader or leaders must first extinguish rivals, but they must also establish their own legitimacy. This is done by raising the level of social control and by attacking nonconformity.[14] Under certain circumstances (coronations on the one hand, or civil disorder on the other) this raising of the level of visible control may be inten-sified to that of a moral panic. There are many examples of this extreme type of cleansing operation after changes of regime in African kingdoms. A European example is that of the Scottish witch-hunt which accompanied the arrival and coro-nation of Anne of Denmark in 1590. The lower, more sustained level of attack on deviance both of behaviour and opinion is characteristic of new regimes such as China in 1949 and, more recently, Vietnam and Cambodia. It was true also of the increasingly autonomous states of early modern Europe. Trevor Roper's sugges-tion that outbreaks of witch persecution followed not only Protestant but also Counter-Reformation victories takes on further significance if the religious forms are seen not only as autonomous belief systems but also as validating ideologies. Populations must not only show their commitment to these ideologies but must behave in a way which reinforces this visible commitment. The punitive treatment of deviance not only demonstrates the control of rulers but also asserts the values of conformists. The advantage of witchcraft over other crimes in this context is that it sums up all forms of non-conformity. Witches are evil. The prosecution of witches is a peculiarly economical way of attacking deviance.

If treating witchcraft as an exception among crimes limits that range of appro-priate analysis, so too does treating it as an optional sub-section of the belief structure of the age. Part of the special value of Thomas's work on England lay in the fact that witchcraft was set in the wider context of religion.[15] Indeed, he is the most distinguished English exponent of the *Annales* school and the study of *mental-ités*. In Thomas's view, the English peasantry at the Reformation became deprived of a variety of religious props and practices which they had hitherto been accus-tomed to, and magical beliefs refilled this gap. It has, however, been argued by Delumeau that the peasantry of Europe were effectively Christianized for the first time during the Reformation and Counter-Reformation. Both these movements emphasized the importance of lay personal religion in a way previously unknown. In pre-Reformation Europe, religious belief and practice were matters for the professionals; lay religion was optional. The idea that individuals were responsible for their own salvation transformed the belief structure.[16] The Reformation and Counter-Reformation brought religion, including a sense of sin, to the peasant through preaching and pastoral care. Delumeau relates this to witch-hunting by arguing that the various scourges of famine and disease which afflicted the peasantry began to be seen as the punishments of a just God. The responsibility for sin was seen to lie with the witches. Delameau also argues that there is a basic antipathy between what he calls 'true religion' and magic, and that the witch-hunt was the product of an assault upon the animist mentality of the peasant. Hunting ceased when 'true religion' had been well established at parish level.[17]

This interpretation may underestimate the extent to which official religion propagated rather than opposed a belief in the physical power of demonic forces but it does lay the emphasis on the struggle for minds. The whole concept of the demonic pact is dependent on the idea of personal responsibility. The argument that Christianization was an important element in the witch-hunt is set in a wider framework by Muchembled, who sees both as a by-product of intensified control by the rulers of newly emergent and shifting political entities.[18] He argues that this involved the imposition of urban values onto the countryside, and suggests that the most persistent witch-hunts took place in border areas. Certainly, it was a period when the new ruling classes demanded that official ideologies should receive assent from the populace. Any collisions between these ideologies and the rebellious individuals produced persecutions. *Cuius regio eius religio* was the formula of legitimate government and expressed a movement towards social control more pervasive than mere law and order.

The chronology of the *decline* of religious persecutions and witch prosecutions is a stronger argument for the autonomy of belief systems than is the growth of the hunt for heretics, witches, and non-conformists. The persecutions died within societies which were still predominantly peasant economies. When the last witches were executed, major industrial change had yet to come. The belief in witchcraft was neither overcome by scientific development nor argued out of court. Its political significance faded as that of secular ideologies rose. Those who were opposed to witch-hunting always argued within the context of the belief in God and the Devil. Trevor-Roper has said that it was necessary for belief in the Kingdom of Satan to die before the witch theory could be discredited. It would be less elegant but would not extend this idea too far to say that it was necessary for the positive side of this ideological and political construct, that of the Kingdom of God, also to fade away. Its replacement, however, by a variety of secular alternatives such as the pursuit of liberty, the sanctity of property, or loyalty to the state, has not obviously produced fewer victims.

It was suggested at the outset that it would be premature to survey in detail the archival research now being carried out on witch trials in various parts of Europe. It is possible, moreover, that by the time this kind of exploration has been carried to a point at which a new synthesis of the European witch-hunt might be expected, both such a synthesis and the analyses of local and national witch-hunts will have been overtaken and absorbed by the developing study of early modern criminology. What is likely to prevent this, however, is that while the study of witchcraft is in some ways broadened by being put into a criminal perspective, it is at the same time confined. It may be thrown into particular relief as an element in the administration of law and order but it still needs to reflect the totality of cosmological beliefs held by ruled and ruler in early modern Europe.

Notes

1   *Register of the Privy Council of Scotland*, vol. v, 409.
2   H. C. Erik Midelfort, *Witch-Hunting in Southwestern Germany, 1562–1684*, (Stanford, Calif., 1972), 150–1.
3   B. Lenman, G. Parker and V. Gatrell (eds) *Crime and the Law: the Social History of Crime in Western Europe since 1500* (London, 1980), xx.
4   For a similar argument, see Chapter 10 in this book by Robert Muchembled.
5   J. H. Langbein, *Prosecuting Crime in the Renaissance* (Cambridge, Mass., 1974), 134; Midelfort, *Witch-Hunting*, 22–3.
6   N. Cohn, *Europe's Inner Demons* (London, 1993), 161-3.
7   Soman, *Annales*, and 'The Parliament of Paris and the Great Witch Hunt (1565–1640)', *Sixteenth Century Journal*, 9, 2 (1978).
8   Gilbert Geis, 'Lord Hale, Witches, and Rape', and comment, *British Journal of Law and Society*, 5 (1978); and A. Anderson and R. Gordon, 'Witchcraft and the Status of Women', *British Journal of Sociology*, 29, 2 (1978).
9   E. William Monter, *Witchcraft in France and Switzerland* (Ithaca, NY), 197.
10   E. Nadel, *Nupe Religion* (London, 1954), 163–81.
11   E. Goody, 'Legitimate and Illegitimate Aggression in a West African State', in Mary Douglas (ed.) *Witchcraft Confessions and Accusations* (London, 1970), 240.
12   But see Alice Clark, *The Working Life of Women in the Seventeenth Century* (London, 1919), 2nd edn, 1968; Roisin McDonough and Rachel Harrison, 'Patriarchy and Relations of Production', in A. Kuhn and Ann Marie Wolpe (eds) *Women and Modes of Production* (London, 1958); Sheila Rowbotham, *Hidden from History* (London, 1973); R. Hamilton, *The Liberation of Women* (London, 1978). For a more recent study of women in England, see Anne Lawrence, *Women in England, 1500–1760* (London, 1994).
13   Unpublished research notes by Malcolm Scott.
14   Terrence Morris, *Deviance and Control* (London, 1976), 19–24.
15   K. Thomas, *Religion and the Decline of Magic* (London, 1991), 43 *passim*, but see 76.
16   J. Delumeau, *La Civilisation de la Renaissance* (Paris, 1967), 23, and *Catholicism between Luther and Voltaire* (London, 1977), 155–72. See also A. N. Galpern, *The Religions of the People in Sixteenth-Century Champagne* (Harvard, Mass. 1976), especially 108–10.
17   Delumeau, *Catholicism between Luther and Voltaire*, 170–2.
18   See Chapter 10 in this book

Chapter 16

Brian Levack

STATE-BUILDING AND WITCH HUNTING IN EARLY MODERN EUROPE

DURING THE 1980S AND 1990S a number of historians have attempted to establish a causal relationship between the great European witch hunt of the sixteenth and seventeenth centuries and the development of the modern state. These scholars have claimed that 'the rise of the nation state' is at the very least one of the secondary causes of the witch hunt; that the hunt resulted from the centralisation of royal power; that it is one reflection of the advance of public authority against 'particularism', that it is integrally related to the assertion of reason of state; and that it proceeds from an impulse towards both absolutism and state sovereignty.[1] The general impression one gets from this line of argument is that witches were in a certain sense victims of the advance of that emerging leviathan, the centralised, bureaucratised, secularised modern state. The purpose of this chapter is to examine this line of argument and to suggest some limitations to it. It will also test some of these theories about the connection between state-building and witch hunting with reference to one country in which it is alleged that they are especially apparent, the kingdom of Scotland.

The argument consists of four separate but related strands. The first deals with judicial and administrative centralisation, which is incontestably one of the most salient features of state development. Here the argument is that the growth of the state involved the advance of central, i.e. royal, jurisdiction, as a result of which areas which had enjoyed a large measure of autonomy, especially those on the geographical periphery of royal domains, came within the ambit of central government control. The ideal after which rulers strove was 'a centralized authority with a perfect bureaucracy, consisting of local official bodies that were merely executive powers'.[2] This attack on localism and particularism, so, it is claimed, led to an increase in the prosecution of witches, as the state enforced witchcraft edicts from the central government and instructed local authorities about a crime they were ill prepared to prosecute. No matter where prosecutions occurred, they reflected the inexorable process by which the juggernaut of the state imposed its authority on subordinate units.

The second strand of the argument deals with both the officialisation of judicial power and its enhancement through new methods of repression, especially judicial torture. The rise of large-scale witch hunting was facilitated by the adoption of inquisitorial procedure, according to which governmental officials conducted the entire legal process by themselves and used physical force to compel men suspected of secret crimes to confess. Inquisitorial procedure was improved during the fifteenth and sixteenth centuries, mainly by involving the state more and more in the initiation of cases, and by the seventeenth century it had become one of the main features of the absolutist state. When witches were subjected to this procedure they became entrapped in what is referred to as the state machine, from which, so it is argued, there was little hope of escape. It is interesting to note in this connection that the justification given for the exercise of these new judicial powers was the doctrine of 'reason of state', which itself reflected the 'secular rationality' of the early modern period.

The third strand of the argument deals with the efforts of the state to reform society and transform it into a godly community. This involved the disciplining of the population or the 'acculturation of the rural world' that Robert Muchembled sees as one of the main characteristics of the absolutist state. This enterprise was undertaken by an entire hierarchy of officials, from the king down to the local judges and parish priests, all of whose authority the state was promoting. The prosecution of witches, according to this thesis, was just one part of this process of acculturation, one in which the state, usually with the assistance of the church, pursued the ultimate objective of destroying superstition, producing a more godly and homogeneous population, and promoting obedience to the 'absolute king and to God'.[3]

The fourth part of the argument concerns the relationship between church and state. One of the main indications of the growing power of the state during the early modern period was that it effectively gained control over, or at least secured the support of, the church. In terms of jurisdiction, this meant either the assumption of control by secular authorities over matters previously entrusted to the church, or the use of ecclesiastical courts to provide effective support for secular tribunals. These changes, which took place throughout Europe in the sixteenth century, greatly facilitated the prosecution of witches. The state, with its almost unlimited judicial resources, was much more capable of conducting these prosecutions than the church had ever been. Even more important was the cooperation that developed between church and state, which was especially apparent in a crime of mixed jurisdiction like witchcraft. As that cooperation became more common, the crime of witchcraft was often viewed as treason against God on the one hand and an act of rebellion against the state on the other. The identification of secular and religious crime was deliberate: the state prosecuted witches, so it is argued, in order to legitimise new regimes through the pursuit of religious deviants.[4]

It is not the purpose of this chapter to challenge all these propositions. There is much of value in the historical work that has just been summarised, and historians of witchcraft have used it to deepen our understanding of the phenomenon we are studying. It is, for example, incontestable that the secularisation of witchcraft prosecutions had a dramatic impact on the intensity of prosecutions and the number of executions.[5] It is also incontestable that the use of inquisitorial procedure by temporal authorities facilitated numerous prosecutions that otherwise might have been unsuccessful. There is, however, a danger inherent in this line of thought that we shall view the state, and especially the monarchy and the central authorities that most clearly embodied and represented it, as the dynamic force in witchcraft prosecutions.[6] Nothing could be further from the truth. The active, the dynamic force in most witchcraft prosecutions were local authorities, members of local elites who did whatever they could to gain the sanction of central authorities but who did not serve as their direct agents. The central officers of the state, moreover, did much more to restrain these local authorities than to abet them in their efforts to prosecute witches.

In order to illustrate this point, let us look closely at the Scottish situation. In many ways Scotland serves as the ideal test case for the process we are studying. The witch hunt in that country has been referred to as one of the major witch hunts in Europe, and the intensity of prosecutions was quite high, perhaps twelve times as great as in England, although it did not reach the level of some German states. While by no means one of the most powerful states of Europe, Scotland made sustained efforts throughout the sixteenth and seventeenth centuries to increase the power of the central government, and it is precisely this attempt to strengthen the state that lies at the centre of the argument that has been outlined above. The Scottish parliament proclaimed the imperial status of its monarchy even earlier than did England, and from the fifteenth century onwards its rulers aspired towards absolute power. Scotland also experienced a reception of Roman law and adopted at least some aspects of inquisitorial procedure. Torture was used as part of an effort to repress political dissent and to assist the state in prosecuting crime.

The links between this process of state development and witch hunting appear to be stronger in Scotland than in other European states. The prosecution of witches was secularised in Scotland at a fairly early date, and there was considerable cooperation between church and state in prosecuting the crime. James VI, the king of Scotland during one of the country's most intense periods of witch hunting, not only was a royal absolutist but also wrote a treatise that encouraged the prosecution of witches. There were many efforts made throughout this period to associate witchcraft with political dissent. Finally, and most important, the crime of witchcraft was, according to Christina Larner, centrally managed. It seems therefore that Scottish witchcraft prosecutions can easily be placed within a framework of political development. According to Larner, 'The Scottish witch-hunt spanned a period which began with the rise of the doctrine of the divine right of kings and ended with the decline of the doctrine of the godly state'.[7]

Our inquiry must begin with the passage of the Scottish witchcraft statute of 1563, the law upon which all secular prosecutions were based until its repeal in 1736. On the face of it, this, like other European witchcraft statutes, proclamations or edicts, was an attempt by the state to assume control of a crime that was prosecuted, if at all, under the jurisdiction of relatively impotent church courts. But the statute does not represent any such secular initiative. The witchcraft statute was adopted by a parliament that was under considerable pressure from the church to inaugurate a campaign of moral reform and establish a godly discipline. This pressure marked the beginning of a long campaign by the clergy to encourage secular Scottish authorities to prosecute witches. This pattern is worth noting; the history of witchcraft prosecutions in Scotland is much more the story of a reluctant central government responding to pressure from subordinate authorities, in this case the clergy, than the attempt of a developing state to discipline the population.

Far more important than the 1560s, at least for our purposes, are the 1590s, when intense witch hunting began, apparently under the supervision of the central government. Regarding the crisis of 1590–1 and the subsequent orgy of witchcraft prosecutions much has been written, and there is no question that James VI, who became convinced that he, a divine right monarch who was the chief enemy of Satan, was the target of the witches' activities, played a significant role in it. At one point he personally interrogated the North Berwick witches, who together with the earl of Bothwell were believed to have been involved in treason as well as witchcraft. But it would be misleading to see the government as the inspiration of the large rash of witchcraft trials that took place between 1591 and 1597, much less those that occurred after 1597. It is true that between 1591 and 1597 the privy council issued standing commissions to local authorities to seek out and punish witches in their towns and parishes. These commissions, however, represented responses to local pressures for prosecution, not initiatives taken by the king or privy council. Moreover, the government, having responded to the crisis in this way, discovered that the situation had become out of control, and in 1597 the privy council withdrew the standing commissions. In order to prevent such miscarriages of justice from ever occurring again, it insisted that henceforth all witchcraft trials receive authorisation from the privy council or the parliament. It was this decision that made Scottish witchcraft, in Larner's words, a centrally managed crime, and it was this central management that allegedly allowed large witch hunts to develop in Scotland at a later date.

But how much 'management' did the central officers of the Scottish state exercise over witchcraft prosecutions, and what was the effect of that management? Secular witchcraft prosecutions in Scotland took three different forms. The first was a prosecution in the central criminal court, the court of justiciary, a process that was often initiated by the lord advocate before royal judges. The second was in a circuit court, presided over by a judge from the central courts. The third was by a commission of justiciary, a warrant granted by either parliament or privy council that allowed members of local elites, such as elders and magistrates, to prosecute and execute witches. There was much more central management of the crime in the first two situations than the last. Although the government approved all three types of prosecutions, and to that extent exercised some control over the judicial process, it actually supervised the process only in the central and the circuit courts, in which officials of the central government conducted, or at the very least presided over, the trials. When commissions of justiciary were granted, however, the government virtually abdicated its control, allowing the local authorities to proceed as they wished, without any guidance or supervision from the state.

This failure of the government effectively to 'manage' prosecutions in the localities assumes enormous significance when we learn that a solid majority of Scottish witchcraft prosecutions originated in parliamentary or conciliar commissions of justiciary, while less than one-third took place in the justiciary court or in the circuit courts. Even more significant are the outcomes of those commissioned trials which, on the basis of admittedly limited evidence, resulted in the astonishingly high conviction rate of 95 per cent. By contrast the conviction rate in the central courts was 57 per cent, while in the circuit courts, which did not function effectively until the late seventeenth century, the conviction rate dropped to an even lower 45 per cent.[8] What these figures suggest is that central authorities tended to exercise a restraining influence over Scottish witchcraft prosecutions while the members of local elites took the lead in demanding and obtaining their prosecution and conviction.

It is important to emphasise that the activities of local elites which are reflected in these statistics are not those of private individuals, much less vigilantes. These men were acting by properly delegated authority, and the fact that they went to great lengths to obtain it, sending an agent to Edinburgh and producing sufficient documentation to the proper authorities, suggests that the rule of law was perhaps more firmly established throughout the kingdom than is usually conceded. What we are witnessing, however, is much more the local elite's use of the judicial authority of the state for its own ends than the central government's imposition of its will on subordinate authorities in the localities. The initiative is coming from the periphery, not the centre. The elders and magistrates who conducted these local trials were acting as the rulers of their towns and villages, not as agents of the central government or as executors of a central governmental policy. The role that central state authorities played in the process was minimal. They ensured that there was a basis for the commission, but did virtually nothing after that. They had neither the money nor the personnel effectively to manage these prosecutions, and it is possible that they did not really care that much about tying local justice more closely to the centre, at least during James VI's reign. Nor did central state authorities do anything to facilitate the spread of witch hunts from one area to another, even though they had a mechanism for achieving that effect.

Once we recognise the essentially local dynamic of Scottish witchcraft prosecutions, the role of the central government as a moderating influence, sometimes even as a sceptical influence, on the prosecution of witches becomes clearer. It was the central government, for example, that resisted the demands of the local presbyteries to issue standing commissions again during the 1640s, a time when witch hunting became more intense than it had ever been before. It was the central government that exposed the famous prickers, John Kincaid and John Dick, as frauds in 1662. And it was central justices like Sir George Mackenzie who were most responsible for the decline in Scottish witchcraft prosecutions in the late seventeenth century.

But what about the procedures that were used to try those witches who were successfully prosecuted? Part of the argument that links witch hunting to the growth of state power is the employment of inquisitorial procedure and the use of torture in the prosecution of witches. Both of these developments mark the officialisation and bureaucratisation of the judicial power as well as the replacement of private by public authority. With inquisitorial procedure the state assumes control over, if it does not also initiate, prosecutions, and through methods like torture it acquires the information that it needs successfully to prosecute dissenters and other enemies of the government. In many ways the advent of inquisitorial procedure is the quintessential expression of the new power of the state.

Now it is important to recognise that Scottish criminal procedure was only partially inquisitorial. Scotland never did away with the petty trial jury, for example, an institution that vanished in those countries where the state gained full control of the judicial process. Nevertheless, Scottish courts did employ many features of continental criminal procedure, such as the initiation of cases by information and the creation of a legal dossier, and therefore it is worthwhile to inquire whether those features of Scottish justice contributed to the intensification of witch hunting. A strong case can be made for the fact that they did not.

The main consideration here is that anything resembling inquisitorial procedure was utilised only in the court of justiciary and on circuit, where trained judges could oversee the judicial process, and it was precisely in these tribunals that witch hunting was greatly restrained. The lord advocate, to be sure, did initiate cases that might not have otherwise reached the courtroom. But once the case began, the officialisation of the Scottish criminal process worked to the advantage of the witch, resulting in a surprisingly high percentage of acquittals, almost as high as in England. One reason for this was the fact that in these central trials the witch was often granted a defence counsel, a luxury denied to her southern English neighbour.

The relative moderation of central Scottish witchcraft trials can also be explained by the infrequency of the administration of judicial torture. Here we come to one of the great misconceptions in the history of Scottish witchcraft, one which also helps to explain the severity of local prosecutions. Contrary to widely held assumptions, Scottish courts did not have authority to use torture as an ordinary instrument of criminal prosecution. The Scottish law of torture was in fact almost the same as its English counterpart. Torture could be administered only by a warrant from the privy council or parliament and only when the members of those bodies considered information from the accused to be vital to the state. For this reason, the great majority of English and Scottish torture warrants dealt with crimes of a political nature: treason, rebellion, sedition, attacks on prominent statesmen and religious subversion.

Considering the large amount of information we have regarding the use of torture in Scottish witchcraft cases, one would expect to find a large number of warrants dealing with that crime. This is not the case. Between 1590 and 1689 the Scottish privy council issued only two warrants to torture suspected witches: the famous trials of 1591 in which James VI was the intended victim, and the trial of six men for murder by poison, witchcraft or some other 'develische' practice in 1610.[9]

If the official authorisation of torture in Scottish witchcraft cases occurred so infrequently, how then do we account for its reported use in numerous other witchcraft prosecutions? How, for example, do we account for the report published in England in 1652 that six Scottish witches had been whipped and their feet and heads burned by lighted candles while hanging by their thumbs with their hands tied behind their backs? The answer is that local magistrates were using torture illegally, a practice that central Scottish authorities only periodically tried to curb. In the case just cited, officials of the kirk were accused of having applied the torture before referring the case to the civil magistrate. In fact, almost all the evidence we have regarding the use of torture in Scottish witchcraft cases indicates that local magistrates or clergy, not central judges or councillors, were administering it without warrant, usually during the interrogations that took place shortly after apprehension.[10] Even the well-known torture of Alison Balfour, who was tried before the court of justiciary in 1594 after having been kept in the caspieclaw for forty-eight hours, appears to have been conducted by local authorities without warrant.

In many instances the torture took the form of pricking the witch with a needle or 'brod' in order to discover the Devil's Mark, which according to demonological theory was insensitive to pain and could not bleed. This task, which was often entrusted to a professional pricker and which was technically legal, could easily develop into a form of torture, in which a suspect could be pricked repeatedly until she confessed. It appears that many of the confessions elicited during the great Scottish witch hunts of 1649 and 1661–2 were the result of torture administered under this pretext.

It appears therefore that the growth of state power and the officialisation of the judicial process did very little to intensify witchcraft prosecutions in Scotland. Indeed, it was the failure of the state to control local authorities and to supervise local justice, that led to the great prosecutions of the seventeenth century. These local authorities figured how to use the power of the state to their advantage, mainly by obtaining commissions that entitled them to proceed. Once they started that procedure, however, they virtually ignored the rules regulating the administration of justice that the state had established, and illegally used one of the most terrifying instruments of state power, judicial torture, to secure convictions. No wonder that Sir George Mackenzie, one of the most ardent royal absolutists in Scottish history, a lawyer who struggled for the elimination of juries and the implementation of a fully inquisitorial system of criminal procedure, should have deplored the actions of these ignorant 'country men' in the provinces. It is also important to note that Mackenzie, who had participated in some of the witch trials of 1661 in Midlothian on special assignment by parliament, distinguished himself as the greatest critic of witchcraft prosecutions in his country, one whose brilliant defence of the witch Maevia has a prominent place among his published pleadings.[11]

The attitude of Mackenzie also suggests two other conclusions. The first, certainly not new among witchcraft historians, is that scepticism developed more quickly at the centre, especially among members of the ruling elite, than in the localities. That argument can even be extended to James VI, whose scepticism, which allegedly originated in England, can actually be backdated to his days in Scotland.[12] Whether the scepticism of central authorities can be explained by their uninvolvement in the hysteria that often surrounded local witch hunts or by their commitment to high standards of judicial impartiality is uncertain, but the pattern is clear. The second conclusion is that the process of decriminalising witchcraft, in which Mackenzie took an active part, always began in the centre, not on the periphery.

Leaving Scotland for the moment, let us ask whether we can extend this argument regarding state power to other European countries. It would seem that England, the country with which Scotland is most frequently compared, would completely destroy the argument and provide strong negative support for those who see links between absolutism and state power on the one hand and intense witch hunting on the other. The low number of witchcraft convictions in England is widely known, and it is tempting to attribute this, at least in part, to the country's low level of 'stateness'. It should stand to reason that a country with such limited central power, the great hold-out against the inexorable tide of absolutism in Europe, the home of the common law which had resisted the officialisation of the judicial process and prohibited the use of torture, should have had a relatively mild and short-lived witch hunt. The problem here is that we tend to confuse what Michael Mann has referred to as despotic and infrastructural state power.[13] England may have resisted the impulse towards absolutism, and its central government may have been both small and constitutionally restricted, but its judicial system was highly centralised, and the central government was able to run the country quite effectively. Indeed, if we measure stateness by the effective judicial power of the central government, England, a country with a common law and a national circuit court system, was one of the most powerful states in Europe. There is no better illustration of the effects of this strength than in the prosecution of witches, which was undertaken locally and without central governmental initiation but which was supervised quite closely and effectively by central judges at the semi-annual assizes. It was this supervision, which was almost absent in local Scottish trials until the late seventeenth century, which ensured that the English prohibition of judicial torture would be enforced and the rules of evidence applied. The process did not, of course, prevent convictions and executions, especially when a witch-hanging judge like Sir Edmund Anderson was presiding, or when the judge failed to instruct the jury properly, as in Exeter in 1682.[14] But the overall effect of central super-vision on the intensity of prosecutions and the rate of convictions and executions was negative.[15]

The importance of central supervision in English witchcraft prosecutions can be illustrated by the effects of its failure in the 1640s, when England experienced the largest witch hunt in its history. Between 1645 and 1647 the self-defined witch-finders, Matthew Hopkins and John Stearne, acting with considerable support and encouragement from towns and villages in the southeastern part of the country, discovered and assisted in the prosecution of large numbers of witches. In their work of detection they used procedures of highly questionable legality, including the torture of forced sleeplessness. Under normal circumstances the justices of the assize would have prevented the use of such evidence at the trials. At the Essex assizes in the summer of 1645, however, where most of the early convictions in this witch hunt took place, the circuit judges from Westminster were not in atten-dance. Instead, the court was convened under the presidency of the earl of Warwick, a legally untrained nobleman who represented military authority. Without the participation of judges from the central court, the justices of the peace who pros-ecuted the cases were given much more latitude in the use of evidence than they would have otherwise received.

A second illustration of the absence of central judicial supervision comes from the English colonies in North America, where there was no circuit court system and where men without legal training served as judges. The danger inherent in such an arrangement became evident in Massachusetts in 1692, when 156 persons, most of them from Salem Village and Andover, were charged with witchcraft, a relatively large witch hunt that led to 19 executions. The judges who presided over these trials failed to enforce the fairly strict standards of judicial proof that had been applied both in English witchcraft trials and in those held in New England prior to the Salem episode.[16] They also tolerated the use of both physical and psychological pressures in order to obtain confessions, thereby violating one of the most important procedural safeguards in Anglo-American criminal law. It is interesting to note that these legally untrained men all came from the general vicinity where the accusations originated and were affected, therefore, by the highly charged emotional atmosphere that developed during the early stages of the hunt. Thus the Salem judges had more in common with the elders and lairds who served as local commissioners of justiciary in Scotland than with the central judges who went on circuit in England.

A final illustration of the role of central authorities in English witchcraft prosecutions comes from the one court in which the state could proceed by information, the central court of Star Chamber. In that conciliar court we find the government using its special judicial powers not to prosecute witches but to take action against their accusers. Indeed, the first trial in England in which the state actively prosecuted the accusers of witches for fraud was the Star Chamber case of Anne and Brian Gunter in 1606–7, an action initiated by the attorney general, Sir Edward Coke. The action followed the acquittal of two women at the Berkshire assizes in 1605 for having allegedly caused the demonic affliction of Anne, a teenage girl.[17]

Crossing the channel to France, we find ourselves in a very different political environment, as both contemporaries like Sir John Fortescue and subsequent historians have never failed to point out. Here it seems we might expect to find the strongest support for the 'state thesis', if we may call it that. In France the prosecution of witches has been associated not only with 'centralising absolutism' and an attack on particularism but with the efforts of the state to discipline the population. Robert Muchembled has seen witch hunting as part of a larger attack on popular culture that was conducted by agents of state and church and was inspired by both the Counter-Reformation and a programme of royal absolutism. Now if we consider the 'state' to comprise all 'natural rulers' from the king down through the hierarchy of provincial and local officials to parish priests and fathers within families, as Muchembled does, and if we consider absolutism to have entailed an assertion of power by all these authorities, then it is hard to deny that witchcraft prosecutions, which usually involved the exercise of power by elites over their inferiors, were the result of the rise of the absolutist state. The difficulty arises only when we attribute the inspiration of these witchcraft prosecutions to those royal officials who stood at the top of this hierarchy and when we see these trials as part of a policy of centralisation. It is true that most of those prosecutions took place in the peripheral regions of the kingdom, outside 'royal' France, but it is difficult to see this as part of an effort to destroy particularism. Indeed, the main reason why prosecutions flourished in these outlying regions was the failure of the government to supervise the judicial process. Local elites in these areas, to be sure, did everything they could to use state power to their advantage, just as they did in Scotland, but they did not prosecute witches as part of some centrally managed or centrally inspired campaign.

Further evidence for the negative role of the French absolutist state in witchcraft prosecutions comes from the work of Alfred Soman on the decriminalisation of witchcraft in those areas which came under the jurisdiction of the parlement of

Paris. According to Soman, the source of the parlement's policy of obligatory judicial review of all witchcraft convictions, which was proposed in 1588, enacted in 1604 and reenacted in 1624, was a local panic in the Champagne-Ardennes region in 1587–8. In this episode, which was not unlike the Scottish panic of 1591–7, local officials were swimming suspected witches, using the courts to settle personal disputes, and executing suspects in summary fashion, sometimes by lynching. The process of establishing control over these local panics was a delicate one, but it eventually succeeded. Part of this process, it should be noted, was the effort of the parlement to restrict the administration of torture to itself, just as the Scottish privy council had tried to do.[18]

The important consideration for our purposes, however, is the fact that the process of state-building, the process of controlling the periphery, indeed the process of establishing anything more than the most tenuous links between the centre and the periphery, had nothing to do with the encouragement of prosecutions and everything to do with its restraint. The effect of judicial centralisation in France was that the higher courts could monitor the actions of local judges, as they did frequently between 1580 and 1650, and even bring criminal charges against those who used abusive procedures in trying witches. It has been argued that one of the reasons for the high incidence of witchcraft prosecutions in the outlying regions of France was precisely the fact that they did not fit into the centralised judicial system of the absolute state and therefore did not have an automatic review or appeals process.[19]

When we turn our attention to Germany, we find ourselves in a somewhat different political world. Here we have difficulty identifying the central state authorities. Should they be the officials of the large and amorphous empire or those of the 350 smaller political units that it comprised? If we decide upon the former, the main argument of this chapter finds strong, albeit negative, support. Even though the famous imperial law code of 1532, the Carolina, included a provision for prosecuting witches, imperial authorities did not actively pursue witches or encourage subordinate officials to do so. Even if they had, their task would have been difficult since imperial power was exceptionally weak.

That of course is the reason why the smaller political units within the empire were able to prosecute witches with such freedom. However much the emperor might have wished to emulate the national states of Europe in restraining witchcraft prosecutions, he had virtually no jurisdictional weapons with which to act. He had no intendants, no viceroys, no circuit judges. He had a central imperial court, the Reichskammergericht, but no method of making appeals to it mandatory. In fact the only provision that imperial authorities could make for local witchcraft trials was the requirement that law professors from nearby universities provide instruction in a crime about which local authorities knew little. This provision, of course, had a devastating effect on witchcraft prosecutions, since it was these very jurists who provided local magistrates with demonological theories as well as a certain amount of procedural training.[20]

As we turn from Germany to Spain, the terms of the argument change once again, since many witchcraft cases were heard before the tribunals of the inquisition, which was of course an ecclesiastical institution. It was, however, also a royal institution, under the control of the king, and therefore can legitimately be considered as part of the state apparatus. Indeed, the inquisition has been referred to as 'an instrument of royal policy, an agent of centralisation', and a defence against the 'centrifugal forces' in Spanish politics. The extent to which the inquisition served to restrain the process of witch hunting, mainly by controlling the various tribunals through the central supreme council in Madrid, helps to illustrate how little witch hunting can be considered the result of centralisation or, more gener-ally, the process of state-building.[21] Further support for this thesis comes from the evidence we have of intense witch hunting in the local municipalities, such as in the towns of Catalonia in 1618, which were sometimes able to evade strict control from the centre.

Witch hunting in Italy, where most historians contend that the development of the modern state began, had much in common with the prosecutions that took place in Spain. In Italy, as in Spain, most witchcraft prosecutions came under the control of the inquisition, and as in Spain the judicial record is one of almost aston-ishing restraint. The main point to be made here is that it was in the courts of the Roman inquisition that inquisitorial procedure was perfected, and where the interest of the state in prosecutions was most boldly asserted. Yet that highly developed procedure, as John Tedeschi has shown, worked constantly in favour of the accused witch, certainly as much as the highly touted common law procedure that prevailed in England.[22]

The final country in this survey, Denmark, is especially relevant to our concerns, since that kingdom, like Scotland, had a monarch who developed a personal commitment to witch hunting. Christian IV (1588–1648), duly alarmed by a witch hunt that took the lives of eleven women in Koge in 1612, apparently was instrumental in the promulgation of the famous ordinance of 1617, which defined the crime of witchcraft for the first time and reserved the penalty of burning only to those who had made pacts with the Devil. Since prosecutions increased dramatically after 1617, it is tempting to see them as the result of actions taken at the centre, especially since accompanying legislation against adultery and fornica-tion suggests a broader policy of state-sponsored discipline.[23] Once again, however, appearances are deceptive. Whatever the role of King Christian in these trials – and it has not been established that there was any at all – his government can certainly not be assigned responsibility for the hunt that occurred. Quite to the contrary, the impulse to witch hunting came from below, from the district courts, whereas the role of the central government was to ensure the adherence to estab-lished procedures, and to guarantee that all convictions from the lower courts be appealed to the county courts and, if necessary, to the supreme court. It is instruc-tive to note that just under 90 per cent of the cases heard at the district level, where trials were held by juries that knew the accused, resulted in convictions, whereas the proportion at the royal county courts was approximately 50 per cent.[24] These percentages, it should be recalled, come remarkably close to those in Scotland, and in both cases the local courts proceeded by jury trial, whereas in the higher courts inquisitorial procedure prevailed.

Some of the conclusions that emerge from this study of witch hunting may not be all that startling. It has long been recognised that local courts pursued witches more aggressively than central courts; that many witchcraft convictions were reversed on appeal; that scepticism appeared first in the central courts. What is not often recognised, however, is the role that state-builders played in this whole process. However much they may have wished for a more homogeneous population, however much they may have desired to discipline the lower classes and help the church wipe out superstition, they also were firm advocates of what has come to be called the rule of law, and that often meant adherence to strict legal procedure. These two goals, of social control and judicial restraint, came in conflict with each other, especially in cases of witchcraft, and the state found itself regulating over-zealous local authorities who exceeded the bounds of royal justice. If we wish to speak about reason of state and absolutism in connection with witch hunting, we should look less at the celebrated introduction of state-sponsored prosecutions and the application of judicial torture, and much more at the central regulation of local justice.

Notes

1   For the argument that witch persecutions were a consequence of the extension of public authority, see Chapter 10 by Robert Muchembled. Christina Larner argues that there was a link betwen state-building and witch persecutions in Chapter 15, and also in *Enemies of God: The Witch Hunt in Scotland* (London 1981), 193. Joseph Klaits also suggests that witch hunts were encouraged by the extension of central power in *Servants of Satan: The Age of the Witch Hunts* (Bloomington, Ind. 1985), 131–47.

2   Hilde de Ridder-Symeons, 'Intellectual and Political Backgrounds of the Witch Craze in Europe', *La Sorcellerie dans les Pay-Bas* 86 (1987), 37–64.

3   See Chapter 10. Also, R. Muchembled, *Popular Culture and Elite Culture in France, 1400–1750* (Baton Rouge, La 1985), 224–30, 235–78.

4   Christina Larner argues in Chapter 15 that when Christianity became a political ideology in the sixteenth century, religious crimes like heresy and witchcraft became political crimes.

5   B. P. Levack, *The Witch-Hunt in Early Modern Europe* (London 1987), 77–84; Larner, *Enemies of God*, 66.

6   The definition of the state used throughout this chapter is a formal and autonomous political organisation under one sovereign and final authority, the officers of which have the legally sanctioned authority to require obedience from the inhabitants of a large and usually contiguous territory over an extended period of time.

7   Larner, *Enemies of God* 192.

8   In each calculation the author considered only those cases whose outcomes are known. He also excluded those cases classified as 'miscellaneous' since they were never fully tried, the accused having escaped from jail. The conviction rate for the circuit courts is especially low, since those courts heard cases only very late in this period, by which time the hunt was declining. The statistics for the trials authorised by commission receive confirmation from Sir George Mackenzie, who claimed that 'scarce ever any who were accused before a Country Assize of Neighbours did escape that trial': *The Laws and Customs of Scotland in Matters Criminal* (Edinburgh 1678), 88.

9   In one sense the warrant of 1591 authorised an 'indiscriminate witch-hunt', as Larner has argued, since the commissioners were given the power to examine

and torture 'all and sundrie persons' who had been, or would be, accused. The warrant did not, however, authorise indiscriminate witch hunting in the localities. It did not delegate the authority to torture to any other individuals besides the six commissioners, and it specifically reserved to the Council the decision whether to put the interrogated suspects to the knowledge of an assize.

10   See for example the report of locally administered torture in 1652 in B. Whitelocke, *Memorials of the English Affairs* (London 1652), 522. One of the main reasons for the use of torture at the local level is that the Council required a confession before granting an *ad hoc* commission to try the suspect. See Mackenzie, *Laws and Customes*, 88.

11   Sir George Mackenzie, *Pleadings in Some Remarkable Cases* (Edinburgh 1673), 185–97.

12   See Stuart Clark, 'King James' Daemonologie', in Sydney Anglo, ed., *The Damned Art* (London 1977), 161–4; also H. N. Paul, *The Royal Play of Macbeth* (New York 1950), 90–130.

13   Michael Mann, 'The autonomous power of the state: its origins, mechanisms and results', in John A. Hall, ed., *States in History* (Oxford 1986), 114.

14   On Anderson see Michael MacDonald, *Witchcraft and Hysteria in Elizabethan London* (London 1990), xvi–xix. On the prosecutions at Exeter and the failure of Sir Thomas Raymond to instruct the jury regarding the use of confessions as evidence see Roger North, *The Lives of the Rt. Hon. Francis North; the Hon Sir Dudley North; and the Hon. and Rev. Dr. John North*, ed. A. Jessop, 3 vols (London 1890), 9, 167–8.

15   For the negative effect of Sir John Holt on prosecutions see Wallace Notestein, *A History of Witchcraft in England* (Washington, DC 1912), 320–1. For the action of the judge in the trial of the women accused of causing the possession of Edward Fairfax's children in 1622 see Edward Fairfax, *Daemonologia: A Discourse on Witchcraft*, ed. W. Grainge (1882), 126–7.

16   On the problem of proof in New England see Richard Weisman, *Witchcraft, Magic and Religion in 17th-Century Massachusetts* (Amherst, Mass. 1984), chs 7–10. The main decision of the judges was to accept spectral evidence. The judges also disregarded the two-witness rule, which was part of New England criminal procedure.

17   C. L'Estrange Ewen gives a summary of the case in *Witchcraft in the Star Chamber* (London 1938), 28–36.

18   Soman, 'Decriminalizing witchcraft', 6.

19   Robin Briggs, *Communities of Belief* (Oxford 1989), 13–14, 45–6. Briggs argues that witches were worse off in these outlying regions because 'the local community found it easier to use the legal system for its own purposes, and it is to those communities that we should look for the driving force behind the persecution'.

20   On this practice see Gerhard Schormann, *Hexenprozesse in Nordwestdeutschland* (Hildesheim 1977), 158–9.

21   See E. W. Monter, *Frontiers of Heresy* (Cambridge 1990), 69, for the tightening of controls over the local inquisitors, who in the earlier period were 'virtually a law unto themselves'.

22   John Tedeschi, Inquisitorial law and the witch', in Bengt Ankarloo and Gustav Henningsen, eds, *Early Modern European Witchcraft* (Oxford 1990), 83–118.

23   J. C. V. Johansen, 'Denmark: the sociology of accusations', in Ankarloo and Henningsen, *Early Modern European Witchcraft*, 345–6.

24   Ibid., 349–50.

PART SIX

Witchcraft, Possession and the Devil

A LATE MEDIAEVAL WOOD CARVING in Malvern priory church in England depicts a lively confrontation between a monk and the Devil. The viewer is left in no doubt about who is having the best of the encounter: wearing a gleeful expression, the monk pokes the thin end of a pair of bellows into the fiend's anus and squeezes the handles with all his might. This grotesque image captures some of the qualities often attributed to the Devil in the late Middle Ages. First of all, the evil one is depicted as vulnerable: his attempt to torment a pious churchman is plainly doomed to fail. Secondly, the Devil is imagined as a physical creature, with bodily limitations that are crudely underlined by the method of his ousting. Lastly, the fiend is shown as a suitable subject for comedy: the carving's scatological humour is typical of late mediaeval and early sixteenth-century jokes about the Devil, which flourished in popular drama and collections of 'merry tales'.[1] These light-hearted representations were not, of course, the only way in which Satan was perceived. The vivid and ghastly depictions of hell and the Last Judgment that adorned many parish churches in mediaeval Europe were a reminder of the fate awaiting sinners in the life to come. Equally, the surviving accounts of pious Christians who came face to face with the evil one, and poor souls who suffered the pains of demonic possession, testify to the horror that Satan could sometimes inspire. For Margery Kempe, the fifteenth-century mystic and author of the earliest autobiography in the English language, visions of demons 'with mouths all alight with burning flames of fire' were so terrifying that they almost drove her to suicide.[2] But such perceptions of the Devil coexisted with a wide range of different representations. In a multitude of different contexts, the fiend could appear as a figure of comedy or dread, as the mighty 'prince of this world' or a limited creature with little power over God-fearing Christians.

Out of this abundance of diverse images and conceptions of Satan in the late Middle Ages, one particular strain of thought emerged as a dominant pattern among the magisterial classes of early modern Europe. This was a particularly pessimistic view of the Devil's influence in earthly affairs, which tended to portray him as an ever-present threat to the wellbeing of individuals and societies. In Chapter 18, Erik Midelfort describes this process as the 'demonization of the world', in which educated Christians came increasingly to 'describe the apparent chaos of life as a dramatic encounter of good with evil, of angelic with diabolical'. This trend was particularly evident in the second half of the sixteenth century, and expressed itself in a wide variety of forms: the new German literary genre of *Teufelbucher*, which depicted the seven deadly sins as expressions of demonic power; the high profile cases of possession and exorcism in Germany, France and Italy; and the marked tendency among Catholic and Protestant writers to attribute all sinful thoughts and behaviour to the direct inspiration of Satan. In England, this last trend was exemplified in devotional writings and catechisms. In the mid-sixteenth century, for example, Thomas Becon devoted three pages to the temptations of Satan in his exposition of the line 'Deliver us from evil' in the Lord's Prayer, whereas earlier commentators had covered the whole prayer without a single reference to the Devil.[3] In seeking the origins of this trend, it is important to note that it occurred across confessional boundaries, and cannot therefore be attributed to the influence of one particular creed. The 'demonisation' of Europe can probably be explained by the context of religious conflict itself, since this encouraged both sides to appreciate the power of evil in what many believed to be the last days of the world; it might also have arisen from the efforts of state churches to impose new standards of morality and religious belief on their populations, as these standards exposed the myriad imperfections of a nominally Christian society.

While educated Europeans adopted an increasingly narrow and pessimistic view of Satan's activities, it appears that a more multidimensional understanding of the Devil remained prevalent among the wider population. For many humble Christians, the fiend was still a potential figure of dread, but he could also appear in a vulnerable, comic or even benevolent guise. German peasants occasionally thanked the Devil for successful harvests.[4] In English cheap print, the legendary figures of Friar Bacon and Mother Shipton both acquired demonic associations in the course of the seventeenth century, but their characters remained sympathetic and completely unthreatening.[5] Some regional beliefs about the Devil seem so distant from the ideas of the educated that they can only be attributed to folklore, and we can do no more than guess at their original meaning. What can we say, for example, about the story in Chapter 13 of Barbara Striglin, the Austrian woman who fell pregnant to the fiend in 1580, then gave birth to a raven from a wound in her side? While such accounts are baffling on their own, they contribute to the general impression that popular attitudes towards the Devil were more variegated than the beliefs of educated Christians in the early modern period. This point has significant implications for the study of witchcraft, and these are considered in the three chapters in this section.

In Chapter 17, David Nicholls explores the rich imagery surrounding the figure of Satan in Renaissance France. For most ordinary people, he suggests, the Devil was a rather ambivalent creature: he was a source of fear and the ultimate punisher of sins, but also the subject of oaths, a dupe to quick-witted countrymen in folk-tales, and a festive character in popular theatre. Neither completely evil nor irre-sistibly powerful, the fiend 'inhabited the invisible world in which God and the saints could be as frightening as he was'. This outlook was unacceptable to Protestant and Catholic reformers alike, who sought to re-educate the population about the true nature of Satan and to suppress their vulgar ideas about him. Nicholls' work reminds us that the idea of the Devil itself was contested in early modern Europe. The importance of folkloric beliefs about Satan was particularly evident in cases of possession. English familiar spirits were believed to enter the bodies of the witch's victims – and sometimes the witch herself – where they caused swellings and convul-sions, and could manipulate their hosts like parasitic puppet-masters.[6] The similarity between these afflictions and cases of demonic possession tended to blur the distinc-tion between familiar spirits and the Devil. In other respects, however, witches' familiars were quite different from orthodox ideas about Satan: they often took the form of small animals, they could be impeded by physical barriers, and were occasionally caught in bottles.[7] A similar discrepancy between folk beliefs and learned theology is identified by Erik Midelfort in Chapter 18. He argues that cases of possession in sixteenth-century Germany were often 'the product of popular fears, fancies, and images of the Devil or of other spirits', and these attitudes 'were thor-oughly strange to the biblical, classical, or medical minds of the literate'. In some cases, it appears that the concept of witchcraft itself was understood in quite different ways. While German demonologists made a clear distinction between witches and the victims of possession, ordinary people sometimes accused possessed individuals of witchcraft. In both Germany and England, these inconsistencies suggest that confessional states were unable to reform traditional ideas about the Devil, and indicate the importance of popular culture in shaping cases of witch-craft and possession.

While Midelfort considers the phenomenon of possession in general terms, in Chapter 19 Moshe Sluhovsky explores the meaning of the experience for one of its victims. The chapter offers an intimate portrait of Nicole Obry, a 16-year-old French girl possessed by the Devil in 1565, and agues that Obry's affliction provides an insight into the world view and life experiences of ordinary women in early modern France. Obry's possession was partly inspired by feelings of guilt about her own sins, which she was allowed to express freely in the course of her exorcism. These feelings were combined with sexual anxieties that arose from her first experience of menstruation. These components of Obry's condition originated in her own life history, and were not imposed by the churchmen who took charge of her disposs-session. In this respect, Sluhovsky notes, she was 'an active participant' in a social drama, 'not merely a passive victim of the authorities' manipulations'. This reading of Obry's experience resembles the work on witchcraft confessions by Lyndal Roper and Louise Jackson (see Chapters 24 and 26), which highlights the role of personal fantasy in these narratives, and draws attention to the way that individuals could use the figure of Satan to explain their own behaviour and dramatise their psycho-logical conflicts.

Like women confessing to witchcraft, however, the agency of possessed indi-viduals was subject to major constraints. As Sluhovsky points out, the affliction was recognised only when the victim conformed to certain types of behaviour. Moreover, the logic of possession meant that its sufferers ultimately had to submit to the authority of the clergy. The experience was also shaped by wider social and political forces. In the case of Nicole Obry, Sluhovsky argues that the intense conflict between Catholics and Protestants in her native Picardy heightened her awareness of the Devil's power. As a pious member of the Catholic majority in a region threatened by a strong Protestant faction, Obry was aware that satanic forces were infecting her community; and it is likely that this perception, combined with her personal anxieties, encouraged her experience of possession. Once the church had confirmed her condition, she became an effective vehicle for anti-Huguenot propaganda. Speaking through her body, the Devil admitted that Protestants were responsible for the desecration of a local church; and her exorcism was eventually achieved through the power of the mass. The church fully exploited the benefits of this extraordinary spectacle. Obry's dispossession was moved from the church in Vervins to the cathedral of Laon, where huge crowds were able to witness her ordeal; and she was carried in procession twice a day to receive the miraculous remedy of the eucharist.

Religious conflict also helps to explain another remarkable feature of Nicole Obry's story. When the Devil first appeared to her, he took the form of her recently deceased grandfather, who asked the girl and her family to perform a series of religious duties on his behalf. It appears that Obry and her relatives had no doubt about the benign nature of the apparition, and carried out most of his instructions in good faith. It was only when they were unable to fulfil his final request for a pilgrimage to Santiago that Obry fell sick and was taken to a local teacher, who was the first to suspect demonic possession. When a Dominican friar confirmed this diagnosis, Obry and her family suspected for the first time that she was receiving messages from the Devil. All their previous experiences conformed to a well established pattern in late mediaeval religion, in which ghosts guided their surviving relatives to the performance of pious works.[8] As Sluhovsky argues, Obry herself played a role in this transformation; but it is also evident that the intervention of the clergy, and the wider context of religious confrontation in Picardy, helped to reshape her encounter with a ghost into a case of possession. In this respect, Obry's case belongs to the wider pattern of 'demonization' identified by Midelfort. In the wake of the Reformation, both Protestants and Catholics were reluctant to accept the existence of spiritual forces except God and the Devil, or to countenance potentially deviant forms of religious expression.[9] This made it more likely that visionary experiences like those received by Nicole Obry would be viewed as demonic illusions.[10] While this case is extreme, it is reasonable to assume that the same desire to suppress unorthodox religious experiences encouraged the spread of demonic possession in Europe from the mid-sixteenth century. When both Catholics and Protestants denied alternative explanations for mystical experiences, the Devil rushed in to claim them as his own.

Notes

1   For comic representations of Satan, see my *The Devil in Early Modern England* (Sutton 2000), 21–3, 65–8. For humorous depictions of demons in popular theatre, see Chapter 17 in this book by David Nicholls.

2   *The Book of Margery Kempe*, trans. B. A. Windeatt (Penguin, Harmondsworth 1985), 41–2.

3   Thomas Becon, *The Worckes* (1564), vol. I, 323r–324r; for an earlier commentary on the same text, see Richard Whytford, *A Werke for Householders* (1530), B3r.

4   R. Po-Chia Hsia, *Social Discipline in the Reformation* (Routledge, London 1989), 153.

5   Oldridge, *The Devil*, 68–72.

6   The ability of familiars to enter human bodies is also noted by Jim Sharpe in Chapter 22.

7   For an interesting comparison from mainland Europe, see Edmund Kern's account of demons in a bottle in Chapter 14.

8   For an excellent study of the religious context of ghostly apparitions, see Jean-Claude Schmitt, *Ghosts in the Middle Ages: The Living and the Dead in Medieval Society* (University of Chicago 1998).

9   Midelfort provides an example of this in a Protestant context in Chapter 19: Judith Klatten's encounter with fairies in 1578 was interpreted as either possession or fraud. For a similar phenomenon in Catholic Sicily, see Gustav Henningsen, 'The Ladies from Outside: An Archaic Pattern of the Witches' Sabbath', in Bengt Ankarloo and Gustav Henningsen, eds, *Early Modern European Witchcraft: Centres and Peripheries* (Clarendon, Oxford 1993).

10 For a similar process in Italy, see Chapter 6 by David Gentilcore. This notes the similarity between the religious ecstasies of female saints and the effects of witchcraft, and points out that the Roman Inquisition viewed both 'false saints' and witches as deluded by the Devil.

Chapter 17

David Nicholls

THE DEVIL IN RENAISSANCE FRANCE

BENEATH THE DAZZLING ACHIEVEMENTS of Renaissance culture lay a civilisation acutely aware of its own fragility. Many intellectuals thought of their epoch as the 'iron age' in which only learning was 'golden', while for the great mass of the population economic and spiritual insecurity went hand in hand. For even in an expanding economy, such as that of France in the late fifteenth and early sixteenth centuries, destitution or worse always threatened, prosperity and even survival being dependent on the size of the harvests and the vicissitudes of trade. One might expect, therefore, a gnawing anxiety to be one component of both popular and high culture. The French historian, Lucien Febvre, one of the pioneers of the history of mentalities, detected 'fear everywhere, always fear' in Renaissance France, while more recently Professor Jean Delumeau, seeking to reconstruct the mental universe of the Protestant and Catholic Reformers of the sixteenth century, has also detected fear as their primary obsession and motivation. Both these views are exaggerated, especially with regard to popular culture. Anxiety co-existed, sometimes paradoxically, with other more optimistic, laughter-creating elements. This was the age of Rabelais as well as Calvin and many seemingly contradictory features went to make up popular attitudes, some becoming momentarily dominant at times of high religious political and social tension.

Much of the fear and hope felt by men and women of all classes was projected through the existence of powerful supernatural forces. The multi-faceted world of popular religion lived in an uneasy relationship with the dominant Christianity of the established Church, until Reformers of all persuasions launched an all-out assault on what they saw as 'superstition'. Alongside the visible world of everyday existence there existed an invisible world where dwelt occult forces promoting good and evil, and more ambiguous figures who could help or hinder humanity, depending on their whims and on human attitudes towards them. Saints, demons, ghosts, fairies, a whole legion of more or less anthropomorphic figures, inhabited this parallel world and intervened constantly in the visible world as helps or hindrances to struggling humanity. Even the saints, far from being merely paradigms of perfect behaviour dwelling in heaven, inhabited the occult world as distant friends or guardian angels who interceded for mankind with God, but who must themselves be propitiated, lest they turn against humanity and inflict evils upon it. *The idea that saints could and did cause illness was condemned by Rabelais in Gargantua*, but was generally accepted by the mass of ordinary Christians. Underlying the fearful elements of the invisible world lay the ancient figure of Satan who, from the late fourteenth century onwards, became the centre of what Professor Delumeau has called a 'diabolical invasion' of western Europe: a terror-ridden obsession expressed, in the fifteenth and sixteenth centuries, in a flourishing infernal iconography and theological concern with the Devil as the tempter of feeble humanity or even 'lord of this world'. As Olivier de Magny summed up in the 1550s:

> The century in which we live is truly one of iron, and the iron has indeed been brought to us from hell.

Little new was invented, but theologians, preachers, printers, miniaturists and sculptors drew on an eclectic farrago of ancient and mediaeval fantasies which they intensified through sculpture in churches, mass-produced books, emotional preaching, and the various manifestations of an intimate and macabre religious art. The punishments of hell entered the collective consciousness with hitherto unparalleled force, and the traps of Satan lay in wait for the unsuspecting. The streets of Renaissance France were dark with something more than night. And this is not merely a picturesque or curious by-way of history, but is important in understanding the viciousness of religious conflict, participants in which viewed their enemies as Lucifer's agents. Changing views of the actions of the Devil and his agents were to culminate, when combined with the effective propagation of Counter-Reformation Catholicism in the paroxysm of the great witch-hunt, when the malevolent use of magic was identified with Devil worship.

The concrete and emotional religious art which dominated new work in French churches between the end of the fourteenth century and the religious wars was commissioned by the clergy for didactic purposes, and its moralistic narratives and morbid preoccupations percolated into printed books. The Devil and his main opponents – the Virgin Mary and St Michael – played a major role. Demons, the punishments of hell and personified vices covered the walls of churches in a powerful synthesis of triumphalism and morbid piety bordering on the perverse. Francois Villon in his 'Ballade pour prier Notre Dame' paid tribute to its effects on the mind of an old woman:

> I am a poor old woman who knows nothing, unable to read. In my parish church I see Paradise painted with harps and lutes, and hell where the damned are boiled; the one frightens me, the other gives joy and happiness.

The early sixteenth-century stained glass, window in the church of St Vincent at Rouen, known as the 'chariot' window, summed up the whole message. The top part shows the earthly paradise before the fall; under this the triumph of evil is portrayed as a classical triumph, with Satan pulled in a cart by his agents, while in the bottom window the Virgin rides in a similiar triumph after defeating the evil one.

This concrete image of the Devil and the struggle between good and evil for human souls was spread by the new art of printing in little books such as the *Art de bien vivre et bien mourir,* printed by Antoine Verard which demonstrated the manner of good living and good dying and the forgiving goodness of Christ, the Virgin and the Church. Vigorous woodcuts showed the deathbed battle between demons and angels for the soul of a dying man. The demons tempt their prey with reminders of his sins and exhortations to remember his loved ones left alone in this world, but the saints and angels show God's eternal goodness towards those who truly repent and think only of the fate of their souls after death. Needless to say, the forces of good win in the end, but the struggle worked as a powerful reminder of the tricks and temptations of the forces of evil and the necessity of living and dying as a good Christian. Similarly, preachers used descriptions of hell, collected for their use in moral tales and culled from a variety of classical, early Christian, Celtic and mediaeval sources, to try and terrorise their listeners into moral living, while the almanachs known as *Shepherds' Calendars* provided suitably gruesome and sadistic illustrations. The clergy felt that people were more likely to be moved to righteousness by fear than by hope.

But the highly individualised portrait of Lucifer and his cohorts, portrayed in a still familiar manner, was only one aspect of the picture presented to the people by the clergy. For the Devil was also a great illusionist and trickster, capable of assuming a multitude of forms in order to pursue his plans for the capture of souls, and it was a major task of theologians and churchmen to unmask him and dispel popular errors on the subject. St Paul, who imagined demons expelled from heaven living in the dark air immediately above the earth and waging constant war against humanity, St Augustine, who saw a continuing conflict between the City of God and the City of the Devil, and a host of lesser writers were all brought into the fray. The diabolical City or the dark world of the Devil was seen as a constant threat, even by members of the intellectual Elite. Renaissance culture may have been a force of liberation for a Rabelais or a Copernicus, but for many of their contemporaries, as for Luther or Calvin, new or rediscovered knowledge induced feelings of a terrible weakness. The Devil and his demons could not change the universal order of the world, but could create local changes, such as making people ill, rendering men impotent or substituting one object for another by trickery in order to pursue their schemes.

Although in theory it was usually held that the Devil could act only with God's permission and that his schemes formed part of God's overall plan, once this was established his powers were virtually unlimited. In the course of their wanderings on the lookout for vulnerable souls demons could take on a variety of shapes, but usually that of an animal, and could take over the bodies of human beings. Precautions were taken to prevent demons entering houses or fields through ceremonies, and devils were driven out of human bodies through a complicated ritual of exorcism, all of which acted as reminders of the necessity of priests and the Church. For many, as for St Paul, the Devil was the ruler of the world, insofar as it was not truly Christianised, and could wield his power with impunity. Elaborate treatises established the numbers of minor demons and the organisation of the diabolical hordes. The anonymous *Cabinet du roy de France* (1581) counted no less than 7,405,920 demons commanded by seventy-two generals all under the orders of Satan, while an even more extravagant theory held that everyone on earth had his own personal demon, hence the necessity for a personal guardian angel. Many minor demons had their own names (Beelzebub, Astaroth, etc.) taken willy-nilly from pagan gods and the desert demons of the Old Testament; and demons possessing human beings were asked their names and willingly owned up.

The external threat of the Turks was clearly the work of the Devil, but the main threats were internal. The long tradition of Christian misogyny showed that women were particularly susceptible to the enemy's wiles and, consciously or unconsciously, his agents. Here again, old ideas were given unprecedented diffusion by religious art and printing. The ambiguous attitudes of St Paul, St Augustine and St Thomas Aquinas were made even worse by works falsely attributed to these masters.

Augustine had declared that, while all human beings possess a body and a soul, in men the body reflects the soul, but this is not the case with women. Men are therefore fully a reflection of God, but women only through their souls. Women's bodies are an obstacle to their exercise of reason; they are inferior to men and should be subjected to them. Feminine vanity, frivolity and weakness opened the door to the Devil. The popular Franciscan preacher, Olivier Maillard, fulminated at length on this subject. The wearing of long dresses 'completes the resemblance between women and beasts, which they already resemble by their conduct', and 'rich collars and golden chains around their necks' show that 'the Devil holds them and drags them behind him, tied and enchained'. In religious art the Deadly Sins were usually given feminine personifications, while a carving in a choir stall at St Martin-aux-Bois (Oise) shows Satan helping a sculptor to carve the image of a woman: to create a woman, the Devil as well as a man is needed. Only by renouncing their bodies in the image of the Virgin Mary could women defeat the Devil and hope for salvation. But this unremittingly gloomy picture tells only half the story. There *were* confusions in the theological view as simplified for popular consumption. Was evil caused by human weakness, or by the Devil as an autonomous agent, or by the Devil with God's permission as a punishment for mankind? Add to this the difficulties inherent in urging people to resist an all-powerful adversary, and we can see that there was plenty of room for other attitudes. When Rabelais's Epistemon visits hell he chats with Lucifer and has a jolly good time, assuring his earthly friends that devils are good companions. Hell is the world turned upside down: the rich and powerful on earth lead a poor life down below, while philosophers and the poor are great lords. The multi-layered work of Rabelais bestrode the worlds of popular and high culture, but before the Reformation and Counter-Reformation instigated massive changes in all cultural spheres, such a mixture was quite normal.

The century between about 1450 and 1550 was the golden age of a vigorous religious theatre, mixing the Bible story and the lives of saints as told in the *Golden Legend* with broad humour and elements from profane farces and the more abstract sotties and drawing on the traditional parody sermons and services, comic monologues and dialogues, and the cornucopian fount of carnivalesque culture. The forces of reform, Protestant and Catholic, were eventually to destroy this vulgarity as demeaning to the dignity of religion, but the battle was still unresolved before the religious wars. Although banned in Paris in 1548, mystery plays continued elsewhere, in some places even into the 1570s and 1580s. Confraternities within the artisan guilds and sometimes town councils promoted them and minor clerics often took part. The larger towns of the centre, the north and Provence built on the tradition of the 'Feast of Fools' to try and outdo each other in lavish spectacle. (In the south-west plays were almost all in dialect and more narrowly religious.)

Lucifer, devils and hell were stock features of these presentations. The mouth of hell, often in the form of the head of a dragon, showed devils leaping in and out, swapping ribald dialogue, and Satan addressing his hosts, while plays were often preceded by a procession with carts representing heaven and hell. In one such procession at Bourges in 1536 a cart carried a 'hell 14 feet long by 8 feet wide in fashion of a rock with a tower ever burning and belching flames, wherein Lucifer's head and body alone appeared . . . vomiting flames and holding in his hands serpents or vipers which writhed and belched fire'. Devils running through the streets throwing firecrackers created a commotion, as described by Rabelais in the Quart livre:

> The devils were all decked out in the skins of wolves, calves and rams, decorated with sheep's heads, bulls' horns, and large kitchen hooks; with great belts from which hung cymbals and bells making a horrific noise. They held in their hands black tubes full of firecrackers, with others holding long tapers onto which at each street corner they threw handfuls of powdered resin producing horrible fire and smoke.

Their appearance, adds Rabelais, caused great contentment to the people, but frightened the little children. He brings out the ambiguity of these noisy, grimacing figures. The association with farce and the festive air surrounding the staging of these plays weakened any theologically-inspired attempt to inculcate the permanent fear of damnation in the watching crowds. The response to their antics could be fear or hilarity. The devils were as much comic folk-demons as deadly serious enemies of mankind. True, damned souls were dragged screaming off to hell, but the forces of evil were defeated, and in the episode of the Harrowing of Hell, Christ descended into hell to release Adam and his seed from damnation. Satan and all his cohorts were no match for the patron saint of the confraternity presenting the play, aided and abetted by the legions of heaven. Christian comfort was thus made immediate and the threat of hell could even be laughed off.

The Devil in the theatre thus combined theological and popular elements. The folk-Devil, an amorphous figure made up of folkloric and distorted theological elements, was one means of resistance to the mental terrorism of the theologians. In popular oaths, despite frequent, thoroughly pointless condemnations by the Church and civil authorities, the Devil's name was taken as much in vain as was God's. Rabelais saw nothing wrong in verbal cursing if active goodness is displayed: Friar John's swearing by the Devil is better than the pious murmurings of hypocritical monks. Even King Louis XII's favourite oath was 'may the Devil take me'. The popular image of the Devil was unsystematic and not fully individualised. He inhabited the invisible world in which God and the saints could be as frightening as he was. In Normandy, Berry and Maine he led ghostly riders in nocturnal hunts through the sky, an activity associated elsewhere with Charlemagne and other long-dead heroes. He was certainly not the effective 'lord of this world' and it was possible for him to be out-tricked by wily countrymen.

In Brittany, and in a weakened form in the Auvergne and the Pyrenees, ideas of a dualist creation were prevalent. For everything that God created, the Devil tried to go one better and failed. Thus God made the sun, the Devil the moon; God made rain, the Devil hail; and in some areas the Devil made the sea to try and cover God's earth. The Devil's parodies were even found among fauna and flora: thus the Devil's version of man was the monkey, the mole or the bear, while other pairs included sheep and wolf, dog and fox, vines and brambles, cabbages and thistles, carrots and hemlock. Legends associating the Devil with old buildings or natural physical features could also bear witness to his weakness. Many geographical features in Brittany were explained as being results of battles between the Devil and Celtic saints. Giant rocks had often been left by the Devil: usually he was carrying them but was forced to drop them by the sound of church bells or the intervention of a saint. Devil's fingerprints and footprints (or hoofprints) were to be found in many places. For example, he left marks on a hill at St Briac in Brittany when he climbed it to escape the anger of the local inhabitants. Only a few legends associated him with prehistoric monuments, but he was particularly connected with bridges. Several, including the bridge of St Cloud, one at Beaugency, and the Pont du Gard, had been built by the Devil on condition that the first living being to cross it belonged to him, but he was tricked by the inhabitants so that an animal crossed before any of them. He was also the builder of Roman roads and monuments, such as the Chemin du Diable at Toul, the Chaussee du Diable near Charleroi, and the Paves du Diable in the Ardennes. In a few instances he had even built churches for his own worship and had been tricked out of them by saints or the people.

Such folkloric ideas were a part of the 'superstition' which Protestant and later Catholic reformers tried to weed out. In the sixteenth century the main attacks came from the Protestants and, although the attack was never entirely successful (as shown by the persistence of the folk-Devil into the early twentieth century), the Calvinist thrust was influential. For Calvin those who do not serve God serve the Devil, and in his vernacular tracts, destined for a mass audience, he branded popular religious practices and Catholic and Anabaptist doctrines alike as 'diabolical'. Thus the Catholic Mass was 'a sacrilege created by Satan to destroy the sacrament of the holy supper', while the manifold errors of Anabaptists and libertines were 'diabolical dreamings', a trick of the Devil designed to 'render the world stupid' and gain souls for hell. Anabaptist martyrs (whom Calvin was only too happy to create personally) were martyrs of the Devil and victims of their mad obstinacy. Even judicial astrology was a 'diabolical superstition' and 'trick of the Devil'. Calvin deployed common sense, sardonic humour and contempt to attack Devil inspired Catholic practices, but he was incapable of full-blooded Rabelaisian laughter. Someone so utterly convinced of his own rightness (which was not really his but God's) did not laugh at the ruses of the enemy. Like later Catholic reformers, he was a humanist unable to understand popular religion or marketplace humour.

Other Protestant writers, notably Henri Estienne and Pierre Viret, were more wholeheartedly humorous as occasion demanded, but between 1540 and 1570 dogmatic Calvinism grew more and more to dominate the French Protestant movement, and Calvinist certainty gave it great strength in the early religious wars. True, in the long run Calvinism failed to introduce a Reformed society and polity in France, and the inability to understand peasant attitudes to religion was one reason for this. But on the eve of the religious wars Calvinist confidence looked like insufferable arrogance to Catholics. When the wars started, ideas about the Devil contributed to their peculiar ferocity. The other side was made up not just of people with whom one disagreed about points of theology but of conscious or unconscious agents of the enemy of all mankind. From the Catholic point of view, the visible refutaton of Protestant doctrine was one way of puncturing their confidence and arrogance and of winning back waverers and the indifferent. It is, therefore, not surprising to find the Devil being used for this purpose.

In 1565, a young woman from Vervins in Picardy, Nicole Obry, whose grandfather had died without confession or the last rites, was possessed by a Devil during her attempts to deliver the old man's soul from purgatory.[1] The unfortunate Nicole's theatrical performances and the attempted exorcisms attracted large crowds of both religions and were accompanied by theological polemics between Catholic and Protestant. The struggle within her body became the symbol of a divided country. Her Devil, Beelzebub, was scared by the consecrated host, and her eventual successful exorcism in February, 1566, in Laon cathedral, using consecrated bread, caused great joy to Catholics. With Protestantism now retreating into a struggle for survival, the way was clear for even more elaborate views of the power of the Devil and his agents. By the end of the sixteenth century and in the early seventeenth century fantasies of witches as Devil-worshippers left the world of the *Malleus Maleficarum* to invade the consciousness of magistrates and, to a lesser extent, the lower classes. Renaissance obsession with the powers of the Devil and the partial defeat of popular resistance to theological ideas paved the way for the great witchcraze in France and the offensive of Counter-Reformation Catholicism in the seventeenth century.

Note

1   In Chapter 19 Moshe Sluhovsky presents a detailed account of this extraordinary episode.

Chapter 18

H. C. Erik Midelfort

THE DEVIL AND THE GERMAN PEOPLE

O N PALM SUNDAY OF 1574, Judith Klatten, a girl from the Neumark (Brandenburg) village of Helpe, took the holy sacrament as was her wont, but instead of feeling spiritually nourished that day, she felt cold wind rushing around her. Later that Palm Sunday she passed out and was carefully laid in her bed, fully clothed. The coma-like trance into which she fell lasted for weeks, and months, and finally for almost five years. What made her condition even more remarkable was that to all appearances for all this time she ate and drank nothing, and consequently excreted nothing. This supernatural fast roused the suspicions of even her own father who reportedly spied on her to see if she was secretly getting up to take nourishment, but he saw nothing. For five years Judith Klatten hardly spoke, except to respond yes or no when she was questioned. And for years apparently she attracted little attention beyond her village. But in the fifth year of her strange condition, in 1578, the Lutheran pastor Caspar Gloxinus came out from town to visit her, thinking that she might perhaps be possessed by the Devil. But this suspicion, too, was shattered by the fact that now the girl prayed properly and confessed her sins. Even so she still refused food, and Pastor Gloxinus, now suspecting fraud, urged that she be brought into town. And so on August 2, 1578, Judith Klatten was brought the four miles into Arnswalde and placed in the local 'hospital' (or nursing home) where she was to be observed day and night.

Under these new conditions she held out only four days before she admitted that she was hungry. After consuming a wine soup with relish she told her attendant that over the past five years she had indeed eaten, but not in any normal fashion:

> Little tiny men and maids wearing beautiful ornaments (whom she alone of all the family could see) ran about every day under her bed and brought her food from whatever was being cooked at home or roasted elsewhere.

Judith had been sustained over the years by the little people, but they were not simply her benefactors:

> They would have gladly carried her away except that someone dressed in yellow forbade it. Even so they pressed her hard and hurt her in the side and pushed her eyes shut so that she couldn't see how their eyes turned brown.

The pixies or elves helped maintain the appearance of a miraculous fast by secretly carrying off her excreta in a blue-white basin. But in the end their powers turned out to have limits:

> For when they were feeding her for the last time before she was brought into the city, they said amongst themselves that if she stayed on in the village they would gladly bring her food, but they couldn't transport food to her over land.

After making these revelations, Judith resumed eating a little; she now spoke a little and was able to walk, albeit with a limp. Her only fear now was that she might be left at home alone.[1]

There may well be psychohistorians who would undertake to explain what Judith Klatten's visions of the little people may tell us of her mental illness, but for myself I am more interested in what her visions tell us about her culture. Certainly by the 1570s, for example, we know that Germany was experiencing a host of miraculous or fraudulent fasts, examples of the way God gives strength to his chosen faithful or of the way the Devil, in league often enough with crafty and malicious priests, deceives the naive and plunges the innocent into superstition.[2] Among Protestants the latter, diabolical view of the matter had come to prevail, and so it is not surprising that both Judith's father and Pastor Gloxinus suspected fraud and that the pastor, initially at least, suspected demonic possession. But obviously Judith Klatten's condition was not any normal demon possession. What I find especially intriguing is her notion that the little people who sustained her over the years could not help her if she moved into town. Regardless of how we understand what was 'really' happening with respect to her nutrition from 1574 to 1578, Klatten seems to have been aware that some rural spirits could not survive in the atmosphere of a town, or at least that it made for a credible story to assert that her helpers were bound to the village.

Certainly in the sixteenth century many observers agreed that some spirits were bound to particular waters, others to particular mountains or caves or mines, others still to specific crystals or houses or forests. The writings of Paracelsus, for example, abound with nymphs, sprites, kobolds, elves, dwarves and fairies. He and his followers held that nature was full of such spirits. Heinrich Kornmann, for example, published a Latin treatise in 1611, firmly based on Paracelsean principles, in which he undertook to set forth all the kind of spirits that inhabit the fires, airs, waters, and earths of our experience, and his example must stand for many.[3] It is equally well known that the miners of Germany had a rich mythology about the Bergmänn-lein who sometimes helped and sometimes exasperated them in their subterranean labors. The world of ordinary experience in the villages of sixteenth-century Germany was also full of spirits, who might frighten the cattle, spoil the beer, and keep butter from forming in the churn.

It is hard to find out much in detail about these spirits and goblins and elves because literate people usually described such ideas as superstition. For Lutherans and Catholics alike, the world was not full of all sorts of spirits. Instead there were, fundamentally, only two kinds of spirits in the world: good angels and bad; and of the two, devils were far the more active. Indeed, one of the most pervasive processes across the sixteenth century, and not just in Germany, was the growing demonization of the world. The learned and literate found that it made better sense of their world to describe the apparent chaos of life as a dramatic encounter of good with evil, of angelic with diabolical.

The process of demonization has been particularly well studied in the area of Lutheran ethics, for here the process resulted in an entirely new genre of litera-ture, the *Teufelbucher,* in which all the old vices of vanity, drunkenness, gluttony, lust, gambling, and infidelity were transformed. What Sebastian Brant and his gener-ation around 1500 had attributed to folly in the *Ship of Fools* and in the *Narrenliteratur* that sprang from Brant's inspired model was rebaptized and reinterpreted as diabolic, starting in the 1550s with such works as Gorlitz's *Sauffteufel* and Musculus's *Hosentetifel, Fluchteufel,* and *Eheteufel.* By the 1560s the genre had become a publishing fad, with as many as twenty-one 'devils' detected and described by (mainly) Lutheran moralists up to 1569. The odd result of this flurry was not exactly what the authors earnestly intended. If every vice had not just some foolish blindness at its base but a specific Devil, then the Devil himself could begin to seem foolish, consuming his destructive energies in the effort to tempt mankind to wear large ruffled collars, pointed shoes, pleated shirts, and enormous pantaloons, or coaxing would-be Christians into un-Christian dancing, swearing, disobedience to masters, melancholy, and general laziness. It should be more widely recognized that even among the literate and learned the Devil had an amazing variety of shapes, ranging from these faintly ridiculous echoes of the mediaeval vice and folly figures up to figures of full apocalyptic terror. Before we draw too sharp a contrast between the Devil of the learned and the demons of the people, therefore, we should have firmly in mind the fact that even among the learned, and even during the process I have called the demonization of the world, the learned and literate were hardly unanimous in their view of what was meant when it was said that the Devil was everywhere. Even so it would be foolish to deny that popular and learned culture diverged over just such an issue, as the history of witchcraft suggests.

In the history of witchcraft we are now familiar with the consequences of the growing demonization of the teamed and literate world. The studies of Norman Cohn and Richard Kieckhefer suggested that the full European belief in witch-craft (with demonic pact, flight to the Sabbat, and sexual intercourse with the Devil) was a learned fantasy, one that had few if any roots among the supposedly ignorant villagers, whose witchcraft remained concentrated on the practical advantages to be obtained from cunning men and wise women and on the frightful damage that could be wrought through the *maleficium* of harmful witches.[4] Pushed to unacceptable extremes in the work of Robert Muchembled, this model of competing conceptions of witchcraft (learned vs. popular) has nonetheless prompted a great deal of important work.[5] No one can be content any longer with the bland generalizations of fifteen or twenty years ago concerning the common beliefs of 'everyone' or of 'the people'. We need to ask exactly whose beliefs we are studying.

And that brings us back to Judith Klatten. What were her beliefs about the spirits who helped her? Evidently, as a pious girl, she did not share the view that such spirits must be devils; but our source, the *Wider Natur und Wunderbuch* of Andreas Angelus (Engel), does not permit us to say much more about Klatten's understanding of what had happened to her. If we simply applied to her situation the findings of the recent witchcraft scholars, we might be tempted to suggest that the Devil in all his forms was a learned creation, and that ordinary, illiterate people lived in a different, non-diabolical world. This would be, I think, a hasty conclusion, for it would seem to rest on the assumption that if the witchcraft of popular culture was not (or was not until relatively late) diabolical, then it might follow that popular culture had no Devil. And that would be going much too far. In fact, the Devil was a frequent figure in popular speech, in slogans and epithets and aphorisms, and we hear often enough that an ordinary man or woman became demon-possessed after his or her spouse invoked the Devil by way of curse.

By studying the publicly reported cases of demon possession I hope to uncover what the ordinary people of sixteenth-century Germany may have thought of the Devil. I have now read most of the pamphlets, broadsides, *neue Zeitungen,* wonder books, and sermons published before 1600 in which demonic actions of all sorts were reported. I am prepared to claim, moreover, that certain popular views are evident in these reports and sermons, but of course such sources have their obvious weaknesses and limitations as guides to the popular mind.[6] First of all, such books make no claim to list all the cases of possession even for a given town or year. Their authors selected examples in order to illustrate a conclusion, and one can search in vain, for example, for Catholic accounts of unsuccessful exorcisms, even though we know that there must have been many unsuccessful efforts to free the victims of demonic obsession or possession. It was, moreover, never against the law to be demon-possessed, and so we cannot expect to find official registers anywhere of the possessed. Like Judith Klatten, many of the possessed may have lain in obscurity without ever coming to literate attention. We don't know how large the 'dark figure' may have been.

Second, the sources I have read are often pieces of zealous polemic.[7] They can hardly be said to have even tried to present cool-headed, objective observation. When Johann Conrad Dannhauer of Strasbourg described the pitiful case of a ten-year-old daughter of a high noble family in 1654, he recorded such detailed and theologically correct conversations between the girl and the Devil that any modern reader will be drawn to the conclusion that Dannhauer himself composed these dialogues. Similarly, when Tobias Seiler described the possession and liberation of a twelve-year-old Silesian girl in 1605, the Devil apparently entered into such theologically learned arguments with Seiler and with other observers, over several days, that any reader is bound to conclude that Seiler was composing not only his own lines, but the Devil's, too. These are hardly examples of straight reportage. Even so, I think that we can get some real glimpses of what these girls may have actually said, some impression of how they understood their troubles, as distinguished from the theological and polemical interpretation to which they were immediately subjected. For example, Dannhauer's Strasbourg girl spoke so often and apparently so movingly of wanting to die, of being ready to die, and of seeing God, that we can surely regard her as a religiously melancholy child with strongly mystical yearnings. And Seiler's girl seems to have spoken with the voice of the Devil, threatening to leave a terrible stench and warning that he would shit in the pastor's throat to make him hoarse. Such notes, I am suggesting, have the ring of spontaneous reporting. They do not seem to me to be merely the acidulous products of overheated theological zeal, although one should reckon with the possibility that Luther's scatalogical contempt for the Devil persuaded his followers to use rough talk with the Enemy. Even so I believe that Seiler was here providing a reasonably accurate account of this event. It remains true that these sources are colored lenses that distort what they permit us to see, but if we can take the shape and color of the lens into account, we may yet be able to say something of what demon possession was like to the demon-possessed and, more generally, what ordinary people in the German-speaking lands thought of the Devil.

One fact on which both the learned and the illiterate would have agreed was the evident rise in demon possession in the second half of the sixteenth century. Observers at the time were so impressed with this spread of possession that no previous age, with the exception of Christ's own age, seemed to have presented so many frightful examples of the Devil's rage. His attacks were a staple feature of the wonder and prodigy literature of the second half of the century. Job Fincel's *Wunderzeichen,* for example, was entirely conceived in the spirit of proving that the rising tide of monstrous births, fiery signs in the heavens, and devilish interventions in the shape of storms, disasters, and demonic possessions gave proof of the imminent end of the world and the urgent need to repent so long as a few seconds remained before the end. Johann Weyer's famous attack on witchcraft trials, the *De praestigiis daemonum* (1563), endorsed this point of view by claiming that in this, the old age of the world, Satan lorded it over the minds of men as never before. Similarly, when a panel of pastors and theologians investigated the mass possessions at Friedeberg and Spandau in 1593–94, they concluded in their report that such demonic actions were possible only because the second *Advent Christi* was at hand. As in the days of his incarnation, now too the world swarmed with devils and with possessed persons. After all, God had revealed (Revelation 20) that Satan would be turned loose exactly one thousand years after the reign of Gregory the Great: $593 + 1,000 = 1593$.[8] Here we do surely see the learned theological mind at work, but at its base lay the commonplace that there had never been so many possessions before. No work set forth this point of view more successfully than the sturdy treatise by the ecclesiastical superintendent of Mecklenburg, the well-known Lutheran moralist Andreas Celichius, whose *Notwendige Erinnerung Von des Sathans letzten Zornsturm* (1594, 1595) gathered all of these observations and arguments together. In just the last twelve years, Celichius exclaimed, he had himself seen about thirty cases of possession, 'some of whom became possessed and convulsive here, but others of whom have come wandering here from Holstein, Saxony, and Pomerania, presenting such horrible spectacles that modest souls have been thoroughly disgusted'. To understand such sufferings and to learn how to treat the miserably possessed were, therefore, timely, even urgent, tasks.

To illustrate the rise of demon possession I have prepared a table of the publicly known possession cases from *c.* 1490 to *c.* 1650 in the German-speaking lands. At least thirty-two places were touched by possession between 1490 and 1559, a span of seventy years; but the next twenty years (1560–79) found twenty-three places infected; and the last twenty years of the century (1580–99) added a further forty-four locations (and a generous increase in scale as well). I do not think that we should regard this apparent increase as an artifact, a product, let us say, of better publicity or better survival of the appropriate sources. If such factors were important we would have a hard time explaining the apparently dramatic drop in possession cases in the first half of the seventeenth century, a time period during which I record only fourteen publicly known cases of demon possession in the various Germanies.

Therefore we should confront the fact that demon possession cases became common in Germany just as witchcraft was generally assuming the dimensions of an epidemic as well. It is well known that Germany experienced relatively few and small witchcraft trials from *c.* 1490 to 1560, but that from then on the panic began to spread.[9] Were the two sorts of diabolical activity connected? In several well-known cases the answer is definitely yes. One widespread assumption was that witches could cause another person to become demon-possessed, an assumption so widespread that already in 1563 Johann Weyer devoted book 3 of his *De praestigiis daemonum* (this became book 4 in editions of the work published in 1567 and later) to refuting it as an absurdity. His critique went unattended in many cases, such as in the 1583 possession and exorcism of Anna Schlutterbaurin, whose very own grandmother was convicted and executed for causing the granddaughter's possession. Dannhauer's report from 1654 of the miserably possessed girl in Strasbourg contained the same information, and although the girl could not be helped in any dramatic way, at least the witch responsible for her troubles could be eliminated, by burning. Roughly speaking, this was the crime of the witches at Salem, Massachusetts, forty years later, for they, too, were convicted of bewitching the tormented girls of Salem. The problem with proving the guilt of a witch accused of causing the possession of another was that invariably the accusation lay in the mouth of one who was known to be full of the Devil, the very father of lies. From the beginning of the great witch-hunts after 1560, therefore, theologians and jurists repeatedly cautioned against taking the accusations of the possessed as serious evidence. And this caution was so widely heeded that we cannot draw any general connection between cases of possession and the rising tide of witchcraft prosecutions.

This parallel to witchcraft is worth exploring in some detail, for even if one did not regularly cause the other, there are similarities we should not overlook. For example, physicians, jurists, and theologians agreed that women were more likely to fall into the crime of witchcraft, and they cited all the well-known spiritual and physical weakness of women, especially post-menopausal women. In their weaknesses, loneliness, poverty, melancholy, infidelity, uncontrollable fantasies, and general sexual frustration, old women made easy victims for the Devil, who usually offered them comfort, riches, companionship, dances, feasts, and an active sex life.[10] So much for the general theory. The match with judicial reality was surprisingly exact. We know that roughly 80 percent of the persons executed as witches in Europe were women, and that older women were more commonly convicted than younger girls or young married women. What we have hitherto failed to notice is that the very same medical and theological reasons existed for expecting demonic possession to predominate among older women as well. The Devil was keen to exploit the weakness, loneliness, infidelity, and melancholy of old women, and yet here we historians have been trained or misled, especially by a few celebrated French episodes, to think that demon possession was mainly an affair with young women, especially nuns. Medical theory in the sixteenth century did regularly note the mental hazards of celibacy for cloistered nuns, but even for physicians it was old nuns who were most at risk, owing to their excessive dryness. Young women were supposedly too healthy to be regular victims of the Devil, and they constitute therefore a major breach in the link between medicotheological theory and actual cases of demon possession. If we look carefully, however, we will find an even more dramatic breach.

From an examination of Table 1 we can discover that women did indeed predominate in the relatively quiet period before 1560, although even then I have recorded four episodes of mass possession (Geel, Lemgo, Thuringia, and Mechelroda) in which the sexes were mixed (we have no clue as to the proportions within the mixture). The period 1560–79 matches our common expectations most perfectly, with ten individual female cases and five cloisters compared to only two male individual cases, but even in this period there was one mass possession of boys (thirty boys from Amsterdam, 1566) and one mixed mass possession (among the citizens of Hamm). Thereafter, our expected picture runs into even more trouble. For the period 1580–99, male individual possessions ran about equal to the female cases (15 to 17), and we need to add the extraordinary mass possessions from Brandenburg and, to a lesser extent, Saxony. The reports of eyewitnesses in Brandenburg from the 1590s repeatedly stated that the Devil seized people and shook them, sending them off into seizures without respect of age or gender. Some 150 were afflicted in the Neumark town of Friedeberg, and about 40 people fell under attack in Spandau, just west of Berlin. Berlin itself came under siege, as did the towns of Stendal, Tangermande, and the Saxon town of Lindau. Unfortunately, we cannot tell the proportions of male and female in these episodes, but contemporary observers were struck by the promiscuous nature of these assaults. Although there are only a few cases after 1600, the new pattern apparently continued, with 8 men and 5 women coming to public attention between 1600 and 1650.

Table 1 Males and females in German cases of possession, 1490–1650

Dates	Individual possessions			Mass possessions		
	Female	Male	Gender unknown	Female	Male	Mixed genders
1490–1559	19	10	0	1	0	4
1560–1579	10	2	0	5	1	5
1580–1599	17	15	7	1	0	7
1600–1650	5	8	1	0	0	0

I find this deviation from learned theory instructive, for it suggests that theologians, jurists, and physicians of the sixteenth century were in no position to evoke cases of demonic possession in exactly the shapes they dictated or expected. Unlike witchcraft, it was no crime to be possessed, and perhaps this simple difference left possession more in the hands and minds of ordinary people than the crime of witchcraft, which was after all defined, prosecuted, and routinized by the literate magisterial classes of Europe. This means in turn that the actual cases of demonic possession, as we find them in the accounts of publicists of the sixteenth century, were certainly in part, and in some cases in large part, the product of popular fears, fancies, and images of the Devil or of other spirits. Like Judith Klatten's little people, some of the aspects of demon possession as it actually occurred were thoroughly strange to the biblical, classical, or medical minds of the literate.

Let us pursue this question further by looking at the preconditions of possession, as they were commonly understood. Throughout the sixteenth century it was widely conceded that the Devil might possess both the greatest of sinners and the least sinful of all. In order to display his majesty, God might allow a demonic possession only to show how strong the Christian sacraments and sacramentals were. Or of course God could permit a horrible invasion of demons to punish the sins either of the possessed or of another person. Possession could chasten or test the faithful or simply present the power of the Devil, a display often thought necessary in the sixteenth century when pastors thought their congregations full of Sadducees, Epicureans, and self-satisfied worldlings, who refused to recognize the reality of the spirit world. Despite the wide range of options open as victims of the Devil, I have the impression that most theologians in the first half of the century were likely to think of possession as a punishment for the sins of the victim. The theological lexicographer Johannes Altenstaig was content to rattle off four reasons for demonic possession: for the glory of God, for the punishment of sin, for the correction of the sinner, or for our own instruction. And Martin Luther usually thought of demon possession as a punishment for, or an instantiation of, sin.[11] Later in the century the learned personal physician to the Elector Palatine, Johann Lang, was even willing to opine that true piety actually kept the Devil away. This was a sentiment enthusiastically endorsed by the Freiburg theologian, Jodocus Lorich, who held that the best way to secure one's health and to escape the attacks of the Devil was to fear God and lead a pious life, for the Devil flees such persons.

Unfortunately for the theory that the Devil worked mainly as God's jailer and executioner, the published accounts of demonic possession show a very different Devil, one that positively preferred to attack pious young Christians. A good example is the 'gruesome story' from 1559 of the godly girl from Platten, close by Joachimstal. She was chaste and modest, went regularly to church, took the sacrament often, and was said to have learned the gospels by memory. Suddenly at shrovetide she was taken sick with seizures, so that her parents thought she had epilepsy. She lay helpless for four weeks, but after Easter the Devil began to speak blasphemies from her. Moreover she began to display such classic signs of possession as eyes that bugged out of her head, a tongue that would stick out a whole handspan, and a head that was wrenched around to face backwards. After repeated tortures and extended conversations with the attending pastors, the Devil was finally driven out through the congregational prayer and song of some one thousand common people. Before he left, however, he claimed that God had sent him to plague Anna's body (but not her soul) in order to warn people to give up their godless pride, gluttony, and drunkenness. And as he flew out the window like a swarm of flies he was reported to say, 'All who don't go gladly to church and would rather stay at home to read and don't attend the Sacrament, and wallow in gluttony, drunkenness, and usury, are all mine, body and soul'. So here was another reason for possession, one that the pastors and theologians had not dreamed of: this Devil allowed a simple smith's daughter to take up the position of the authors of the *Teufelbucher*, to preach virtue while at the same time giving vent to her most blasphemous and irreverent ideas. It is possible that these words and indeed the whole account were corrupted by our pastoral reporter, but I think it more likely that this girl was pious and *did* say something of the sort.

Hers was not an isolated case. When Veronica Steiner was seized by the Devil in 1574, in the castle Starnberg in Lower Austria, she too possessed two voices, one the deep, coarse, manly voice of the Devil, and the other her own tender, reasonable, modest, Christian voice. With her own voice she prayed, praised God, admonished others to pray, sighed over her own sins, and accepted the Catholic faith. But with her devilish voice she cursed and barked, spat against the Catholic religion and its adherents, and sang unchaste drinking songs and perverted Psalms. She too seems to have found in demon possession a way of expressing the two violently contradictory ways she felt about religion.

Or take the case of the eighteen-year-old maid from Meissen, who fell down in fits in 1560, but on recovery would launch into extraordinary prophecies. God had been good to everyone, she reminded her listeners, but no one showed a proper thankfulness and so God's punishment was coming. Girls must give up their vanity, married persons their adultery. Woe to the rich who did not help the poor; woe to parents who did not discipline their children; and woe to all Germany for constant drunkenness, gluttony, pride, and the deliberate ignoring of godly sermons. This girl fell repeatedly into trances in which she saw God, angels, and hell. Suspicious of this behavior, Hieronymus Weller (the well-known student of Luther) examined her and had to admit that 'it is nothing but Scripture that I heard, and a serious sermon of repentance, which should move us as directly as if it were a good angel's voice'. Here was a girl who would certainly have been labeled demon-possessed at other times or in other places, but her piety prevailed in this case. She was allowed to preach in this odd way.

When the noble lady Kunigunde von Pilgram was seized by the Devil in 1565, one of the signs of her possession was that she wanted to pray but was forcibly restrained by the Devil. Both the accounts by Melchior Neukirch of a possession case from Braunschweig in 1595–96 and that by Johann Conrad Dannhauer with respect to the noble girl from Strasbourg (1650–54) allow us to make the same point, but with even more pathos. In the Braunschweig case, Appolonia, the daughter of Heinrich Stampken, was known to all for her piety. She loved her catechism, using it in her prayers both morning and night; she attended sermons eagerly, took the Lord's Supper and absolution gratefully, and was altogether too good. One day she fell into weakness and depression, a debilitating combination that lasted three-quarters of a year, but then she broke out in fully demonic gestures and speech. With loving pastoral care she arrived at lucid intervals and admitted that the beginning of her troubles had been when she had heard someone curse her and wish the Devil into her. From then on she had had horrible doubts that perhaps she was not a child of God, maybe she was not of the elect. These religious doubts had prompted her depression, which in turn opened the door to the Devil. Neukirch mobilized the whole congregation of Saint Peter's and others as well, with repeated prayers and hymns that were printed up so that all of Braunschweig could pray at once for her release. Most dramatic and peculiar of all are the prayers composed by Appolonia herself, long stanzas of rhymed verse of which I give only two examples:

> The Devil uses great force
> And plagues me horribly in many ways.
> Seizes me in all my members,
> Rips me and pains me greatly.
> O Lord help me from this torture.
> Preserve my body and soul.

> God's Son must win the battlefield
> and drive you, Devil, from his house
> Do your worst for God is with me
> I fear you not at all.

Here was surely a girl who had taken in rather too much of the Lutheran teachings to which she had been exposed, or perhaps it would be safer to say that she experienced Luther's *Anfecktungen* but had them drawn out over months at a time.

Dannhauer's noble girl of Strasbourg (1650–54) was just ten when she fell to the Devil, but the odd thing about her condition was that while her body and her 'outer and inner senses' were tortured, her mind remained clear and Christian, and she was able, apparently, to curse Satan herself and order him to leave her. She was persuaded firmly that she was a child of God, no doubts on that score, but she assured others that it would be better for the godless to experience her pangs in this world. 'For they give themselves over to godless gaming, gluttony, and drinking, to whores and lovers, and forget all about God. But how will it turn out for them in the end?' God will punish those who have not borne crosses in this world. She was not content to echo the sermons of the moralizers, however, for this pre-adolescent also had a strong urge to die. She went on and on, in words that Dannhauer must have put in her mouth; but the basic message may well have been hers: 'I'll gladly die if Thou wilt, if it be Thy fatherly will. O dear God I thank you from the bottom of my heart that you are giving me the strength still to escape'. In some of her visions she saw God and his angels.

Here then were demon possessions that produced revival sermons and angelic visions. These afflicted souls may have been using the cultural idiom of demon possession, but they were surely extending it well beyond what the theological wisdom of the sixteenth century had led anyone to expect. By the 1570s this was plain to observers such as Georg Walther, pastor of Halle, or even earlier to Veit Dietrich, the short-lived pastor of Nuremberg, both of whom commented on the pious, modest Christianity displayed by the possessed (or at least many of them) when they were given a little respite from the assaults of the Devil.

In these deviations from official expectation I think we can see what ordinary people were able to make of the cultural idiom of demon possession. In another area a sort of popular confusion arose. In high legal theory as it developed in the sixteenth century, the difference between the crime of witchcraft and the condition of demonic possession was clear. Witches were those who entered into a pact with the Devil while the possessed were those who passively, involuntarily endured the external and internal assaults of the Devil. What could be clearer?

But is it clear what happened to Anna Roschmann in 1563? At the age of twenty as she lay in her Augsburg bedroom, the evil spirit came to her and asked her to be his, 'whereupon she began to act very strangely and as if she had lost her reason.' Soon she was showing the symptoms of full, raging possession, but we must note that it had begun with an invitation from the Devil. Or what shall we think of Anna Barbara of Stein am Rhein, whose very mother had cursed her and caused her to be possessed? Many common folk thought of her as a witch. Truly confusing is the case of Hans Schmidt, a smith's apprentice from Heidingsfeld, near Würzburg. In 1589 at the age of nineteen, Schmidt fell in with bad company, and got hold of a book that contained the secrets of the magic arts. Realizing its dangers, Schmidt finally burned the book, but he suffered further temptations. Satan offered him money on one occasion and on another tempted him to hang himself, but Schmidt resisted these advances until he was finally possessed by a highly frustrated Devil. Here the story began as many a witchcraft seduction tale began, but because of his powers of Christian resistance the youth was possessed. Indeed by the late sixteenth century many a suicide attempt was attributed to demon possession.

To take another example, Appolonia Geisslbrecht was confronted first, in 1583, by a Devil who offered her plentiful food, drink, and dance. In this case she actually accepted the Devil's offer but was then at once possessed. Instead of witchcraft, this case turned confusingly into demonic obsession. Pastor Nicolaus Blum told a similarly confusing story from his parish in Dohna. In 1602 it appears that God permitted a noble student from Prague to be possessed as punishment for the sin of 'Zauberey,' that is, the crime of magic, for which women were being executed by the hundreds at just that time. Here again it may have been the youth's resistance to Satan that made the difference, but it could also have been his noble and student status. We know of other adventurous students who signed actual pacts with the Devil, for example, without having to pay the ultimate penalty for their indiscretions. So it was with the desperate twenty-five-year-old woman whom Tobias Wagner tried to help in 1643. In a deep depression and eager for money, the young man made a pact with the Devil, who then prompted him to attempt suicide. When he was saved from death by his wife, he merely fell into a deeper and more demonic melancholy.[12] Why was this case not treated as witchcraft? Perhaps because of the suicide attempt, perhaps because of the evident depression and desperation. But also perhaps because ordinary people were having trouble keeping the supposedly clear categories of witchcraft and possession clearly separate. Certainly that would seem to be the case with the famous Christoph Haizmann, the painter whose demonic possession in 1677 was studied by Sigmund Freud as an example of 'diabolical neurosis'.[13] Haizmann, too, had a pact with the Devil, or perhaps two pacts, but he was not treated as a witch; instead, a pilgrimage and repeated exorcisms liberated him from the Devil and from his pacts.

So here too we have a cloudy area where the jurists and theologians had taught clarity. I take these cloudy areas to be indirect evidence of the independent will-fulness and indocility of popular culture at certain points. We would be very wrong to think that ordinary people did not have a notion of the Devil, but my examples of pious demoniacs and of those who curiously made a pact with the Devil or dabbled in magic or were suicidal only to become possessed suggest areas of resis-tance to or ignorance of the official word of jurists and pastors. I would be reluctant to describe the method I am using here as a form of 'higher criticism,' for these pamphlets and wonder books were far from being canonical texts; but there is a certain vague similarity in that we need to develop what I would call 'educated surprises' in order to imagine what may lie behind a text.

Another old approach, and one still worth using, is that of simple geography. Many things seem noteworthy on the maps I have drawn, but I find it especially significant that only thirty-nine towns and villages south of the Main River had cases of demon-possession and only one of these was a true obsessional epidemic (Eichstatt). In contrast, northern Germany had over sixty-five separate towns with cases of actual or suspected demon possession, and several of these episodes, espe-cially in the northeast or northwest, were massive outbursts of demonomania. A surprising number of these northern cases came from Lutheran Saxony and Brandenburg, a fact that may be connected to the great Gnesio-Lutheran contro-versy over exorcism at baptism.[14] And only a tiny number appear in the great lands of the Counter Reformation, Bavaria and Austria. Proud as he was of the miracles performed by Our Lady of Altotting, Dr Martin Eisengrein, writing in 1570, listed only one dispossession of demons in his almost 200-page-long treatise on that famous pilgrimage shrine. Demon possession does appear now and then, but rarely, in the Bavarian and Franconian miracle books; and so it seems that southern Germany, and especially the southeast, was surprisingly lacking in demon possessions and famous exorcisms.

I do think it is important to notice the frequency of demon possessions among nunneries and among the most Gnesio-Lutheran areas, for in both situations the attempt to live an ever more perfect life may have led to stronger temptations than those felt in other parts of Germany. This would help to explain the account from Brandenburg in the 1590s in which the Devil was said to have strewn coins all over the streets, but whoever picked up a coin became instantly (but not permanently) possessed. Perhaps only a region where the demonic vices of greed, usury, pride, and vanity had been censured for over a generation and with increasing apocalyptic fervor could have generated such a story. And that in turn suggests that when we speak of popular ideas of the Devil, we cannot mean only those ideas that literate, educated people did not share. By the late sixteenth century the German people generally believed that demon possession was on the rise, and they may even have taken the rise as a sign of the imminent end of the world. But while accepting this learned interpretation of what they saw around them, ordinary people also knew how to shape the idiom of possession to some of their own ends.

In a collection of papers on cities and their culture, it will not escape notice that my discussion of demon possession has not concentrated mainly on cities. The Devil was equally active in towns and in the countryside. It is true that Judith Klatten's little people were symptomatic of a rural, not an urban, view of things.

The spirits and goblins of Germany had no really urban form; but perhaps the classic Devil was a townsman. Certainly his opponents were. Time and again, when a demon proved impossibly difficult, a demoniac would be brought into town because there the spiritual resources of a region were often concentrated, whether in the priests and relics of many a Catholic town or in the large congregations of Lutheran towns, whose Lutheran hymns became the Protestant substitute for exorcism. And so the history of demon possession may tell us something, after all, about cities and their culture in the Renaissance.

Notes

1   For full citations of the German sources on which this chapter is based, see the original version in Steven Ozment, ed., *Religion and Culture in the Renaissance and Reformation* (Sixteenth Century Journal Publishers, Kirksville, MO. 1989), 99–119.

2   On the general phenomenon, see Rudolph M. Bell, *Holy Anorexia* (University of Chicago Press, Chicago 1985).

3   On this body of writing, see Allen G. Debus, *The Chemical Philosophy: Paracelsan Science and Medicine in the Sixteenth and Seventeenth Centuries*, 2 vols (Science History Publications, New York 1977); for a short introduction, see Lynn Thorndike, *A History of Magic and Experimental Science*, vol. 5 (Macmillan, New York 1941), 617–51.

4   For the work of Kieckhefer and Cohn, see Chapters 1 and 2 in this collection.

5   Robert Muchembled, *Popular Culture and Elite Culture in France, 1400–1750*, trans. Lydia Cochrane (Louisiana State University Press, Baton Rouge 1985). See also Chapter 10.

6   See Steven Ozment, 'The Social History of the Reformation: What can we learn from Pamphlets?' in Hans-Joachim Köhler, ed., *Flugschriften als Massenmedium der Reformationszeit* (Klett-Cotta, Stuttgart 1981). Ozment seems to ignore some of the chief weaknesses of these sources as windows into the popular mind while proving their usefulness for other kinds of social history.

7   The polemical nature of much possession literature is noted by Sluhovsky in Chapter 19. On this point, see also D. P. Walker, *Unclean Spirits: Possession and Exorcism in France and England in the Late Sixteenth and Early Seventeenth Centuries* (Scolar, London 1981).

8   See Robin B. Barnes, *Prophecy and Gnosis: Apocalypticism in the Wake of the Lutheran Reformation* (Stanford University Press 1988), for a discussion of this sort of Lutheran numerology.

9   Brian P. Levack, *The Witch Hunt in Early Modern Europe* (Longman, London 1987), 152–68.

10   There are examples of such seduction scenes in my *Witch Hunting in Southwestern Germany, 1562–1684: The Social and Intellectual Foundations* (Stanford University Press 1972).

11   This topic is far too complex to be passed over in a sentence. Perhaps Luther was so persuaded that the Devil *spiritually* possessed every unregenerate person, inspiring him or her to sinful thoughts and deeds, that he transferred this prejudice to those cases of *physical* possession that he dealt with. In practice with real people, however, Luther could act sympathetically and without this prejudice. See Heiko A. Oberman, *Luther: Man Between God and the Devil* (Fontana English

edn, 1993); Jeffrey B. Russell, *Mephistopheles: The Devil in the Modern World* (Cornell University Press, New York 1986).

12   On this case, see H. C. E. Midelfort, 'Catholic and Lutheran Reactions to Demon Possession in the Late 17th Century: Two Case Histories', *Daphnis* 15 (1986), 623–48.

13   For a fascinating account of the case of Christoph Haitzmann, and Freud's interpretation of his experiences, see Roy Porter, *A Social History of Madness* (Weidenfeld and Nicolson, London 1987), 83–9.

14   See Bodo Nischan, 'The Exorcism Controversy and Baptism in the Late Reformation', *Sixteenth Century Journal* 18 (1987), 31–51.

Chapter 19

Moshe Sluhovsky

A DIVINE APPARITION OR DEMONIC POSSESSION?

O N N O V E M B E R 3 , 1 5 6 5 , I M M E D I A T E L Y following All Souls' Day, Nicole Obry (Aubrey), a sixteen-year-old, recently married girl, encountered a spirit.[1] Nicole was born in the village of Vervins in the diocese of Laon in Picardy. She was the daughter of Pierre Obry, a well-off butcher, and his 'very energetic and intelligent' wife, Katherine Willot (Vuillot). Nicole was a pretty, pious, and good-natured girl but not very intelligent, as her teachers at the convent of Montreuil-les-Dames testified. She could recite the seven penitent psalms and a few prayers but could not write or read, not even her Book of Hours, and this despite her ten years at the convent. At the time of the encounter with the spirit, Nicole was a recent resident of the city of Laon, to which she had moved three months after her marriage to the tailor Louis Pierret. The couple had just settled into their 'petit mesnage a part eulx' when Nicole complained for the first time that one evening while she prayed in the local church near the cemetery where her grandfather Joachim Willot was buried, the spirit of the recently deceased grandfather appeared to her. In this vision and in a number of visions during the following days, the grandfather told Nicole that he was suffering in purgatory because he had died suddenly before he had time to confess and to keep certain vows which he had taken before his death. He then asked Nicole to mobilize his family to pray for his soul and to give charity on his behalf. More specifically, his male relatives were to go on a series of pilgrimages to shrines in Picardy and Flanders, and to Santiago de Compostela in Spain. Nicole's husband, one of her uncles, and a third relative left for the local shrines. Nicole, from her parents' home in Vervins, followed their journey in detailed visions. She heard their conversations and 'even envisioned what they were served to eat'. She recounted the details to her parents, and upon their return the pilgrims confirmed the accuracy of these visions.

But Nicole's family could not fulfill the last request, the pilgrimage to Santiago, and Nicole started to suffer from involuntary seizures. She threatened that the grandfather's spirit would turn her mute, deaf, and blind unless his requests were fulfilled. She further claimed that her suffering was a direct result of the family's disregard of the grandfather's request. The family consulted the village priest, the local teacher, and a Dominican friar. The teacher, who was troubled by Nicole's suffering and temporary paralysis, was the first to suspect that the spirit was not the grandfather's ghost but rather an angel or a Devil. He interrogated it and rejected the spirit's attempt to deny that it was, in fact, inside Nicole's body and not next to it. He proceeded to observe that 'it is not the habit of good Angels to torment other creatures'. By establishing that the spirit was an evil one and that it resided inside Nicole's mouth, the teacher cleared the way to declare that Nicole was, in fact, possessed by the Devil. Friar Pierre de la Motte, who was well respected around the diocese and was in Vervins to deliver Advent sermons, was then invited to examine Nicole. Alarmed by the girl's physical gesticulation and suffering, La Motte immediately declared: 'A Devil possessed this body'. He confirmed that the spirit was not the grandfather's ghost but a Devil and that Nicole's revelations resulted from possession and not from apparitions. La Motte then conversed with the spirit in Latin and forced it to confess that, indeed, it was the Devil himself.

After the identification of the grandfather as a masked Devil, the friar and the bishop of Laon began exorcising the evil spirit from Nicole's body. The first exorcism took place on November 27, 1565, two days after the first Advent sermon. The ceremony first took place in Vervins, but the number of visitors forced it to move to the cathedral of Laon, where 10,000 (or, according to the *Manuel*, 150,000) people watched the proceedings. According to church manuals, exorcism should not take place in public, and the bishop tried to move it to a more private space, but the Devil himself opposed it. The Devil threatened not to exit Nicole's body unless the exorcism was public and God's benevolence was manifested for all to watch. This well suited the exorcist's plan to turn the exorcism into a major spectacle of the Catholic doctrine. For the next two months, twice a day, Nicole's convulsions, seizures, and paralysis stopped only when she was fed with the Eucharist. Throughout this time she was carried twice a day in religious processions, first to the local church in Vervins and after the transfer of the exorcism to Laon, to the cathedral of this city. (Before too long, Laonnais Protestants got the governor of the province to put an end to this part of the ceremony.) Nicole was then put on a stage which was erected especially for the occasion next to the main altar. From her bed/altar, she responded to questions addressed to her in Flemish, German, French, and Latin. She answered always in French or Flemish, her voice gruff and frightening. She also revealed people's secrets and sins and brought them to confess.

Nicole's exorcist chose to use the most powerful magical instrument in his possession, the Eucharist, as the means of exorcism. Holy water, crosses, and saints' relics were more commonly used by exorcists and were recommended in professional manuals. La Motte himself also tried to use them, but they were proven not powerful enough to cast out Nicole's demon. Clearly, by relying on the Eucharist, the exorcist and the Catholic Church manifested to eyewitnesses that their theology of transubstantiation was right and that Catholic priests were invested with a unique power to use this instrument. The people who gathered in Laon witnessed the Devil in Nicole's body trying to resist the Holy Sacrament. The Devil even confessed publicly that he feared the Sacrament because it was the 'Real Presence' of God, as Catholicism maintained, and not just a sign of it, as Huguenots had it. He further admitted that his name was Beelzebub and that he was a Huguenot leader. He promised that with the Huguenots, whom he called his 'bons amis', he will do Christ more evil than the Jews did. For the next few weeks, Nicole was fed with a growing quantity of consecrated Hosts, their number increasing as the exorcism met with fierce resistance by the Devil. The latter also bolstered his force. He called for help, and Nicole's body became possessed by more than thirty additional evil spirits. Some of Nicole's possessing spirits were cast out during a well-publicized and well-attended pilgrimage to Notre-Dame-de-Liesse. These spirits left Nicole's body but not before they announced that they were returning to Geneva, their headquarters. The remaining demons left during a final exorcism at the cathedral on February 8, 1566.

Impressed with this drama, nonbelievers confessed to their sins, and Protestants converted back to Catholicism. 'And many families from our pious Picardy owe their return to the true religion to this prodigy', exclaimed the local royal notary, Guillaume Gorret. King Charles IX himself was impressed by Nicole's purity and honesty. He stopped in Laon to witness the miracle and then invited Nicole to visit him at his chateau de Marchais, where he stayed during pilgrimages to Notre-Dame-de-Liesse. There he gave her ten écus d'or as a sign of his gratitude for her role as 'a living witness of the Catholic faith'.

Jean Bodin, who was a royal prosecutor in the subalternate court at Laon at the time, Agrippa d'Aubigne, Guillaume Postel, and Florimond de Raemond, who converted to Catholicism following the event, all wrote about the 'Miracle of Laon', as the case became known. This case, in turn, set the tone for numerous other cases of spirit possession in early modern France. Four separate cases of possessions in Soissons in 1582 were modeled on it, and the same Devil who possessed Nicole Obry later possessed Laurent Boissonnet of Soissons and Marguerite Obry of Beauvais. When a Devil entered Marthe Brossier of Romorantin in 1598, in the most famous case of its kind in the century, eyewitnesses testified that she had read accounts of the Miracle of Laon. Her Devil even admitted that he was the same Beelzebub who had attacked Nicole thirty years earlier.

In this chapter I want to use Nicole Obry's possession (with references to three additional cases from northern France) to suggest a new interpretation of spirit possession in sixteenth-century France. Together, these four cases represent a specific stage in the development of the phenomena of spirit possession and exorcism in this period. Unlike the famous outbursts of demonic possession in French convents in the seventeenth century (Aix-en-Provence, 1609–1611; Loudun, 1632–1640; Louviers, 1643–1647), the protagonists in these cases were lay individuals. Unlike later cases, these possessions did not contain accusations of *maleficium*, and the exorcisms did not evolve into witchcraft trials. This last distinction between possession with or without *maleficium* is significant. Possession is an involuntary interaction between a human being and a possessing entity, and its termination is dependent upon a successful ritual of exorcism. Witchcraft, on the other hand, involved a voluntary pact with the Devil, usually signed not by the possessed person but by a third participant. A resolution of the case was achieved when the diabolic pact ended, usually through the physical elimination of the culprit. Only then was the possessed healed and reintegrated into his or her society. These two distinct phenomena, however, have sometimes been conflated since the late sixteenth century and in much of the recent literature on the topic. This conflation erases the richness and complexity of spirit possession and its unique character as both subversive and reaffirming religious idiom, as both culturally constructed behavior and madness. By focusing our attention on early French cases of spirit possession without *maleficium*, we can better understand the theological distinction between the two phenomena. These cases also unveil the psychological dynamics that led people to become possessed by evil spirits, a topic that is rarely addressed in the current literature on the topic.

In the following interpretation, the possessed individual becomes an initiator of the drama, a participant in the processes of diagnosis and of definition of the behavior as possession, of prognosis, and, finally, of recovery. Possession was a complex and recognized syndrome. Possessed people had to exhibit a set of well defined manifestations of 'abnormal' behavior in order to be determined possessed. These included the ability to understand foreign languages, to manifest unnatural physical strength, to react with horror to sacred objects, and to suffer from involuntary convulsions, gestures, seizures, vomiting, fits, faintings, and paralysis. It was not easy, therefore, to fake possession; neither was it easy to cure it, and contemporaries debated alleged fakeries in numerous cases. Most of the existing historical explanations of spirit possession in early modern Europe ignore this complexity and emphasize instead the political and ecclesiastical circumstances that determined the exact nature of the authorities' intervention in the final stage of the drama, the exorcism. It has been argued convincingly that rituals of public exorcisms were orchestrated by the Catholic Church in France (and in other parts of Europe) to exhibit the Real Presence of God in the Holy Sacrament and to demonstrate the unique power of Catholic priests to combat Satan and to administer cures to their co-religionists.[2] As such, exorcisms were used as efficient visual propaganda in the religious conflicts following the Reformation. While these explanations are undoubtedly true, the focus in the following pages is on an earlier stage in the process, the possession itself, and on the possessed woman. My use of the term 'woman' to describe the possessed person's gender is not accidental. I have so far found eighteen cases of demonic possession of individual laypersons in sixteenth-century France. All but two of the cases I examined (and most of the reported European cases of possession) occurred to women or young girls, and the gender of the possessed was, as we shall see, an integral and important part of the syndrome.[3]

In the following reading, the possessed woman becomes the agent rather than the prey of her possession; she is an active participant and not merely a passive victim of the authorities' manipulations. This last argument, however, should not be pushed too far. The state of being possessed was not desired by the demoniacs, as Michelet romanticized it; neither was the possessed woman a feminist warrior fighting for her rights in a patriarchal society, as some recent interpretations of the European witch craze portrayed her.[4] Possessed people operated within very constrained boundaries, which were defined by the Church. They had to convince clerics, inquisitors, exorcists, doctors, and lay viewers that they were, indeed, possessed and not witches, melancholic, epileptic, or simply mad. Theologians and doctors in the sixteenth century tried continuously and unsuccessfully to delineate clear distinctions among these different manifestations of supernatural interventions. Adherence to strict rules of conduct determined the demoniac's fate; if her behaviors deviated from what was accepted and defined as spirit possession, she was in danger of being uncovered as a witch or being silenced as insane. The few possessed women who managed to remain within these very narrow restrictions acquired a voice which allows us to hear some of their concerns, anxieties, and tensions. The Miracle of Laon, as we shall see, is a rare opportunity to hear just such a voice. Implicit in this last argument is the assumption that the religious and political authorities did not maintain a monopoly over the right to define or to diagnose. The healing agency, the Church, entered the scene only after a woman (in our case Nicole) had exhibited and acted out specific symptoms which attracted attention and which brought about the suspicion that her deviant behavior could derive from possession by evil spirits. The possessed woman and the Church then had to collaborate to achieve their joint goal: the demoniac's recovery.

What follows is a three-layer analysis of Nicole Obry's possession. I first argue that religious ferment motivated Nicole's original message and that during the early stages of her possession she did not regard herself as possessed by demonic powers. This religious context is then supplemented by plausible psychological motivations for her encounters with the spirit. Together, these two readings emphasize the personal dynamics that led to the outbreak of Nicole's symptoms. But spirit possession cannot be explained merely as a personal behavior. It was a cultural idiom and must also be explained as such, in a broader cultural setting. The third layer of analysis suggests two contexts to Nicole's possession. First, I suggest viewing Nicole's behavior within the European tradition of female ecstatic spirituality. Finally, a political-religious context connects Nicole's possession and exorcism to specific religious and political developments in Picardy and northern France in the second half of the sixteenth century.

The use of Nicole Obry's possession for Catholic anti-Protestant propaganda is all too obvious. Exorcism, in fact, was as old as the Church itself and served as a proof of authenticity for religious messages from the days of the early Church until the nineteenth century. Throughout the Middle Ages, routinized exorcisms were performed by priests during the baptism service and by professional exorcists whose job was to do just that: expel demons from human beings, from animals, and from the fields. Picard Protestants were also aware of the Catholic Church's attempt to publicize and to prolong Nicole Obry's exorcism, and they tried to stop it. They ridiculed the event in combative poems against the Catholics and against coreligionists who believed in the miracles, whom they compared to asses. They also petitioned their patron and protector, Louis de Bourbon, the governor of the province, to put an end to the public ceremonies, and the latter even arrested the girl for a fortnight. Catholics, too, were conscious of the propagandistic victory.

The governor of Ile-de-France, the Marechal de Montmorency, intervened and ordered the authorities to put an end to the 'spectacle' which threatened the shaky Peace of Amboise. But Boulaese, among others, rushed to record the miraculous events that took place in Laon. He published a short pamphlet, *Le Miracle de Laon,* the first in a series of publications.

Instead of dwelling on the religious and political dimension of the case, let us focus our attention on Nicole's behavior before the authorities' first intervention and before the definition of these behaviors as demonic possession. We should distinguish the theological and polemical interpretation to which Nicole's possession was subjected from her own understanding of the events. Prior to the ecclesiastical intervention, Nicole never made any reference to the Eucharist or to the contemporary debate on the Real Presence, two issues that became the center of the exorcism ceremony. Even during the earliest exorcisms other sacramentals – holy water, the sign of the holy cross, and invocations of saints – were used to cast out the demon from Nicole's body. Similarly, in a series of possessions and exorcisms in Soissons in 1580 to 1582, the Sacrament as an anti-Huguenot symbol and as the means of exorcism was introduced by the exorcists only in a later stage of the proceedings. The possessed themselves addressed other religious concerns. Before the Dominican friar forced Nicole's spirit to confess that it was actually the Devil, the spirit had insisted and sworn that it was 'a messenger of God, the spirit and the soul of Joachim Willot', Nicole's grandfather. Nicole herself recognized him as such, and her family, which was familiar with the circumstances surrounding the grandfather's death, never doubted Nicole's identification of the spirit or her explanation of the events which led the grandfather to reappear as a ghost. Furthermore, in the early stages of the examination, there was no mention of the spirit's entering into Nicole's body. In fact, Nicole's encounter with her grandfather could and should be viewed as an apparition and not a possession. As we recall, Nicole was in the local church at Vervins when the deceased's spirit appeared to her and asked her to fulfill religious vows so that it could be moved from purgatory to heaven. Similar requests characterized what was unique about apparitions. The sixteenth-century French theologian Noel Taillepied explained: 'When the spirits that appear to us command us to perform good deeds, it is probable that these are wandering souls or good and saintly spirits'.[5] From Nicole's perspective there was no apparent reason to suspect that this entity was a masked Devil. Nicole had a series of additional apparitions which further confirmed her status as a divine messenger or a seer, not as a possessed woman. Before the Dominican intervention, Nicole, her family, and the spirit all agreed that the latter's intentions were devout and that Nicole was serving as a vessel of communication between the dead ancestor and the living relatives. A special mass was even celebrated in Vervins to mark the return of Nicole's relatives from their pilgrimages and the confirmation of Nicole's visions. Thereby, the local ecclesiastical authority confirmed Nicole's apparitions.

But Nicole's body told a different story. Her pains, involuntary seizures, and catatonic relapses increased daily even before the official recognition of her state as possession. She exhibited the physical signs of possession, and her 'apparitions' could also be regarded as the clairvoyance capabilities of possessed people. In other words, while Nicole's words claimed visionary powers, she was clearly ambivalent about these powers, and her body expressed a rejection of this responsibility. During the exorcism itself, Nicole responded to questions addressed to her in Flemish, German, French, and Latin. The ability to understand foreign languages was defined in the church manuals as the sine qua non of spirit possession. Unlike witches or people who get possessed voluntarily, 'those who are possessed . . . speak diverse foreign languages', explained sixteenth-century French barber-surgeon Ambroise Pare.[6] Admittedly, Nicole started to understand foreign languages only after her behavior was defined as possession and while she was already being exorcised in public ceremonies. At this stage of the exorcism, she had an obvious interest in collaborating with the exorcists. Only her cure by means of exorcism would enable her integration into her society and, more importantly, put an end to her suffering. The original characterizations of her power as visionary was replaced with a definition of possession. By speaking in tongues, Nicole affirmed the new diagnosis of her behavior as possession by either the Holy Spirit or evil spirits. It was left to the authorities to determine the nature of the possessing spirit and to decide how to treat it.

Nicole's original apparition revealed her grandfather's unfulfilled religious vows. In the following weeks, Nicole (and the devils who spoke through her) recalled other sinful incidents from her childhood and from the family's recent past. Years before, Nicole had lost her sister's rosary and Nicole's mother, in anger, had cursed her: 'Let the Great Devil carry you away'. It was also revealed during the exorcisms that throughout her childhood Nicole stole money from her grandfather and mother's coffers, as well as towels, linens and sheets, dishes, a candelabra, meat, wood, butter, cheese, and tallow. Nicole now blamed the Devil for seducing her to commit these petty thefts. It is clear that her transgressions and those committed by her mother and grandfather disturbed Nicole for numerous years. Similarly, the young boy Laurent Boissonnet became possessed in Soissons in 1580 to 1582 because of a sin he had witnessed years before, when he saw his uncle stealing a mouton from one Pierre de Roy. His Devil further revealed that the boy's aunt did not pay for masses for her deceased husband's soul. When the young Nicole le Roy became possessed in the village of Nampcet (diocese of Soissons) in 1582, her Devil justified his possession of her body by alluding to an unnamed sin 'which she reminded her that when she was six, she had stolen some raisins and that when her father chased her, she scratched him'. Finally, the famous demoniac Marthe Brossier, in 1598, attributed her behavior to a religious transgression by a family member, her father's sin of not attending mass.[7] Like Nicole Obry, all of these possessed people identified their possessing agent as a messenger who appeared from the dead to demand stricter obedience by family members to religious precepts. In all of these cases, young women (and in one case, a young boy) used their encounters with spirits (whether we define them as apparitions, as they seemed originally to be, or possessions, as the authorities determined) to confess their or their immediate relatives' sins and to mobilize their families to improve their Christian conduct.

Nicole Obry, Nicole le Roy, Marguerite Obry, and Marthe Brossier were, of course, not the only young and pious girls who got possessed. In fact, most of the demoniacs in early modern Europe were young women. All of these possessed women exhibited what ethno-psychiatrists and anthropologists call 'altered states of consciousness', a culturally specific syndrome of deviant behaviors which are both idiosyncratic and structured. Altered states of consciousness serve societies to establish contact with the 'beyond', to predict the future, and to interpret events. They can occur to any member of the community regardless of his or her position in the society (as was the case with the demoniacs in early modern France) or be restricted to professionals: shamans, prophets, mediums, oracles, etc. Most societies recognize and define altered states of consciousness as legitimate (normal, permitted, 'nondeviant') conditions and institutionalize them, which is to say incorporate them into the cultural system as legitimate behaviors.[8] Cross-cultural studies have clearly indicated that young women are recognized in many societies as especially efficient agents for this role. They can be defined as prophetesses, visionaries, magic practitioners, voodoo performers, etc. By entering into a trance, these women bring messages to their societies. By arguing that someone else is speaking within them, these women expand the narrow space they have in traditional societies to speak out on religious matters and to participate in their society's theological dialogue and spiritual quest. By being in trance or possessed, they disclaim responsibility for the content of their messages, attributing it to a higher (and usually masculine) power. By disclaiming their voice, they gain a hearing. Nicole Obry and her contemporary possessed women, I suggest, also needed to express a religious message that, due to psychological dynamics or societal limitations, they could not address explicitly. The encounters with spirits allowed them to verbalize their messages. The definition of these encounters as demonic possessions enabled them to disclaim authorial responsibility for the content of their spoken words.

So far we have argued that spirit possession in the case of Nicole Obry and in similar cases in early modern France was the means whereby young women acquired a voice to express their religious concerns. This explanation, however, is incomplete. Many more women, we may assume, experienced and witnessed religious transgressions, and most of them never became possessed. Most women used more common means, such as confessions and gossip, to express similar worries. A satisfying explanation for demonic possession should also supply a more immediate cause for the outburst of this unique behavior. This personal psychopathological dynamic, I argue, had to do with the possessed women's sexual anxieties.[9] While lack of specific data concerning the demoniacs prevents us from overpsychoanalyzing them, it is apparent from the sources that spirit possession was gendered as analogous to heterosexual intercourse and that sexual metaphors played a major role in the construction of the idiom. Most of the possessed laywomen in early modern France were at about the age when they menstruated for the first time, got married, and/or lost their virginity. Nicole Obry herself first encountered the spirit at age fifteen or sixteen, the age of menarche in early modern Europe.[10] Furthermore, Nicole's mother testified to a team of doctors and Catholic and Huguenot theologians that her daughter became possessed a month after she menstruated for the first time. Immediately following her encounter with the spirit, when Nicole first showed signs of sickness, her parents assumed that she was pregnant, and the Devil himself explained that he 'entered her womb that he caused to swell, as if she were pregnant with a child'.[11] The Devil further associated Nicole with sexual images by calling her a 'whore' and a 'prostitute'. Nicole le Roy first got possessed seven months after her own marriage and during her first pregnancy. In the following months and while she was lactating, her right breast swelled and became hard as a stone. Sexual expressions and metaphors, explicit sexual gestures, accusations, and fantasies also characterized the numerous cases of multipossessions in French convents in the seventeenth century.[12] Often, I argue, possessed women projected their unvoiced sexual anxieties and equated their personal notions of sexual impurity with parallel familial and/or communal dangers. Menstruation and pregnancy were two charged periods in the lives of early modern European women. They highlighted the Christian mistrust of the body in general and of the female body in particular.[13] Both events also associated the female body with malediction and uncleanness.

In constructing their deviant behavior in accordance with a recognized syndrome, the demoniacs invited the religious authorities to define their oracular intervention as possession. This allowed the possessed women to express their anxieties, to disclaim responsibility, and to hint at the cure. In the first stage of their possession, they gained a voice to express their sexual, familial, and religious concerns. In the second stage, the exorcism, they distanced themselves from the content of their messages, asked for help, and were reintegrated into their society. This argument does not claim that there was a conscious manipulation on behalf of the possessed women to disclaim any responsibility for the content of their messages or for their transgression of gender role by voicing religious concerns, but neither was it totally unconscious. In a famous letter written sometime between 1152 and 1157, the mystic Hildegard of Bingen instructed her follower and student Elizabeth of Schonau not to speak 'of her own accord but from the serene light', to authenticate her visions by making herself 'a mirror' or 'a trumpet which only renders the sound and does not produce it unless another breathes into it in order to bring forth the sound'.[14] Hildegard expressed the need of female visionaries or seers to unvoice their messages in order to gain a hearing, their need to speak as somebody other than themselves. Similar concerns and even similar musical metaphors were used in the sixteenth century by the Spanish mystics Lucrecia de Leon and Juana de la Cruz. In the twelfth century, some contemporaries doubted the source of Hildegard and Elizabeth's vision, and suspected that they were possessed by evil spirits, as was the case with the Cordovan nun Magdalena de la Cruz in 1546. Teresa of Avila and some of her followers in the second half of the century were equally suspected.[15]

Admittedly, Nicole Obry and the other possessed laypeople in early modern France had little in common with these female visionaries, most of them religious women of high standing in their communities and with powerful patrons to protect them. Unlike the female mystics and seers, the demoniacs whose cases concern us here did not try to acquire religious authority. Their goal was much more limited and immediate: to voice a spiritual concern that had direct impact on their lives. Nevertheless, during their possessions the possessed women from northern France attained some degree of religious authority, which resembled the much more eminent public role female visionaries gained through the tradition of female ecstatic piety.

Our explanation of Nicole Obry's possession has so far accounted for the religious transgressions and the psychopathological dynamics that initiated her possession. I have suggested that a personal or familial religious transgression was equated in the possessed women's (un)conscious with their own sexual impurity. In a final layer of analysis, I suggest that the religio-political context in Picardy contributed to the women's religious anxiety and to the metaphors of impurity and penetration of the body social by unclean agents.

Religious ferment, both institutionalized and ecstatic, was widespread in early modern Picardy. The region was influenced more than other parts of France by the Beguine piety and mysticism of the fifteenth century. This could have created a tradition of lay piety that legitimized Nicole Obry's original apparitions. In the early sixteenth century, the province became a fertile ground for French humanism and biblicism, and suffice it to mention that Lefevre d'Etaples, the translator of the first French edition of the Bible; Francois Vatable; Olivetan; Louis de Berquin, one of the first Protestant martyrs; and of course, John Calvin were all Picards. In the 1550s and 1560s, reformed ideas spread fast in the province. Educated women of aristocratic stock played a dominant role in directing the religious sentiments of their families. But Catholic believers also mobilized, and Picardy witnessed and was the geographical center of a penitential movement. In the early seventeenth century, Picardy was known for its mystical movement *of Illuminés,* and contemporaries feared that they were as many as sixty thousand *Illuminés* in Picardy and northern France in the 1620s: men and women who claimed to have divine visions and inspiration.

During the Wars of Religion and the League period, Picardy was divided between a Catholic majority and a powerful Protestant minority led and protected by Louis de Bourbon, the prince of Condé. Condé served in the early 1560s as the governor of Picardy and lived in his chateau de La Fere, near Laon.[16] Nicole Obry's possession in 1565 followed an epidemic in 1556 and the battle of Saint-Quentin in 1557, when King Philippe II's army, led by Emanuel Philibert of Savoy, defeated the French army. The remains of the defeated army escaped to Laon, only to be further devastated by the mass desertion of the unpaid German mercenaries. During the 1560s many Protestant refugees from the Low Countries arrived in Picardy, people who escaped Spanish religious persecutions and enjoyed the protection of Louis de Bourbon. In September 1565, just two months before Nicole's encounter with the Devil, the church of Saint-Pierre-le-Viel in Laon was broken into, and a ciborium containing Hosts was stolen. Protestants were immediately blamed for the profanation, and expiation ceremonies followed soon. Nicole probably knew about this event. The Devil who possessed her certainly did, and, speaking through her mouth, named the Protestants who were culpable of the sacrilege. Similarly, the four possessions in Soissons in 1582 followed soon after the recovery of the city by the Catholics following the Calvinists' seizure of the city the previous year. A similar correlation between the timing of possessions and 'infections' or 'penetrations' of the body social by Protestantism were also typical of other cases of spirit possession: Aix-en-Provence, Agen, and Loudun, where multiple possessions took place in 1611, 1619, and 1638, respectively, were all cities with religiously divided populations. As Lyndal Roper has recently argued about religiously divided sixteenth-century Augsburg, in all of these cities 'the disturbance in the religious realm . . . was thus expressed somatically'.[17] In all of these cases, I believe, possession was an expression by pious Catholic women of religious ferment. These women witnessed communal and religious transgressions. They equated them with their own fears over their and their family members' religious conduct. They further projected personal sexual anxiety onto the communal threat. Nicole Obry, Nicole le Roy, Marguerite Obry, and other possessed women either in witnessing apparitions or by becoming possessed, acquired a voice for themselves to address these issues and to draw their society's attention to the transgressions. But by using the cultural idiom of spirit possession, they also directed the religious authorities to relieve them of the tension and the responsibility that awareness of these religious transgressions entailed.

Notes

1   The account of Nicole Obry's possession in this chapter is based mainly on the following texts: Jean Boulaese, *Le Thresor et entière histoire* (Paris 1578); Jean Boulaese, *L'Abrégée histoire* (Paris 1573); Jean Boulaese, *Le Manuel* (Paris 1575); Christophle de Hericourt, *L'Histoire de la Sacrée Victoire* (Laon 1569). References for specific details in the narrative can be found in the original version of the chapter, published in *Sixteenth Century Journal* 27, no.4 (1996), 1039–55.

2   On spirit possession as religious propaganda in the early modern period, see D. P. Walker, *Unclean Spirits: Possession and Exorcism in France and England in the Late Sixteenth and Early Seventeenth Centuries* (Philadelphia, Pa 1981); 'Demonic Possession Used as Propaganda in the Later Sixteenth Century', in *Scienze, credenze occulte, livelli di cultura* (Florence 1982), 237–48; Jonathan Pearl, 'Demons and Politics in France, 1560–1630', *Historical Reflections* 12, no. 2 (1985), 241–51; Ottavia Niccoli, *Prophecy and People in Renaissance Italy* (Princeton, NJ 1991); Philip M. Soergel, *Wondrous in His Saints: Counter-Reformation Propaganda in Bavaria* (Berkeley and Los Angeles 1993), 99–158.

3   While most historians agree that women were more likely to get possessed than men, H. C. Erik Midelfort argues in Chapter 18 of this book that in the German cases he examined men were just as likely to get possessed. In France, however, in all but two of the sixteenth-century cases examined by Sluhovsky, the possessed were women and not men. Interestingly enough, all of Midelfort's own examples discuss possessions of women.

4   J. Michelet, *La Sorcière* (Paris 1862); Carol Karlsen, *The Devil in the Shape of a Woman: Witchcraft in Colonial New England* (New York 1987).

5   Taillepied is quoted in Jean Delumeau, *La Mort des pays de Cocagne* (Paris 1976), 167–8. See also William Christian, *Apparitions in Late Medieval and Renaissance Spain* (Princeton, NJ 1981), esp. 6–7.

6   It is not clear from theological and medical treatises on spirit possession whether the ability to speak in tongues refers to *glossolalia* or to *xenoglossia* (the ability to understand foreign languages). While most writings on the topic emphasize the knowledge of foreign languages, many possessed people (including Nicole Obry) were incapable of conversing in foreign languages and had only a passive knowledge of languages spoken in their surroundings.

7   Charles Blendec, *Cinq histoires admirables* (Paris 1582), fols 5r, 7r, 60v, 67v.

8   Erika Bourguignon, 'A Framework for the Comparative Study of Altered States of Consciousness,' introduction to her collection *Religion, Altered States of Consciousness, and Social Change* (Ohio State University Press 1973), 3–35.

9   For the predilection of women for spirit possession, see Ioan M. Lewis, *Ecstatic Religion: An Anthropological Study of Spirit Possession and Shamanism* (Harmondsworth 1971), 30–5; B. Beit-Halahmi, 'The Turn of the Screw and the Exorcist-Demoniacal Possession and Childhood Purity', *American Imago* 33 (1976), 296–303.

10   Peter Laslett, 'Age at Menarche in Europe since the Eighteenth Century', in *Marriage and Fertility: Studies in Interdisciplinary History*, ed. Robert R. Rotberg and Theodore K. Rabb (Princeton, NJ 1980), 285–300.

11   Nicole Obry resurfaced in historical records in May 1577, when she arrived on a pilgrimage to Andens to invoke Saint John the Baptist, whose head was a relic in the possession of the local cathedral. According to an appendix to Boulaese's *Thresor*, Nicole had lost her sight a few weeks earlier and was advised by her

doctors to pray to the saint for a cure. With the twenty-six-year-old Nicole was her only son, Pierre Pierret, who was ten at the time of his mother's pilgrimage. This means that Pierre was born sometime in 1566 or 1567, shortly after Nicole's possession. Was she already pregnant with him at the time?

12 For good discussions of the sexual context of these cases, see de Certeau, *La Possession de Loudun* (Paris 1980). In Jewish early modern cases of spirit possession, the possessing spirits admitted that they had penetrated the women through their vaginas. No similar cases have been found in Christian Europe, where the evil spirits tended to enter and exit the body through other orifices.

13 On menstruation, see Patricia Crawford, 'Attitudes to Menstruation in Seventeenth-Century England', *Past and Present* 91 (1981), 47–73. For the prevalence of the connection between psychological distress and gynecological or obstetrical problems, see also Michael Macdonald, *Mystical Bedlam: Madness, Anxiety, and Healing in Seventeenth-Century England* (Cambridge 1981), 38.

14 The letter is included in Kathryn Kerb Fulton and Dyan Elliott, 'Self-Image and the Visionary Role in Two Letters from the Correspondence of Elizabeth of Schonau and Hildegard of Bingen', *Vox Benedictina* 2 (1985), 221–2.

15 On Hildegard and Elizabeth, see B. Newman, 'Hildegard of Bingen', 171–4. On Magdalena de la Cruz and Teresa of Avila, see Alison Weber, 'Saint Teresa, Demonologist', in *Culture and Control in Counter- Reformation Spain,* ed. Anne J. Cruz and Mary Elizabeth Perry (Minneapolis 1991), 173–87.

16 On the Wars of Religion and the devastation they brought on Picardy, see David Potter, *War and Government in the French Provinces: Picardy, 1470–1560* (Cambridge 1993), 200–32.

17 Lyndal Roper, *Oedipus and the Devil* (Routledge 1994), 176.

PART SEVEN

Witchcraft and Gender

B URIED AWAY IN THE TURGID, relentlessly misogynistic pages of
the *Malleus Maleficarum* (1486) is a story so surreal and comic that it is
impossible to forget. Interrupting their discussion of the witch's power to cause
impotence in men, Kramer and Sprenger invite their readers to consider the
following information:

> And what, then, is to be thought of those witches who . . . sometimes col-
> lect male organs in great numbers, as many as twenty or thirty members
> together, and put them in a bird's nest, or shut them up in a box, where
> they move themselves like living members, and eat oats and corn, as has
> been seen by many and is a matter of common report? . . .
>   For a certain man tells that, when he had lost his member, he
> approached a known witch to ask her to restore it to him. She told the
> afflicted man to climb a certain tree, and that he might take whichever
> member he liked out of a nest in which there were several members.
> And when he tried to take a big one, the witch said, 'You must not take
> that one,' adding, 'because it belonged to a parish priest'.[1]

At one level, this strange anecdote can be read as a testament to male anxieties
about the sexual power of women.[2] At another, it is noteworthy because it resembled the content of contemporary jestbooks, and probably owed more to popular
culture than learned theories about the nature of witchcraft. The inclusion of
such material in the *Malleus* indicates the willingness of its authors to incorporate
the widest possible range of sources, each of which added weight to their central
arguments about the existence of witches and the dangers they posed. The fact
that such material was available suggests that the stereotype of the female witch
was by no means confined to the learned elite. On this point the demonologists were

at one with ordinary villagers: they assumed that the majority of witches were women.

This assumption is reflected in the surviving records of witch trials. The best recent estimates suggest that three-quarters of those executed for witchcraft in Europe were women, though the figures varied considerably from place to place. Men and women appear to have been equally vulnerable to accusations in parts of France, while men outnumbered women as witchcraft suspects in some countries on the periphery of the continent like Iceland and Estonia.[3] These figures were outweighed, however, by those from Germany and Scotland, where some 70 per cent of the accused were women, and regions like Hungary, Denmark and England, where 90 per cent of witches were female. The potential influence of sexual stereo-types on prosecutions was illustrated in a list of 'presumptions against witches' drawn up for justices of the peace (JPs) in Yorkshire in 1592: the first presump-tion was 'that they are most comonly weeke women'.[4]

Such records have obliged historians to evaluate the relationship between witch-hunting and gender relations in the early modern period. But despite the considerable attention paid to this issue, there is still no consensus among academics in the field. One important interpretation, represented in Chapter 20 by Christina Larner, holds that accusations were aimed primarily against *witches* rather than women as such, though the social position of women made them unusually vulnerable to prosecu-tions. According to Larner's famous formulation, witchcraft was 'sex-related' but not 'sex-specific', since it was never denied that men as well as women could be guilty of the crime. She argues that attempts to explain witch-hunts in terms of the suppression of women by men distract historians from the wider political and religious context of the persecutions: it is necessary first to explain why Europeans came to accept the reality of satanic witchcraft, then to consider why women were especially vulnerable to accusations. This approach complements Larner's wider argument – represented in Chapter 15 of this book – that the politics of the Reformation encouraged ruling groups to investigate 'secret crimes' against the family, including sexual offences, infanticide and witchcraft. In each of these areas, women were more exposed to accusations than men.

Marianne Hester offers a stimulating criticism of Larner's work in Chapter 21. She argues that withcraft involved characteristics that were socially constructed as 'feminine', such as vengeance, lust and pride; and this meant that the crime was always closely identified with women. This argument complements the views of Louise Jackson, who points out in Chapter 26 that accusations of witchcraft involved a reversal of accepted female roles: witches were poisoners instead of providers of food, harmers instead of healers, and child killers instead of child protectors. Thus a typical witch was the mirror-image of a 'good woman', while possessing an excess of archetypally female vices. All of this suggests that the idea of witchcraft strongly implied female culpability, even though it was possible for men to be involved as well. Hester suggests that villagers and magistrates might have been looking for witches rather than women, but their understanding of the crime inclined them to look for female suspects. Moreover, the social circumstances of women were not enough in themselves to account for their targeting as witches. In some instances, women and men could engage in identical types of behaviour but with very different outcomes: women who asked their neighbours for food and were turned away could subsequently be accused of *maleficium*, while this was less likely to happen to men. For Hester, the witch trials of the early modern period were part of a wider movement to reconstitute gender relations during a time of social change. They had the effect of marginalising women involved in certain trades – such as brewing – and allowing men to assume more authority in expanding areas of the economy.

One objection to Hester's work is that it tries to explain witch trials as the outcome of a single cause: the restructuring of gender relations during a period of change. Like all monocausal explanations, it is open to the charge of overgeneralisation: did the economic circumstances that allegedly encouraged gender conflict in England apply to other countries that experienced persecutions? As Larner points out in Chapter 20, any interpretation of witch trials as 'woman-hunting' forces its proponents to explain 'why women appeared particularly threatening to patriarchal order at this time, and why they ceased to be so threatening about 1700'. This is a difficult task, since persecutions took place in so many different social and political contexts. The same objection could, of course, be levelled against Larner's own view that the prosecutions arose from the 'politicisation of religion' in the early modern period (see Chapter 15). Both interpretations involve a considerable degree of generalisation; and readers will have to decide which, if either, of these generalisations they find most convincing.

An alternative, less ambitious approach is to examine the records of specific witch trials for evidence of gender conflict in particular social circumstances. This is the method employed in the remaining chapters in this section. In Chapter 22, Jim Sharpe explores a familiar theme in the debate: the role of women in the prosecution of other women as witches. He suggests that women in England were unusually active in the prosecution of witchcraft in comparison to other crimes. Women featured often as accusers and victims of witches; some also played the specialist role of 'searchers', persons appointed by the courts to examine the bodies of those accused for hidden teats used to suckle familiar spirits. Licenced midwives, with their specialist knowledge of female anatomy, were often employed in this capacity, thus reversing the popular idea that midwives were commonly accused of witchcraft.[5] Sharpe's argument challenges the view that English witch trials represented an attempt by men to control independent women, and seeks to relocate the prosecutions in the context of the female community in early modern villages. It was in this world of female relationships, he suggests, that anxieties about *maleficium* were most frequently expressed.

The themes raised in Sharpe's chapter are reviewed in Chapter 23 by Clive Holmes, who acknowledges that ordinary women frequently voiced concerns about witchcraft, and were often prominent in village-level attempts to deal with the threat of harmful magic. For Holmes, however, women's encounters with witches normally stopped short of taking formal accusations to the courts. Like Robin Briggs in Chapter 3, he emphasises the informal efforts that individuals made to placate and coexist with those suspected of *maleficium*: the witches at Pendle in Yorkshire, for example, were appeased by their neighbours for decades before their activities reached the attention of local magistrates. Holmes argues that women were generally less inclined to move beyond this strategy of accommodation and seek legal remedies than men. He points out that female witnesses in trials often testified about misdeeds that had occurred many years before the prosecution itself, suggesting that these acts were not instrumental in the proceedings against the accused. Men, on the other hand, described more recent acts of *maleficia*. He concludes that it was men rather than women who took the lead in prosecuting witches: they were the primary actors in the legal drama, and made the crucial decisions about who should be tried for the crime. By taking this into account, Holmes seeks to return our attention to what he calls 'the misogynous dimension of witchcraft'.

All the chapters in this part concentrate on the accusation and trial of alleged witches by other members of their community. This approach is essential for understanding the social dynamics of persecutions; but there is a danger that it obscures the experience of the witch herself, and depicts her as the passive victim of forces completely beyond her control. As the chapter by Clive Holmes suggests, however, women suspected of *maleficium* could play an active role in the formation of their own reputations. Indeed, the idea of witchcraft provided a cultural resource for those who fell under suspicion of the crime as well as their accusers: the supposed powers of the Pendle witches probably afforded them more influence in their community than they would otherwise have enjoyed. This idea has been developed by Geoffrey Scarre, who argues that the constraints imposed by patriarchal culture meant that women were more likely to resort to magic than men:

> For men, there were usually more direct methods for attaining their ends or revenging themselves on their enemies; and it is possible that the complaints of a man against harsh or uncharitable treatment would have been listened to, just because he was a man, more sympathetically than those of a woman. Witchcraft may have held more appeal for women than for men not because, as contemporaries thought, women were more wicked and more easily led than men, but because their social and economic position imposed greater constraints on their possibilities of action.[6]

Scarre's interpretation restores the agency of women who thought themselves to be capable of *maleficium*, but places this in the context of wider social restraints. A similar picture has emerged from the study of witchcraft confessions in recent years: these texts reveal how some women came to internalise the idea of witchcraft as an act of self-definition, but did so in a culture that allowed them only a limited range of alternative models by which to understand their own feelings and actions. The study of this material provides a further insight into the relationship between gender and witchcraft; and this will be picked up in Part 8.

Notes

1   Heinrich Kramer and James Sprenger, *Malleus Maleficarum*, trans. Montague Summers (1928; repr. Dover Publications, New York 1971), 121.

2   It should be noted, however, that the *Malleus'* preoccupation with female wickedness was absent in most later demonologies, though there was a consensus among later writers that women's weaknesses made them more susceptible to the Devil's temptations. Allegations of causing impotence were comparatively rare in witch trials.

3   For a survey of data on the sex-distribution of witchcraft suspects, see Robin Briggs, *Witches and Neighbours* (HarperCollins, London 1996), 260–2.

4   Archives of the Yorkshire Archaeological Society, DD146/12/2/10.

5   The idea that midwives were commonly accused of witchcraft was originally encouraged by the excessive reliance of historians on the *Malleus Maleficarum*, which claimed that midwife witches abducted infants for ritual sacrifices. Surviving trial records suggest, however, that midwives were not particularly prone to accusations. See David Harley, 'Historians as Demonologists: The Myth of the Midwife-Witch', *Social History of Medicine* 3(1), (1990), 1–26; Lyndal Roper, *Oedipus and the Devil: Witchcraft, Sexuality and Religion in Early Modern Europe* (Routledge, London 1994), 201.

6   Geoffrey Scarre, *Witchcraft and Magic in Sixteenth and Seventeenth-Century Europe* (Macmillan, London 1987), 53.

Chapter 20

Christina Larner

WAS WITCH-HUNTING WOMAN-HUNTING?

WHEN THE ORGANISERS of an unemployment rally suggested 'Ditch the Witch' [Margeret Thatcher] as a banner slogan, it was left to a schoolgirl member of the local Labour Party to protest that this was sexist. They changed it to 'Ditch the Bitch', and the schoolgirl gave up. The same week the death of an elderly woman from starvation was reported in the press. It was noted that she had been the bane of the social work department for years, refusing offers of help, asserting her privacy and independence, and abusing all those who came near her. The report also noted that the local children called her 'the witch'. Only the children? And what do Margaret Thatcher and a pauperised escapee from the welfare state have in common?

The stereotype witch is an independent adult woman who does not conform to the male idea of proper female behaviour. She is assertive; she does not require or give love (though she may enchant); she does not nurture men or children, nor care for the weak. She has the power of words – to defend herself or to curse. In addition, she may have other, more mysterious powers which do not derive from the established order. All women threaten male hegemony with their exclusive power to give life; and social order depends on women conforming to male ideals of female behaviour. The identification of any woman as a witch will, therefore, set against her not only males, but also conforming females and their children.

To what extent, then, was the European witch-hunt (between the late Middle Ages and the beginning of the eighteenth century) a response to a perceived threat to the social order through some change in the status or power of women? During those years, several thousands of people, mostly peasant women, were put through a complex judicial process administered by men, and executed for witchcraft. Was this a thinly disguised attack on women as such?

The case that the witch-hunt was a woman-hunt is a strong one. In the first place, the stereotype of a witch in Christian Europe has always been that of a woman. In twelfth-century Russia, the authorities in one district became anxious about the prevalence of witchcraft and began to round up the entire female population. In 1492, in Langendorf in the Rhineland, they arrested all but two of the adult women. On the island of Coll, off the west coast of Scotland, a man claimed to have been attacked by a witch who had turned herself into an angry sheep. He said that, if all the women in Coll were placed together in a pen, his dog would be able to sniff out which of them was the witch. If you are looking for a witch, you are looking for a woman, and it could be any woman.

Whether anonymous or publicly identified, a witch threatens the established order. It was not for nothing that Margaret Lister of Fife was described in her indictment in 1662 as 'a witch, a charmer and a libber'. The last term seems to have had much the same pejorative meaning it carries today: a liberated woman who insists on making an issue of it. Witches are conspicuous. The women who went to the stake during the witch-hunt went cursing, often for the crime of cursing.

The ratio of females to males put on trial for witchcraft reinforces the theory that the witch-hunt was part of the sex war. The actual number of those involved is permanently inaccessible, but reliable figures for particular criminal archives suggest that in areas at the centre of the witch-hunt, in Germany, France, Switzerland and Scotland, 80 per cent of the accused were female. For areas on the periphery – in England and Russia, for example – the proportion of females was nearer 95–100 per cent.

While I am considering dubious but not quite pointless statistics, it might be worth adding that witchcraft (the ultimate in human evil) was sex-related to females in just the same proportion as sanctity (the ultimate in human good) was sex-related to males during the 'sanctity epidemic' of the later Middle Ages.

When the witch-hunt is put into its criminal context, the idea that the authorities in the sixteenth and seventeenth centuries consciously sought to terrorize and intimidate women gains further strength. Up to this period, women tended to be regarded in law as the responsibilities of their fathers or their husbands. In the sixteenth century, certain activities of women were made into crimes for the first time.

While older women were coming into the courts for witchcraft offences (including unofficial healing) and for keeping disorderly houses, younger women were being prosecuted for infanticide and prostitution. The criminalization of younger women came in the wake of new punitive attitudes to sexual activity. Women with children, lacking the male escape routes of mercenary fighting or urban labouring, were also particularly vulnerable to the new laws against vagabonds. There is much to suggest that in the law-and-order crises generated by the new regimes of early modern Europe, women were a prime symbol of disorder.

So what is the case for arguing that the witch-hunt was not directed primarily by men against women? One line of argument is that, since women accused other women and were frequently chief witnesses in the courts, there was nothing misogynous about witch-hunting. Male judges were simply responding to pressures from below; pressures which came largely from women. This line of reasoning is based on a failure to recognize that a patriarchal social structure divides women. Dependent for their livelihood on the goodwill of men, most women will not only conform, but also attack women who by their nonconformity threaten the security of conformist women.

At village level, nevertheless, many accusations of witchcraft were between women. Where men might use knives, women used words. When Janet MacMurdoch was defending herself against the accusations of Jean Sprot in Dumfries in 1671, she argued that Jean should not be accepted as a witness since she was as great a witch herself. She could tell fortunes from the way a person walked.

A more absurd argument which has been floated suggests that, since male suspects appear to have been treated with the same harshness as females once they reached the courts, no bias against women can be detected in the authorities. This ignores the crucial process through which those who were put on trial were selected in the first place. It does, however, draw attention to the more substantial objection that the crime of witchcraft, while sex-related, was not sex-specific. About 20 per cent of suspects were male.

There are other reasons for doubting whether the witch-hunt was a straightforward, thinly disguised woman-hunt. Those who were prosecuted for witchcraft were not, except during certain mass panics, randomly selected (any more than males who were prosecuted for crimes of violence in this period were randomly selected).

The cursing and bewitching women were the female equivalent of violent males. They were the disturbers of social order; they were those who could not easily cooperate with others; they were aggressive. Witches, like male bullies, were not 'nice people'. 'And when I gave my malison [the opposite of benison]', one Scottish witch said at her trial, 'it always lighted'. From this perspective, the pursuit of witches was no more a persecution of women than the prosecution of killers and maimers was a persecution of men. The parallel is not exact, but it is not absurd.

The prime interest of the authorities at the time was the pursuit of witches as such. A witch to them was a person who had renounced Christian baptism, given his/her soul to the Devil, and was in conspiracy with other witches to overthrow the social order. The purpose of a witch-hunt was the prising out of dangerous persons who were enemies of God, the state and the people. The fact that these ideological enemies turned out to be 80 per cent female could have added fuel to the misogyny of the age rather than be a direct consequence of it. Despite the long-term stereotype, sixteenth century demonologists spent much time puzzling over why women were so much more wicked than men.

The objection to viewing witch-hunting simply as woman-hunting is that it leads us to ask too narrow a range of questions about it. We must ask why women appeared particularly threatening to patriarchal order at this time, and why they ceased to be so threatening about 1700. Was it because of a rise in their status and independence? Was there a superfluous female population? Was it (paradoxically) because the Christianization of the peasantry through the Reformation and Counter-Reformation increased the individual responsibility of women for their spiritual lives? Was it because the religion so diffused was relentlessly patriarchal?

The thought that witch-hunting was actually witch-hunting, however, opens out a further range of questions about the function of Christianity as a political ideology in this period, the role played by witch-hunting in law and order crises, and the legitimacy of parallels with other great, less sexually-specific persecutions and purges of past and present.

Marianne Hester

PATRIARCHAL RECONSTRUCTION
AND WITCH-HUNTING

O NE OF THE MOST CONSISTENT yet least understood aspects of the
early modern witch-hunts is how accusation and persecution for witchcraft
came to be largely directed against women, throughout Europe and the so-called
New World.[1] In an attempt to question why the greater proportion of those accused
of witchcraft were women, this chapter seeks to move beyond Keith Thomas's
analysis in *Religion and the Decline of Magic* (1971) and also beyond the dichotomy
of 'sex-related versus sex-specific' set up by Christina Larner's work.[2] Focusing
mainly on English material, it argues that in our quest to understand the phenomenon of the witch-hunts we have to see male–female conflictual relations as an
integral part of the process of accusation and persecution. The accusation of women
was not merely a reflection of an age-old stereotype, nor merely the by-product
of a patriarchal society; the witch-hunts were a part of, and one example of, the
ongoing mechanisms for social control of women within a general context of social
change and the reconstruction of a patriarchal society.[3] It is generally recognised
that Europe in the early modern period experienced a variety of major changes in
terms of demography, ideology, economy, religions and political systems. Levack
has rightly pointed out that change is not a feature unique to this period, and that
'change' alone cannot explain the witch-hunts at this time.[4] Nonetheless, during
the sixteenth and seventeenth centuries, Europe experienced changes and a restructuring of society which created many uncertainties, ambiguities, tensions and
conflicts – not least with regard to male–female relations.[5] Within this context
witch persecution served – in a dynamic rather than functional sense – as a means
of recreating the male status quo in the emerging social order. This chapter examines some of the evidence for the relationship between witchcraft and patriarchal
reconstruction, in particular links between 'the female' and the witch, the gendering
of expectations and meanings and male–female conflict with regard to resources.

Keith Thomas, talking of course primarily about the English context, states
that 'the judicial records reveal two essential facts about accused witches: they
were poor, and they were usually women'.[6] He places witchcraft within its social

environment, arguing that the answer to who the witches were can be found at the village level where allegations arose. Essentially, Thomas argues that witchcraft accusation was related to failure to carry out some hitherto recognised social obligation; a poor woman would ask for charity or to borrow essential supplies (often from another, slightly better off, woman), but denied and eventually, if misfortune happened to the one who had denied her, would be accused of using witchcraft to cause the misfortune. This classic model of witchcraft accusation has since been shown to have a wider application than merely for England,[7] although one might question whether it actually explains why it was women who predominated amongst the accused. For Thomas, this scenario of social relations in a context of changing, conflictual, moral obligations does explain why the accused were older, poor and often widowed women. He points out that during the late Tudor and early Stuart period, when formal witchcraft accusation was at its height, village conflicts around neighbourliness grew especially acute. The erosion of the manorial system with loss of customary tenancies and common land created poverty while at the same time breaking up old cooperative village communities. Widows were particularly adversely affected by these changes leaving them vulnerable to witchcraft accusation. Thomas, like Macfarlane, clearly shies away from seeing this outcome for women as in any way related to male–female conflict. He argues that because the misogynistic or 'blatantly sexual aspects' of witchcraft common in continental literature such as the *Malleus Maleficarum* were not a feature of English trials, and especially because the accusations were often from one woman to another rather than between women and men, 'the idea that witch prosecutions reflected a war between the sexes must be discounted'.[8] Thomas thus presents a complex analysis of possible links between early modern social relations at the village level, beliefs about witchcraft and neighbourliness, and social change which incorporates women's position as dependent poor and especially as poor widows. But, despite his claims to the contrary, he does not actually manage to explain why it should be women rather than men who are in this position of vulnerability, of dependency and poverty. This is because his somewhat positivistic approach to the material detailing the accused and victims of witchcraft does not allow him to examine the process of gendering of the social relations he otherwise so eloquently describes.

Since *Religion and the Decline of Magic* was first published in the early 1970s the work of Christina Larner has probably had the greatest impact on historians' perceptions of why it was largely women who were accused of witchcraft during the early modern period. Larner argued that the witch-hunts in early modern Europe (and especially in Scotland, the area of her researches) were sex-related with regard to women but not sex-specific. Larner did not give precise definitions for these terms, but indicated that the term 'sex-related' meant that witch-hunts were 'one degree removed from an attack on women as such'. 'Sex-specific' would be applied only if all the characteristics of the witch were attributable to women, and in practice, she argued, this is not the case because 'the two principal characteristics of the witch, that is malice and alleged supernatural power, are human rather than female characteristics'. She concludes that while the vast majority of those accused amid those prosecuted for witchcraft were women, the witch-hunts were not actually about women hunting, but were more to do with the imposition of a Christian political ideology. It was the age-old gender stereotype of the witch that made them sex-related. There are, however, some problems with Larner's dichotomy of sex-related versus sex-specific. For a start, Larner's own work is actually more ambiguous than the dichotomy that has arisen from it suggests. As she says when discussing the link between witchcraft and the type of person accused, there is some evidence to suggest that the relationship is direct: 'Witch-hunting is women hunting or at least it is the hunting of women who do not fulfill the male view of how women ought to conduct themselves'.[9]

Secondly, defining 'sex-specific' by reference to a set of characteristics which can seemingly apply to only one sex ignores the possibility of change in the perception and interpretation of any characteristics attributable to men or women. Neither sex has a monopoly on any characteristics or behaviour – except as constructed and specified at any particular time. With regard to the early modern period there is some evidence to suggest that the principal characteristics of the witch were being perceived increasingly as female characteristics, including a perception of malice and use of supernatural power as more likely to be female characteristics.[10]

This leads us to another related problem, that of placing as central to witch-hunting the imposition of a Christian political ideology and the argument that the sex-relatedness of accusations is separate from this and merely to do with the age-old stereotype of the witch. This misses the point (otherwise implicit in the quotation from Larner) that gender relations are an integral part of Christian political ideology, constructing and being constructed by this. It is not enough, to use Scarre's words, 'to say that more women than men were tried for witchcraft because the stereotypical witch was a woman'.[11] Finally, Larner's use of the dichotomy of sex-related versus sex-specific has unfortunately set up a dualism which it is often difficult to look beyond – where historians tend to concur emphatically with her argument of sex-relatedness, while not thinking beyond this and merely ridiculing and marginalising the argument that the witch-hunts were indeed sex-specific.

If we *are* to use the terms 'sex-related' and 'sex-specific' at all, then we should use the terms to reflect a more complex situation. I would suggest that the witch-hunts were not merely sex-related or merely sex-specific, but – at different times and at different levels – both related to and specific to women. We may, for instance, consider beliefs amongst the learned elite and the development of a legal framework for dealing with witchcraft, especially prior to the witch-hunts, as sex-related; while at a local level, amongst the peasantry, beliefs and activities against witches were – in most European countries – sex-specific. If we focus on the development of the witchcraft construct amongst the learned elite in the centuries leading up to the witch-hunts, we see that unequal male–female social relations were also reflected in and constructed by the emerging notion of the witch. One of the results, a sexual double standard with female sexuality presented as inferior to that of men, is obvious in texts such as the *Malleus Maleficarum*.[12]

But in this pre-witch-hunt period the focus of persecution was those persons considered by the Catholic church as 'heretics', including both men and women; although at a local and informal level, persecution of those deemed to be witches was probably more specific to women even then. Cohn, for example, documents instances of local lynchings, supposedly of witches, that all appear to be of women.[13] In most of the countries affected by witch-hunts we see an orientation of persecution away from men, and also away from the elite, towards women and in particular poorer, older and often widowed women during the sixteenth and seventeenth centuries. Formal witch accusations change from being merely sex-related to being more sex-specific at this time.[14]

We need to move beyond the dichotomy set up by Larner's work so that we may develop a more sophisticated analysis of why the majority of those accused of witchcraft during the sixteenth and seventeenth centuries were women, and this requires a deeper look at male–female relations (or gender relations) during this period than most historians have so far attempted.[15] If we are to understand how a *female* witch stereotype developed, and how and why witch-hunting was directly linked to sex/gender, we must take into account that European society prior to, as well as during, the witch-hunts was male dominated or patriarchal, with a resultant gendering of social relations, social structures and discourses at many different levels. We need in particular to take into account the dynamic nature of patriarchy, where continuity of inequality between men and women relies on changing forms of oppression over time. As I have pointed out elsewhere, societies that are male dominated rely on constructions of 'the female' which present women as both different and inferior to men; and sexualisation, or eroticisation, of 'the female' in a variety of ways over time, is particularly important in constructing, and thereby maintaining, this difference.[16] Where the early modern witch-hunts are concerned we have much evidence of this sexualising process, where it was particularly female sexuality that was perceived to make women different from men. Male sexuality was not discussed in a similarly negative manner. Women were considered sexually insatiable and prone therefore to sinful and deviant behaviour, by contrast to the 'norm' which was construed as heterosexual, procreative sex under male control.[17]

In recent years there has been a tremendous development in the theorising of the process involved in what Thomas terms the 'war between the sexes', that is the oppressive relations, structures and discourses that characterise patriarchy for women. Hobby, talking specifically about women's activities within the patriarchal context of seventeenth-century England, has outlined the many ways women's lives were curtailed by comparison to those of men, but also how women acted within this context as subjects making choices, albeit limited ones: 'Women find ways of coping with their oppression and ways of resisting it, but this capitulation or resistance is not free or self-determined: it can normally only occur within the limits and on the terms of the framework set by the dominant group, men'.[18]

During this period of the witch-hunts, the patriarchal ideal for women was that they should be quiet (not scolds) and subservient to their husbands (not cuckolding the latter). Marriage, as the site of a heterosexual, procreative sexuality under the control of men, was – as expressed in many sermons, pamphlets and other literature at the time – deemed the only appropriate place for any sexual activity to take place.[19] These ideas were expressed most obviously by the middle and upper classes, but they were also reflected in attitudes towards and decisions about the behaviour of women from the lower classes as exemplified by church court cases: many women were punished through these courts for bearing an illegitimate child and for fornication, that is, heterosexual intercourse outside marriage.[20] Witchcraft accusation must be seen in this context of widespread fears that women were by no means complying with the ideal of the quiet compliant wife.

The women accused of witchcraft may be seen as victims of the witch-hunts, but the construct of the female as an actively sexual, hence sinful being, upon which accusation of witchcraft relied, shows us that women were by no means considered passive or compliant. Women were perceived to be morally weak by comparison with men, but this could also make them appear ultimately stronger than men. Women's supposedly insatiable and immoral sexuality was likely to lead them into allegiance with the Devil who could fulfill their sexual desires even better, so it was feared, than mere mortal men. In the English trial material this allegiance was explicit with some of the later trials such as the 1645 trials in Essex involving Matthew Hopkins, but also implicit in the symbolism of the familiar and the witches' marks in other trials.[21] Clive Holmes notes that Thomas Cooper, in a text of 1617, 'made an explicit attempt to conflate the familiar's sucking blood from the witch with the continental discussion of the coven and the witch's relationship with Satan'. Bernard's *Guide to Grand-Jury Men,* a decade later, provided a fully argued theory of this link. And sexualisation of the witches' mark was made especially apparent after 1630, with the publication of the fourth edition of *The Country Justice* by lawyer and JP, Michael Dalton. In this, Dalton cites Bernard 'with enthusiastic approval', but also changes Bernard's insistence that witches' marks may be found anywhere – although in 'very hidden places' – to a more explicit focus on the genitals. Thereafter, magistrates recommended that the pre-trial body search for witch's marks be 'focused upon the genital area'.[22]

In the circular, self-fulfilling, gender discourse of the witch-hunt period women were perceived as more likely to be sexually deviant than men because women were by definition (like Eve in the garden of Eden), sexually deviant. And deviance, in a God-fearing and deeply superstitious society, was construed as witchcraft. James VI of Scotland (later also James I of England) wrote, for example, in his D*aemonologie*:

> The reason is easie: for as that sexe is frailer than men is, so it is easier
> to be intrapped in these grosse snares of the Devill, as was well proved
> to be true, by the Serpents deceiving of Eve at the beginning, which
> makes him the homelier with that sex ever since.[23]

Here we have a direct example of the link between the construction of 'the female' as different and inferior to men and 'the witch'. It was men who stood to gain by the linking of witchcraft and 'the female' because it provided them with a greater moral and social status than women, and also, as I shall discuss further below, because it probably allowed them greater access to resources and potentially lucrative crafts and trades than women. The belief in witchcraft, as found during the sixteenth and seventeenth centuries, must be seen as a gendered ideology serving the material interests of men within patriarchal relations, and not merely, as Thomas suggests, as a means of dealing with guilt after 'unneighbourly' behaviour.

The age-old female stereotype of the witch does not, as both Thomas and Larner indicate, in itself explain why women predominated amongst the accused during the early modern period. We have to look to the general context of male–female relations, conflict and discourse to gain a better understanding of how the construct of 'the female' became synonymous with the witch. The process of gendering is of central importance: that is, the process of construction and positioning of women (by themselves, other women and men) as inferior and subordinate to men, and the many subtle or not so subtle pressures underlying such constructions and positioning. General beliefs about witchcraft in the early modern period were linked to sex/gender in such a way that it was expected that women and not men would use witchcraft for retribution and to cause harm – that is, there was a gendering of expectations and meanings.

Delphy has pointed out, with regard to social relations in French peasant society, that it is the sex of the individual that determines how a task is perceived rather than the nature of the task itself.[24] We can see this process clearly in trial material from England, Europe and New England, where men and women might carry out similar activities but only women end up accused of witchcraft, or where it is women who end up accused of men's misdemeanours. One pattern we are all familiar with from the trial material involves the suspect asking someone from another household, usually a woman, for food, other household items and even money. When refused this, the refuser or her/his family subsequently suffers death or illness. The woman making the demand is then accused of witchcraft. But if a man makes demands of a woman then it still the woman who is accused of witchcraft – as in the case of John Chaundeler and Elleine Smithe at the 1579 trial in Chelmsford. The pamphlet for the trial tells us that Elleine Smithe inherited some money from Alice, her mother, which Alice's widowed husband, John Chaundeler, then demanded for himself. It transpires that John and Elleine have fallen out over his demand for the money. Subsequently John Chaundeler dies, and before his death states that Elleine bewitched him so that he was unable to eat or digest meat. The result is that she ends up as the accused.

In another instance, from the same trial, it is Thomas Prat who takes Mother Staunton's grain but it is Mother Staunton who ends up accused of witchcraft. The pamphlet for the trial describes Mother Staunton walking past Thomas Prat's house with some grain. He wants some for his chickens and takes it from her. He has previously equivocated about whether or not she is a witch, stating at one time that she is not but having on another occasion 'raced her face with a Nedle' and subsequently believed himself bewitched.[25] When his chickens eat Mother Staunton's grain three or four dozen of them die, supposedly providing evidence that *she* has bewitched them.

I have already indicated that Thomas in *Religion and the Decline of Magic,* amongst others, does not agree that the witch-hunts may be linked directly to male–female conflict or sex struggle. Since we find from the trial material, both English and other European, that women who were accused of witchcraft largely used witchcraft against other women, and that accusations were often directed by women against women, Thomas argues that this shows there was a conflict *between women* rather than a struggle between the sexes. Others have more convincingly attributed this situation to women's position and general lack of power in a patriarchal society, where apparent use of witchcraft became an alternative for women 'incapable of using the more normal or socially approved means of revenge such as physical violence . . . or recourse to law courts', that is, unable to use the means usually employed by men.[26]

Larner, echoed by Sharpe, has also suggested that while men use physical violence, women are more likely to use verbal violence as represented by cursing. Thomas gives numerous examples of cursing leading to an accusation of witchcraft, but, although his examples are almost exclusively of women, he makes no mention of this fact. He quotes Thomas Cooper's 'stock pattern' of the link between cursing and witchcraft accusation: 'When a bad-tongued woman shall curse a party, and death shall shortly follow, this is a shrewd token that she is a witch'.[27] Yet while Cooper clearly takes a gendered view of the curser, Thomas does not take this up, instead concluding in gender-neutral terms that cursing 'was a means by which the weak and defenceless tried to avenge themselves upon their enemies'.[28]

Seeing witchcraft as a form of negative power available to women in a particular inegalitarian context is an overall picture of the witch-hunts, but we must also be careful not to lose sight of the complexity of male–female relations that such use of witchcraft by women entails. It is too easy to end up by focusing on women's accusations against one another as a problem related largely to women and women's communities, that is as women's problem, rather that as an outcome of a wider patriarchal context. Holmes provides some interesting evidence of men's and women's relative social positioning and the process of formal witchcraft accusation suggesting that women's accusations against each other were indeed secondary to men bringing the cases to court. Using data from the English home circuit, he argues that it was primarily men who brought charges of witchcraft, while women played a more ancillary role.[29] We need to consider that women's social position made them vulnerable to becoming witches, but also vulnerable to 'possession' and to becoming bewitched. Furthermore, women were often the ones in charge of the domestic goods the witch requested, and it was between women that the related transactions of lending and borrowing were likely to take place. Material from other societies and periods also gives us some important clues about the role women may have in relation to other women. We find that within patriarchal societies, women are often placed in the position of moral gatekeepers who socially control other women, and that there are various ideological, material and psychological pressures on them to do so. By acting as moral gatekeepers they may feel valued or at least have some power, even if their actions at the same time place both themselves and other women more firmly within patriarchy. The role women have in contemporary and historical Middle Eastern and North African societies, for instance, of carrying out clitorectomies on other women is a case in point. Nawal El Sadawi explains how older female relatives (mothers, grandmothers) are the ones who have the 'privilege' to carry out these operations, which reinforce women's inferiority and sexual servitude to men.[30]

Within the particular patriarchal context of early modern Europe, then, use of witchcraft was a means (albeit negative) by which women could increase their power. There are examples in the trial pamphlets and records of women using witchcraft to better their situation in many different ways. When we look more closely at witch trial material, it is also apparent, however, that witchcraft beliefs were by no means hegemonic among the women accused of witchcraft, or those providing evidence. In the trial pamphlets from Essex we find that, while some of the women probably did believe that they had or could have used witchcraft, others are described as not sharing this belief and appeared to be much more sceptical about witchcraft. For example, at the 1566 trial at Chelmsford one of the accused,

Elizabeth Frauncis, appears to believe that she could and did use witchcraft to procure, amongst other things, sheep and a wealthy husband via the cat-familiar Satan. By contrast, in a 1582 trial at St Osyth, Elizabeth Bennet (who is said to deny that she herself used witchcraft) is shown to attempt to explain how she thinks an accusation against another woman, Ales Newman, can be understood in more 'rational' terms without recourse to witchcraft. She is recorded as saying that Ales was merely angry at Johnson, the collector for the poor, because he did not give her the handout she required, although what she says ends up being tied into the evidence against Ales, because the words she uses to signify anger — 'harded speeches' — are at the same time constructed as a sign of women's misdemeanour, as cursing, and hence witchcraft. We see here an example of the gendering not only of language and meanings, but of expectations about women's behaviour.[31]

At a local level we thus see women using the means available to them to improve their condition, but we also see how the constructs which led them to use witch-like behaviour at the same time constructed them as witches — whether they wanted this or not. At a local level, use of witchcraft can be seen as a part of the day to day activities of the 'women's community' but — crucially — relying on wider patriarchal gendered notions of the witch, and elite ideas about the unruliness of women and the need to control them. Witchcraft accusations may therefore, to a large extent, be situated (as Thomas situates them) within the women's community, but they were integrally linked to and served to reinforce — or reconstruct — the male status quo.

Finally I want to look at the male–female conflict around resources that formed a part of the contextual background to the early modern witch-hunts, as already hinted at by the case of Elleine Smithe's inheritance and John Chaundeler's claims on it. There appears to be a link between male–female relations, economic change and witchcraft accusation — even if we cannot always establish a direct link between individuals accused of witchcraft and specific instances of male–female conflict around resources and livelihoods.

In taking early modern England as our example, we have to think of a society with a rapid increase in population, and resultant pressure on resources; with women outnumbering men, yet with decreasing means of livelihood for women. Convents had been closed during the Reformation, and women were being excluded from crafts and trades such as weaving and brewing as well as from the guilds; enclosure of common land (already happening in Essex at this time) exacerbated the difficulties of a growing mass of landless peasants, amongst other effects removing the space for grazing for women's livestock.[32] Thomas, as indicated earlier, does link some of these economic changes to the impoverishment and dependence of certain lower-class women, and especially widows. This may also be understood by the more widely acknowledged concept of the feminisation of 'poverty' — a concept that also applies within the present global economic context.[33]

A number of historians have documented how the period of pre-capitalism and early capitalism, that is, the early modern period, saw a deterioration of women's role in production.[34] Moreover, Chris Middleton indicates that it was specifically men who became predominant in the occupations which were foremost in the development of the emergent capitalist production (as had also been the case in the development of the earlier feudal production). He argues that capitalist production developed 'at the expense of sexual equality', that is, at the expense of women.[35] Sylvia Walby suggests in addition that when there are changes in the economic sphere, such as changes in production methods, conflict around male–female power relations takes place in order to ensure male dominance.[36] We can indeed find some evidence of a realignment of male–female power relations in the sixteenth and seventeenth centuries due to the major changes taking place in the economy at that time. Evidence of women's work, in areas such as brewing and weaving, suggests that there was a struggle between the sexes around making a living, which also had the effect of ensuring that men rather than women obtained the better positions in, and thus control of, the emerging capitalist economic structure. Overall, patriarchy was maintained within the developing economy, and women's relative dependence on men ensured.

The case of brewing provides an interesting example. Brewing is acknowledged as an important industry in the early modern period, because beer, and in particular ale (brewed without hops), was the staple drink of men, women and children at most meals. Women did the brewing of ale needed for immediate consumption by the household, and prior to the sixteenth and seventeenth centuries women also brewed ale for sale. Judith Bennett has documented how the exclusion of women from brewing took place over a considerable period, but it was during the sixteenth and seventeenth centuries that brewing finally changed from a female to a male occupation. Excluding women from brewing occurred alongside the separation of brewing (by men) from the sale (by women) of beer, a policy pursued by the government with the aim of imposing stricter regulation and supposedly simplifying the collection of taxes, as well as improving the quality of the beer brewed. Bennett concludes:

> All of these changes were very slow and uneven, proceeding over the course of several centuries and affecting different regions of the country at different times and in different ways. But their overall effect was clear; by 1700, brewing, which had been a home-based trade dominated by women four centuries earlier, was becoming a factory-based industry controlled by a steadily shrinking group of wealthy males.[37]

Alongside the other economic changes mentioned by Thomas, the changes to the brewing industry must seriously have reduced the earning capabilities of village women.[38] It was only widows who retained access to brewing through inheritance from their husbands. Michael Roberts documents how the *selling* of ale became an occupation informally reserved for poor widows during this period.[39] Sue Wright similarly points out that in the urban environment of Tudor and Stuart Salisbury there were numerous women, especially widows, who were licensed as alehousekeepers (the poor end of the market) but few as innkeepers (the richer part of the market).[40]

With regard to the discussion in this chapter there are a number of important issues which arise from the example of the brewing industry. These include: the construction of women as incapable of brewing; the link of this construction to the witch; and the position of widows as both brewers and ale-sellers.

Bennett shows convincingly how the popular and also negative representation of the alewife, in prose, poetry, ballads, drama, carvings, sculpture, and drawings

(p. 169) was linked to her demise. For instance the early sixteenth-century poem, *The Tunning of Elynor Rummying* depicts the alewife Elynor Rummyng as a grotesque and ridiculous old women, who is of dubious religious and sexual virtue, and a highly unscrupulous tradeswoman (p. 170). She is almost a stock figure in misogynistic literature: 'a grotesque old witch-like woman', but also a corrupt tradeswoman who sells her customers adulterated drink at hard driven prices in a disgusting atmosphere (p. 171). Bennett argues that such popular representations undermined the position of the alewife by questioning her general trustworthiness, while at the same time allowing men to be seen in a much more positive light. The construction of the alewife as different and inferior to the male brewer often relied, like the construction of the witch, on her sexualisation or eroticisation, and, we find, in the example of Elynor Rummyng, allusions to her also being associated with witchcraft: she entertained a customer who 'seemed to be a witch', she dressed up 'after the Saracen's guise' and like an Egyptian', and 'the Devil and she be sib' [like brother and sister] (p. 170). It is difficult to tell whether alewives or women who brewed beer were accused of witchcraft directly.[41] Yet the construction of the alewife and the witch relied on similar terms, and both served to justify the social control of women and the maintenance or reconstruction of the patriarchal status quo – securing men's dominant position within the social order, and also opening up new areas for male control.

For women during the early modern period financial independence was generally linked to their marital status. Women on their own, particularly widows, were more likely to be financially independent than married women because married women were deemed subordinate to their husbands (as reflected in the law) and under their husbands' control financially. Widows might inherit their husbands' land, property and/or craft or trade, and unmarried women might occasionally inherit their fathers' land and property or engage in other productive activities.[42] Thus during the period of the witch-hunts women's work was largely defined by the institution of marriage. For example, a woman could only practise a craft alongside her husband, taking on his craft, or in her own right as a widow or as a single woman living in her father's household.[43] Where the example of brewing is concerned, Bennett suggests that the masculinisation of the brewing trade had the effect of changing the economic balance between husbands and wives, the wife becoming more dependent on her husband. Unmarried women were also very badly affected: 'They became less and less able to compete with men or married couples for customers, licenses and economic legitimation'.[44] The women, likely to be widows, who were still able to be brewers might therefore pose a threat to the increasingly male monopoly of the trade. They were vulnerable to misogynistic attack or possibly witchcraft accusation as a result.

By looking at material concerning socio-economic changes in the sixteenth and seventeenth centuries we find that the picture regarding witchcraft accusation and women becomes more complex. On the other hand, women accused of witchcraft tended to be those, as identified by Thomas, who were among the most vulnerable in the economy, that is, labouring women, widowed and possibly older, and poor. But they might also be amongst those in competition with men for work in lucrative areas such as brewing, that is, women carrying out a craft or trade, and more specifically, widows, who were more able to do so. Dependent or in competition, either way they might be seen to pose a threat. Women were gener-ally in a less advantageous situation than men within the changing economy, especially within the peasantry and amongst artisans and traders – the areas that were particularly relevant to the emerging capitalist economy and also the group amongst whom witchcraft accusations predominated.

To conclude, by examining the processes involving gendering of social rela-tions, expectations and disclosures concerning the witch in the early modern period we may surmise that witch-hunting became sex-specific at this time, serving as one means of maintaining and reconstructing male dominance and male power *vis-à-vis* women. Patriarchy, potentially under threat in the rapidly changing society, was merely reconstructed to maintain the status quo. Our understanding is enhanced by consideration of the conflictual and dynamic male–female relations at the time, and by taking a deeper look at the context of male–female relations than historians have often tended to pursue with regard to this period and topic.

Notes

1   In Chapter 5 of this collection, for instance, E. William Monter suggests that sex remains the most important feature of most witchcraft accusations.

2   See Chapter 20 for Larner's distinction between 'sex-specific' and 'sex-related' witchcraft.

3   Monter suggests that acts such as infanticide were also a focus for prosecution of women in the early modern period to a greater extent than had been the case previously. It thus appears that during the sixteenth and seventeenth centuries there were a variety of attempts to control sexual behaviour in particular and women specifically, through both formal witchcraft accusation and by legal retri-bution against other sexual deviance.

4   B. Levack, *The Witch-hunt in Early Modern Europe* (London 1987), 139–42.

5   See S. D. Amussen, *An Ordered Society* (Oxford 1988), and J. Klaits, *Servants of Satan* (Bloomington, Ind. 1985).

6   Keith Thomas, *Religion and the Decline of Magic* (Harmondsworth 1973), 520.

7   J. P. Demos, *Entertaining Satan* (Oxford 1982); A. M. Walker and E. H. Dickerman, 'A woman under the influence: a case of alleged possession in sixteenth-century France', *Sixteenth Century Journal,* 22 (1991), 534–54.

8   Thomas, *Religion,* 562, 563.

9   C. Larner, *Enemies of God* (London 1981), 92.

10   Klaits, *Servants,* 58–9.

11   G. Scarre, *Witchcraft and Magic in Sixteenth and Seventeenth Century Europe* (London 1987), 51.

12   H. Kramer and J. Sprenger, *Malleus Maleficarum* (Nuremberg 1496). See also C. Merchant, *The Death of Nature* (London 1980).

13   Norman Cohn, *Europe's Inner Demons* (London 1975).

14   Klaits also appears to document this change from sex-related to sex-specific, although without using these terms. He attributes the increased focus on women as the accused during the early modern period to 'a dramatic rise in fear and hatred of women during the era of the Reformation' (p. 52).

15   For a good example of an approach to the witch-hunts that takes male and female

relations into account at the heart of the discussion see C. Karlson, *The Devil in the Shape of a Woman* (New York 1988).

16   M. Hester, *Lewd Women and Wicked Witches* (London 1992).

17   See Amusen, *An Ordered Society;* M. Hester, 'The dynamics of male domination using the witchcraze in sixteenth and seventeenth century England as case study', *Women's Studies International Forum*, 13 (1990); Hester, *Lewd Women.*

18   E. Hobby, *Virtue of Necessity* (London 1988), 8.

19   See Amusen, *An Ordered Society*; S. Shepherd, *The Women's Sharp Revenge* (London 1985); L. Woodbridge, *Women and the English Renaissance* (Urbana, Ill. 1986); L. B. Wright, *Middle Class Culture in Elizabethan England* (Chapel Hill, NC 1935).

20   Martin Ingram provides extensive examples and interpretations of such cases from the church courts: *Church Courts, Sex and Marriage in England 1570–1640* (Cambridge 1987); and P. E. H. Hair lists many original indictments and outcomes: *Before the Bawdy Court* (London 1972).

21   See Sharpe, *Instruments of Darkness*, ch. 5; Klaits, *Servants*, 56.

22   See Chapter 23 in this book by Clive Holmes.

23   Cited in Larner, *Enemies of God*, 93.

24   C. Delphy, *The Main Enemy: A Materialist Analysis of Women's Oppression* (London 1977).

25   Hester, *Lewd Women*, 173–40. Laura Gowing, in her discussion of women's slander litigation in early modern London, describes how scratching the face and especially the nose of a woman was a punishment indicating that she was a whore. See 'Language, power and the law', in J. Kermide and G. Walker, eds, *Women, Crime and the Courts* (London 1994). We can speculate that to 'race [Mother Staunton's] face with a nedle' similarly symbolised that she was being presented in sexualised terms; women accused as witches were often presented as sexually deviant.

26   See Monter, Chapter 5.

27   Thomas, *Religion*, 512. See M. Ingram, 'Scolding women cucked or washed', in Kermode and Walker, *Women, Crime and the Courts*, p. 48, for a discussion of cursing and in particular scolding as a specifically female offence.

28   Thomas, *Religion*, 512. The punishment of women convicted specifically of scolding appears to parallel witchcraft accusation in that it became more severe in the same period as witchcraft became a major female crime, that is, from the mid-sixteenth to the mid-seventeenth century. See Ibid., 57; Underdown, 'The taming of the scold', in A. Fletcher and J. Stevenson, eds, *Order and Disorder in Early Modern England* (Cambridge 1985), 116–36.

29   Holmes presents this argument in Chapter 23. See also Demos, *Entertaining Satan*; Karlson, *The Devil in the Shape of a Woman.*

30   N. El Sadawi, *The Hidden Face of Eve* (London 1981).

31   Hester, *Lewd Women*, 166–7, 183–4.

32   See Amussen, *An Ordered Society.*

33   H. Scott, *The Feminisation of Poverty* (London 1984).

34   See I. Charles and I. Duffin, eds, *Women and Work in Pre-Industrial England* (London 1985); J. Kelly, *Women History and Theory* (Chicago 1986); A. Clark, *Working Life of Women in the Seventeenth Century* (London [1919] 1982).

35   C. Middleton, 'The sexual division of labour in feudal England', *New Left Review*, 113–14 (1979), 147–68; and 'Women's labour and the transition to pre-industrial capitalism', in Charles and Duffin, eds, *Women and Work*, 181–206.

36   S. Walby, *Patriarchy at Work* (Cambridge 1986).

37   M. Bennett, 'Misogyny, popular culture, and women's work', *History Workshop Journal,* 31 (1991), 169.

38   Clark, *Working Life,* 228.

39   M. Roberts, '"Words they are women, and deeds they are men": Images of work and gender in early modern England', in Charles and Duffin, eds, *Women and Work,* 122–80.

40   S. Wright, '"Churmaids, huswyfes and hucksters": The employment of women in Tudor and Stuart Salisbury', in Ibid., 100–21.

41   Macfarlane gives the occupation of one husband of an accused witch (out of forty-nine known for Essex) as a beer brewer. See Hester, *Lewd Women,* 162.

42   S. L. Watkins, 'Spinsters', *Journal of Family History,* 9 (1984); Charles and Duffin, *Women and Work.*

43   See Amussen, *An Ordered Society,* ch. 3.

44   Bennett, 'Misogyny', 182.

Chapter 22

Jim Sharpe

WOMEN, WITCHCRAFT AND THE LEGAL PROCESS

T HE PROBLEM OF GENDER is one that has only recently begun to attract the attention of historians of crime, of the law, and of the operation of legal systems. There have, of course, been a number of works that have demonstrated the potential fruitfulness of various lines of approach: the different participation rates of the two sexes in various types of offence; male and female involvement in litigation, perhaps most notably in church court slander cases; and on such gender related (or indeed gender specific) matters as infanticide and scolding.[1] Yet it remains clear that considerable work needs to be done both in charting the statis-tical contours of such matters as prosecutions brought against men and women, and the punishments inflicted upon them, as well as in using court records to help to understand gender as a social construct, as a bundle of assumptions or attitudes about how men and women should behave.[2] The difficulties in following such a course are, unfortunately, more severe when women are under consideration. The English legal system was run by men, the statutes it enforced were drawn up and promulgated by men, and the English common law seemed designed to constrain the rights of women as much as possible.[3] At first sight then, it would seem that historians studying the relationship between women and the legal process in the past have had their task restricted to doing little more than cataloguing the ways in which women were disadvantaged.

Nowhere would this premise, again at first sight, seem more conspicuously true than when considering the prosecution of witchcraft in Tudor and Stuart courts. As is well known, around 90 per cent of persons indicted for witchcraft at the Home Circuit assizes between the passing of the Elizabethan statute in 1563 and the abolition of laws against witchcraft in 1736 were women.[4] Work on compa-rable sources suggests that this rate was fairly usual for the indictment of malefic witchcraft in England.[5] Yet even the first step that might be taken beyond this simple counting exercise exposes complications. Reworking the figures for Essex, we discover that the 236 presentments for witchcraft or related matters made before the Archdeacons of Essex and Colchester between the 1560s and the 1630s reveal a male participation rate of 29 per cent.[6] Further complications arise when we examine cunning men and women, those 'good' witches who attracted so much hostility from the writers of English demonological tracts, but whose services were so eagerly sought by the population at large. Whereas over 90 per cent of those accused at the Essex assizes for witchcraft were female, two-thirds of the cunning folk whom Macfarlane was able to identify in his Essex study were men.[7] These figures suggest that we will have to refine our standard notions of the connection between women and witchcraft at some future point. For the present, however, it seems safe to take as our starting point that the overwhelming majority of persons accused of malefic witchcraft were women, and that a study of witchcraft cases could offer a potentially fruitful approach to the study of women's involvement in the legal process in early modern England.

We must, however, pause to consider what we mean by the term 'legal process'. To understand the operation of the law in its full context, it is necessary to go beyond the courtroom and the strict rules of legal procedure, and even to speculate about what was going on outside areas covered by the legal record. The English criminal legal system was an accusatory one, and, in large measure, the prosecution of witches, along with other felons, was dependent on the initiative of the person offended against – the victim. As I have argued elsewhere, on the strength of Northern Circuit assize depositions, women showed no reluctance in accusing other women of being witches, or of giving evidence against alleged witches.[8] Indeed, in both these areas female participation in the legal system seemed to be at least equal to that of men. In this chapter I should like to take things further, and seek other points at which we can delineate a distinctive female contribution to the prosecution of witches: the role of women in searching for the witch's mark; wider evidence about female involvement as winesses in witchcraft cases; the behaviour of both witches and their accusers in court; and the subsequent behaviour of condemned witches on the gallows. A consideration of these topics, based as it must be on imperfect and at times contradictory materials, can only lead to very tentative conclusions. What it does demonstrate is that witchcraft prosecutions cannot be interpreted purely as the oppression of women by a male dominated legal system.

One area where women were of unique importance in the judicial trial witchcraft was in their being used to search for the witch's mark. The mark was seen as a method of establishing guilt in some fifteenth-century Continental trials, although the then current custom of shaving body hair from the suspects to facilitate the search does not seem to have been followed in England.[9] The first pamphlet account of a witchcraft trial in England, published in 1566, stressed the importance of the mark as a means of establishing proof, and as English trials progressed its importance remained central. It also seems that it gradually became accepted that the mark, with women, most commonly took the form of a teat-like growth in the pudenda, from which it was thought that the witch's familiar sucked blood. Contemporary usage dictated that if the discovery of such a mark was thought vital for proving witchcraft, the search for it should be made by women. The earliest known reference to appointing women for this task comes, perhaps a little unexpectedly, from the court leet of Southampton in 1579. The wording of the relevant order suggests that the practice was already a familiar one. The leet jury directed that half a dozen honest matrons should be appointed to strip widow Walker and to determine if she had 'eny bludie marke on hir bodie which is a comon token to know all witches by'.[10] That the practice was widely known at this time is confirmed by a tract describing the prosecution of several women in Essex in 1582.[11] This incident involved the searching of a number of suspected witches by local women, including the alleged victims of witchcraft, one such group of searchers being described as 'women of credite'.[12]

The actual mechanics by which women were appointed to search witches varied enormously. Edward Fairfax, a Yorkshire gentleman who thought two of his daughters were being bewitched, recorded how in 1621 the suspected women were 'by appointment, at the house of widow Pullens, at Fuystone, searched for marks upon their bodies', which suggests a degree of official sanctioning of the process. Some years later, in another Yorkshire case, Dorothy Rodes, another parent who thought her child to be bewitched, noted how the suspected witch, Mary Sikes, was 'searched by weomen appointed by a justice of peace'. A male witness recorded how he went with one of Rodes' sons to Henry Tempest, a Riding justice who seems to have been much involved in witch cases, 'to procure a warrant for searching the said Mary Sikes and Susan Beaumont'. Six women, three married and three widows, were appointed. Another Yorkshire witness, Alice Purston, told in 1655 how she and other women were appointed to search Katherine Earle on the direction of the constable of their township who was himself acting under direction from a justice. Four years earlier, in another Yorkshire case, the direction seems to have come simply from the local constable.[13] The decision to search seems, therefore, to have involved an interplay between official attitudes and the demands of the local community, whose members were aware of the need to search for the mark. This suggests that the legitimation for searching operated at both an official and a popular level.

Perhaps the most remarkable evidence we have of the dynamics of the search for the mark comes from the case of Elizabeth Sawyer, executed after trial at the Middlesex Sessions in 1621. Sawyer's trial was rather hanging fire, with neither the judge nor the jury apparently having much idea of what to make of the evidence before them. At that point a justice who had taken considerable interest in the case, Arthur Robinson, intervened. He told the court that 'information was given unto him by some of her neighbours, that this Elizabeth Sawyer had a private and strange marke on her body, by which suspition was confirmed against her'. 'The Bench', we are told, 'commanded officers appointed for those purposes, to fetch in three women to search the body of Elizabeth Sawyer'. One of these was Margaret Weaver, 'that keeps the Session House for the City of London, a widdow of honest reputation'. She was joined by 'two grave matrons, brought in by the officer out of the streete, passing there by chance'. Sawyer resisted the searchers, behaving 'most sluttish and loathsomely towards them, intending thereby to prevent their search of her', but the women continued in their efforts, each of them deposing separately to court about the results of the exercise. They found a teat 'the bignesse of the little finger, and the length of halfe a finger', which looked as though it had recently been sucked. This evidence proved decisive and swung the jury against Sawyer.[14]

As this case suggests, the credentials needed by women searchers were those resulting from good character rather than technical expertise. Some other cases, however, suggested that women with some type of knowledge might be favoured.

Midwives were, of course, uniquely qualified to comment on irregularities in the female genitals. The exceptionally rich documentation provided by the Matthew Hopkins trials of 1645–7 shows a number of them in action. A midwife named Bridget Reynolds searched one of the Essex witches, Elizabeth Harvey. Five women gave evidence against Joan Salter, one of those accused on the Isle of Ely, and deposed how they found three teats in her privy parts 'which the midwife and the rest of these informants have not seen the like on the body of any other woman'.[15] Later in the century, again in Essex, we find a midwife being appointed to search the body of a suspected witch 'in the presence of some sober women'. This she did, and informed the author of the narration of the case

> that she never saw the like in her life: that her fundament was open like a mouse hole, and that in it were two long biggs, out of which being pressed issued blood: that they were neither piles nor emrods (for she knew both) but excressences like to biggs with nipples which seemed as if they had been frequently sucked.[16]

Some midwives clearly felt themselves able to give expert evidence in witchcraft cases.[17]

Others might claim a more general expertise. Hence, again during the Hopkins trials, Anne the wife of Thomas Savory of Upwell in Norfolk was examined by 'some that were there who p[re]tended to have skill in the discovery of witches' who 'sayd that some of the divles impes had sucked her'.[18] The Hopkins episode also saw the emergence of a woman who clearly attained a regional reputation as a searcher for the witch's mark, Mary Philips. Philips was involved as a witness in some of the early Essex trials in the spring of 1645 and, for reasons which remain elusive, seems to have acquired a wider repute as a finder of the witch's mark. Certainly, she was brought in by the authorities of Aldeburgh in Suffolk to supervise other women searching suspected witches there, and was paid for such duties and also received expenses.

Not all of the women searched, as the case of Elizabeth Sawyer suggests, submitted willingly, while several of them offered those searching them explanations for those physical peculiarities which risked being identified as the witch's mark. Joan Salter explained to an investigating justice that 'the markes that she hath about her are not the markes of a witch but caused as it pleaseth God she beleaveth by child bearing'. Mary Armitage, a Yorkshire witch, was searched by four women in 1658, and a suspicious hole a quarter of an inch deep was found on her right shoulder. The suspected witch attributed this to an injury sustained while carrying a bundle of thorns, one of which penetrated her shoulder. She explained that the thorn 'continewed there about a yeare before itt could be gott out and caused a great swelling and since that tyme there hath beene a little hole upon her shoulder'. Something of the experience of the search for the witch's mark is conveyed in the examination of another Yorkshire witch, Katherine Earle. Earle asked

> why she did not tell the woemen that searched . . . of a marke betweene here thighs as well as that of behind her eare she at first answered that she did not know of it, whereat the women laughing she p[re]sently after said it came by a burne and she had it 36 yeares.

The frequency of references in surviving depositions to women searching for the mark suggests that the practice, existing as it did on the peripheries of the legal process, was widespread and culturally familiar. This point is reinforced by a remarkable case from Oxfordshire in 1687. Joan Walker of Bicester, the widow of a gentleman, petitioned the bench in that year, to the effect that despite her good reputation and good conduct,

> severall wicked & mallicious persons enveing the good name, fame, credit & reputacon of your peti[tioner] have uniustly & without any ground or collo[u]r of reason given out in speeches that your peti[tioner] is a witch which odious name yo[u]r peti[tioner] utterly abhors & detests & all the works of the devill.

To clear herself, widow Walker requested that the bench should order that she 'may be searched by foure & twenty honest sober iudicious matrons & make report of their opinions at next sessions', and that the persons abusing her should be bound over to appear there. By this time, and at this social level, the attention of the jury of women searchers was clearly recognized, while Walker's suggestion that she should be searched by 'foure & twenty' women is instructive. A criminal accusation at the sessions or assizes typically would be screened by a grand jury of twelve or so men, and then tried by a trial jury of another twelve. Walker obviously desired that the search that was intended to clear her name should mirror proper legal process as far as possible.

   This last case reminds us that the female searchers officially sanctioned to search women were but one of a number of types of juries, or near juries, of female experts who were called in to adjudicate in a number of legal matters, both criminal and civil. The English mediaeval ecclesiastical courts had sought female assistance in cases of annulment of marriage on the grounds of the husband's impotence, when the accuracy of the plea was tested by 'honest women' who, by baring their breasts and kissing or fondling the man, attempted to arouse him sexually.[19] This practice seems to have been discontinued by the sixteenth century, but the operation of the church courts still made occasional use of women as experts in sexual cases. Thus when, in 1595, a man from Barking in Essex was presented for incest with his daughter, it was reported that the suspicion was not founded merely on 'common report', but also 'upon the assertion of honest women, who have had the examinacion of the young wench'.[20] Although the point needs further investigation, it seems certain that similar searches, sometimes with official sanction, would be made by women in infanticide and rape cases. Most familiar, perhaps, was the use made by female juries in examining women who claimed to be pregnant after conviction for felony, and who hence hoped to delay or evade being executed.[21] Together, this use of female juries or less formal groups of female investigators constitutes a part of the legal process that must modify the general assertion that women were excluded from official participation in it. They did not serve as magistrates or jurors but the authority derived from the crucial evidence of their 'special knowledge' was a dramatic reversal of their generally powerless roles as petitioners, witnesses or parties to litigation.

   Women were also frequently involved as witnesses against witches. The Home

Circuit assize records reveal that there were 1207 calls for witnesses at witch trials between 1600 and 1702. Of these, 631 (or 52 per cent) involved men and 576 (or 48 per cent) women, a nearly even split. In isolated cases, there might be a heavy preponderance of women witnesses: 14 women to 3 men in Kent in 1657, 10 women to 5 men in Surrey in 1664, 8 women alone in Essex in 1650. Such cases would seem to support the conclusion advanced elsewhere, on the strength of Northern Circuit assize depositions, that women felt no qualms about giving evidence against female witches.[22] The Home Circuit records also suggest that the proportion of women witnesses increased over the seventeenth century, from 46 women to 80 men in 1600–09, to a preponderance of women witnesses in the 1660s and 1670s. The importance of these figures is emphasized when we compare them to the gender ratio of all witnesses called to give evidence in felony cases in Hertfordshire between 1610 and 1619. In that decade 572 men and 36 women were called to give evidence in felony cases at the Hertfordshire assizes, a ratio of over twelve male witnesses to each female.[23] In the same decade, taking the Home Circuit as a whole, there 92 men and 82 women were called to give evidence in witchcraft cases. On these figures, women were over 11 times more likely to act as witnesses in witchcraft trials at the assizes than they were in all felony cases. We return to the notion that the connection between women and witchcraft lay not only in the gender of the accused, but also in a much wider, much more complex, and as yet barely investigated web of assumptions about gender, female power, and female interaction in early modern England.

It is possible to push beyond statistics occasionally, and to reconstruct something of the experience of women in the courtroom. Such instances throw light on what is still one of the problem areas of English legal history: the very basic issue of how trials were actually conducted, of what happened in the push and shove of a court in session. The official documentation engendered by an English criminal trial in this period rarely sheds much light on these matters. The indictment is a notoriously arid document, while depositions, although invaluable for illustrating other matters, were essentially pre-trial documents that by their very nature usually tell us nothing of what happened in court. Other sources can be more revealing and, as we shall see, something can be constructed from pamphlet accounts of trials, and from isolated references in letters, diaries, memoirs, and such like. The general point to be made is that court proceedings were more disorderly, more ramshackle, and less seemly than those obtaining in a modern court of law. Some notion of typical conditions can be gained from the case of Mary Spencer who, at her trial for witchcraft, complained that 'the wind was so loud, and the throng so great, that she could not hear the evidence against her'.[24] John Aubrey noted that at the trial of a witch in 1653 'the spectators made such a noise that the judge could not hear the prisoner nor the prisoner the judge, but the words were handed from one to the other by Mr R. Chandler, and sometimes not truly reported'.[25] Sometimes the throng in the court during a witchcraft trial might be so oppressive, and demonstrate its hostility to the accused so forcefully, that, as Roger North recorded of one post-Restoration case in the south-west, the judge might be pressured into convicting against his inclinations.[26]

All this was bad enough for the accused, but even giving evidence could be a stressful experience. The century which witnessed the judicial style of judge Jeffreys in 1685 was not one in which witnesses might usually expect indulgent attitudes from judges, and witnesses, male and female alike, were often browbeaten or ridiculed by the judiciary. In 1712 there occurred the last known assize trial for witchcraft in England, the accused being a Hertfordshire woman named Jane Wenham. One of those giving evidence against her was Elizabeth Field. She told how Wenham had bewitched a child of hers about nine years previously. The judge asked why she had not prosecuted Wenham immediately after this incident, to which she answered 'she was a poor women, and the child had no friends able to bear the charges of such a prosecution'. The judge, who was sceptical, and who was subsequently to reprieve Wenham after conviction, asked sarcastically if Field had now grown rich.[27] Conversely, there were signs of women witnesses being treated with politeness. In 1702 Richard Hathaway was tried as a cheat for accusing Sarah Morduck of witchcraft. Elizabeth Willoughby was one of those giving evidence on Hathaway's behalf before the sceptical Chief Justice Holt. Holt asked her what skill she had in matters of witchcraft, and she replied that she had been bewitched as a child, and that this experience had given her insight into such matters. An obviously unconvinced judge Holt was very restrained in his subsequent questioning about this claim.[28]

If the treatment of women witnesses varied, so did that of the women accused of witchcraft. Low conviction rates at the assizes suggest that throughout the period of the operation of the English witch statutes, judges were, broadly speaking, sceptical about, if not the abstract possibility of witchcraft, at least of the guilt of the individual old women brought before them.[29] By the later seventeenth century, when convictions were very rare, judges must have played a major part in helping accused witches evade execution. Yet in other instances women accused of witchcraft in the confusing and hostile environment of the court might find themselves under heavy pressure. In many cases the accused were elderly women who had been cowed by the experiences of community hostility, examination by justices and mob pressure on the way to the place of trial. Such women were unlikely to mount much by way of a coherent defence against the charges levelled against them. Nevertheless, scattered evidence suggests that a few women were able to defend themselves in court. Thus in 1586 Joan Cason, a widow of Faversham in Kent, was tried at the borough sessions for invoking evil spirits and bewitching a child to death. Seven women and one man, poor people but her near neighbours, gave evidence against her. Cason, while admitting contact with what may have been familiars, denied bewitching the child to death, claiming that her adversaries were maliciously accusing her and that there were existing differences between them in which her accusers had already done her wrong. Her arguing convinced the Recorder of Faversharn of her innocence, although a bungle over legal technicalities led to her execution.[30]

Other cases of what amounted almost to defiance were recorded. Anna Trapnel, the Interregnum religious visionary, recorded how during her travels in Cornwall she was investigated as a witch, and that a clergymen helped to frame an indictment against her, 'but though he and the witch-trying woman looked steadfastly in my face, it did no way dismay me'.[31] Margaret Landish, one of the Essex witches accused in 1645, alleged malice and an old grudge against her at her trial, and at one point made 'a strange howling in the court to the great disturbance of the whole bench'.[32] Temperance Lloyd, one of three witches executed at Exeter in

1682, although confessing her witchcraft at her trial, was 'perfectly resolute, not minding what should become of her immortal soul, but rather impudently at, as well as after her tryal, so audacious'.[33] Another distraction to the court was offered by Anne Ashby, tried at Maidstone in 1652. Ashby confessed to copulation with the Devil, and in open court 'fell into an extasie before the bench, and swelled into a monstrous and vast bigness, schreeching and crying out very dolefully', and on her recovery claimed that her familiar had entered her body.[34]

More commonly, the progress of witch trials was disturbed by sufferings of this last type on the part of the alleged victims of witchcraft. One of the recurring themes of English witchcraft was the possession of young people by spirits sent by a witch, or by curious diseases inflicted on them by witchcraft. The accounts of the sufferings of such possessed persons, frequently involving fits and convulsions, are some times very long and very harrowing. What is striking, however, is the number of occasions when such behaviour occurred in the courtroom, sometimes being regarded (at least by the accusers) as evidence of bewitchment. Although people of either sex might be possessed, it seems that most of the cases of fits and convulsions occurring in court of which details have come down to us involved young women. Frequently these took the form of dramatic interventions on the part of the alleged sufferer when the supposed witch entered the court or was first noticed by the supposedly possessed girl.

Thus in one well documented case we find Mary Glover, daughter of a London shopkeeper, who was thought to be bewitched in 1602, falling into a fit when she was called to give evidence in court. The three strong men who carried the girl out of court declared that they had 'never carried a heavier burden'. The Recorder of London and other officials tested the genuineness of her fit by burning her hand until it blistered: the girl remained insensible.[35] In another case, tried at the Berkshire assizes at almost the same time, Anne Gunter, a gentleman's daughter, similarly went into fits at the trial of two of the women who had allegedly bewitched her, one witness referring to the 'gogling of hir heade & eyes, the turning of her armes and hands, the dubling & swelling of hir body' in court. Two decades later two other daughters of the gentry, Helen and Elizabeth Fairfax, likewise 'fell into a trance before the judge, and were carried out'. Justices present followed the girls out, and 'made experiments to prove if they counterfeited or not'. The girls' father noted that 'report said that it was not so civil as I expected from such men, yet their curiosity found nothing but sincerity in my children'.[36]

The theme of the possession of adolescents is a major one in the history of English witchcraft in this period, and is too complex to go into here. What is obvious is that being possessed, whether in the courtroom or not, gave adolescents a unique opportunity to cast off their characteristically submissive and repressed role, and indulge in bad behaviour that was not only licensed, but also made them the centre of attention.[37] Given the probability that girls were more likely than boys to be deeply socialized into submissiveness, their behaviour when possessed attracted considerable comment from contemporary observers, and indeed may have been regarded as a deeper affront to social norms than that of young males.[38] Something of the divergence in the normal expectations of a young woman's behaviour and that of the possessed adolescent girl in the presence of a judge can be

glimpsed in the account of the sufferings of yet another daughter of the gentry
Margaret Muschamp. The girl and her mother were attempting to persuade a sceptical judge to prosecute the persons suspected of witchcraft, and the girl fell into
fits before the judge, at one stage, as was typical in such cases, vomiting foreign
bodies. But when she came out of her fits, she 'did not know what was past, as all
the beholders did see onely an innocent, bashfull girle, without any confidence at
all when she was out of her fits'.[39] When examining gender as an aspect of witchcraft, it is clear that being possessed and launching a witchcraft accusation gave
many an 'innocent, bashfull girle' the chance to become the centre of attention
and to exercise power over adults.

After trial and condemnation the witch, like any other felon, would be prepared
for death. Appropriately enough, this process would be entrusted to a clergyman.
Hence Henry Goodcole worked on (to use the contemporary phrase) Elizabeth
Sawyer in 1621 to accept her sinfulness and the death by hanging that it had drawn
upon her, and to make a full confession. It was desirable that the condemned witch,
like other convicted felons, should 'make a good end', and die penitently and with
dignity. In Sawyer's case, Goodcole officiated at the execution, and at the gallows
read to her the confession that she had made earlier, which she declared to be true
'in the hearing of many hundreds'.[40] Sometimes this sort of clerical pressure could
be excessive. Joan Peterson, executed at Tyburn in 1652, was, at the place of
execution, exhorted nine or more times to confess by the Ordinary of Newgate.
At this point the executioner commented that 'the Ordinary might be ashamed to
trouble a dying woman so much', to which the clergyman responded that 'he was
commanded to do so, and durst do no otherwise'. This story does at least demonstrate that convicted witches could be obdurate at the gallows.[41] Ideally, however,
as with Elizabeth Sawyer, an execution would involve the convicted witch making
a 'good end' and behaving in an appropriately edifying fashion. Thus when Joan
Cason died at Faversham in 1586 she made a gallows speech accepting that her fate
was the result of divine justice, and made so godly an end that many who had
previously been her enemies lamented her death.[42]

But not all died so edifyingly. Ann Bodenham, executed at Salisbury, was worked
on by a minister named Foster, 'who comforted her to bear death Christianly, boldly,
and chearfully'. He managed to bring her 'to that pitch as to promise him she would
goe a true penitent to her place of execution, and to die as a lamb'. She refused,
however, to confess the matters for which she had been convicted, adding 'that she
wrongfully suffered death, and did lament extremely, and desired to die quietly'.
Her execution was, in fact, less than edifying. According to the pamphlet account,
she was 'very desirous for drink, and had not Mr Undersheriffs prudence been such
as to restrain her from it she would have died drunk'. As she walked to the gallows,
'by every house she went by, she went with a small piece of silver in her hand, calling for beer, and was very passionate when denyed', while she was also, for unclear
reasons, very annoyed when the sheriff told her she could not be buried at the
gallows. In fact, at the gallows she refused to confess, and

> being asked whether she desired the prayers of any of the people, she
> answered, she had as many prayers already as she intended, and desired

> to have, but cursed those that detained her from her death, and was
> importunate to goe up the ladder.

She then tried to turn herself off on the gallows, but was restrained by the executioner, who asked her forgiveness, as was the custom. 'She replyed forgive thee?
A pox on thee, turn me off, which were the last words she spoke'. 'Thus', concluded
the account of her trial, 'you have her wicked life, her wofull death. Those that
forsake God in their lives, shall be for saken of him in their deaths'. Those who
have argued that witchcraft accusations were a means of controlling women can at
least take consolation in Bodenham's case as one of hegemony's failures.[43]

     This chapter has concentrated on witchcraft and the secular criminal law courts.
But before moving to any conclusions on the evidence presented by this connection, we should remind ourselves that there were other tribunals involved with
witchcraft cases, notably the ecclesiastical courts. Less serious forms of witchcraft,
sorcery and charming might be presented before these courts, while, more importantly for our immediate purposes, defamation suits involving allegations of
witchcraft might be pursued there. Ecclesiastical law gave women greater opportunities for litigating than did the common law, and some of the better documented
cases reveal clearly how witchcraft accusations might form part of a wider body of
tensions and conflicts between women.

     One such case was tried before the Chester Consistory Court in 1662. It arose
from problems between Mary Briscoe and Ann Wright. Wright's daughter, aged
about twelve, had fallen ill, and 'was very sadly afflicted and in a strange manner
by fitts', during which time 'she would many times say that Mary Briscoe pricked
her to the heart with pins and would have her heart and the like, and she did swell
much in the body and soe dyed'. In consequence, as a witness named Cicely Winne
deposed, 'the said Mary Briscoe was suspected by many neighbours to be the cause
both of her afflictinge and likewise of a brother of hers who was sadly afflicted
before that & dyed in a strange manner'.

     Thus we have a case which resembles so many others: the strange death of a
child, the allegation of witchcraft, the neighbourly evaluation, the focusing of suspicion, the defamation suit in defence of good name. Unusually, however, the
surviving documentation allows us to piece together something of the background.
Neither woman had an unblemished reputation. Briscoe was described as a 'very
troublesome and wrangling woman among her neighbours', or as a 'very wilfull
high spirited woman amongst her neighbours'. Indeed, her husband, worried about
the suspicion of witchcraft against his wife, had discussed the problem with Cicely
Winne, and told her 'he was much troubled at it but he could not rule her, and
he was very much afraid that she would come to the same end as her Moth[er]
did'. But Wright herself had given birth to an illegitimate child just after the
Restoration, had refused to identify its father to the midwife and had refused to
do penance for it. One witness, interestingly, deposed that Wright claimed Briscoe
had bewitched her at the time of the child's conception. She also complained at
about the same time of being compelled 'to be a witness against her husband for
speaking treason against the king'. Another women, Margery Whishall, claimed
that Wright had slandered her for adultery. With Wright and Briscoe we obviously

have two rather contentious women, who had, in fact, already been locked into a dispute over a house in which Wright had dwelt, 'which the said Mary had a great mind of'. This dispute had already provoked a suit which had been arbitrated by a justice of the peace. This case, which ended in Wright performing public penance in her parish church, demonstrates how the ecclesiastical law helped women to become agents in legal matters. Wright and Briscoe were clearly not victims of a patriarchal legal system, but rather two women who were willing to use the law to pursue their own ends.

This assertion reminds us of the problems of determining a specifically female experience before the courts and legal process. We are examining witchcraft, a crime which, correctly, has been regarded as having a peculiar connection with women. But much of what seems to have happened to women involved in witch-craft cases, whether as accused, accusers or witnesses, seems very similar to what happened to their male counterparts: men accused of felony, and male witnesses giving evidence in court, might be hectored or pressured by aggressive judges, and men convicted of felony, like women convicted of witchcraft, were 'worked on' by clergymen before their execution in hopes that they might produce a model speech from the gallows. However, we must keep our minds open to the possi-bility that although women might have shared with men the experience of going through various stages of the judicial process, the quality of that experience and the reactions and emotions it might provoke could have been very different for them.

There were, however, aspects of the prosecution of felony which were either specific to or more marked in trials of witchcraft. The most obvious of these, as I have stressed, was the use of groups of women to search suspected witches for the mark. Another recurring theme in accounts of witchcraft cases was the frequent occurrence of something amounting to mob action, or at least popular pressure. Of course, the phenomenon of crowd action or popular attitudes towards crimi-nals or at executions was not limited to witchcraft cases; but the frequency of references to hostile mobs is striking, especially since they were on the fringes of the legal process. Suspected witches might be subjected to swimming, scratching or other forms of popularly licensed violence. Further research into this issue might lead to some useful insights into attitudes to gender, given that most of the people towards whom such violence was directed were women.

The willingness of other women to act against alleged witches is also a constant theme. As I have suggested elsewhere, materials from Yorkshire demonstrate that witchcraft accusations were not simply foisted onto women by men, but rather were frequently generated from tensions between women, often arising from such traditional female concerns as childrearing, and were often formulated and refined in the world of female sociability, gossip among women, and female concern over reputation.[44] This creates problems for those investigating constraints on female behaviour in early modern England. Many witchcraft accusations, I would argue, reveal a social arena where channels of female force, female power, and female action could run. The high level of participation of women witnesses in witchcraft cases, and the ready participation of women in searching for the witch's mark, were areas in which women could enter the male dominated milieu of legal process, and in which women, perhaps within parameters dictated and maintained by men, could carve out some role for themselves in the public sphere. This would seem to be a line of investigation well worth pursuing.

This leads us to a final point. It is a commonplace that early modern England was a patriarchal society in which issues of gender, like everything else, were viewed in hierarchical terms, and in which women, not least in their status before the common law, were disadvantaged. This is especially relevant when we consider witchcraft, an offence which, even if we eschew some of the women's movement writings on the subject from the 1970s, is somehow connected with the male domination of women. Yet in the preceding pages we have seen women acting strongly: defying judges and executioners; accusing other women as witches; giving evidence against suspected women witches; and suing each other for defamation arising from allegations of witchcraft. Even though contemporary attitudes to gender probably made those experiences different for the women involved, they nonetheless establish women as active participants in the legal system. Like all of us, these women found themselves in a real world that imposed constraints upon them. Yet within those constraints and limitations, in the legal process and before the courts as elsewhere, they were historical actors.

Notes

1   For participation rates, see C. Z. Weiner, 'Sex roles and crime in late Elizabethan Hertfordshire', *Journal of Social History*, 8 (1975), 18–37, and J. M. Beattie, 'The criminality of women in eighteenth-century England', Ibid., 80–116; for defamation litigation, J. A. Sharpe, *Defamation and Sexual Slander in Early Modern England: the church courts at York,* Borthwick Papers, 58 (York 1980); for infanticide, P. C. Hoffer and N. E. Hull, *Murdering Mothers: infanticide in England and New England 1558–1803* (New York 1981); for scolding, D. E. Underdown, 'The taming of the scold', in *Order and Disorder in Early Modern England,* eds A. Fletcher and J. Stevenson (Cambridge 1985), 116–36.

2   Gender as a social construct has so far received little attention from historians of early modern England. For an important preliminary discussion, see S. Amussen, 'Gender, family and the social order, 1560–1725', in Fletcher and Stevenson (1985) 196–218. The themes raised here are discussed further in S. Amussen's *An Ordered Society* (Oxford 1988).

3   For a contemporary introduction to women and the common law, see *The lawes resolution of womens rights* (London 1652).

4   For a list of these indictments see C. L'Estrange Ewen, *Witch Hunting and Witch Trials: the indictments for witchcraft from the records of 1373 assizes held for the Horne Circuit AD 1559–1736* (London 1929), 117–265.

5   Cf. materials for the Western Circuit printed in C. L'Estrange Ewen, *Witchcraft and Demonianism* (London 1933), appendix L, 439–46.

6   A. Macfarlane, *Witchcraft in Tudor and Stuart England* (London 1970), 278–93.

7   Ibid., 117–18.

8   J. A. Sharpe, 'Witchcraft and women in seventeenth-century England: some northern evidence', *Continuity and Change,* 6 (1991), 179–99. For a somewhat different perspective on these issues, see Chapter 23 in this collection by Clive Holmes.

9   Ewen, *Witchcraft and Demonianism*, 63.

10   *The examination and confession of certain wytches at Chensford in the countie of Essex before the queens maiesties judges, the xxvi day of July anno 1566* (London 1566).

11   *Court leet records*, vol. 1, part 2, AD 1578–1602, eds F. J. C. Hearnshaw and D. M. Hearnshaw, Southampton Record Society, I (Southampton 1906), 187.

12   *A true and just recorde of the information, examination and confession of all the witches taken at S. Oses in the countie of Essex, whereof some were executed and others treated according to the determination of the law* (London 1582), sig D4.

13   W. Grange, ed., *Daemonologia: a discourse on witchcraft* (Harrogate 1882), 78.

14   H. Goodcole, *The wonderfull discoverie of Elizabeth Sawyer* (London 1621), sig B2v.–B3v.

15   *A true and exact relation of the severall informations, examinations and confessions of the late witches arraigned and executed in the county of Essex* (London 1645), 26.

16   J. Boys, *The case of witchcraft at Coggeshall, Essex, in the year 1699* (London 1909), 21–2.

17   For the absence of midwives among witchcraft suspects, see Chapters 3 and 6 in this book. For a slightly different perspective, see Chapter 14 by Gary K. Waite.

18   For full citations of the archival sources used in this chapter, see the original version in Jenny Kermode and Garthine Walker, eds, *Women, Crime and the Courts in Early Modern England* (UCL Press, London 1994), ch. 5.

19   For a case of this type see R. H. Helmholz, *Marriage Litigation in Medieval England* (Cambridge 1974), 89.

20   P. Hair, *Before the Bawdy Court* (London 1972), 189.

21   This practice is discussed in *A Calendar of Assize Records: introduction*, ed. J. S. Cockburn (London 1985), 121–3. See also J. C. Oldham, 'On pleading the belly: a history of the jury of matrons', *Criminal Justice History*, 6 (1985), 1–64.

22   These figures are based on an analysis of abstracts of assize cases given in Ewen, *Witch Hunting and Witch Trials*, 187–264. For analysis of the Northern Circuit Depositions, see Sharpe, 'Witchcraft and women'.

23   These figures are derived from abstracts of indictments given in *A calendar of assize records: Hertfordshire indictments James I*, ed. J. S. Cockburn (London 1975), 70–223.

24   *Calendar of State Papers, Domestic 1634–5*, 79.

25   Ewen, *Witchcraft and Demonianism*, 125.

26   R. North, *The lives of the right hon Francis North, Baron Guildford; the hon Sir Dudley North; and the hon and rev Dr John North*, 3 vols (London 1890), vol. 3, 130–1 describes this case, where the judge was 'a mild, passive man, who had neither dexterity nor spirit to oppose a popular rage'.

27   *A full and impartial account of the discovery of sorcery and witchcraft practisd by Jane Wenhant* (London 1712), 28.

28   *The tryal of Richard Hathaway* (London 1702), 20.

29   Ewen, *Witch Hunting and Witch Trials*, 99, shows that of 513 persons accused of witchcraft at the Home Circuit assizes, 112 (or 22 per cent) were executed. Many others, of course, suffered lesser penalties.

30   The contemporary account of this case is printed in B. Rosen, *Witchcraft* (London 1969), 163–7.

31   Trapnel, *Anna Trapnel's report and plea* (London 1654), 24.

32   Ewen, *Witchcraft and Demonianism*, 256. Landish was sentenced to death.

33   *The tryal, condemnation and execution of three witches* (London 1682), 4.

34   *A prodigious and tragicall history of the tryall, confession and condemnation of six witches at Maidstone, in Kent* (London 1652), 4.

35   Ewen, *Witchcraft and Demonianism,* 197. Materials relating to this case are brought together in M. MacDonald, *Witchcraft and Hysteria in Elizabethan London: Edward Jordan and the Mary Glover case* (London 1990).

36   Fairfax, *Daemonologia,* 123–4.

37   This phenomenon is perhaps most familiar in the context of the trials at Salem, Massachusetts, in 1692. For a work which, although now somewhat dated, does focus on this issue, see M. L. Starkey, *The Devil in Massachusetts: a modern enquiry into the Salem witch trials* (New York 1950).

38   For the relationship between possession and gender, see Chapter 19 in this collection by Moshe Sluhovsky.

39   M. Moore, *Wonderfull news from the North* (London 1650), 15–16.

40   Goodcole, *Wonderfull discoverie of Elizabeth Sawyer,* sig D2v.

41   Ewen, *Witch Hunting and Witch Trials,* 276.

42   Rosen, *Witchcraft* ,166–7.

43   E. Bower, *Dr Lamb revived or witchcraft condemn'd* (London 1653), *passim.*

44   Sharpe, 'Witchcraft and women', 192–5.

Chapter 23

Clive Holmes

WOMEN: WITCHES AND WITNESSES

THE ROLE PLAYED BY WOMEN in the legal process against witches, as accusers or witnesses, has been frequently cited in the course of skirmishes about the question, as posed by Christina Larner, 'Was witch-hunting women-hunting?' Keith Thomas has argued that 'The idea that witch-prosecutions reflected a war between the sexes must be discounted, not least because the victims and witnesses were themselves as likely to be women as men'. This argument is mirrored by that of Alan Macfarlane, and has been followed, in relation to the New England trials, by John Demos.[1] Feminist scholars, like Larner, Carol Karlsen and, most recently, Marianne Hester, have found such reasoning 'simplistic'.[2] Yet Karlsen's acknowledgement that the role of women as accusers remains one of the most baffling questions about witchcraft does suggest the need for further discussion, and an essay by J. A. Sharpe, examining the involvement of women in Yorkshire prosecutions, displays some of the potential of the subject.[3] An examination of the process of witnessing – a process, as I shall argue, of considerable cultural complexity – will illuminate a number of issues raised by the witchcraft prosecutions: the shaping role of the legal system, the dynamic interweaving of elite theology and the concerns of the populace and, not least, the misogynous dimension of witchcraft.

We may distinguish three ways in which women might participate in the trial procedures against witches. Two of these are very distinctive. First, women might testify as 'possessed' victims of the witch's malice; control of their minds and bodies had been seized by the Devil at the instigation of the witch. Secondly, women might report the results of physical searches that they had been instructed to conduct upon the witch's body, designed to discover the incriminating physical characteristics that indicated her complicity with Satan and his minions. In both instances the female deponents appear to acquiesce in and reinforce theories of witchcraft, developed by theologians and lawyers, which emphasize female weakness – the greater susceptibility of women to satanic temptation; their greater sensual depravity. Before discussing these instances, it will be necessary to examine a third group of women involved in criminal prosecution: those who testified simply to their experience of the witch's *maleficium* – to children lamed or killed, to stock or crops blighted, to the interruption of agricultural or domestic procedures. This kind of testimony is more inchoate than the other two categories; it lacks their conceptual clarity and sophistication. Yet, because it is the basic form of female engagement in the courts, both involving the greatest number of deponents, and rooted in popular rather than elite beliefs, it must be examined first.

I

The sources available for the study of witnessing can be divided into two categories. First, transcriptions of the testimony proffered to the examining magistrates or in court. Such evidence survives in a multiplicity of forms: in the private papers of JPs and ministers; in the official files of the clerks of assize and of the peace, and of the functionaries of the ecclesiastical courts; in published works – academic treatises and popular broadsides; even plays and ballads. Rich in detail, such testimonies certainly display the involvement of women in the process of accusation. And they indicate the concerns that exercised female witnesses, though these are, of course, refracted through the pens and the assumptions of their elite, male interlocutors. But the survival of these various sources is so random that any attempt to undertake a quantitative study, to calculate, for instance, the proportion of male and female deponents in witchcraft cases, would be misleading. Any statistical exercise, an essential ground base to a discussion of witchcraft testimony, has to be undertaken from the second of the available sources: the assize indictments. The latter, though highly formulaic and consequently opaque in terms of any substantive detail concerning the cases that they record, do have the virtue of surviving in a sufficient chronological series, at least for the Home Circuit, to permit a preliminary analysis.

In the 1590s the clerk of assize for the Home Circuit began to endorse some of the indictments upon which the accused were tried with the names of the witnesses in the case, and this was uniformly practised after 1600. In the course of the following century some nine hundred and seventy witnesses were recorded on witchcraft indictments: almost half of these (47.68 per cent) were women.[4] The endorsements also suggest that women were becoming proportionally more involved in witchcraft accusation in the course of the period. In the last years of Elizabeth's reign (1596–1602) 38.2 per cent of witnesses against witches whose names were endorsed on the indictments were women; 43.4 per cent in the reign of James I. However, after the Restoration female witnesses were in the majority (52.9 per cent) in the counties that formed the Home Circuit. They were also in a majority in this latter period in indictments emanating from the assize courts of the Northern Circuit (56 per cent), though not in Norfolk Circuit cases (43 per cent).[5] The apparent rise in the proportion of female witnesses is not merely the product of a change in the recording practices of the clerks of assize. Early in the seventeenth century the clerks did not, in any of the indictments for major criminal offences, invariably annotate the document with the names of all those who were expected to testify at the assizes; in later records such omissions seem less frequent. However, there does not appear to be any gender bias in the determination of names for endorsement on the earlier indictments. The rising proportion of female deponents in witchcraft cases in the course of the seventeenth century is not an optical illusion induced by changing clerical practice.

Why did this significant shift in the proportions of male and female deponents occur in the century after 1590? The phenomenon is paralleled by an increase in the involvement of female deponents in all cases before the assizes. Women formed only 10 per cent of the witnesses in non-witchcraft cases in a sample of sessions of the Essex assizes between 1596 and 1625; after the Restoration the proportion had more than doubled (22 per cent).[6] But this shift reflects, not any change in the courts' readiness to accept female testimony, but simply the fall in the number of property offences coming to the attention of the assizes. Property crimes – larceny, burglary, housebreaking – had dominated proceedings from the 1590s until the end of the reign of James I; they declined markedly after 1660.[7] And in these prosecutions the bulk of the testimony was provided by men. As the numbers of property offences brought before the assize courts waned in the course of the century, so too did the proportion of male witnesses attending at Chelmsford.

The rising percentage of women witnesses in witchcraft cases is also related, though tangentially, to offences against property. In the reigns of Elizabeth and James 36.8 per cent of all witchcraft cases coming to the attention of the assizes involved an indictment alleging that the accused had damaged stock; in 14.3 per cent of incidents, stock-damage formed the sole charge. Indictments of stock-damage, either alone or in conjunction with other acts of *maleficium,* dropped to 15.8 per cent in Charles I's reign, rose slightly to 25 per cent in the Interregnum, then plummeted to a mere 2.9 per cent after the Restoration. And in indictments concerning malefic damage to stock, as in all property crimes, the testimony of men predominated: men formed 80.8 per cent of witnesses to these charges. As the crime of witchcraft was increasingly perceived as involving mysterious human ailments and death; as indictments, like that against Margery Stanton of Wimbish in 1579, alleging the destruction of *'unum spandonem* (gelding) *colons white',*[8] disappear from the record, so the proportion of female witnesses increased. Women, attendant at the sick-bed of the victim, were well placed to describe the mental anguish and mortal physical torments inflicted by the witch.

Here, then, is the explanation for the growing proportion of women formally testifying in witchcraft cases in the course of the seventeenth century. Women were simply better placed than men to describe the incidents and activities that conformed to the altered perception of the nature of witchcraft as a criminal offence. The shift in the conceptualization of the offence was instigated by the legal elite. After 1660 the local justices and the courts were reluctant to admit charges of witchcraft except in cases of mysterious and terrifying illness leading to death or, more rarely, where the accused was directly alleged to be involved in diabolic practices. This restructuring of the offence by magistrates and lawyers certainly does not indicate any fundamental change in the nature of popular belief concerning witchcraft. The ancillary material produced in the official investigation of the late seventeenth-century cases demonstrates that at the local level witches were still believed to exercise their powers in the destruction of stock or the interruption of agricultural and domestic procedures. But the legal elite, unlike its Elizabethan predecessors, now refused to entertain formal accusations based on this kind of evidence. So, for example, at the Suffolk assizes in 1694 four indictments, three for killing by witchcraft and one for entertaining evil spirits, were preferred against Philippa Munnings of Hartest but, though no charges were formally levelled, her neighbours also believed her to be guilty of destroying stock and spoiling brewing.[9] The case of Jane Wenham, found guilty at the Hertford assizes in 1712 for diabolic dealings, revealed longstanding popular suspicions of a traditional kind that had little to do with the elite concerns that informed the language of the indictment. One Walkern yeoman believed that he had lost stock to the value of £200 through her maleficence over the years; another local farmer's sheep had died mysteriously after he threatened Wenham for stealing his turnips.[10]

The Wenham case deserves further discussion. It clearly displays the complex process which attended the transformation of local concerns into formal legal procedure. Suspicion against Wenham had festered for years, and was reinforced in 1711 by the mysterious behaviour and illness of a possessed maidservant. The girl's affliction was studied and the charge of witchcraft against Wenham engineered by local Anglican clergymen, eager to use the opportunity to assert the reality of witchcraft in the face of growing intellectual scepticism. The case, for them, was a skirmish in the wider battle against deism and agnosticism. But when the divines sought to indict Wenham for 'wasting and consuming' her victim, the clerk of assize insisted that 'he neither could, nor would, lay it so'; an indictment for witchcraft required either the death of the victim or proof of diabolic practices. This was, as the clerical prosecutors complained, an odd reading of the Jacobean legislation, but it was one that had begun to be favoured by the judges in the 1630s, and which was revived after the peculiar circumstances of the Civil War and Interregnum cases. Hence, in the Wenham case, the odd, sardonic form taken by the indictment – 'conversing familiarly with the Devil in the shape of a cat' – ostensibly bringing the offence within the compass of the clause of the statute that made it felony 'to entertaine employ feede or rewarde any evill and wicked spirit'.

In the Wenham case the manipulation of popular concerns and belief by elements of the elite, both the Tory divines crusading against infidelity and the cynics of the legal establishment who derided and sought to frustrate their efforts, is very apparent. Local suspicions and concerns had to be moulded to the requirements of legal categorization and procedure and, beyond these, to the political and theological concerns of the elite which informed and shaped the juridical forms. But such transmutation was not peculiar to the post-1660 cases in which it emerges most clearly. It was a permanent feature of the formal prosecution of witchcraft. From 1563 suspicions rooted in folklore had to be orchestrated to accommodate them to the machinery and the values of the elite. This raises a critical point concerning the analysis of the role of witnesses, male and female. We must consider: first, how local fears and suspicions were drawn to the attention of the magistracy; secondly, how far the authorities tailored the evidence to the constraints imposed by the changing assumptions of a system in which the witnesses were, in some measure, only marginal participants.

II

It is difficult to make confident assertions about the nature and patterns of popular beliefs about witchcraft. All the sources are, in some measure, distorted by refraction through the conceptual framework of the elite. Yet we may suggest a couple of its features salient to this enquiry. First, the mysterious powers that constituted witchcraft would normally be possessed by women. There is little of the sophisticated misogyny, a powerful brew of biblical and Aristotelian emphases on female inferiority, developed by elite commentators obliged to explain the substantial plurality of women in prosecution.[11] In so far as any attention was paid at the popular level to questions of the origin of this power, it appears that it was thought to inhere in matrilineal lineage: 'by discent . . . from the grandmother to the mother, and from the mother to the children'. Secondly, men and women shared a fear of witches. From a sample of the cases coming to the attention of Richard Napier, minister of Great Linford and astrological physician, between 1601 and 1627, Ronald Sawyer has noticed the plurality of women both among those named as witches (94.7 per cent), and among Napier's patients, a group of 109 persons, who believed themselves the victims of witchcraft (59.7 per cent). Sawyer's figures further suggest that women were quicker to nominate those they held responsible for their sufferings: 45.5 per cent of Napier's male patients were ready to name the witch persecuting them; the figure for female patients is 58.2 per cent. Women seeking the protection of the ecclesiastical courts against the damage to their reputations, occasioned by abuse or rumours that suggested that they were witches, name men and women in almost equal numbers as their slanderers.[12]

But a general fear of a local woman possessing the formidable powers attributed to witches does not automatically transmute into legal prosecution. Confronted by power-wielding women, villagers at first instance might seek to ensure that they were not the victims of such power, perhaps to control and deploy it for their own purposes. The witch, in consequence, might be treated with an elaborate if cautious deference. Edward Fairfax noted that the inhabitants of Knaresborough Forest coexisted with the witch-clans in their midst, and that the head of one of the latter 'had so powerful hand over the wealthiest neighbours about her, that none of them refused to do anything she required, yea, I unbesought they provided her with fire, and meat from their own tables'.[13] A similarly dense and long-standing network of social relations is apparent in Pendle Forest between the rival witch-families, headed by their respective matriarchs, Old Chattox and Old Demdyke, and the villagers. The latter not only tolerated the petty thefts, begging and extortion of the suspected witches, but employed them routinely both in domestic industry and as healers. They sought protection from the witches' power both by paying blackmail and by recourse to counter-magic.[14]

How did villagers who may have co-operated, if uneasily, with the suspected witch come to testify against her? In both Knaresborough and Pendle that transformation was accomplished by the direct intervention of members of the elite. Fairfax's engagement in the prosecution of the Knaresborough witches stemmed from the mysterious illness of his daughter, Helen, who eventually attributed her condition to their maleficence. In Lancashire the zealous magistrate, Roger Nowell, 'a very religious honest gentleman, painefull in the service of his Countrey', was moved by local rumours to launch an investigation. Nowell's intervention, while spurred by local suspicions and tensions, swiftly transformed them. Relentless interrogation of one of the accused – the boy attempted suicide – eventually elicited the required confession of diabolic activities. Such examples of direct elite orchestration are, however, rare. In the bulk of cases the decision to bring a witch to the attention of the authorities appears to have been undertaken entirely within the neighbourhood, and the process of transmutation, whereby suspicion became prosecution, is opaque. Yet a few cases provide significant indicators concerning that process.

Brian Darcy's self-congratulatory account of his short but spectacular career as a witch-hunter in north-eastern Essex in 1582 permits some discussion of the local instigation of prosecution. Darcy, like Roger Nowell, was well versed in the continental theories concerning the satanic dimension of witchcraft, and he proved a vigorous and inventive inquisitor; in cases from St Osyth, Darcy's home, and its immediate vicinity, local beliefs hinted at in the earliest depositions were quickly swamped by a plethora of importations from the current theology of witchcraft. However, not all the 1582 cases were generated directly by Darcy's inquisitorial techniques or refracted through his rich imagination. His activities acted as a catalyst, encouraging the villagers of Oakley and Walton to voice their long-held suspicions of their neighbours, Annis Heard and Joan Robinson, to the authorities. Darcy, dedicating his energies to the pursuit of the St Osyth's coven, seems to have made little attempt to shape primary testimony from these peripheral communities. All witnesses concurred that to cross these women, to refuse to lend or sell them implements or goods, to demand the return of borrowed articles or payment, could be dangerous. Agricultural and domestic routines had failed; stock had sickened, died, or acted unnaturally (Thomas Rice's goose, 'that hath been as good for the bringing foorth of her broode as any goose in Walton', had refused to hatch her eggs). Illness, occasionally mortal, had afflicted their enemies. Yet, as in Knaresborough and Pendle, social relations were maintained with the witches. The villagers, if they did fall foul of Heard or Robinson, had recourse to counter-magic – heating a bewitched spindle to get it to work again; burning the ears of an afflicted pig to cure it; using a red-hot iron to get milk to churn and wort to brew. Men and women concurred in suspecting Heard and Robinson of witchcraft, but female experience of their maleficence tended, not surprisingly, to concentrate on the interruption of domestic routines. Women also seem readier to deploy, or perhaps merely to acknowledge their use of, counter-magic to frustrate the witch. The suspicions against Heard and Robinson, generally held, were obviously of long duration; they came to the attention of the authorities because the villagers were inspired and educated by Darcy's crusade at neighbouring St Osyth. But the effective decision to transmute village suspicion into official testimony, and to organize their neighbours for this, was taken by local *men*. Edward Upcher had long suspected Robinson for the death of his wife. He visited the gaoled St Osyth woman, Ursley Kemp, who, under Darcy's relentless questioning, had become his star witness, confessing satanic practices and naming a wide coven of accomplices; she readily confirmed Upcher's suspicion, and he led the Walton prosecution. In Oakley, John Wadde, a yeoman who had suffered heavy stock losses for several years, was the first formally to denounce Heard, initially to the ecclesiastical court, then, encouraged by the St Osyth's investigation, to Brian Darcy.[15]

   The role of local men in organizing the process whereby suspicion and gossip were transformed into formal accusation, as in the 1582 Oskley and Walton denunciations, is apparent in other cases, admittedly few, where we can reconstruct a narrative with some confidence. In 1682 Temperance Lloyd was convicted for afflicting Grace Thomas of Bideford; the bulk of the testimony was provided by women who had attended the girl during her long sickness, but the accusation was driven on by her brother-in-law, Thomas Eastchurch, a respected local merchant. He had sought the advice of a number of eminent physicians on Grace's behalf. Once the witchcraft diagnosis had been suggested, he pursued Lloyd's destruction with equal vigour.[16] Ten years before, a local JP had reported that Widow Peacock of Malmesbury was 'of very bad fame and very terrible to the people', yet 'nobody will eyther be at the charge to prosecute her, or run the hazard of her revenge if she be acquitted . . . except such a person as this Mr Webb'.[17] With Robert Webb, a wealthy member of the Malmesbury elite, we have another figure like Upcher, Wadde and Eastchurch: a man with wealth, standing and confidence. These characteristics were essential, given that prosecution was time-consuming and expensive and its failure might leave accusers hostage to the malice of the witch, if a complaint was to be brought to the attention of the authorities. Yet the energetic prosecutor would not stand alone; his immediate complaint against the witch would be backed by corroborative testimony from his neighbours, both men and women.

   It is significant that the women who became involved in the process often retailed older grievances and suspicions that had festered but previously gone unremarked to the authorities. John Swettson, a Cambridge apothecary, indicted Margaret Cotton for the death of his infant daughter in the summer of 1608; two poor women joined him in the prosecution, complaining of mysterious deaths in their families eighteen months before. Samuel Pacy, a Lowestoft merchant, held Amy Duny and Rose Cullender responsible for the mysterious illness of his two daughters, and he and other members of his family testified to their afflictions at the assizes. They were joined by eight additional witnesses. Three testified concerning the ailments of their children, subsequent to, but mirroring, the torments of the Pacy girls. Three, two men and a woman, deposed concerning the interruption of agricultural routines that they attributed to the witches; Anne Sandeswell recalled an incident seven or eight years before, while the men referred to occasions 'not long since'. Of the witnesses, only Dorothy Durent blamed the witches for a death, that of her daughter five years before, and she also testified concerning her infant son's illness, for which she had sought help from a cunning-man, in 1657.[18] In some cases the ancillary testimony offered by women deals with incidents so remote as to rouse the court's suspicions concerning the witness's motives in coming forward. When Elizabeth Field testified that her child had died many years ago upon Jane Wenham's touching it, the judge asked 'why she did not prosecute . . . immediately?' Her artless reply – she appeared now, 'the Opportunity presenting itself', and had not done so before because 'she was a poor woman, and the child had no friends' – drew from the judge a stinging and insensitive retort: 'was [she] grown rich since?'[19] Yet her experience, drawn into the court to supplement a case orchestrated by others, may have been typical of that of many women. In several cases in the Home Circuit in the Elizabethan and Jacobean period a witch would be charged on a number of indictments, some alleging maleficent acts undertaken years before; so, in 1572 at Chelmsford assizes, Agnes Francys was arraigned on four indictments; two alleged recent incidents of murder and the destruction of stock; the other two dealt with murders respectively three and six years earlier. In 1596 at Hertford, Alice Crutch was arraigned upon two indictments for the recent destruction of the stock, and upon a third indictment for murder by witchcraft four years previously; in this case two men testified to their losses, while a woman deposed concerning the earlier death. This latter case is not untypical of those involving several indictments in which the names of witnesses are listed: women formed a higher proportion of the witnesses to the charges of earlier maleficence than to those of more recent provenance.[20] One further pattern that emerges from the Home Circuit indictments may reinforce the suggestion that women were being mobilized by men, who were the driving force behind the decision to bring local suspicions and fears to the attention of the courts. In 27.7 per cent of the witchcraft accusations between 1596 and 1642 men alone acted as witnesses, while in 67.7 per cent of them men and women testified together; only in 4.6 per cent of the cases did women testify against an accused witch alone.

Men and women believed that their female neighbours could deploy maleficent powers. They treated such witches warily, guarding themselves by seeking to avoid conflict, by elaborate deference, and, when necessary, by erecting a protective shield of counter-magic. However, another response had been made available by the legislation of 1563. This strategy, prosecution, was usually pursued by substantial men in the community who would lay the charge, and solicit the confirmatory testimony of their neighbours, often women. Yet the elite who controlled the judicial machinery had their own agenda, and cases emanating from local tensions and suspicions would have to be adjusted, and might be transformed, when brought to the attention of magistrates and ministers. These groups were concerned, not with the trivia of stock-loss or the interruptions of domestic and agricultural processes, but (as in the case of Smith) with diabolism, or with mysterious ailments and death. The development of this latter emphasis in the course of the seventeenth century explains the preponderance of female witnesses in later cases.

Women, despite their numerical involvement, were largely passive actors in the formal legal process against witches in the bulk of the cases that came to the attention of the judiciary. Does this argument also hold for those women whose depositions, on the face of it, suggest far more engagement in the concerns of the elite? Women also witnessed against witches in two more distinctive, if rarer, contexts: first, as victims of diabolic possession through the instigation of a witch; secondly, as examiners for the physical marks which were increasingly seen as key evidence in prosecution. Such testimony, it seems, reflected and confirmed intellectual edifices – of witchcraft as diabolism; of the inferiority of women as indicated by their greater susceptibility to satanic temptation – constructed by the elite.

Protestant divines sought to transform the gross popular superstitions that emerged in the witchcraft trials. Their missionary efforts, apparent in the interrogation of Mary Smith and the triumphant publication of her eventual confession of diabolism, were designed to insist on their theological conceptualization, that satanic covenant was the essence of the offence. Their treatises, sermons and editions of confessions, often explicitly designed for 'the capacity of the simpler sort', were reinforced by works that were more obviously popular – chapbooks, broadsides and ballads – and by the theatre of the court and the gallows. By the Civil War their educational efforts appear to have borne fruit. In confessions from eastern England in 1645–7 the Devil figures prominently: he appears in human guise, contracts directly with his acolyte, and has carnal relations with her. This extensive group of depositions is a tribute, in part, to Matthew Hopkins's acquaintance with continental theories, his skill as an inquisitor, and his own prurient fantasies. But many of the confessions are far from stereotyped, particularly the accused's artless accounts of their discussions with Satan: so Elizabeth Southerne, a Dunwich pedlar,

> met the divell midsomer last like a black boy 10 years old by a whitethorne as she went to Westleton and there he promised her 2s 6d and he had it not then but said she shold have it the next time she came that way but he fayled of his promise, he met her indeed, but complayned of the hardnes of the times.[21]

The idea that a direct relationship with the Devil is the foundation of the witch's power, largely absent in early depositions, seems to have become more generally understood by the mid-seventeenth century.

We could simply argue that the testimony of women in possession cases or as searchers, in which they repeated and confirmed elite theories, is another indication of the general transformation of popular belief engineered by the divines. However, a detailed analysis suggests that a more complex process of cultural construction was involved, in which ministers and lawyers played a direct and immediate role.

III

The most spectacular testimony in witch-trials, which, in consequence, is over-represented in the published accounts, was provided by those who, it was claimed, were possessed by the Devil through the agency of a witch. Nine women were convicted at Leicester assizes in 1616 upon the testimony of the thirteen-year-old Edward Smith; his fits during the trial, 'in the syght of all the greatest parsons here, as dyvers knyghts and ladies and manny othars of the bettar sort', were 'most terrible to be tolld'. Horror might be punctuated by moments of didactic piety. William Avery, after raving in the presence of the judges, 'came to his perfect understanding, and . . . spoke very discreetly, Christianly, and charitably to every point'; Jane Throckmorton, upon the witch's courtroom confession, emerged from her fit, kneeled and asked her father's blessing.[22] Cases of diabolic possession through the agency of a witch presented the maximum opportunities for an edifying and cathartic drama in the court They also emphasized the diabolic origins of the witch's power upon which the divines so pertinaciously insisted. As in New England, women, particularly adolescents, preponderate among 'possessed' accusers.[23] The degree of involvement of these girls who in their testimony so comprehensively reinforced academic theory, deserves discussion.

Most of the published accounts of possession cases provide a narrative which describes the victim's confrontation with the witch as the first act of the subsequent drama. Thomas Darling inadvertently farted as he passed Alice Gooderidge; William Perry failed to salute Joan Cocke with sufficient courtesy when they met; Mercy Short, when an accused witch held in Boston gaol begged her for a little tobacco, 'affronted the hag': all were subsequently subjected to fearful physical and mental torments.[24] But, by the time it was employed by Cotton Mather in his accounts of the possession of the Goodwin children and of Mercy Short, this was simply the formulaic convention of a substantial literary genre. The actual process whereby the sufferer's affliction was recognized as possession, and the witch-inter-mediary nominated, involved far more complex transactions. A few documents enable us to see this process directly. According to a pamphlet of 1612 Mrs Elizabeth Belcher, 'a vertuous and godly gentle-woman', struck Joan Vaughan, the daughter of a notorious local witch, after Joan had made an obscene gesture at her: a few days later Elizabeth was possessed, crying out in her fits, 'Heere comes Joane Vaughan, away with Joane Vaughan'. A manuscript offers a very different account. Elizabeth had been sick for fifteen months; physic was unavailing, as were the efforts of the local practitioner of astrological medicine, Richard Napier. Belcher's friends suspected witchcraft, but she refused to entertain this suggestion. Then, when Elizabeth was in her fit, those attending her began to nominate suspects; all were rejected until they named Joan. 'Hath she done it?', the sick woman asked; the bystanders named Joan again: Elizabeth responded, 'Did she?', and from that moment never ceased to accuse Joan, testifying at Northampton assizes where the witch was condemned.[25] In other cases, the conventional format of the narrative barely conceals the more diffuse reality. The orthodox beginning of the account of the possession of the daughter of Lady Jennings – her fear of an old woman 'who suddainly appeared to her att the dore and demanded a pin of her' – seems quite irrelevant to the subsequent story. The girl nominated witches only after a severe illness of four months during which desperate medical remedies had been unsuc-cessfully attempted, and there had been much discussion among the family and visitors of the possibility of witchcraft. If the possession-through-witchcraft diag-nosis is the product of a dialogue involving many actors, so too was the subsequent behaviour of the victims, culminating in their courtroom performances. A basic pattern of language and gesture, gaining definition in the century after 1590, was learned by the possessed, largely in response to the expectations of those who gath-ered about them to offer consolation and to participate vicariously in the conflict with Satan. Michael MacDonald, analysing Dr Stephen Bradwell's account (1603) of the possession of Mary Glover, shows how her symptoms, initially 'undistinc-tive', 'strengthened and changed over time, so that they confirmed with increasing clarity' a diagnosis of possession through witchcraft.[26] Dr John Cotta, writing in 1619, complained that the actions and accusations of the possessed 'ordinarily' involved 'the abusive impression of some indiscreete whispering about the sick', while in several cases paradigms of appropriate behaviour, in the form of earlier possession narratives, were available in the sickroom.[27] The behaviour and testi-mony of the possessed were thus entangled with the interests of various other participants in the drama, chiefly from their own family networks, but also of medical professionals and divines.

The possessed themselves were not simply malleable puppets articulating the concerns of others in a process of social ventriloquism. The witchcraft-possession identification might prove seductive to those whose symptoms bewildered medical experts, their families and neighbours, and, crucially, themselves. The victim became the focus of an intense attention, often, as with Katherine Wright and Anne Gunter, demonstrably absent from their previous affective relations. The behavioural traits of possession, while conforming to a basic pattern, could be individually shaped to provide an outlet for personal feelings that would not otherwise achieve sanctioned expression – sexual fantasies, religious doubts, rage at parents, frustration with the constrictions imposed by social and gender roles. Nicholas Starkey's children, aged nine and ten, delighted in 'filthie and unsavoury speeches'; they scoffed at Scripture as 'bible bable, bible bable'; the boy bit his mother and called her 'whore'; Margaret Byrom, a poor kinswoman who lived on the Starkey family's charity, 'nicknamed and taunted' her benefactors.[28] But while the possessed were appropriating language and behaviour in ways that were intensely personal and liberating, the structure to which most accusations conformed, including the assertion of the responsibility of a witch for the victim's experience, was the product of a social process in which key roles were played by adults and males. The possessed adolescents were the tools of the divines; their dramatic performances reinforced the witchcraft-as-diabolic-covenant theology, with its ancillary emphasis upon the frailty of the 'weaker sexe' in the face of satanic temptation.

IV

A similar analysis is also appropriate in discussion of the evidence of the third group of female witnesses, those who testified to the physical marks that were thought to characterize a witch. They too confirmed, if more tangentially, suppositions concerning both the diabolic nature of witchcraft and female inferiority. And equally it is the element of elite construction and manipulation of their testimony that is most apparent.

At Lancaster assizes in 1634 some twenty people were convicted as witches. The accusation, levelled by a ten-year-old boy, was firmly rooted in long-standing local suspicion: it was corroborated by evidence of the witch-marks on the accused. Four men and sixteen women were accused; thirteen of the women were found to have marks or paps, and these were located in the genital area of eleven of them. The Lancaster case provides the first instance of the fully developed, officially sanctioned, search for the witch's mark in England, and their usual discovery in the pudenda. Lancaster should also have been the last instance of the presentation of such evidence in court. The 1634 convictions troubled some of the authorities and they sought a respite of execution while further investigations were undertaken: these, sanctioned by the Privy Council, included an evaluation of the physiological evidence. Four of the convicted women were brought to London and re-examined. Ten London midwives 'made diligent search and inspeccion of those women' in the presence of a panel of distinguished physicians headed by William Harvey. They reported that one of the women had unusual but explicable marks; on the other three they found 'nothing un naturall neyther in the secrets or any other partes of theire bodyes, nor any thinge lyke a teate or marke, nor any signe that any suche thing haith ever beene'. Yet despite this critique, and further questions concerning the reliability of the search procedure during the wave of prosecutions in East Anglia in 1645–6, pre-trial examination of the accused by 'ancient skilfull matrons and midwives' continued as a feature of the witch accusations in England and the American colonies into the eighteenth century.[29]

The testimony of these 'knowing women' resulted in the condemnation of a number of individuals. Moreover, with its emphasis upon the female genitals, it reinforces the gender-oriented dimension of the academic theory of witchcraft, and resonates with the more overt continental discussions of women's insatiable lust as a major element in their compact and relationship with Satan. As with the possessed adolescents, however, a full understanding of the context in which their role as witnesses developed allows us to see the matrons and midwives as marginal particants in procedures originating in the concerns of exclusively male professional groups: the clergy, again, and the magistracy.

Academic writers were frequently embarrassed by aspects of the popular beliefs about witchcraft that emerged in accusations. Yet 'that which by experience is found to be true' could not simply be dismissed, and consequently had to be read or shaped in a way that permitted its incorporation into their theoretical constructs – hence the misogynous explanations developed by the divines to account for the plurality of female witches that emerged from popular accusation. That the accommodation of popular belief and intellectual theory often proved awkward, and the resultant synthesis uneasy, is very apparent in the divines' wrestling with the problem posed by the witches' familiars. These creatures, which according to popular belief were kept by the witch and employed to execute her designs, were almost unique to English folklore. In consequence they were often the butt of the jibes of sceptics, and divines were taxed to explain their presence in terms of their theology of witchcraft. Gifford set out the difficulty: Satan was the efficient cause of the witch's maleficence; Satan and his minions were described in Scripture 'to be mightie terrible spirits, full of power, rage and cruelties'. Why, then, were they masquerading as 'such paltrie vermin, as cats, mise, toads and weasils'? Having posed the problem, Gifford sketches an answer, 'it is even of subtiltie'. The devils adopt these base guises so as not to terrify their dupes by revealing their horrendous forms and power.[30] This early answer is fleshed out by later writers into a more detailed narrative of the witch's transaction with Satan that assimilates further 'odd performances', as Joseph Glanvill ingenuously described them, from the popular belief system.[31] It appears in the earliest trials that it was commonly thought that the witch housed and fed her familiars:

> Ursley Kemp lodged her two cats, a lamb and a toad in a large wool-lined pot, maintaining them on beer, cake and white bread. The diet seems ordinary enough, if extravagant, but it was occasionally supplemented with the witch's blood. So, after accomplishing Mother Waterhouse's fell purposes, her familiar, a cat, was rewarded with a chicken and a drop of her blood; this she gave him by pricking her hand or face and putting the bloud to his mouth whyche he sucked.[32]

Decontextualized and analysed in isolation, this blood-gift bore some affinities to the idea of Protestant continental theorists, that Satan, after making the covenant, clawed his new disciple, drawing blood with which to sign the compact and leaving an insensible scar as its tangible symbol. From this structural resemblance, the English commentators developed a syncretist theory, combining continental concepts and insular folklore. The witch enters a covenant with Satan who marks her and draws blood; the Devil then provides a familiar who regularly sucks blood from the resulting wound, drawing it into a teat; this inverted Eucharist is designed to 'put her in mind of' the original transaction, 'the more to aggravate the witch's damnation'.[33]

The work of the academics had been to incorporate local 'experience' emerging from the substrate of popular belief into a general theory, while still maintaining the coherence of the latter. Their theories were to be reinforced, and developed, by another group: lawyers and magistrates.

By the early seventeenth century some local officials were clearly troubled by the evidential problems posed by the usual form of witchcraft accusation. Accounts of the victim's sufferings that followed a curse, reinforced by various dubious bits of confirmatory counter-magic, increasingly seemed insubstantial. Accordingly, in the absence of a confession, magistrates sought tangible proof of the witch's status. Their quest took a number of directions. In 1612 the Northamptonshire JPs, faced with a difficult case, experimented with the water-ordeal as practised on the Continent and approved by King James; the three accused witches all floated, and 'the suspition that was before not well grounded, was now confirmed'.[34] So effective a litmus test proved attractive to other magistrates before the Civil War, and the technique was used extensively in the 1645–6 witch-hunt in eastern England. However, its lavish employment by Hopkins and Stearne hardened objections that had already been expressed by a number of clerics, notably the influential William Perkins, who denounced the practice as unwarranted by Scripture, and thus merely a form of illicit counter-magic. In 1646 Judge Godbolt halted the use of the water-ordeal by Hopkins and his entourage and, although it survived as a vigorous element in the popular response to witchcraft, its official employment ceased save in very remote jurisdictions.

The discovery of the physical peculiarities thought to mark a witch provided, as did the water-ordeal, the desired positivistic test of guilt. And, like the ordeal, it was an importation from continental practice, though reworked to accommodate parochial experience. European commentators asserted that at the making of the covenant the Devil clawed or branded his neophyte, leaving an insensible scar; proper physical examination could reveal such satanic stigmata and, by 1600, their discovery by qualified experts was essential for conviction in some jurisdictions. A few English theorists follow their continental counterparts in describing the anaesthetic mark, but in other writings and in local police practice the test was transformed, duplicating the English account of the covenant by an emphasis on the familiar. In England, the discovery of the sucked teat becomes an appropriate demonstration, equivalent to the search for the insensible brand in Scotland or Geneva, of the witch's pact with Satan. The search was employed intermittently before 1634: the earliest surviving instance is the demand of a Southampton leet jury in 1579 that Widow Walker should be searched for any bloody marks 'which is a comon token to know all witches by'; Brian Darcy had suspects searched in the 1582 St Osyth investigation, as did the Derbyshire JPs in 1597.[35] But the practice was not universal: in 1593 Mother Samuel's mark was discovered after her execution, and in 1621 a JP had to press his colleagues on the Middlesex Bench to institute the search of a suspect; in this case two of the three women who examined Elizabeth Sawyer were 'brought in by the Officers out of the streete, passing there by chance'.[36] Nor, in these early examples, was the search so concentrated on the genital area. The key event behind the 1634 Lancaster proceedings with their emphasis on female sexuality, and the frequent appearance of similar 'paps or marks in her secrets' in the findings of the searchers thereafter, is the publication of the fourth edition of *The Countrey Justice* by Michael Dalton, lawyer and Cambridgeshire JP, in 1630. Dalton revised his influential vade-mecum for local magistrates in the light of the 1627 *Guide to Grand-Jury Men* by the divine, Richard Bernard, which sets out the full-fledged theory expressing the role of the familiar in terms of the diabolic compact. Dalton cites Bernard with enthusiastic approval and emphasizes the utility of the discovery of the marks as incontrovertible proof – 'maine points to discover and convict . . . for they prove fully that those witches have a familiar and made a league with the Devil'. Yet Dalton also transforms his source in a key respect. Bernard insists, with copious citation of the available English cases, that the mark may be anywhere, but that, since it is likely to be in 'very hidden places', the search must be diligent. Dalton, in his summary, shifts the language of Bernard's argument: the teats, 'these the Devil's marks . . . be often in their secretest parts, and therefore require diligent and careful search'.[37] Fortified by Dalton's confident pronouncements, magistrates after 1630, confronted by the evidential difficulties that typified all witchcraft accusations, employed the recommended body search as a routine aspect of pre-trial procedure. And the search focused upon the genital area, as Dalton's misreading of his source proved equally authoritative.

The role and self-perception of the women who participated in the search procedures do not admit of easy analysis. It has been suggested, in the colonial context, that a particularly active part was played by midwives who, given an official distrust of their profession and the suspicions of witchcraft that focused on their presidency over the enclosed process of birth and their use of charms, were protecting their own precarious positions by associating themselves with orthodox belief.[38] But this hypothesis cannot survive David Harley's demonstration that its essential premise, the vulnerability of midwives to witchcraft prosecution, is a myth.[39] Certainly some midwives were prepared to assert categorically that physical marks were unnatural, and to denounce those they searched as guilty of diabolic relations. In 1645 Bridget Reynolds of Ramsey searched three local women, diagnosed their marks as suspicious, and testified against them at the assizes. In 1653 another midwife, Mrs Odill of Fairfield, Connecticut, authoritatively silenced those women who, in a macabre scene beneath the gallows, had examined the corpse of an executed witch and argued that the genital marks were 'such as other women might have'. Yet, while some midwives affirmed and reinforced the search procedures that had been shaped in the intersection of theology and jurisprudence by divines and lawyers, others were more wary, using a neutral, even ambiguous, language in their depositions. When Ellen Garrison of Upwell was searched in 1647, 'some that were there that pretended to have skill in the discovery of witchcraft sayd that some of the deviles impes had sucked her'; but, despite this weighty professional opinion from Stearne and his circus, then touring the Isle of Ely, the local midwife was far more circumspect in her testimony. Some, like the London midwives in 1634, were prepared to exculpate individuals, or to question the validity of the entire procedure; John Hale, minister of Beverley, Massachusetts, reported the doubts of 'a skilful midwife' concerning the witch's mark.[40]

The laconic references in the English records, and even the fuller verdicts of colonial juries, hardly permit any exhaustive analysis of how the 'Ansient and Knowing Women' perceived their marginal role as searchers. In particular, those searches in which no incriminating marks were found, thus exculpating an accused witch, leave few traces in the English records, though such occasions may have been frequent. It is tempting to fill the lacunae by introducing a comparative discussion of the other related activities where women played a role in the penumbra of the legal system. While women were appointed to conduct physical examinations in civil and criminal cases turning on virginity or pregnancy, they were most frequently employed on juries empanelled to test the claim that a woman convicted of a capital felony was pregnant. In the event of a positive determination execution was delayed, and the respite usually became a reprieve, even in those cases where the jury's 'pregnant' verdict was subsequently proved incorrect. J. S. Cockburn, considering the frequency with which such 'mistakes' were made, has argued that the jury of women embodied the sentiment of the court and the wider community in favour of mercy in a particular case.[41] A similar argument may explain some of the determinations in searches for the witch's marks; they were simply expressions of local sentiment concerning the innocence or guilt of the accused. Searchers were often prepared to testify not only to the accused's physical marks, but to her reputation as a witch, or to their own experience of her maleficence. Frances Ward, with three other women nominated by the constable of Heath, found incriminating marks on Margaret Morton. Yet Ward was hardly a neutral observer: she attributed the deaths of two of her children to Morton, and reported that the accused, her mother and her sister were 'all a long time suspected' of witchcraft. Yet longstanding popular suspicions did not invariably lead to the discovery of the conclusive physical evidence; the search of the Widow Coman of Coggeshall, generally supposed to be a witch, found no discovery of that nature.[42] The searchers obviously took their responsibilities seriously, and this might lead to arguments among them resulting from their doubts in individual cases or about the procedure in general.

The searches were an unstable creation that juxtaposed the conceptual schemes of the theologians with a pragmatic response by the magistracy to increasingly troubling evidential problems. Those women, midwives and others, who affirmed that their searches had revealed the Devil's mark reinforced, often unwittingly, ministerial theories concerning the satanic dimension of witchcraft and the inferiority of women. But arguments among the searchers and the ambiguous language with which they often hedged their findings may equally have led to elite concern regarding both the efficacy of the test and, beyond that, the intellectual viability of the demonological speculation upon which it rested so uneasily.

V

The prosecution of witches in early modern England, and thus the role of women as witnesses, is a process of considerable cultural complexity. It involved a continuous but shifting dialogue among a variety of social and professional groups. Popular belief, shared by men and women, was that the mysterious, harmful power that constituted witchcraft would inhere in certain women. The response to this power, to the threats that it posed to life, to health, to property, and to domestic routines, was essentially instrumental: to placate or 'curry favour' with the witch; to secure an effective counter-magic against assaults. In 1563 the elite, following the example of their continental counterparts, constructed a machinery of prosecution and so added a new weapon in the armoury against witchcraft. Victims could now choose to destroy their assailants through the formally sanctioned procedures of the courts. The opportunity created by the legislation was employed by both men and women, but men, usually those of some status in their communities, were the more engaged participants. It was they who brought charges and who orchestrated the prosecution, organizing their neighbours to testify to earlier experiences of the accused's malice. Women, though active in the creation of local suspicions through gossip, and in the deployment of the traditional protective therapies and techniques that ratified accusation, were ancillaries in the formal procedures of quarter sessions and assizes.

Those who chose to employ the official machinery against witches were obliged to shape the local fears and rumours from which the prosecution emanated to the formalities of the law as defined by the statutes and to the reading of these by magistrates and judges. The changing concerns of the latter groups explain the growing proportion of female witnesses in witchcraft trials, apparent in the 1630s and after 1660. The judiciary were no longer prepared to entertain indictments for stock-damage, to which men had testified; fearful mortal illness or mental anguish alone would sustain a prosecution and women, attendant at the sickbed of the victim, were better placed to give evidence. The concerns of the legal elite also explain the involvement of women in the searches for those physical characteristics which indicated conjunction with diabolic familiars. Lawyers, troubled by the absence of evidence that met increasingly strict norms for conviction, experimented with a number of procedures that might provide tangible proof of guilt or innocence. The search for the witch's mark by committees of women, approved by the leading practical manual for local magistrates, proved the most enduring of these official confirmatory tests. Its justification lay in the developing theories of the other major professional group involved in witchcraft prosecution, the divines.

Witchcraft prosecutions after 1563 placed the clergy, well read in the continental theory of the essentially diabolic origins of the offence, in a quandary. Much of the popular belief that emerged in the courts seemed to trivialize witchcraft and to give ammunition to sceptics. In consequence, engaged divines used every opportunity to educate the populace concerning their witchcraft-as-heresy formulation, to transform popular belief with, to judge by the mid-seventeenth-century evidence, some success. Yet in this process aspects of popular belief were incorporated into the theories of the divines. The features of witchcraft that emerged regularly in the trials could not easily be dismissed, and had to be accommodated to theological presuppositions. So the animals who frequently attended the witch were diabolized as familiar spirits or emanations of Satan himself. From this theological reading of folklore emerged the test of the witch's mark in its insular English form, and with it the committees of women who searched the accused.

All witnesses, but particularly those girls who described their possession and the matrons who discovered the genital marks, ratified the misogynous rationalizations proffered by the divines to explain the preponderant numbers of women accused of witchcraft. Their testimony apparently confirmed that women were the weaker sex, more easily seduced by satanic temptation. But the machinery in which they became involved, often at the instigation of men, was created, controlled, and ultimately discarded by the magisterial and clerical elite. And it was they who read local experience in terms of a particular intellectual scheme. The construction of a prosecution was a complex, dialogic process, involving many actors, and the intersection of divergent and shifting systems of ideas. We can show that female participation as witness in the English trials was extensive and, proportionately, growing in the seventeenth century. But the social meaning of these figures is not so easily read. They certainly do not eliminate 'gender' or 'misogyny' as key categories for any discussion of witchcraft beliefs and prosecutions.

Notes

1   Keith Thomas, *Religion and the Decline of Magic* (London 1971), 568. See also Alan Macfarlane, *Witchcraft in Tudor and Stuart England* (London 1970), 160; John Demos, *Entertaining Satan* (New York 1982), 64.

2   See Chapter 20 in this book by Christina Larner; also Carol F. Karlsen, *The Devil in the Shape of a Woman* (New York 1987), 226; Marianne Hester, *Lewd Women and Wicked Witches* (London 1992), 201.

3   J. A. Sharpe, 'Witchcraft and Women in Seventeenth-Century England: Some Northern Evidence' *Continuity and Change*, 6 (1991), 179–99. See also Sharpe's Chapter 22 in this collection.

4   C. L'Estrange Ewen, *Witch Hunting and Witch Trials* (London 1929), provides synopses of all the assize indictments.

5   For full citations of the archival sources used in this chapter, see the original version in *Past and Present*, 140 (1993), 145–79.

6   The sample consists of those assizes at which Essex witchcraft cases were determined; twenty courts between 1600 and 1624; six between 1660 and 1675.

7   For a general discussion of the 'fall in the levels of indictment for property offences', see J. A. Sharpe, *Crime in Early Modern England* (London 1984), 58–60.

8   Transcribed in Ewen, *Witch Hunting and Witch Trials,* 81.

9   Francis Hutchinson, *An Historical Essay Concerning Witchcraft* (London 1720), 59–60; PRO, ASSI 35/135/14.

10   For the local conflicts surrounding this prosecution, see Phyllis Guskin, 'The Context of Witchcraft: The Case of Jane Wenham', *Eighteenth Century Studies*, 15 (1982), 48–71.

11   For further discussion of this issue, see Clive Holmes, 'Popular Culture? Witches, Magistrates and Divines in Early Modern England', in S. L. Kaplan ed., *Understanding Popular Culture* (Berlin 1984), 94–5.

12 Based on an analysis of the Essex defamation cases listed in Macfarlane, *Witchcraft in Tudor and Stuart England*, 278–301.

13 Edward Fairfax, *Daemonologia*, ed. William Grainge (Harrogate 1882), 32–5.

14 Thomas Potts, *The Wonderfull Discoverie of Witches in the Countie of Lancaster* (London 1613), sigs C, E1v, E2v.

15 W. W., *A True and Just Recorde, of the Information, Examination and Confession of All the Witches, at S. Oses in Essex* (London 1582). The text is reproduced in Barbara Rosen, *Witchcraft in England* (University of Massachusetts 1991), 103–57. This 'anonymous' tract is obviously Darcy's own work.

16 *A True and Impartial Relation of the Informations against Three Witches* (Exeter 1682), esp. 17–23.

17 Letter of an anonymous Wiltshire JP of 1672, published in the *Gentleman's Magazine*, 102 pt 1 (1832), 492.

18 *A Tryal of Witches, at the Assizes Held at Bury St Edmonds* (London 1682).

19 Francis Bragge, *A Full and Impartial Account of the Discovery of Sorcery and Witchcraft* (London 1712), 28.

20 Ewen, *Witch Hunting and Witch Trials*, 127, 185.

21 Ibid., 299.

22 John Nichols, *The History and Antiquities of the County of Leicester*, 4 vols (London 1795–1811), ii pt 2; Ewen, *Witchcraft and Demonianism*, 209–12; *The Most Strange and Admirable Discoverie of the Three Witches of Warboys* (London 1593), sig. Ov. This last text is reproduced in Rosen, *Witchcraft*, 239–97.

23 The author calculates that in English cases that were believed to involve possession through the agency of a witch, just over 80 per cent of victims were female. In New England the figure is 86 per cent. See Chapter 19 in this book for the relationship between possession and gender in France.

24 I[ohn] D[enison], *The Most Wonderfull and True Storie, of a Certaine Witch Named Alse Goodenige* (London 1597), 3; Richard Baddeley, *The Boy of Bilson* (London 1622), 46; Cotton Mather, 'A Brand Pluck'd out of the Burning', in *Narratives of the Witchcraft Cases, 1648–1706*, ed. G. L. Burr (New York 1914), 259–60.

25 *The Witches of Northamptonshire* (London 1612), sigs B2–C1. This text is in Rosen, *Witchcraft*, 344–56. See Michael MacDonald, *Mystical Bedlam: Madness, Anxiety and Healing in Seventeenth-Century England* (Cambridge 1981), 212.

26 Michael MacDonald, *Witchcraft and Hysteria in Elizabethan London* (London 1991), xxxvi; see, in general, xxxiii–xxxix.

27 John Cotta, *A Short Discoverie of Severall Sorts of Ignorant Practisers* (London 1619), 69. The account of the possession of the Throckmorton children, published in 1593, was made available to the demoniac William Sommers at Nottingham in 1597–8, and to Ann Gunter in Berkshire in 1604. Samuel Harsnet, *A Discovery of the Fraudulent Practices of J. Darrell Concerning the Pretended Possession of W. Somers* (London 1599), 93.

28 John Darrell, *A True Narration of the Strange and Grevous Vexation by the Devil, of 7 Persons in Lancashire and W. Somers: Wherein the Doctrine of Possession and Dispossession of Demoniakes is Applyed* (London 1600), first pagination, 2, 3, 9, and second pagination, 10; George More, *A True Discourse Concerning the Certaine Possession and Dispossession of 7 Persons in One Familie in Lancashire* (Middleburg), 45.

29 The search was employed in a Virginia case of 1706 and in the accusation against Jane Wenham of Walkern in 1712.

30 Gifford, *Dialogue Concerning Witches and Witchcraftes*, 22–3.

31   Joseph Glanvill, *Saducismus Triumphatus,* 2nd edn (London 1682, Wing G823) pt 1, 17–23.

32   W. W., *True and Just Recorde,* sig. A3; Ewen, *Witch Hunting and Witch Trials,* 319.

33   Matthew Hopkins, *Discovery of Witches* (1647), 3.

34   *Witches of Northamptonshire,* sig. C2. For more general discussion of the water-ordeal, see Robert Bartlett, *Trial by Fire and Water: The Medieval Judicial Ordeal* (Oxford 1986).

35   Ewen, *Witchcraft and Demonianism,* 75; W. W., *True and Just Recorde,* sigs C3, D3.

36   *Most Strange and Admirable Discoverie,* sig. O4; Henry Goodcole, *The Wonderfull Discoverie* (London 1621), sigs B2–B3.

37   Michael Dalton, *The Countrey Justice,* 4th edn (London 1630), [273]: second pagination, after 276.

38   Sanford Fox, *Science and Justice: The Massachusetts Witchcraft Trials* (Baltimore, Md 1968), 83–90; Richard Weisman, *Witchcraft, Magic and Religion in 17th-Century Massachusetts* (Amherst, Mass. 1984), 88, 101–3.

39   David Harley, 'Historians as Demonologists: The Myth of the Midwife-Witch', *Social Hist. Medicine,* 3 (1990), 1–26.

40   John Hale, *A Modest Enquiry into the Nature of Witchcraft* (Boston, Mass. 1702), 72.

41   S. Cockburn, *Introduction to the Assize Calendars* (London 1985), 122. There is a very useful discussion of the various court-appointed bodies made up of women in James C. Oldham, 'On Pleading the Belly: A History of the Jury of Matrons', *Criminal Justice Hist.,* 6 (1985), 1–64.

42   Gilbert, 'Witchcraft in Essex', 211, 215.

PART EIGHT

Reading Confessions

IF WE ARE TO BELIEVE THE CONFESSION of Ellen Driver, one of the women accused of witchcraft in Suffolk in 1645, an extraordinary wedding service took place in her parish some sixty years earlier. It was then that she married the Devil in the shape of a man, who subsequently lived with her and gave her two children, which turned out to be 'changelings'. Driver's infernal spouse 'enjoined her before [their] marriage to deny God and Christ'; and on their wedding night he 'had the carnal use' of her body, but she found him to be 'cold'. As they lay in bed together 'she felt of his feet and they were cloven'. Their relationship lasted for two years, and ended only when her mysterious lover died. In all this time, however, Driver claimed that 'she did not know that any of his neighbours did ever see him'.[1]

It is tempting at first sight to dismiss this testimony as the product of mental illness or coercion. This temptation grows stronger when one considers the context in which the old woman's disclosures emerged. She was kept awake for two nights by 'watchers' before she confessed; and this deprivation of sleep, combined with Driver's age and the immense psychological pressure she was under, probably explain her willingness to do so. These factors cannot, however, explain all the details in her account. The concepts of marriage and cohabitation with Satan were comparatively rare in cases of witchcraft, and were possibly fantasies based on her life experiences; and the details about the Devil's appearance and his changeling children seem to derive from folk tales. Since the surviving account of Driver's admissions is very brief, and hardly anything else is known about her, we can never piece together the personal sources for her confession; but this is not the case with some other alleged witches. In a small number of cases, sufficient evidence survives to permit a detailed analysis of the stories they told. As Lyndal Roper argues in Chapter 24, this material suggests that a person's confession to witchcraft was not 'merely a conduit' for the beliefs of their accusers. Rather, a witch fantasy had to persuade its hearers of its truth. Indeed, the interrogation was a lengthy process because the authorities had constantly to assure themselves of the witch's veracity, summoning witnesses to confirm details and checking punctiliously for inconsistencies in her account. The fantasy had to be created by an individual witch out of the elements of fantasy available to her, from what her culture knew of the Devil and his ways, and what she selected had a logic.

The three chapters in this section examine the logic of witchcraft confessions, and consider the implications of these documents for our wider understanding of witch persecutions.

In Chapters 24 and 25, Lyndal Roper and Malcolm Gaskill explore the fantasy worlds of two individual witches. Roper's piece is based on the confession of Regina Bartholome in Augsburg in 1670. Like Ellen Driver, Bartholome claimed to have taken the Devil as her husband. Unlike Driver, however, her admissions to satanic witchcraft appear to have been largely voluntary, and can be readily traced to other experiences in her life. Roper applies ideas from psychoanalysis to explain Bartholome's testimony, and argues compellingly that she used an imaginary relationship with Satan to express feelings about her father and her unsatisfactory experiences with other men. The narrative of this relationship was shaped in the context of her interrogations, but its main elements came from Bartholome herself. In Gaskill's chapter, the voluntary confession in 1647 of the Cambridgeshire witch, Margaret Moore, is subjected to a similar analysis. Avoiding the pyschoanalytical language employed by Roper, Gaskill suggests that Moore's confession described the fantasies she experienced after the death of her first three children. It was the imagined spirits of these children that visited her one night and asked for her soul, before assuming the shape of witch's familiars. Subsequently, Moore appears to have convinced herself that she could use these spirits to bring harm to her enemies, a belief that was, perhaps, understandable given the impoverished and powerless circumstances in which she lived.

The work of Roper and Gaskill raises problems about the relationship between the present and the past. By using the methods of twentieth-century psychoanalysis to explain the mental world of a seventeenth-century woman, Roper invites the charge that her approach is anachronistic. She is alert to this problem, and counters it by pointing out that *all* historical inquiries rely on the assumption that people in past cultures were in some respects similar to those living today: 'historical interpretation as we undertake it day by day nearly always depends at base on the assumption of a measure of resemblance: how else can we make sense of historical actors?' If we accept that this is the case, it seems that the only consistent response to the charge of anachronism is to abandon the study of history altogether. A more specific criticism of Roper's work concerns the validity of psychoanalysis itself. The correctness of psychoanalytical theories is by no means taken for granted by academic psychologists, and the effectiveness of such theories in the interpretation of human behaviour is the subject of much debate.[2] Given that psychoanalysis is not necessarily a reliable tool for understanding subjects in our own age, its validity to early modern historians is at least open to question. In the particular case of Regina Bartholome, Roper makes an impressive case that some of the ideas central to psychoanalysis – the relationship between parents and children and the use of fantasy to resolve feelings of guilt – could lead to confessions of witchcraft. The relevance of these themes in other situations, and the usefulness of psychoanalysis to explain them, must await the outcome of further research.

Malcolm Gaskill addresses the relationship between the past and present in a rather different way in Chapter 25. He warns against the danger of viewing witchcraft from a late twentieth-century perspective, since this can impede our understanding of the true meaning of the crime to early modern people. Instead, he advocates a 'more self-consciously past-centred approach which seeks to insert the speech and action contained in recorded accusations back into the fluid structure of the mentalities that shaped them'. It is in this context that Margaret Moore's confession is important: it reveals the perceived reality of witchcraft to an individual who was herself accused of the crime. Like Roper, however, Gaskill accepts that phenomena observed in the present can shed light on the past. It is common today, for example, for bereaved persons to experience visions of the dead, and such people often accept the objective reality of what they have seen. These incidents are strikingly similar to the one described by Moore in 1647, and they probably constitute a persistent feature of human experience. The interpretation of such events, however, depends on the wider culture in which they take place. As Gaskill points out, Moore's experience 'remains an important event historically because of the specific form of the vision, and the manner in which she interpreted and described it'. In seventeenth-century England, the appearance to a grieving mother of her deceased children could be easily incorporated into the interpretative framework of witchcraft; and Moore's perception of the children as familiar spirits was, perhaps, further encouraged by pre-existing suspicions among her neighbours that she was a witch.

The cultural context of witchcraft confessions is explored persuasively by both Roper and Gaskill. Though they base their work on the testimonies of individual subjects, they relate these testimonies to the beliefs and fears of the communities to which they belonged. For Roper, the narrative created by Regina Bartholome reflected – and was partly shaped by – the anxieties of the ruling elite in Augsburg about the stability of family life. This concern was both moral and political, since the city fathers regarded the household as a microcosm of society as a whole: an attack on one undermined the other. Roper notes that witchcraft 'exposed the yawning possibility that an individual might attack paternal authority and, with it, society, the community of Christians which the city constituted'. Since Bartholeme used her confession of witchcraft to express anxieties about her own father, and the town council perceived itself as a paternal authority, there was a lethal understanding between the witch and those conducting her prosecution. In the case of Margaret Moore, Gaskill suggests that the suspicions of her neighbours might have encouraged her to assume the role of a witch, and to interpret her own experiences in these terms. This led to a vicious circle of 'deviant' behaviour on both sides, until Moore came to accept completely her ability to inflict *maleficium* on her accusers.

One aspect of the social context of witchcraft that is touched on by Gaskill and Roper is the role of gender. Gaskill points out that witchcraft fantasies could empower individuals who had few other means to exercise control over their lives; and this insight is, perhaps, particularly relevant to early modern women. Roper's work draws attention to anxieties about the family in this period, and the ways in which women understood their socially constructed roles as daughters or mothers. In Chapter 26, Louise Jackson picks up the same theme to support the contention that witch-hunting was 'woman-hunting'. In order to make this case, Jackson moves beyond the study of a single confession to examine a series of depositions from Suffolk in 1645. These texts suggest that women were using the concept of witch-craft to help them deal with situations in which they experienced emotional traumas. These traumas, Jackson argues, arose from circumstances that were largely deter-mined by the gender assumptions of seventeenth-century society. Susanna Stegold, for example, appears to have convinced herself that she was responsible for the death of her abusive husband because of the 'ill wishes' she had for him. Tormented by guilt when he died from a sickness with no obvious explanation, she came to believe that she had killed him with *maleficium*. In other cases, women who acted in ways that offended against gender stereotypes – such as failing to care for their children because of post-natal depression – resolved their feeling of guilt by attributing their actions to demonic intervention. Since they perceived their own behaviour as 'unnatural' and evil, it was relatively easy for such women to believe that they had entered a pact with the Devil.

Jackson makes a powerful case that witch beliefs could provide a psycholog-ical resource for early modern women in times of personal distress, but the use of this resource was ultimately destructive. There is a striking parallel here with the experience of some puritan women in seventeenth-century England, who used the idea of satanic temptation to overcome feelings of guilt they experienced as a result of unhappy marriages. In an anonymous spiritual autobiography of 1652, a London woman described the hatred she felt for her drunken and abusive husband when 'the Devil set his foot into my heart'. When she identified the demonic origin of these feelings, however, she called on God to help her vanquish the evil one and live contentedly with her unreformed spouse.[3] Testimonies of this kind can be viewed as the mirror image of the witchcraft confessions discussed in Jackson's chapter. It seems that for some women the attribution of 'ill wishes' to the Devil allowed them to cope with the material frustrations of their lives by joining battle with Satan; but others appear to have succumbed to the belief that they were guilty of witchcraft. Both outcomes, however, had the practical effect of reinforcing the authority of men.

Notes

1   The details of Driver's confession are hazy. She claimed that 'it was sixty years since the Devil wooed her to marry him', though she was aged sixty at the time of her statement. The text is reproduced in C. L'Estrange Ewen, *Witch Hunting and Witch Trials* (Heath Cranton, London 1929), 303–4.

2   The literature on psychoanalysis is huge, and a comprehensive account of the subject is beyond the scope of this book. For a critical introduction, see Alex Howard, *Challenges to Counselling and Psychotherapy* (Macmillan, London 1996) and Anthony Stevens, *An Intelligent Person's Guide to Psychotherapy* (Duckworth, London 1998).

3   Vavasour Powell, ed., *Spirituall Experiences of Sundry Beleevers* (1652), 160–91. For more examples, see my *The Devil in Early Modern England* (Sutton 2000), 101–4.

Chapter 24

Lyndal Roper

OEDIPUS AND THE DEVIL

I

IN 1670, REGINA BARTHOLOME CONFESSED that she had lived with the Devil as man and wife. Aged 21 when she was interrogated by the Augsburg Council, she had met the Devil five years before. She recalled that the Devil was clad in silken hose with boots and spurs and that he looked like a nobleman. They enjoyed trysts twice weekly at a tavern-bakery in Pfersee, a nearby village where Jews lived. The Devil ordered lung sausage, roast pork and beer for her and the two ate with relish alone in the inn parlour. He promised her money, but she had received barely 6 Kreuzer from him, and even that had turned out to be bad coin. In return for this meagre reward, Regina had signed a pact with the Devil for the term of seven years. She had forsworn God and the Trinity, and she had taken the Devil – her lover – as her father in God's stead.

This story, dramatic in its simplicity, begins to make more sense when related to the life-story which she also provided. Regina's father, a poor man, worked for the council as a day-labourer. Around the time Regina first encountered the Devil, and having just reached puberty she had embarked on her first sexual liaison with a man some years her senior, Michael Reidler, who worked as a prison overseer. At about the same period, her mother had initiated an adulterous affair with a young man, Regina's cousin, who boarded in the house. Mother and cousin had also travelled to the village of Pfersee, where her mother pawned the occasional item with the Jews. Regina's mother's affair ended in disaster: Regina's mother was publicly exhibited in the stocks and humiliated, she was banished forever from the city and her young lover fled the town and died 'of drink' not many years after. Regina, left alone with her father, cooked and kept house for him: 'when he came home from his hard work there was no one else who could cook him something warm so that he could restore himself', as her father put it in a petition to the council on her behalf. So far as practical matters were concerned, Regina had taken her mother's place.[1]

Bartholome took in another lodger, this time a young man named Jacob Schwenreiter who was engaged to be married and who worked, like him, as a day-labourer: the two men, Schwenreiter and Bartholome, shared the marital bed. Regina, now parted from her first lover, fell passionately in love with this new male presence, bringing him brandy, bread, cheese, soups and sitting on his bed. She told him she knew a ruse to get money from the Jews at Pfersee, and promised him a share in the proceeds. But her feelings were not returned. Schwenreiter soon brought his bride to the house, fondling her for hours, so Regina believed. Meanwhile, Regina's plot to swindle the Jew at Pfersee and thereby win the young man's affections had misfired: she had accused a Jew of having sex with her (a relationship which would have offended against the taboo on intercourse between Jews and Christians) but her target was a man of unimpeachable character and her accusations failed to stick. She was lucky to escape with a mere censure and brief imprisonment for perjury. She lost her young man Schwenreiter forever when he married, and about this time, so Regina claimed, another young man, a furrier, sought to gain her affections by plying her with a love potion.

The ensuing quarrels in the Bartholome's house finally brought the whole household, including the newly-weds, before the council's disciplinary officer, the mayoralty. Once there, Regina's publicly-uttered threat to kill the new bride was enough to guarantee her incarceration, and thus began the process of criminal interrogation which was to lead both to her confessions of involvement with the Devil and the revelation of her own history which I have provided here in brief.

How can we explain the fantasy of Regina Bartholome, the woman who came to believe herself to be the Devil's lover, daughter and wife? What is the relation between the different narratives she supplied, diabolic and – in our terms – realistic? In this chapter, I shall argue that the fantasy of witch-hood is created in a project of collaboration between questioner and accused, and that the dynamic by which it progressed can indeed be usefully explained psychoanalytically. My claim is not only that, despite what seems at first acquaintance their exotic mental landscape, early modern people have recognizable subjectivities, evincing patterns with which we are familiar. I shall attempt to show that the logic of the interrogations and the process of constructing a full-blown witch fantasy can be illuminated by considering them in psychoanalytic terms.

This may seem a perverse procedure for a historian to adopt. After all, in reaction to some bold early attempts to apply psychoanalytic interpretation to historical characters, historians of early modern Europe have mostly advocated caution. They have insisted upon the radical psychic difference between early modern people and ourselves, pointing to the historical embeddedness of such concepts as family, individual and subjectivity. As Natalie Zemon Davis has reminded us, early modern people characteristically presented their subjectivity in relation to others – family, guild, town.[2] Honour, so many historians have urged, was the substance through which early modern people conceptualized their own identity – and honour is an intrinsically social notion. In an honour society, people derive their sense of self-worth from that of the group to which they belong: the dishonour of one member imperils not the individual alone but the whole. David Sabean has suggested that conscience, which psychoanalysis would see as an inherent part of superego formation, was actually a late child of seventeenth-century Protestantism.[3] Stephen

Greenblatt has argued that psychoanalysis depends on a notion of the self which was itself only in the process of creation in the early modern period: consequently, we cannot apply psychoanalytic theory to people who conceived of the subject in a radically different fashion.[4] Early modern people are held to lack that conviction of individuality we take to be central to self-understanding: modernity consists in the chasm which separates us from them. Though psychoanalytic notions may yet flavour the textual interpretation we offer, a commitment to the historical seems to entail that psychoanalysis cannot be adopted by historians as a serious interpretative theory.

While it is certainly true that early modern people thought differently about the relationship between mind and body, held that dreams could aid diagnosis of physical, rather than mental disturbance, believed that the Devil was active in the world and classed as 'real' phenomena which we would reckon to the world of fantasy, such arguments push caution too far. It is striking that it is the distinctive nature of early modern people to which historians point when ruling psychoanalysis out of court, so that what is modern is defined by a change in the notion of the self; a radical imputation of otherness which, however, is parasitic on our own determination to historicize subjectivity by providing a strong narrative of the birth of the self. Yet at the same time, historical interpretation as we undertake it day by day nearly always depends at base on the assumption of a measure of resemblance: how else can we make sense of historical actors? It does not, I think, endanger the status of the historical to recognize that some of its features are enduring: the importance of fantasy, the unconscious, the centrality of parental figures to psychic life, the way in which symbols or objects invested with deep psychic significance seep into more than one sphere of an individual's life. As psychoanalysis insists, identity is tenuous and is formed in part through identification with and separation from others, a feature which does not set the early modern period apart. Honour, it seems to me, was not the only or even primary way in which early modern people made sense of their predicaments: their rage at being dishonoured, their defence of reputation against insult, their fear of shame gave expression to what was felt as an attack on them in which the psychic and the bodily were indistinguishable – after all, a woman's honour was to do with her body. We would do better, I think, to relate honour to other features of the psychic and emotional lives of early modern people than to seek to explain their behaviour in terms of a reified notion of honour. A phenomenon such as witchcraft in which mental and emotional events have physical effects, in which the individual agency of both the witch and her victims is of the essence, in which we are confronted with the gripping nature of the lurid phantasms of the witch-craze, demands explanation not only in sociological but in psychological terms. When historians are drawn to apply psychoanalysis to the study of the witch-craze, they generally use it to derive conclusions about an entire society: here, however, I intend to draw on psychoanalytic ideas in order to reconstruct the mental life of an individual.

Regina Bartholome was not generally reputed to be a witch. No one accused her of witchcraft, although people concurred that she was 'strange'. The history of witchcraft has often taken women to be victims, scapegoats for the anxieties of a society. Yet one of the troubling features of a case such as this is the witch's own self-destructive capacity. Regina precipitated her own imprisonment. She first embarked on the highly risky strategy of accusing a Jew of having an adulterous relationship with her, an imputation which she could not prove, and which threatened her own reputation as it undermined his. It also embroiled her in a dangerous criminal investigation from which she was lucky to escape with a short term of imprisonment. Her history is littered with false accusations. She accused the young bride of Jacob Schwenreiter (the young man who was the object of her affections) of stealing something from her – as indeed she had; but it was her bridegroom, not her 'tin pan, bedstead and half a measure of corn' that she had stolen. When Regina cited her before the authorities and then, in the chancellery itself, threatened to kill her, she secured her own imprisonment.[5]

The momentum of Regina's trial derived in part from her own drive to accuse herself, to punish herself and to uncover the truth of a crime she felt herself to have committed. Under interrogation the witch faced two council representatives and ultimately the torturer, who would be her executioner. It is easy to see their exercise of power over their victim: they stood for the power of the council, and they were armed with the instruments of torture. It is less easy, and less comforting for the historian, to see the witch's own manipulation, however unsuccessful, of the situation or to discern the ways in which the sadism of the questioning process may have gratified the needs of the witch.

But how do we interpret what she confessed? The content of witch fantasy is difficult territory for historians, trained as we are to look for verification or to construct social meaning. How can social meanings be derived from material which seems to us both patently unreal and recalcitrantly personal? The most illuminating interpretations have examined witch confessions as a collective psychosis, whose features are best outlined in terms of historical development. The historian's task is to trace the gradual appearance of such motifs as the witch's dance, the pact with the Devil, the satanic mass. These are explained as the production, in the mouths of the persecuted, of the fantasies gradually elaborated by their interrogators. Looking from the other end of the telescope, Carlo Ginzburg has viewed these fantasies as the creation of the people, not of their elite interrogators, interpreting their features as the eruption of older, pagan patterns of belief.[6] He uncovers their mythic structures, tracing their elements back to their folkloric avatars. This is a process in which the fantasies of particular witches play little part: witches themselves, less significant than the culture they inhabit, are not Ginzburg's primary subject of concern.

Both these approaches, however, concur in locating the source of fantasy outside the witch herself. She is merely a conduit either of the traces of a vanished primitive religion, or of the witch beliefs of her interrogators. But a witch fantasy had to persuade its hearers of its truth. Indeed, the interrogation was a lengthy process because the authorities had constantly to assure themselves of the witch's veracity, summoning witnesses to confirm details and checking punctiliously for inconsistencies in her account. The fantasy had to be created by an individual witch out of the elements of fantasy available to her, from what her culture knew of the Devil and his ways, and what she selected had a logic. In Regina Bartholome's account, there was no clutter of diabolic characters to distract from the central focus of the tale, the relationship between Regina and the Devil. There were no sister witches, no accomplices, no apprentice witches whom Regina had seduced, no nocturnal gatherings. Instead, this pared-down form of testimony allowed the themes of her own psychology to emerge more clearly.

II

How did the witch fantasy emerge? The summary of Regina Bartholome's relations with the Devil with which I began this chapter was not a free initial admission. It emerged, with considerable resistance, over the course of eight sessions of inter-rogation both with and without torture and its threat. During these she provided four different accounts of her relations with the Devil, each time moving the moment of her initial encounter with him further back into the past, and each time attaching the moment of his initial appearance to a different love relationship in her own short life.

First she told how the Devil appeared after she was given a love potion by the young furrier who she believed was trying to force her into marriage. This was an extraordinary, voluntary admission, not a response to a question. It was Regina herself who brought the Devil into the story, explaining how he had visited her in her cell when she had first been imprisoned by the council: diabolic interpretation was not the consequence of the council's own determination to construct her story in this way. Once introduced, however, the Devil's role became a joint concern as her interrogators sought to make sense of her behaviour. Regina's first account soon gave way to the story that the Devil had appeared to her some months earlier, when she was involved in bringing the accusations against the Jew of Pfersee, at the time when she was hoping to persuade the young day-labourer Jacob Schwenreiter to be her lover. In a later interrogation, Regina confessed she had known the Devil long before, and dated the time of her diabolic seduction to the period when her mother began the adulterous affair which was to end in her banish-ment. And finally, in a last burst of revenge, she made this period more precise, associating it with her very first affair with Michael Reidler, the prison overseer. Why was he not punished as she had been, she demanded? This man, her first seducer, 'may well have been the Devil himself'. As Regina well knew, this was an accusation which, if the council had believed her, would surely have led to his being incarcerated and tortured just as she was.

Each new version of the story elicited in response to the council's questions thus progressively traced back the moment of her own departure from the Christian community to a prior period in Regina's own psychological history, stopping only when she reached puberty. We might note in passing that it parallels the explana-tory logic of psychoanalysis, where the patient is encouraged to explore themes from his or her early life in order to understand subsequent conflicts and relations; and it was a logic of explanation shared by both council and witch. As with the life narratives offered in psychoanalysis, it is not, however, a 'realistic' narrative which can be abstracted from the diabolic narrative, but a whole story which offers meaning. Along the way, Regina introduces us to the characters who populated her own life history. But there is something odd about this seemingly real 'life'. All the stories, apart from the first love potion story, reveal the same theme of love and rejection. Even the first story is an inversion of this pattern, for this time it is Regina who plays the part of the rejector, a role which, we might observe, she is also attempting to play (by means of the interrogation) in relation to the Devil, freeing herself from his power and attempting to rejoin the Christian community. And we might notice that the retelling of her stories in interrogation allows Regina to take revenge, to retaliate against those who rejected her, a dynamic which reaches its culmination in her accusation that her first seducer was the Devil himself.

Here we might make use of Joyce McDougall's helpful image of the 'theatres of the mind', which she employs to describe the use individuals make of other people to play the split parts of the person's own inner world, so that it is the individual's inner conflicts which are projected into fantasy and acted out in relations with others. Because these conflicts are intolerable and unresolved, they are constantly repeated and re-enacted.[7] Interrogation for witchcraft, we might say, conferred the accused a theatrical opportunity to recount and restage these linked conflicts and what better audience than the rapt ears of the council's representatives and the executioner?

But what are the themes of these dramas? The images which Regina chose and the narratives which she offered are littered with Oedipal themes. At its most basic, the logic of her account apparently suggests that she felt herself to have succeeded in gaining her father's love and stealing her mother's position by cooking and keeping house for her father. It was as if, by a terrible retribution of fantasy, her forbidden Oedipal desires seemed to have been fulfilled. No wonder she felt herself to be worthy of punishment. It is important, here, to note that these transactions occurred at the level of fantasy: there is no evidence that we are dealing with a case of incest, an observation which does not, however, diminish the importance of the theme. Oedipal themes also recurred in the relations she recounted with others. Her first lover appeared just as her mother took a new lover, deserting her father. Regina herself was aged only 12 at the time. This was in seventeenth-century eyes a precocious sexual affair with a man her social superior, senior to her in age. Ominously enough, Reidler seems to have worked as a prison overseer. If her first lover evinced some paternal characteristics, older than she, and a Landsmann of her father's, the second man with whom she fell in love, Jacob Schwenreiter, was yet more closely associated with her actual father. He shared not only her father's trade but even his bed. His inaccessibility and the cruel manner in which he flaunted his new wife only served to underline Regina's failure to establish an independent love-relationship: indeed, he allowed her to repeat the Oedipal drama, this time against a mother-figure who refused to be dislodged. And when Regina attempted to blackmail the Jew at Pfersee for engaging in sexual relations with her, her revenge displayed a similar retaliatory logic. He, too, was an older, married man. She had pawned goods with him just as her mother had pawned goods with the Jews at Pfersee, yet neither had he given her more money nor had he returned her goods. He had right and the law on his side: her revenge therefore had to take the form of an extreme and dishonest assault on his sexual reputation. In the kind of symbolic repetition that typifies Regina's story, she accused him of breaking a taboo akin to the taboo on incest, the taboo on sexual relations between Jew and Christian. Pfersee was, of course, the setting for the idyll between her mother and her nephew. And in a 'return to the scene of the crime' so characteristic of Regina's interrogations at every turn, it transpired in the end that Pfersee was the locale of her own seduction by the Devil. In the very same tavern, she finally claimed, the Devil and she regularly stole away to a side room where she did his will, a scenario, incidentally, which neither the bemused keeper of the inn, his wife nor his servant could bring themselves to substantiate.

There is no mileage, I think, in the usual historical strategy of teasing out the 'real' from the fantastic elements in this account. We cannot isolate the point at which events which we know to be 'real', her mother's affair, her relationship with the prison overseer, end, and where the fantastic begins. Indeed, discarding the fantastic would be an inappropriate strategy because what is important are the elements which Regina chose to make sense of her life. Her narration of one set of events, whether real or fantastic, does not so much indicate the cause of the events which occurred later as display the same pattern of meaning: in this case, multiple incest. This is not, of course, to claim that trauma does not leave its mark upon the psyche. But we cannot simply 'read off' the real event from the page of the interrogation. It is important first to uncover the psychic logic of her tale, a story which inter-weaves diabolic with sexual themes, before we can guess at its meaning. So far, the patterns I have described are rather like the patterns which might be expected to be evoked by a kind of free association. But interrogations were not conducted as analytic discussions. The threat of torture, even when it was neither threatened nor carried out, was implicit in the interrogation and when there were specific points on which the council was not content with its subject's answers it would, after consultation, authorize the exhibition and then use of the instruments of torture. In Regina's case, actual torture was resorted to only once, after the sixth interrogation, when she was suspended from the rack with empty weights for two sessions. The application of torture, however comparatively mild in this case, does not in itself explain what the witch confessed, why she provided the particular narrative she did or how she persuaded the council of its truth: the council knew that pain sometimes led people to false confessions.

And there is another salient feature of difference in seventeenth century witch narratives: the role of the Devil. To us, the fantasies which surround him seem clearly part of the realm of the imaginary, more definitively unreal than the material I have been describing. But to them he was part of the real world. In talking about the Devil, therefore, Regina was not engaged in an activity different in kind from the rest of the confession she gave. This observation is helpful in considering how we ought to interpret diabolic material. Diabolic fantasy as it appears in interrogation is not, I would argue, to be equated with some kind of hallucinatory activity or treated as any more part of the world of the imagination than the rest of her confession.[8] Instead, I think it should be interpreted as part of the whole narrative that the witch offered. In the figure of the Devil, the witch had available to her a character who could dramatize psychic conflicts with extraordinary clarity.

There were good reasons why, in seventeenth-century Germany, confessing oneself to be a witch might involve supplying both a life history and a story about the Devil. The Devil whom witches encountered was not an abstract force or a symbolic figure of evil. Though he appeared in different guises he was, first and foremost, on each occasion a character with whom one had a relationship. Regina, for instance, discovered he shared her taste for lung sausage and beer. His dashing clothes placed him as a nobleman in contrast to her drab workaday world. His appearance, his gestures and his attire always had to be specifically described by the witch, even while she drew from a possible repertoire of familiar elements with which to describe him. Becoming a witch meant engaging in an intimate relationship, usually sexual, with the Devil as a character, and consequently, its discovery entailed the analysis of the wellsprings of the witch's own personality, motives and emotions. Interrogation therefore aimed at the construction of an account of the individual's own history and his or her relations with others which could explain how someone could come to sever human attachments, choosing instead to cleave to the Devil in a kind of perversion of the soul.

The diabolic elements of Regina's interrogation thus echoed the themes of the life history with precision. As the formula of renunciation of Christ which Regina provided had it, she had forsworn God and taken the Devil as her father. He, too, was her lover. She even imagined the possibility of giving him children: whether these were sired by him or by her other lovers, the Devil had told her she must surrender them to him. In this way, we might say, the story of the Devil allowed her to develop the Oedipal narrative yet further so that she might in imagination provide her father with the phallic compensation of children; but so powerful and persecuting was this father-figure that she was not even to be allowed to keep these children. Of course no seventeenth-century court would have interpreted her story in this way. But her seventeenth-century hearers would have invested the diabolic narrative with a similar epistemological importance. For them, the diabolic narrative helped explain the life history, and the life history, the relationship with the Devil. It was because Regina listened to the Devil that she had acted as she had; it was because she wanted money and because she was lascivious that the Devil was able to seduce her.

III

The Oedipal elements were not, however, restricted to the motifs of the narrative Regina provided. Her narrative was the product of a conversation. If we look at the interaction in the interrogation, we notice that much of it dramatizes relations between fathers and daughters. Regina began her interrogation by appealing to her interrogators to be allowed 'to return to her father', and throughout the course of the interrogation, she made this appeal again and again: 'She pleads for God's mercy, that my lords should send her out again soon, so that she should return to her father.' 'Oh you poor father, shall your child never come to you again? If they were to do anything to her, they would be killing her and her father.' Return to her own place becomes equated with return to her father, an image she expresses in the compound word 'fatherland', as she begs with ominous prescience: 'My lords should let her die in her fatherland, so that she could only return to her father again'; 'if she were to be exiled they would be killing her, let them allow her to die in her fatherland'. At the end of her very last interrogation she stated, half begging, half ruefully remarking 'if for God's sake one had only granted her life, for her old father's sake'. Claiming to love her father and desiring to return to him, her pleas implicitly contrast him with the powerful, cruel council and show the council to be another powerful father-figure: 'She begs that my lords should behave to her as fathers, and should not drive her out of her fatherland'. Repeatedly she rails against the council, castigating it for its lack of mercy, crying that 'she could not sense that there was a gracious authority here, because they were trying to drive her out into misery'. Here she is rejecting the council's own claim to be a benevolent paternal authority, the vision of itself which it so tirelessly repeated in its steady stream of ordinances and public pronouncements. Behind the council, sanctifying its power, loomed another paternal authority: God. For Regina, he, too, was a father who failed her, and in his stead she said she had adopted the Devil as her father. As she put it in her rendition of her blasphemy against God, she admitted that 'she said because God was no longer her father, she would take the Devil as her father, he should be her father'.

Regina's rage against paternal figures is uncontainable: against the council, whom she blames for her mother's exile, against God, who will not hear her. Her anger is expressed in her constant threats of suicide, the blame for which she lays at the council's door: 'if my lords were to shame her and to banish her then she would throw herself in the water. They had sent her mother away in the same way, let it rest on their consciences'. 'My lords should not drive her out into misery, for otherwise she would drown herself or hang herself, and then my lords would be responsible'. Seventeenth-century people, who viewed suicide as a crime and a sin, had perhaps a livelier awareness than we do of the aggressive logic of killing oneself.[9] This rage is also expressed through the vehicle of a fear of public mockery. Public humiliation, her mother's fate, was the outcome she claims constantly to fear; and yet her own behaviour precipitated her interrogation and ultimately the most lurid, public form of shaming imaginable, a public account of her sexual exploits with the Devil, read out for all to hear at the moment of her execution.

It is evident that Regina's world is populated with good and bad fathers. We might say, following Melanie Klein, that by splitting her mental universe up into 'good' fathers, who offered protection and love, and 'bad' fathers, who did not care for her, Regina was able to contain a 'good' image of her own father while projecting the 'bad' father on to other figures.[10] This was an assignment of values which was highly unstable: the Devil, the 'good' father who offered her sausage, money and love, proved unreliable and maltreated her, giving her false coin, failing to prevent her imprisonment and beating her in her cell. The cost of Regina's perverse reassignment of moral values was immense. Her pact with the Devil excluded her from Christian society, and made her unable to recite the Lord's Prayer. It left her suffering from a rage and anger against others which made it impossible for her to live peaceably with her neighbours. Paradoxically, the interrogation thus offered her the chance of reconciliation and reintegration with the community of Christians in the town, with the council, in acceptance of its just power and in submission to its decrees about her faith in God, in conversion before her execution. By the fourth interrogation, after about six weeks of being unable to recite an Our Father, she found she was once more able to pray.

Regina's perverse reassignment of moral values had protected her image of her father as good and protective and kept her anger alive. When this mental organization began to crumble, so too her unacknowledged hatred of her father whose inability to prevent the affair or prevent her banishment had after all, in a sense, caused her mother's downfall began to emerge. In the sixth interrogation she began to distance herself yet further from the Devil, saying, in response to the council's question about whether the Devil was not comforting her, 'Yes, he comforted her, but the comforting was no use. He was letting her stick in it. It would have been better if she had called to God, God would have helped her overcome'. This was eventually to lead, under torture, to her own terrible admission, later in the same interrogation, that she had bought a little yellow powder from the apothecary with which to poison her father. But in the very next interrogation she explained how she had mixed the powder in with broth she made for him, a revelation she at once attempted to modify, saying the Devil had only told her to give it to her father, and denying that she knew the powder was poison thereby informing the council, of course, that it was. Until the sixth interrogation, Regina had not confessed to any acts of malefice and her crime had concerned her pact with the Devil, not any use of sorcery to harm man, woman or beast. But now she confessed to attempting to set two houses on fire, to having attempted to poison the bride of the young man with whom she was in love, to having 'ridden the beasts' naked at Goggingen, causing them to sicken, and to having tried to commit parricide, a transgression against natural affection and social order.

Witnesses were called to cross-check these latest admissions. The supposed victims of arson rejected all talk of sorcery out of hand; the shepherds at Goggingen could find nothing amiss with their herds. The young bride had noticed no ill effects but did express fear of Regina. But when Regina's father, Hans Bartholome, was interrogated, he faltered. He explained that he had no idea that his daughter had attempted such a thing. Seeking to defend himself from the imputation of fatherly irresponsibility, he stated that 'He could not say that on a single day of his life he had ever sensed that the Evil One came to her, as he only now heard, she was supposed to have had dealings with him [the evil one] at Pfersensteg'. He explained that his daughter had been 'aggressive in the head' since her youth, but was not able to supply a forthright denial of the possibility that his daughter was a witch, or even to deny that she might have felt hatred for him. Regina ended her final confession beseeching the council to let her return to her father: tragically, he was in the end unable to protect his daughter. Like his wife before her, he was compelled to deliver Regina to the council's justice.

IV

To this point, we have explored the dynamic of Regina Bartholome's confession. But why should the council have believed that she was a witch? The answer to this question is not as straightforward as one might expect. For the council did have available to it an alternative explanation of Regina's behaviour: namely, that she was of unsound mind. Indeed, when she was at first tried for her accusation against the Jew of Pfersee, the council agreed with the assessment of her neighbours that she was simply 'a bit touched', and sent her on her way recommending that good care be taken of her. In the second trial, the council took care to have its own medical experts examine Regina to see whether she was mentally imbalanced: they determined that she was of sound mind and that her melancholic tendencies were to be explained, as she herself did, by the conditions of her incarceration.

Just twenty years later, two other supposed witches' lurid confessions of involvement with the Devil did not faze the council: in each case, it concurred with its own medical advisers that the woman was suffering from melancholy, and freed her.[11] And about the time that Regina met with execution for her whoredom with the Devil, Regina Schiller was failing to convince authorities in Augsburg and all over southern Germany that she was indeed, as she claimed, bound to the Devil by a diabolic pact written in blood. Regina Schiller's diabolic confessions were more elaborate and more riveting than those of Regina Bartholome: she could even produce the scrap of paper on which she had signed her baptismal birthright away in blood. Why then did the council suddenly change its mind about Regina Bartholome and embark on a trial for witchcraft?

These disquiets led me back to the role of the interrogators: of the council, who formulated the questions and who voted on guilt; of the questioners, the council's representatives who interrogated Regina over eight sessions and who coaxed her answers from her; and the executioner. Their role as questioners was to tie in the threads of Regina's narratives, discarding what they took to be false or irrelevant. Their questions supplied a logic of motive for her admissions: why did she make a pact with the Devil? To whom did she feel hatred and envy? What had the Devil whispered to her? Some motives they held to be not further analysable, and greed was foremost among these: when Regina several times claimed she summoned the Devil 'for the sake of filthy money' they adopted this as a primary explanation of her sin in the final condemnation. Similarly, they elicited material about paternal relations and not about maternal ones because women's relations with men fitted their own explanatory paradigm of witchcraft, women's seduction by the Devil.[12] Of course, we face particular difficulties here because we are dealing with a collective character, the council, not with a discrete individual. It is hard, moreover, to do more than guess at the psychic investments which underlay their interest. Of necessity our information must be indirect, derived from the question structure itself, its turns of phrase and its dynamic: interrogators put questions, and are not subject to them. None the less, asking questions is never an innocent activity, and questions shape narratives. That the councillors were able to elicit this material seems likely to have been in part because of their own unconscious investments in the elements of her tale.

Regina posed no real threat to the power of the council, but her extreme behaviour gave voice to an insubordination towards authority, secular and divine, which her audience of councillors found at once appalling and compelling. At her very first interrogation in the second trial her questioners demanded to know 'whether she did not have to realize and admit how kind the authority had been in punishing her so graciously', proceeding to ask her how she dared to claim the council was acting unjustly; in the fifth interrogation they again asked, as Regina repeated her complaints, 'what she had to complain about, that one treated her too severely, since she had well deserved this many times before'; and in the sixth

interrogation they once more asked her why she had said in the previous questioning session that she had an ungracious government, trying, with the following
question, to bring her to confess that they were generous rulers.

In part for this reason, the question script compiled on behalf of the council
focused at first upon the pact Regina made with the Devil. It was not only that
belief in the pact characterized elite beliefs in witchcraft, though this was clearly
important as the council strove to make sense of the confrontation of its own
demonological beliefs with the plethora of fantastical empirical evidence which
Regina supplied. The pact was so significant because it gave documentary form to
the transgression the council perceived to lie at the root of witchcraft: the rejection of the good, just and paternal authority and its replacement with its inverse,
the Devil. By her eighth and final interrogation, Regina had surrendered herself
utterly to the council's authority:

> she had not been able to pray, but now she could pray; She asked my
> lords for God's sake, that one might yet grant her life if it could be
> . . . If they should want to take her life, so let it be in God's name; if
> she were to be pardoned, she would have God and her government to
> thank.

Witchcraft exposed the yawning possibility that an individual might attack paternal
authority and, with it, society, the community of Christians which the city constituted. But it also made evident the fact that reintegration into the community was
sanctioned, in the last analysis, by force: it secured Regina's acceptance of its
'gracious' authority by the relentless questioning and threats of torture of which
she complained. This violence at the heart of the benign paternal relations of
authority offered an arresting allegory of the psychic dimensions of the councillors'
own power as fathers.

Witchcraft interrogations involve two parties, the witch and her interrogators.
Both are required for the production of fantasy. It was her interrogator's relentless questioning and ruthless eye for detail which encouraged the fantasy from the
witch, and supplied the connections to motive and guilt. Both had psychic investments in its content. At times, as the process of interrogation continued, the
collaborative drive between witch and interrogator could become so intense that
the questioners elaborated on the script of questions they had been given: it was
her interrogators who suggested to Regina that she must have lived with the Devil
as man and wife, a formulation which made deep psychological sense, and which
she was willing to adopt as a description of her own behaviour.[13]

V

Historians have long puzzled why so many more women than men were the targets
of witchcraft accusations. I have argued elsewhere that the prevalence of women
among witches cannot be explained in terms of the sociological characteristics of
women as a group: only a tiny proportion of women were interrogated for witchcraft, and they were often accused by members of their own sex.[14] But it can,

I think, be related to dilemmas surrounding the psychic identity of womanhood. Elements in the interaction between the witch and her persecutors allowed the fantasy of witchcraft to unfold. The psychic conflicts attendant on the feminine position, whether Oedipal or related to motherhood, provided the substance of the psychic drama of the witchcraft interrogation, and supplied the material on which their interrogators could work in fascinated horror, developing in turn their own fantasies about femininity, about fatherhood and about diabolic activity. Most women, of course, managed the psychic conflicts of femininity without falling prey to morbid diabolic temptation. Not every case of witchcraft furnished interrogations displaying an emotional engagement with the Devil, nor did all witches produce witch fantasies. But in those few cases of women witches who did, the possibilities present in a culture obsessed with the power of the Devil, of fathers and of women, enabled a combustion of interests to occur, flaring up into interrogations under torture and the production of those sadistic, masochistic stories which so whetted their contemporaries' appetite for tales of the relation between women and the Devil.

Notes

1   For full citations of the German sources for this chapter, see the original version in Lyndal Roper, *Oedipus and the Devil: Witchcraft, Sexuality and Religion in Early Modern Europe* (Routledge, London 1992), ch. 10.

2   Natalie Zemon Davis, 'Boundaries and the Sense of Self in Sixteenth-Century France', in Thomas C. Heller, Morton Sosna and David F. Wellbery, eds, *Reconstructing Individualism: Autonomy, Individuality, and the Self in Western Thought* (Stanford, Calif. 1986).

3   David Sabean, *Power in the Blood* (Cambridge 1984), esp. 171.

4   Stephen Greenblatt, 'Psychoanalysis and Renaissance Culture', in his *Learning to Curse* (New York and London 1990).

5   This took place on 22 July 1670. Here it is worth noting the corresponding investments of Regina's accusers in the fantasy of witchcraft. Just four years later, Maria Schwenreiter was among the witnesses against Anna Bruhler and her husband in another case of accusations of sorcery. This time, she claimed that Bruhlerin's husband had told her that Bruhler had caused Schwenreiter, her husband, to lose his 'manhood', condemning her to a childless marriage. Maria Schwenreiter thus saw not only Regina Bartholome executed, but also Anna Bruhler exiled for ever from the town: she, too, was caught up in a repetitive cycle of witchcraft accusation, tending to identify the sources of her misfortune in others.

6   Carlo Ginzburg's thesis is set out in Chapter 8 in this collection. For a longer exposition, see his *Ecstasies: Deciphering the Witches' Sabbath* (London 1990).

7   Joyce McDougall, *Theatres of the Mind: Illusion and Truth on the Psychoanalytic Stage* (New York 1985).

8   For this reason, attempts to 'explain' the phenomenon of witch fantasy physiologically, by appeal to the effects of grain fungus, mushrooms, etc. seem unhelpful, because they do not explain why the specific fantasies developed in the way they did, why they employed particular elements, nor why they were of interest to the authorities. See, however, G. R. Quaife, *Godly Zeal and Furious Rage: The Witch in Early Modern Europe* (London 1987).

9   See Michael MacDonald, *Mystical Bedlam: Madness, Anxiety and Healing in Seventeenth Century England* (Cambridge 1981), 132ff.

10   Interestingly enough, he also changed colour, appearing first dressed in white, then in black, as if reflecting his moral fluctuation.

11   In October 1696 Anna Bohm was found to be not *integra mentis*, although she did evince all sorts of evil. In July 1699 Anna Scheifeihut was found to be suffering from *melancholica* and her tendency to curse and blaspheme was held to be aggravated by loneliness. Her relatives were admonished not to leave her alone. We seem here to have practical examples of the way in which the currency of the views of witch sceptics like Johannes Weyer or Reginald Scot that witch fantasies might be the melancholy productions of old women could coexist with the belief that there were none the less real witches.

12   The author has followed the evident themes of the interrogation in concentrating on paternal themes in this case. However, Regina also called to Mary the Mother of God, and accused the council of having punished her mother unfairly. She does not apparently evince the same splitting processes in relation to female figures, although this may be implicit in her appeal to Mary.

13   See Louise Jackson's contribution to this book (Chapter 26) for examples of a similar process in seventeenth-century England.

14   See Stuart Clark, *Thinking with Demons* (Oxford 1997), ch. 8; and Robin Briggs, 'Women as Victims? Witches, judges and the community', *French History* 5 (1991), 438–50.

Chapter 25

Malcolm Gaskill

WITCHCRAFT AND POWER IN EARLY MODERN ENGLAND

The case of Margaret Moore

A WITCH-HUNT, INSTIGATED by Matthew Hopkins, the self-appointed Witchfinder-General, took place in East Anglia in the years 1645–7, and claimed the lives of around two hundred women and men.[1] This chapter examines the case of just one victim of the trials, in the light of some of the ideas which have emerged from historical studies of witchcraft in early modern England. It explores the possible meaning of a single supernatural occurrence in the broader context of popular beliefs and mentalities, with a view to understanding how ordinary people might perceive power – its limitations and its extension – in an extraordinary manner.

I

In later sixteenth- and seventeenth-century England, opportunities to live according to individual preference were rare, and for most people the pattern of life was determined by adverse economic conditions over which they had little or no control: population increase; land hunger; inflation; dearth; and, as a result, competition for power, space and resources. Under such harsh conditions, it is easy to imagine that an atmosphere of fear and insecurity might form the backdrop to the daily life of many communities, and that charity and good neighbourliness existed as unrealized Christian ideals as much as they faithfully mirrored social relations in the period.[2] In many instances of conflict, often between close neighbours, and especially where disputants were too poor to engage in protracted litigation, impotence prevailed and a tense state of deadlock emerged. Equally, for many, life was a struggle not only with other people, but with the impersonal obstacles put up by the social and economic environment: poverty, disease and mortality. Women were particularly powerless, and therefore resorted to (or were believed to resort to) other means of overcoming hardship and opposition; the use of words to compensate for the lack of more direct female power, for example, has been suggested.[3]

In such straitened circumstances, personal frustration and despair encouraged the belief in some individuals that magical power might be harnessed as a means of extending the boundaries of terrestrial power. This is a familiar explanation of sorcery and cunning magic, where a consensus of belief usually existed between witch and client, but it is less commonly encountered in discussions of *maleficium* or diabolic communion because the witch trials have been inextricably linked to the history of persecuting societies – an approach which mutes any agency on the part of the witch. However, belief in an act of harmful magic was also potentially shared by accused and accuser alike. Viewed together, a physical world marked by hardship, and a mental world which permitted the possibility of witchcraft, provided fertile psychological ground either for delusion and desire in the witch, and/or paranoia and hostility on the part of the witch's victim. Struggles with neighbours and nature alike could be elevated to an imaginary, supernatural plane, and ultimately resolved (on the part of a victim) in the material world of the criminal legal process. In this way, a dramatic paradigm was applied to real life, and depositions containing accusations and confessions might be seen, in modern terms, to overlay reality with fantasy as a conscious or subconscious means of influencing a court. Such documents constitute, then, a real and powerful 'fiction in the archives'.[4]

II

The lives of ordinary individuals in early modern England flicker for a moment before the eyes of historians fumbling in the darkness of the past, and then disappear as quickly as they appeared. The life of Margaret Moore is a case in point. She lived in the first half of the seventeenth century in Sutton, a comparatively large village in the hundred of Witchford in the south-western corner of the Isle of Ely, Cambridgeshire. Then, as now, Sutton was dominated by a central street, at the eastern end of which stood the parish church, and behind which the village sloped away to the south, overlooking a large expanse of fenland towards the village of Haddenham. Until the eighteenth century this lowland was flooded, but elsewhere rich arable land was to be found, and Sutton was noted for its cherry orchards. Moore had a husband, who may not have been present at the time she was accused of witchcraft, but was almost certainly still alive (she is consistently referred to as the wife of Robert Moore). At some point in her life she had four children, three of whom died in infancy – a fact which, it will be argued, is crucial to a proper understanding of the story. Various clues from the surviving documentation suggest that she was poor, although she was probably not among the poorest since she kept animals.[5] At present, this is virtually all that is known of her for certain prior to her apprehension as a witch in May 1647.[6]

Some time before this date, in the parish of Witchford just over three miles to the east of Sutton, three farmers suffered misfortunes which were attributed to the witchcraft of Margaret Moore. Thomas Maynes and Jo Foster both lost cattle, and Thomas Nix fell sick and died. According to Matthew Hopkins' associate, John Stearne, who mentions Moore specifically in his memoir of the witch-hunt, her murdered victim (presumably Nix) sold her a pig for 2s 2d but she paid him only the two shillings. So after coming to her door one day, either to collect the debt or reclaim the pig, he became ill and, thinking of his debtor Moore, summoned her, pleading that 'he could not depart this life, untill hee had spoken with her'. At first, she refused to go but finally was forced to attend by Nix's friends just prior to his death.[7] It is unusual that the approximate date of the bewitchings is not stated either in the depositions or in Stearne's account, and both narratives accordingly give the impression of a rapid transition from crime to apprehension, examination and trial. However, there are good reasons for believing that these events occurred as much as a decade earlier; e.g., the will of a Thomas Nyx, husbandman of Witchford, was proved at the consistory court at this time. Witchcraft prosecutions occurring so long after the fact were by no means unusual, and may reflect the gradual accretion of suspicions and feelings of hostility against an individual over a period of time. By the time well nursed grudges spilled over into formal accusations, a long litany of alleged offences might be stored in the collective memory of the community.

If either Maynes or Fisher, or the family and friends of Thomas Nix, gave evidence against Moore, it does not survive. What is certain is that, some time after the alleged bewitchings, she was apprehended and examined informally by two gentlemen of Sutton, Benjamin Wyne and Perry Jetherell, before whom she confessed herself to be a witch and guilty of the charges laid against her.

The first witness, Benjamin Wyne, deposed that Moore had told him that she had surrendered her soul to the Devil 'because shee would save the life of on[e] of hir Children which upon the Contract he would save & to doe for hir what she should Command'. A familiar spirit named Annis was sent to her, which she allowed to suckle before sending it to bewitch Thomas Nix, who died soon afterwards. Jetherell elaborated on this story relating that Moore had confessed that one night, soon after the death of her three children, the following strange and poignant event had occurred:

> she herd a voyce Calling to hir after this Manner, Mother Mother to which the said Margeret answered sweet Children where are you what would you have with me & thay demanded of hir drincke w[hi]ch the said Margeret Answered that she had noe drincke then theire Came a voyce which the said Margeret Conceaved to be hir third Child & demanded of hir hir soule, otherwise she would take a-way the life of hir 4th Child which was the only Child she had left to which voyce the said Margeret made answer that rather then shee would lose hir last Child she would Consent unto the giving a-way of hir soule & then a spirit in the liknes of a naked Child appeared unto hir & suckt upon hir Body.[8]

Moore herself confessed before the magistrate that 'she hard ye voyce of hir Children whoe had formerly died Calling unto hir in these words mother mother good sweet mother lett me in'. She arose at once to open the door, and although she could see no one, the voice continued, 'good mother give me some drincke', to which she answered that 'she had noe drincke but water'. She closed the door, returned to her bed, but the voice started again, closer to the bedside this time: 'mother mother Give me yo[u]r soule & I will save the life of yo[u]r 4[th] Child w[hi]ch is now livinge w[i]th yow'. Moore immediately agreed, sealed the covenant and then suckled her two spirits, Annis and Margaret, which she sent to Witchford to kill Thomas Nix, three of Thomas Maynes' bullocks and John Foster's cow. She ended by saying that she had performed many other acts of witchcraft, and that she was very sorry for all she had done.

If Hopkins' and Stearne's motivations (and those of their clients) seem obscure, knowledge of their methods is perhaps more enlightening for explaining Moore's confession. Illegal torture, such as sleep deprivation followed by leading questioning (a favourite method of Hopkins and Stearne), cannot be ruled out in the case of Moore and the other Sutton witches. One contemporary described these methods:

> Having Taken the suspected Witch, shee is placed in the middle of a room upon a stool, or Table, crosse legg'd, or in some other uneasie posture, to which if she submits not, she is bound with cords, there is she watcht & kept without meat or sleep for the space of 24 hours.[9]

Hopkins denied that this was a means of extracting confessions (adding that forced confessions were worthless for establishing guilt), and argued that 'they being kept awake would be more the active to cal their Imps in open view the sooner to their helpe'.[10] But Hopkins and Stearne contrived to justify this practice. In modern times extremes of fatigue have proved to be a highly effective means of extracting the most outlandish confessions from detainees without recourse to physical force.[11]

Conspiracy and malice against individuals cannot be ruled out as motivations for the accusations, especially when one considers that Moore's case was not isolated. On the same day that Moore was examined and committed, two other accused witches from Sutton, John Bonham and William Watson (Bonham's wife having been taken into custody five days earlier), also confessed and were sent to Ely for trial. It is perhaps significant that the depositions for the three Sutton witches taken on this day consisted solely of the accused's confession and Wyne's brief and unsubstantiated information. The Bonhams were certainly unpopular in Sutton, and were prosecuted (unsuccessfully) at least twice for the suspected murder of their son – in 1636 and 1662; witchcraft was not mentioned in either prosecution. Watson's and Bonham's confessions were relatively simple in content, and did not specify what the suspects had to gain from their diabolical pact. Both confessed that the Devil appeared to them as a large mouse and a mole respectively, and both fed their familiar on blood pricked from their finger, before it set off to inflict damage on local livestock. But the case of Margaret Moore is different. Accusations made against her may well have been malicious, but, as with the other cases, this is very difficult to demonstrate. Of greater interest than the sincerity of the accusers, is the style and content of Moore's confession, because it concerns imagined power, and therefore has implications for the way in which an ordinary person might view his or her place in the world.[12]

III

Even if Margaret Moore was the victim of torture, there are grounds for thinking that her story was not concocted by her tormentors, but constructed in her own

mind from desire, emotion, experience and beliefs. Neither did the story necessarily originate at the time of her examination: long before that she could have
believed that she had actually seen the spirits and given her soul to the Devil,
thereby making her testimony a faithful account of an experience which, when challenged by her neighbours, she confessed out of a sense of remorse. In Continental
trials, it was common for the suspect's adherence to a confession to last only as
long as the torture under which it was extracted.[13] Moore, however, confessed
three times before different audiences: to Wyne and Jetherell; to Casten; and to
an assize court, suggesting the possibility of genuine belief in her own guilt. It is
possible that accumulated vocalized suspicions, rumours and accusations of witchcraft suggested to her that she actually possessed the powers attributed to her by
others. In criminological terms, 'primary deviation' might have been succeeded by
'secondary deviation' occurring when a suspect begins to accept his or her own
allotted role as a social deviant.[14] In this circular fashion, Moore could have assumed
the mantle of witch laid out for her by neighbours suspicious of her conversation
and behaviour.

Regardless of the influence exerted by her neighbours, delusions of the kind
described by her would have been understandable considering the loss of three children and her natural concern for the life of the last surviving child.[15] A modern
study of hallucinations experienced by the bereaved revealed that almost half the
subjects studied experienced visions of the dead, while their mental state remained
otherwise normal. Moreover, it is apparently common for such persons to believe
in the objective reality of what they have witnessed, and to feel comforted by the
experience.[16] Illusion and delusion deserve to be seen in the context of contemporary beliefs, since apparitions and fantasies, such as those experienced by Moore,
were formed in an area between universal human anxieties and aspirations on the
one hand, and specific cultural traits on the other.[17] Even if her experience can be
attributed to psychological behaviour recurrent over the centuries, it remains an
important event historically because of the specific form of the vision, and the
manner in which she interpreted and described it.[18]

The same recommendation would apply if Moore's vision was, in fact, a
dream.[19] It was common in this period for the sources of dreams to be identified
as carnal, divine or diabolic, and for their content to be interpreted in one of three
ways: as an excursion of the soul into the spirit world; as a symbol or as an apparition – a real encounter with a spirit.[20] Social anthropology provides an interesting
parallel here: in his famous study of modern African witchcraft, Evans-Pritchard
offered the following insight:

> It must be remembered that a bad dream is not a symbol of witchcraft
> but an actual experience of it. In waking life a man knows that he has
> been bewitched only by experiencing a subsequent misfortune or by
> oracular revelation, but in dreams he actually sees witches and may even
> converse with them. We may say that Azande see witchcraft in a dream
> rather than that they dream of witchcraft.[21]

Many sixteenth- and seventeenth-century sources include references to persons who
suffered nightmares attributed to the malign practices of witches.[22] But, as Moore's

case might suggest, dreams of witchcraft could also invade the sleep of the witch, and therefore a functionalist assessment (such as that of Evans-Pritchard) could be extended to allow for a greater consensus of belief between accuser and accused. Some studies of early modern witchcraft have even described opponents playing out conflicts at the dream level, with both witch and victim dreaming their respective roles.[23]

Boundaries separating the physical and the metaphysical, the natural and the supernatural, were drawn differently in the seventeenth-century mind,[24] and it has been argued that because the material world limits the possibilities open to the individual (in a way that the dream world does not), it is understandable that our ancestors were slow to dismiss the dream experience as an illusion. As one student of the subject has expressed it: 'if the waking world has certain advantages of solidity and continuity, its social opportunities are terribly restricted'.[25] If Moore's communion with the spirits of her children was indeed a dream – and it is no accident that this and similar visitations in other depositions occurred at night in the bed chamber – then considering her desperate condition, it may well have been an event of fundamental importance in her life, a perceived chance to enter an overlapping sphere between the worlds of life and death to alter the course of her fate.[26]

Seen in the context of prescientific mentalities in general, and her viewpoint in particular, Moore's witchcraft becomes just another form of power: defensive and offensive magic employed by a woman with limited comnmand of the resources of the natural world for the benefit of her family. The power to inflict *maleficium* might even be seen as a skill towards which some men and women actually aspired.[27] Whatever misfortunes the farmers of Witchford might have seen fit to explain by witchcraft, arguably Moore was fighting her own battle with adversity, and her words can be interpreted as reflecting her desire to conquer it. Although in many ways it is true that this explanation simply takes refuge in traditional functionalism, it does at least return a greater measure of human agency to the equation and the individual actions that constitute a witchcraft accusation can be seen to have been determined by personal belief and choice, rather than generalized patterns of behaviour shaped by impersonal forces. In other words, Moore could have been accused of witchcraft not simply because she looked and behaved according to a popular stereotype (the classic anthropological reduction), but because, for her own reasons, she herself believed that she was a witch.

There are obvious parallels between her case and the Faust myth: a transaction with the Devil in which the soul could be exchanged for material gain. This familiar fictional paradigm pervaded high literature, cheap print and folklore throughout mediaeval and early modern England, but is less commonly encountered in real English witchcraft trials. Faustian temptation played a part in the Lancashire trials of 1634, during which one suspect confessed that she was 'in greate passion & anger & discontented & w[i]thall oppressed w[i]th some want', and the Devil appeared and offered her all she needed in return for her soul. Overall though, the East Anglian examinations of the mid-1640s are unusual for the explicit presence of the Devil, and his offers of assistance to the poor, financial and otherwise.[28] Adam Sabie, for example, one of the suspects from Haddenham, confessed that a spirit had visited him in the form of a child and had comforted him with the words:

'ffeare not Sabie for I am thy God' and then told him to go to Lady Sandys' house where he would be given £20 – a substantial sum to a poor fenman. This pattern appears in the examination of suspects in other counties. In the Suffolk trials of 1645, one man was offered a deal by the Devil, 'he beinge at plowgh curseinge &c'; another was promised an annual income of £14 in return for his soul.

These confessions, forced or voluntary, took the form that they did because it was (and remains) common for poor or otherwise oppressed people to fantasize about the reversal of their predicament – Margaret Moore's specific fantasy, as we have seen, concerned resisting the domination of death and poverty.[29] One anthropologist has written: 'Witchcraft is in many respects the classical resort of vulnerable subordinate groups who have little or no safe, open opportunity to challenge a form of domination that angers them'.[30] In Moore's case though, as in many cases from the 1640s, the deployment of witchcraft by the poor and vulnerable person to resist domination serves constructive, personal ends at the expense of harm caused to others, not just causing harm for purposes of revenge.[31] It is specially noticeable in Moore's confession (and in others similar to hers) that the story turns from a description of personal powerlessness to a situation where the witch is issuing commands, at the precise moment the diabolical compact is sealed. Furthermore, it must be significant that one of Moore's familiar spirits shares her name, suggesting a more powerful alter ego, a supernatural version of herself, able to perform her will on earth in a way that she could not otherwise manage (the familiar of one of the other Sutton witches, John Bonham, was named John). In context, surrendering her soul for the sake of her child can be equated with a metaphysical extension of the principle of laying down life for love, and therefore represents an extension of power, whereby the soul is reified in an imaginary sphere as something with which she is able to bargain.

This chapter has not sought to explain the events which occurred at Sutton in 1647, still less to establish a new model of witchcraft prosecutions in early modern England as a whole. Rather, it has offered one interpretation among the many required to accommodate the wide variety of circumstances behind individual accusations – variety that more schematic interpretations can overlook. To this extent, neither argument nor example are intended to be in any way typical. On the other hand, an attempt has been made to readdress the more general problem of the functional value of witchcraft, by looking at a case where both accuser and accused offer their views on, first, the potency of magic and, secondly, the occasions on which such magic might have been used. Each of these areas of thought has an important implication for the long-term history of mentalities as a whole, and of witchcraft specifically. In the first place, participants in this drama demonstrate explicitly that they inhabit the same mental universe, a universe in which the boundary between the realms of the natural and supernatural was yet to be fixed. Second, it is possible to see that witchcraft accusations might be explained in terms of developing social and economic competition, without tying the dynamic to any particular aspect of this change. Together, these conclusions suggest that, until such time as developments in religious and scientific attitudes 'disenchanted' the world, and mounting pressure of population against resources was relieved by more favourable economic conditions, overlap between the material and invisible worlds would continue to offer not only a means of explaining misfortune – as for Margaret

Moore's accusers – but also a potential source of power with which the weak might seek to free themselves from the constraints of daily life and take control of their destinies.

Notes

1   For the best modern account of this extraordinary event, see James Sharpe, *Instruments of Darkness: Witchcraft in England 1550–1750* (London 1996), ch. 5. The exact number of executions in 1645–7 is unknown. Sharpe estimates that at least a hundred alleged witches were killed and 'the real total may have been comfortably over that figure'.

2   On the role of fear and insecurity in witchcraft accusations, see Chapter 3 in this book by Robin Briggs.

3   See for example, C. Z. Wiener, 'Sex roles and crime in late Elizabethan Hertfordshire', *Journal of Social History*, 8 (1975), 46–9; D. E. Underdown, 'Taming of the scold: the enforcement of patriarchal authority in early modern England', in A. Fletcher and J. Stevenson, eds, *Order and Disorder in Early Modern England* (Cambridge 1985), 116–36.

4   N. Z. Davis, *Fiction in the Archives: Pardon tales and their tellers in sixteenth-century France* (Stanford, Calif. 1987).

5   For full citations of the archival sources used in this chapter, see the original version in Jenny Kermode and Garthine Walker, eds, *Women, Crime and the Courts in Early Modern England* (UCL Press, London 1994), 125–45.

6   The parish register of Sutton indicates that on 10 May 1641, Robert Moore married Margaret Holland. This name cannot be found elsewhere in the Sutton register, but there was a Holland family in nearby Stretham, to whom a daughter, Margaret, was born 17 July 1586. This is probably too early to be Moore, but it is interesting that the verso of the 1647 deposition gives her parish as Stretham rather than Sutton.

7   J. Stearne, *A Confirmation and Discovery of Witchcraft* (London 1648), 219.

8   None of the three children were found in the parish register under the name of Moore, suggesting either Civil War under-registration, that they died before they could be christened, or that they were christened elsewhere.

9   Gaule, *Select cases of conscience,* 78.

10   Hopkins, *Discovery of Witches*, 5, 7.

11   See, for example, A. Koestler, *Darkness at Noon* (London 1940).

12   Lyndal Roper makes the point that, in spite of the stereotyped form of confessions, witches added their own personal inflections, and constructed their own narratives. See Chapter 24 in this collection. For a historian who is more pessimistic – where judicial sources are concerned – of the ability to 'unsnarl ordinary beliefs from the manipulative processes in which they were embedded', see R. C. Sawyer, "Strangely Handled In All Her Lyms": Witchcraft and healing in Jacobean England', *Journal of Social History*, 22 (1989), 462–3.

13   Brian P. Levack, *The Witch-Hunt in Early Modern Europe* (London 1987), 193, 196.

14   E. Lemert, *Human Deviance: Social problems and social control* (Englewood Cliffs, NJ 1972), ch. 3. See also Chapters 24 and 26 in this collection.

15   The emotionally charged issue of the lives of children could provide the key to other accusations in 1647. One of the Haddenham witches confessed that although she agreed to signing a pact with the Devil, she refused to surrender the life

of her child. In the early seventeenth century a high proportion of the cases of 'disturbing grief' encountered by the physician Richard Napier were bereaved mothers. See M. MacDonald, *Mystical Bedlam* (Cambridge 1981), 82.

16   W. D. Rees, 'The hallucinations of widowhood', *British Medical Journal*, 4 (1971), 37–41; E. Parish, *Hallucinations and Illusions: A study of the fallacies of perception* (London 1897), 36; W. E. Matchett, 'Repeated hallucinatory experiences as a part of the mourning process among Hopi Indian women', *Psychiatry*, 35 (1971), 185–9. See also J. Wertheimer, 'Some hypotheses about the genesis of visual hallucinations in dementia', in C. Katona and R. Levy, eds, *Delusions and Hallucinations in Old Age* (London 1992), 201–8, esp. p. 207, where it is stated that visions of the bereaved manifest 'the hallucinatory realization of the desire to rediscover the departed, and fantasized ambiguity of the absent presence'.

17   E. R. Dodds, *The Greeks and the Irrational* (Berkeley, Calif. 1951), 103–4, 116–17.

18   On the difficulty of separating universal and specific components of mentalities, see G. E. R. Lloyd, *Demystifying Mentalities* (Cambridge 1990), 135–6.

19   For a seventeenth-century ballad where, in different circumstances, starving children calling for food and drink haunt the dreams of the woman responsible for their death, see *The Midwife's Lamentation* (London 1693), in *The Pepys Ballads*, 8 vols, ed. H. E. Rollins (Cambridge, Mass., 1929–32), vii, 194–6.

20   Thomas, *Religion*, 151–3, 176, 286, 768–9; A. Macfarlane, *The Family Life of Ralph Josselin* (Cambridge 1970), 183n; H. J. Rose, *Primitive Culture in Greece* (London 1925), 151–2. The ancient Greeks did not speak of 'having' dreams, but of 'seeing' them. Dodds, *Greeks and the Irrational*, 105. Visions in early modern England were also described as waking dreams: in the 1680s Francis North explained the confessions by witches in these terms. R. North, *The Lives of the Norths*, ed. A. Jessopp, 3 vols (London, 1890), iii, 152. On the symbolic meaning of dreams, see Macfarlane, *Family Life of Ralph Josselin*, ch. 12.

21   E. E. Evans-Pritchard, *Witchcraft, Oracles and Magic among the Azande,* abridged edn (Oxford 1976), 230.

22   For some sixteenth-century examples of this, see C. L'Estrange Ewen, *Witchcraft and Demonianism* (London 1933), 70, 75–6.

23   See Chapter 8 in this collection by Carlo Ginzburg. Also relevant is Gustav Henningsen, *The Witches' Advocate: Basque witchcraft and the Spanish Inquisition* (Nevada 1980), which describes the dream aspect of sorcery and counter-sorcery in the Basque country in the early seventeenth century.

24   Macfarlane writes of 'reciprocity: associations of thought and event which worked across the artificial boundaries demarcating the social, physical and spiritual worlds'. *Family Life of Ralph Josselin,* 195.

25   Dodds, *Greeks and the Irrational*, 102.

26   D. H. Lawrence once wrote: 'When anything threatens us from the world of death, then a dream may become so vivid that it arouses the actual soul. And when a dream is so intense that it arouses the soul – then we must attend to it'. *Fantasia of the Unconscious* (London 1923; Penguin edn 1971), 165.

27   In 1632 an Essex woman was presented before the archdeacon's court for wishing herself to be a witch so as to be revenged on a neighbour with whom she had previously fought in the street. Macfarlane, *Witchcraft*, 286.

28   On the relationship between Faustian tales in cheap print and English witchcraft allegations, see D. Oldridge, *The Devil in Early Modern England* (Sutton 2000), ch. 7.

29   A petition from 1649 suggests that this was a time of high mortality, unemploy-
      ment, and poverty in Sutton, and called for redress for its inhabitants 'soe they
      may not all perish by famine in time of plentie as many allreddie doe'.

30   J. C. Scott, *Domination and the Arts of Resistance: Hidden transcripts* (New Haven,
      Conn. 1990), 36–44.

31   In the 1660s a poor Lancashire woman confessed to having been a witch since her
      mother died 30 years earlier. The mother had nothing to bequeath, and so left her
      daughters a pair of familiars. T. Heywood, ed., *The Moore Rental,* Chetham Society,
      Old Series, II (1847), 59–60.

Chapter 26

Louise Jackson

WITCHES, WIVES AND MOTHERS

Witchcraft persecution and women's confessions in seventeenth-century England

Introduction

IN AUGUST 1645 A SUFFOLK WOMAN Anna Moats was judged guilty of witchcraft at a special court of Oyer and Terminer held in Bury St Edmunds. Magistrates were told she had confessed, within two hours of her arrest, to having 'imps' or evil spirits and that the Devil had first appeared to her 'when she was alone in her house and after she had been curseing of her husband and her children'.[1] Branded as a scold and a witch, Anna had been persecuted for her failure to conform to the accepted norms of female behaviour – instead of fulfilling the expected role of a 'good' wife and mother she had been cursing and shouting at her husband and children. Anna was just one of over 100 individuals, mostly women, who were the victims of Hopkins, the remaining details of whose cases I shall be examining here. I shall try to show, through my examination of the remaining source material, not only that witch-hunting was woman-hunting – a way of sifting out subversive females – but that the women accused, in their confessions, were judging themselves in their role as neighbours, wives and mothers. Indeed it seems to be the case that some accused witches were, within their court confessions, contextualising their own insecurities and experiences within the linguistic framework of demonology.

The main primary source for my investigation of the 1645 trials is a manuscript account of the Suffolk depositions, now in the British Library, and which was transcribed and published in full by historian C. L'Estrange Ewen in the 1920s.[2] Ewen wrote that these depositions 'from their rough nature bear the appearance of having been taken down at the time of the examinations on three separate occasions or perhaps at their reading in the Court at the trials'.[3] The depositions name 91 accused witches and vary in length from a name, to a line to a paragraph. However, they are extremely useful, both qualitatively and quantitatively, since a large number contain details of what the witch was alleged to have told her confessors and how freely this information was given. These have been supplemented through the use of a tract written by Hopkins's assistant, John Stearne, in 1648 which gives further names and details about executions.[4] Ewen has estimated that a total of 124 witches can be traced who appeared in the Suffolk court in 1645 and it seems that 68 of these were executed.[5] At least 80 per cent of these 'Suffolk witches' were women.[6]

Many problems arise in using documents relating to witchcraft trials in general and these confessions in particular as source material. We have no records left directly by the women themselves. All written reports take the form of court records or pamphlets containing material selected by a male intermediary such as a court scribe. However, it is important to try to analyse the processes involved in the witchcraft confession because it can help lead us to a greater understanding of women's subjectivities and experiences in early modern England. To ignore these would be to draw a complete blank which would serve little other function than perpetuating the exclusion of women from history. Moreover, if we look at the source material carefully we can indeed find hints and clues as to what was happening for the women themselves. The confession text is a layered one – leading questions were asked of the women, sleep deprivation was sometimes used as a method of physical coercion, and the influence of witnesses and accusers is very apparent. However, there is still some input from the women themselves as they speak about their lives within the context of witchcraft belief.

Most major studies of the phenomenon have tended to concentrate on the power dynamics of the witch-hunts and have given political or economic analyses of the relationships between accusers and accused, church and state, or elite versus popular culture. Most recently, Marianne Hester has used a revolutionary feminist framework to analyse the witch-craze as part of the ongoing attempt to assert male supremacy over women through mechanisms of violence.[7] My aim is to approach the witch-hunts from a very different level: to try to examine what was happening from the perspective of the women who were themselves accused of being witches. This is not to say that the issue of power dynamics will not be taken into consideration, but that my central focus will be gauged at the level of the personal, and I will be mostly concerned with an attempt to put the experiences of the 'witches' themselves into our picture of events.

The process of confession

Christina Hole wrote that 'the problem of voluntary confessions has troubled many who share the widely held modern belief that all condemned witches were innocent victims of credulity and ignorance'.[8] In other words, why on earth did some women condemn themselves to death through their own utterances? Of course confessions were, in many cases, the result of ill-treatment; however, it is undoubtedly the case that some of the alleged witches do seem to have been quite ready and prepared to make confessions and statements that they had bewitched their neighbours. Witch trial sceptic Reginald Scot, writing in 1584, was clearly bothered by the incidence of voluntary confession; he decided the women concerned must be suffering some form of madness or delusion. Using contemporary medical terminology, he suggested that their over-vivid imaginations were brought on by an excess of the humour 'melancholy' in their bodies: 'If our witches phantasies were not corrupted, nor their wits confounded with this humor, they would not so voluntarily and readily confess that which calleth their life in question'.[9]

I do not believe pathology provides a sufficient explanation for the women's behaviour – can there really have been that many mad women in Suffolk and why should they all have thought they were witches? Nor do I believe, like Margaret Murray, that the women who claimed they were witches were actually members of some highly organised Dianic cult inherited from a pagan past.[10] Although a few of the women implicate others whom they worked with as witches, most do not. Most of the women, as I shall show in my examination of the Suffolk material, seem to have been very isolated in their role as witches.

Witchcraft, throughout the period, was treated as a 'secret crime'; this meant that, similar to poisoning, it was likely to be committed in private or behind closed doors. No one except the witch herself, could know about her meetings or compacts with the Devil. From a rationalist twentieth-century viewpoint it was also an 'impossible crime' – the criminal potential of witchcraft was completely dependent upon a belief in the spirit-world which had to be shared by victim, witnesses, judge and jury alike. Demonic possession, for example, was only possible in a society which believed it could actually happen. The implications of all this for an alleged witch were that many forms of evidence were accepted as proofs which would, at a later date, fail to stand up in a court of law. It was accepted that the appearance of familiars, the presence of witch-marks, even the abatement of an affliction after an alleged witch had been 'scratched', were all clear signs of proof.

When a case came before the court, evidence was given by four different categories of witness – accusers (often neighbours who claimed they were the victims of witchcraft), interrogators (such as Stearne and Hopkins who questioned the accused), watchers, and searchers. The watchers were employed to observe the witch in her home or in prison to see if her imps appeared. The searchers checked the woman's body for witch's marks, teats or paps from which her imps suckled. Most of the watchers and searchers mentioned in the text are women and often the same individuals performed both functions. Prissilla Brigs, for example, was employed to search Thomazine Ratcliffe and she told the court she had found two teats on her body. Abigail Brigs (her sister?) told the court that Thomazine had been in custody for 6 days and that during this time she had confessed to Abigail that she had killed her husband; Stearne, who also questioned Thomazine, expanded on her statements. All in all a total of 13 women and 45 men are actually named as court witnesses in the manuscript depositions. This gender ratio of one female to every four male accusers appears to represent a totally different pattern to that discovered by Clive Holmes in his analysis of Home Circuit witch trials. Holmes has discovered that nearly 50 per cent of witnesses were women in the Home Circuit counties during the seventeenth century. However, rather than seeing this as evidence of an equal involvement of men and women in the witch trials, Holmes goes on to show that leading men in the community instigated the legal process of prosecution and then mobilised their neighbours, often women, into giving confirmatory testimonies. It was the male elite, therefore, who set the legal ball rolling.[11] I do not think the picture in Suffolk was very different. Most of the 13 named women were watchers and searchers, involved in the court process, rather than individual informants. There are, however, several instances in which male witnesses refer to the 'bewitching' of their wives, to their comments and actions. It seems that in Suffolk, although women made informal allegations about other women in the village, their husbands may well have acted alone as official informants when the matter came to court.

Physical and mental pressures explain to a certain degree why a substantial number of women accused of witchcraft made the confessions they did; the amount of bullying and harsh treatment that was used against them must not be underestimated. However, this does not provide the whole picture. Some women clearly believed they had met the Devil and he had persuaded them to use witchcraft; their motives for believing this can only be unravelled by working towards an understanding of their material and psychological experiences.

The confession records show a great attention to detail and an interesting mix of popular elements of witchcraft belief (the Devil, imps) with localised, individualised aspects. There are interesting references in the Suffolk depositions to local topography (meetings with the Devil at named places in the neighbourhood) and domestic objects and food items (apples, butter) within a broader symbolic framework of a widely accepted demonology.[12] There is clearly an interaction taking place in the confession-making process; between the accused, her accusers and her interrogators; between a widespread witchcraft belief and individual experience. We need to treat the confession text as a palimpsest made of different layers of detail and interpretation, added one on top of another as different people became involved in the process of accusation and confession. An alleged witch may have told earlier versions of her story before she came into contact with the courts. At some point in her career she chose, for some reason, to take on the language of demonology to describe her actions and motives.

Thus production of a written confession was a very complicated and involved process. A real woman's life had been interpreted, altered and filtered through a linguistic system to become written words on a page. There are numerous stages in the process; but the common factor in each is the transforming power of language. Dale Spender has written that 'language is our means of classifying and ordering the world, our means of manipulating reality'.[13] Language is used to interpret and define experience and to give meaning to it. When I use the term 'experience' I am referring to physical and psychic events, how women reacted to them, and how women remembered them. Events become culturally organised experience when they have been labelled and examined within a set framework of belief.

Persecution and gender

The witch trials are significant in the study of gender relations and women's oppression because they are a clear example of organised state violence against women.[14] Although a few men were accused (20 per cent in the Suffolk sample), a significant number of these were associated with another female witch. The key to understanding the witch trials lies in their gender-specificity. The details of the cases refer directly to traditionally defined feminine space – the home, the kitchen, the sickroom, the nursery: to culturally defined female tasks or occupations and their direct opposites – feeding (poisoning), child-raising (infanticide), healing (harming), birth (death). Given the involvement of women in the dairying economy of Suffolk, it is hardly surprising, therefore, that the Suffolk material contains many references to witchcraft in the dairy and the bewitching of cattle. When things went wrong in the domestic world or the farmhouse – the cream curdled, the butter would not set or the child fell ill, witchcraft might be suspected. Women were in a potentially extremely powerful position through their control over child-rearing and feeding; the witchcraft persecutions can be seen as an officially sanctioned bid to control this threat and to reassert male power over women.

Woman were faced with a basic set of role models against which to judge themselves – the good wife, the witch, and the scold.[15] As I shall show, women were very aware of these constructions; both those who were being accused and those women who were participating in watching or making allegations, desperate to prove they were on the side of virtue before someone also tried to label them as witch.

The witch was the stereotypical opposite of the good wife. She was the woman who was trying to act entirely independently of male control, asserting her own powers, sexual and otherwise, to gain financial reward or carry out revenge on her enemies. The witch was a warning to women as to what would happen if they behaved in a way which could be counted as subversive. As I have said, the type of activities associated with witchcraft were a direct inversion of the traditionally accepted roles for women. The position of the 'scold' was a 'halfway house' – she was the woman who was just beginning to break out of control and therefore must be kept in order through the bridle or the ducking stool.

In the production of confessions, coercion was as much cultural as it was physical. Frameworks of belief about women's roles, responsibilities and expectations would lead women to condemn themselves. It is important to remember that it was a popularly held belief during the seventeenth century that the Devil existed as a material phenomenon and that any individual could meet him in a wood or on a country road. Chance meetings with strangers or animals could be explained in such a way. Explanations for both macrocosmic and microcosmic events were similarly sought in terms of God and the Devil. Hence, when Thomas Hudson fell lame and his doctor could find no cause for it he assumed that Ann Ellis of Metlingham had bewitched him; however, the deposition records that 'lately changeing his surgeon he doth now begin to mend' – and Ann was found innocent. The Devil also functioned in the psychological as well as the material world – on mind as well as body. Ann Laurence has shown that seventeenth-century women who gave testimonies to the civil war churches about their conversions referred to extremes of emotion in terms of religion:

> A woman who was convinced that God had ceased to love her because her transgressions reported that 'I had temptation by Satan to drown myself in a Pond', and another woman reported that it was only her unborn child which prevented her from destroying herself. Two other women mentioned suicide among the temptations offered by Satan, which they overcame thanks to God's intervention.[16]

Personal life crises such as suicide attempts and depression were almost always seen as temptations from the Devil; desire to carry out acts which were considered 'morally bad' was associated with evil. What we today might choose to call undesirable thoughts, impulses, or drives were in early modern England seen as external influences on the individual and were associated with the Devil. In shorthand, Satan was everything you did not want to admit to.

The temptations of the Devil were a particular feature of the conversion narratives produced by members of baptist and other sects. Presbyterian Hannah Allen described in her autobiography, which took the form of a religious testimony, how she had battled against the Devil during the dark days of her melancholy to regain her faith and happiness in God: '12th May 1664. Still my time of great distress and sore trials continues. Sometimes the Devil tempts me woefully hard and strange thoughts of my dear Lord which, through his mercy, I dread and abhor the assenting to, more than hell itself'. She also recorded that the Devil had suggested to her that she must die and be with him.[17] Baptist Sarah Davy, in her autobiographical account, *Heaven Realised,* described how her 'distrustful heart' was 'exercised with variety of temptations by the Devil as to distrust the goodness of the Lord'.[18] The language Hannah Allen and Sarah Davy used to describe their emotional despair is not very different, as I will show, from the words attributed to the women of Suffolk in their witchcraft confessions.

Witches, wives and mothers

What I would like to suggest, by looking closely at some of the material in the Suffolk cases, is that women's insecurities as wives and mothers as well as traumas about experiences or events, were being played out through the framework of the witchcraft confession.

Susanna Stegold of Hintlesham was found guilty of using witchcraft to kill her husband. One of the inquisitors, John Easte, read out her confession in court. She had, he said, confessed that the Devil had first come into her after her marriage and that she knew she had special powers because her greediest pig had died when she had wished it would stop eating. The marriage seems to have been an extremely unhappy one for Susanna; she may well have been beaten or ill-treated. She had allegedly confessed that her husband was a 'bad husband' and Susanna clearly hated him. Indeed her strength of feeling was so intense that, when he died mad, she seems to have believed she had killed him through her own evil thoughts:

> Her husband being a bad husband she wished he might depart from her meaning as she said that he should die and presently after he died mad bewitched him or not and said she wished ill wishes to him and what so ever she wished came to pas.

In common law a man was entitled to beat his wife (so long as it was not fatal) and a woman was supposed to accept it as her due – only when a woman's life was actually in danger could the ecclesiastical court intervene.[19] Susanna's husband had obviously made her suffer in some way but it is she who was racked with guilt.

She knew that sickness which had no obvious natural explanation was attributed to the Devil. Hence the framework of belief about gender roles and about the association between witchcraft and illness caused her to feel his death might be her fault. She assumed she was a witch and went on to confess that she had three evil spirits or imps. For Susanna, belief in the Devil seems to have been a way of coping with guilt or hiding the emotional trauma.

Susanna's case is not the only one in which it appears that a victim of abuse may have taken on the language of demonology to explain her feelings or experience. Margaret Benet confessed that 'the divell in the shape of a man . . . carried her body over a close into a thicket of bushes and there lay with her and after scratched her hand with the bushes'. Jana Linstead 'met with the devill in the shape of a man who wold have lyen with her but she denied him whereupon he threatened her but did her noe hyrt'. Widow Thomazine Ratcliffe 'confessed that a month after the death of her husband there came one to her in the shape of her husband and lay heavy upon her and she asked him if he wold kill her and he answered in the voice of her husband no I will be a loving husband'.

Belief in the Devil could provide a framework to describe a situation in which a woman was frightened or felt threatened and which she was unable to articulate in any other way. With no other language available to describe or explain her feelings, belief in the Devil became the only answer. Nazife Bashar has shown that, while rape legislation existed in early modern England, prosecutions were very few.[20] It is likely that in many instances, women did not possess the vocabulary to describe a bad experience as rape. Furthermore, if these are cases of abuse it is very significant that the women should assume they themselves are actually guilty of witchcraft as a result of the experience. As victims they are seeing themselves at fault and blaming themselves for what has happened.

I have chosen to examine next the cases of Susanna Smith and Prissilla Collit since they both contain references to infanticide, a crime which has recently been associated with post-partum psychosis but which, in seventeenth-century England, was seen as the work of the Devil. Again it was a subversion of the normal 'motherly' female role. Suicide, also referred to in these cases, was a great sin according to the church and canon law and was similarly the work of the Devil.

Prissilla Collit of Dunage confessed, after she had been watched in custody for three nights, that the Devil had appeared to her when she was sick some twelve years previously and tempted her to kill her children to escape poverty. She refused to make a covenant on this occasion but did place one of her children next to the fire to burn it. Fortunately another child pulled its sibling away from the fire:

> In a sickness about 12 years since the divell tempted to make away with her children or else should always continue poor, and he then demanded a covenant of her which she did deny, but she carried one of her children and layed it close to the fire to burne it, and went to bed again and the fire burnt the hare and the head lininge and she heard it cry but cold not have the power to help it, but one other of her children pulled it away.

Here the Devil is performing both a practical and psychological function. Firstly, for poor women like Prissilla, who had no economic resources or means of bettering their lives, a pact with the Devil could, they hoped, bring financial security. It was a common cultural belief that the Devil could bring his servants money and other rewards and could help them against their enemies. Indeed Prissilla confessed the Devil promised her 10 shillings for sealing the covenant although she never received it.

Other women, in their confessions, mention similar unfulfilled promises. Elizabeth Hobert, for example, covenanted with the Devil that, in return for her body and soul, she would be avenged of those who angered her and would be furnished with money; he never performed it, however. Women may well have 'turned to witchcraft', through conscious decision, as a solution to poverty and powerlessness. Some of them may even have been open about their activities as a way of achieving status in the village, status which for poor women was impossible to achieve in any other way. Marianne Hester, analysing the 1566 Chelmsford cases of Elizabeth Frauncis, Agnes and Joan Waterhouse, has suggested that all three women were using witchcraft as a 'means of empowerment: to obtain a rich husband and various commodities, to get their own back on their husbands or neighbours or to kill their husband with whom they quarrelled'.[21]

In Prissilla Collit's case the Devil came up with another practical suggestion – killing her children to escape poverty. The links between infanticide and poverty were strong throughout this period: Sharpe, in his study of Essex court cases, has shown that most women accused of infanticide were unmarried mothers, often domestic servants, who could not afford to bring up a child and were forced into the act out of desperation.[22] Of course it is impossible to tell whether prosecutions reflected the actual incidence of the crime – were single domestic servants simply more likely to be suspected than married women? However, although we cannot properly answer this question, it is undoubtedly true that infanticide was, for some women, a solution to poverty and desperation.

In discussing infanticide and the Devil it is important to consider the psychological role of demonic intervention as an explanation of behaviour. Wrightson has shown that certain assumptions were generally made as to what 'normal' maternal feelings consisted of; he quotes the writer William Gouge who, in 1622, praised the 'tender care' of the mother for the child, and argued that God had 'so fast fixed love in the hearts of parents as if there be any who it aboundeth not, he is counteth unnatural'.[23] Although the courts were just beginning to accept illness as mitigation for infanticide in the most exceptional cases, there was no discussion of what we would perhaps now term post-natal depression or post-partum psychosis. Unmarried servant girl Sinah Jones, tried at the Old Bailey in 1668, was sentenced to death for stifling her baby although she said 'she knew nothing of the cloath in the mouth of the child, and that she had not her senses and was light-headed'.[24] Infanticide was considered a crime against God and nature; it was a deviant subversion of the role of the 'godly' mother and therefore likely to be associated with witchcraft. One has only to glance over the pages of *Malleus Maleficarum* to find many references to witches cutting up and eating babies, inducing abortions, and cutting off male reproductive organs.

Murder and harm to children is a common feature of many of the witch trials and the Suffolk material is no exception – approximately 20 per cent of the Suffolk 'witches' were accused of harming or killing children. It is interesting, however, that several of the Suffolk witches confessed to trying to kill their own children rather than someone else's. Generally, as Thomas and Macfarlane have shown, the typical accused witch was the older woman in the village, usually a widow or spinster who lived on her own.[25] However, in the Suffolk material some 24 of the women named as witches are either specifically referred to as *uxor* (Latin, meaning married woman) or wife, or mention is made of a husband. One woman, Elizabeth Deekes, is described as 'a silly young woman'.[26] We know that 10 of the women were widows, but in most cases marital status is not given. Although no ages are given, by no means all the women are post-menopausal since mention is made of young offspring. It could well be that, as a result of the frenzied witch-hunting activity generated through the involvement of Matthew Hopkins, the concept of who was a likely suspect expanded to encompass younger women. Hoffer and Hull have described the growth in persecutions for infanticide and witchcraft at this time as attempts to control deviant young women and deviant old women respectively.[27] In Suffolk in 1645, however, it can be argued, the two crimes were no longer distinctive but were, rather, closely merged; younger women were accused of witchcraft and, furthermore, accused witches of different ages produced confessions of trying to kill their children at the suggestion of the Devil.

Prissilla Collit had clearly been very ill when the Devil appeared to her suggesting she kill her children to escape poverty; she may well have been feverish and confused, light-headed like Sinah Jones, or suffering from psychosis. Lyndal Roper has suggested that mothers who accused their lying-in-maids of bewitching their newborn children in Reformation Augsburg were projecting their own negative feelings towards their infants (perhaps a result of post-partum psychosis) on to others.[28] A similar process may have been taking place in Prissilla Collit's case – she, however, projected her 'evil' feelings against her children on to the Devil, leaving herself in a dangerously complicitous position. It is important to emphasise that concepts of 'self' are historically and culturally specific, framed by structures of language and belief. In the seventeenth century undesirable thoughts, impulses or drives, instead of being seen as the subconscious or unconscious stirrings of the Freudian psyche, were viewed as something separate from and indeed alien from the self. In Prissilla's case the battle against what society told her were normal natural motherly feelings and her own 'sinful' impulses appears to be articulated in terms of God and the Devil. Speaking in terms of the Devil could be a way of trying to exonerate herself from personal blame, although of course this backfired and resulted in a witchcraft accusation.

Prissilla was not the only Suffolk woman who referred to infanticide in her confession. Mary Scrutton, a married woman, confessed that the 'Devil appeared to her twice, once like a bear, once like a cat, and that she tempted her in a hollow voice to kill her child'. It is worth noting that this is the only reference I have come across to the Devil as a 'she' – one can only presume the change of gender occurred because the cat was seen as female. Susanna Smith confessed to Robert Mayhew the day after her arrest that 18 years previously the Devil had appeared to her in the form of a shaggy red dog and tempted her to kill her children. We are told that 'she strove with him 24 hours before he went from her but she would not kill them'. Just as the godly woman was supposed to nurture her offspring, so, in popular eyes, the witch figure destroyed them. If infanticide was the work of the Devil, a woman could be easily led to assume she had the Devil in her if she even questioned her relationship with her children.

The case of Susanna Smith is particularly interesting because the rest of the deposition is based on incidents which took place while she was in prison and therefore tells us much about the state of mind of an accused witch awaiting her fate. Although she began confessing, the questioning had to stop because her throat was so swollen she could not speak, possibly for medical reasons and possibly through trauma. The deposition says that 'being desired to relate further of her witchcraft there rise two swellings in her throat so that she cold not speake'. When Mayhew returned the following day to complete the session Susanna told him the Devil had appeared to her the day before her arrest and told her to fast

> She confessed that the Devil . . . appeared to her in likeness of a black bee and told her that she should be attached [arrested] the next day and that if she confessed anything she should die for it and being demanded why she would eat nothing there being good meat provided for her she said the divell told her she sholde never eate nor drink againe but they then provided and brought her meat and with much trembling she got some down.

Susanna is now describing the traumas she is suffering as a result of imprisonment in terms of the Devil because that is the language she has been given. Mayhew has, presumably, been questioning her for two days about her involvement with the Devil and, in her disordered state, she turns to this frame of reference to describe her emotions. Susanna's personal experience is being shaped and created in terms of demonological language right before our eyes.

Susanna decides to refuse food, saying that the Devil has told her to do so. We can, if we choose, read her fast as a desire to withdraw into herself, to separate her inner self from her body; in a similar way the swelling in her throat cut off all communication with the outside world since she could not speak. In rejecting the food brought to her by her enemies the gaolers, Susanna was perhaps aiming to gain more control of her situation; the interrogator was in a clear position of dominance and she may have been trying to take back some of that power for herself.

Susanna allegedly told her confessors on the next occasion that the Devil had given her a knife so she could kill herself:

> The divell had told her were there a rusty knife in the room where with she might kill herself and they looked in that place and found such an old knife as she described but she said that she cold not kill herself because they was . . . in the next room.

Hatred of her bodily existence and desperate fear of what will happen to her combine to make Susanna contemplate suicide. This is a theme which crops up several times in the Suffolk material and the conceptualisation of suicide as the work of the Devil is very interesting, particularly because of the close similarities in language between the witchcraft confession and the religious testimonies provided by 'the godly' of the civil war churches (as quoted above). Lidea Taylor confessed 'that her imps counselled her to steale and that they counselled her to kill herself'. Ellen Greenehif confessed that her 'mother did send her 3 imps that after she had them she often tempted to kill herself'. Elizabeth Fillet of Wetherden confessed that 'the divell tempted her to kill herself to avoid the scandal of prosecution'. Suicidal tendencies, like those of infanticide, were conceptualised as an external force (the Devil), acting on or overriding a woman's will. Suicide was seen as a sin by the church, preventing proper Christian burial on sacred ground, and was a crime according to the law of the land. Michael Dalton described it in 1626 as 'an offence against God, against the king and against Nature' (like infanticide it was 'unnatural').[29] Those who were alleged to have taken their own lives were tried posthumously by a coroner's jury, and if found guilty of self-murder (as it was usually known) had their goods confiscated and, as popular custom had it, were buried at a crossroads face-down in the grave and with a stake driven through them to stop their malevolent souls from straying.

In their search for personal or spiritual identity (both closely interconnected at this time) both the godly Puritans of the civil war sects and the women who ended up in court as accused witches spoke of battles against the Devil. Both confession and testimony were personalised accounts of experience which followed a very standard stylised format.[30] Both spoke of the influence of the Devil. It was a fine line between saint and witch. It was context which decided how that woman would be labelled – as Hopkins very visibly and openly hunted through Suffolk, it is likely that more and more women began to question their own behaviour in terms of witchcraft. The witch-hunts created the witch; the civil war churches created the mystic conversion of their members.

Although Susanna Smith threatens to commit suicide, she does not do it. Similarly she made a point of refusing food but then ate. To some extent she appears to be playing games with her interrogators. In both instances she is telling them that, although they have locked her in gaol and can ultimately dispense with her if they wish, she still has control over her own body in the meantime – she at least has the power to starve herself or take her own life if she chooses. Susanna is amazingly resilient and resourceful given the limited circumstances; for others it was not so easy.

Conclusion

While historians have, for the most part, concentrated on recreating the political and social agenda within which the witch-hunts were set, it is also important to look at the impact this had on women's lives – particularly those women who were involved in the trials. A couple of recent studies have opened up the discussion on the role of women in the witch-hunts – Roper's analysis of the motivations of mothers as accusers, and Holmes's study of women witnesses.[31] I have tried to add to this discussion by focusing on those women who were the direct targets of the persecution, and by showing that it is possible to carry out a productive examination of the different 'meanings' of their alleged confessions despite the complicated problems surrounding the use of such a source. I have tried to listen for their voices, however faint.

The standard formula of the witchcraft confession provided a set framework of meanings within which the accused witch presented and thereby defined her own experiences. It is important to stress that it has not been my intention to put clear labels on these experiences. Confession texts, as I hope I have demonstrated through my study of the Suffolk material, can be 'read' in a number of ways. However, it *is* possible to use these texts to open different windows on to the lives of the women who said they were witches.

Firstly, we can see that emotional responses to events and concerns were being articulated through the medium of the witchcraft confession; demonological language and the conventions of witchcraft belief were used to cover or explain personal traumas, insecurities or dilemmas. The references to sexual assault and abuse are veiled but present; those to suicide, and 'bad' husbands much easier to find.

Secondly, it is clear that the witchcraft confession was intricately connected with self-identity; it specifically required a woman to judge herself and her behaviour within the constraints of demonological language. For a few women self-definition as a witch could be a form of empowerment. For others, however, who refer to feelings of guilt, remorse and shame, it was very much a negative construct. Margaret Legat allegedly told an informant she was 'a damned creature'; and Elisabeth Warne 'confessed that pride and lustfullness had brought her to this and desired she might be walked apace for she had the Devil within her'.

I have shown how the image or stereotype of the witch had been defined as the opposite of the good or godly woman (particularly in her roles as wife and mother). The Suffolk cases contain many references to nagging wives or lewd women, infanticide and child care. These cases clearly show that the accused women, in their confessions, were judging themselves as wives and mothers – they were judging their angers, their bitterness, their fears and their failures to live up to the expectation of others.

These conclusions also provide us with an answer to Christina Hole's problem of 'the voluntary confession'.[32] The Suffolk women who confessed that they were witches were also confessing that they were 'bad' mothers, 'bad' wives and 'bad' neighbours. The cultural, social and psychological impact of the county-wide witch-hunt cannot be over-estimated – the knowledge that 'witches' existed and were rife at home and abroad may well have caused every woman to examine her life very closely, and some to come forward and confess. Women's insecurities about their roles as wives and mothers were being played out within the context of the witchcraft confession.

Notes

1   C. L. Ewen, *Witch Hunting and Witch Trials* (Kegan Paul, London 1929), 305.

2   British Museum Add. MS. 27402, fos 104–121; Ewen, *Witch Hunting and Witch Trials,* Appendix VI, 291–313. Unless otherwise stated, all quotations in this chapter are from this source.

3   C. L. Ewen, *Witchcraft and Demonianism* (Heath, London 1933), 302.

4   J. Stearne, *A Confirmation and Discovery of Witchcraft* (London 1648).

5 Ewen, *Witchcraft and Demonianism*, 302.

6 It is not possible to attribute sex in cases where surname only is given. The 80 per cent represents those accused known to be women.

7 See Chapter 21 in this collection by Marianne Hester. For a more extensive treatment, see her *Lewd Women and Wicked Witches: A study of the dynamics of male domination* (Routledge, London 1992).

8 Christina Hole, *A Mirror of Witchcraft* (Chatto & Windus, London 1957), 182.

9 Reginald Scot,*The Discoverie of Witchcraft* (Dover Publications, New York 1972), 33.

10 M. Murray, *The Witch-Cult in Western Europe* (Oxford 1921).

11 See Chapter 23 in this book by Clive Holmes.

12 For example, Margaret Benet confessed that 'the Devil met her as she came from Newton' and Margaret Spara confessed that she met the Devil in the wood at Mendam. Katherine Tooley sent her imp Jackly to meet the minister on the road from Celsol to Westleton to strike him and his horse dead.

13 D. Spender, *Man-made Language* (Routledge and Kegan Paul, London 1980), 30.

14 See Hester, *Lewd Women and Wicked Witches*.

15 See S. Amussen, 'Gender, family and social order 1560–1725', in A. Fletcher and J. Stevenson, eds, *Order and Disorder in Early Modern England* (Cambridge University Press 1985).

16 A. Laurence, 'Women's psychological disorders in seventeenth-century Britain', in A. Angerman, G. Binnema, A. Keunen, V. Poels and J. Zirkzee, eds, *Current Issues in Women's History* (Routledge, London 1989).

17 Hannah Allen, *Satan his Methods and Malice Baffled* (1683), extracts printed in E. Graham, H. Hinds, E. Hobby and H. Wilcox, eds, *Her Own Life: Autobiographical writings by seventeenth century women* (Routledge, London 1989), 202–4.

18 Sarah Davy, *Heaven Realised* (1670), extracts printed in Graham, Hinds, Hobby and Wilcox, eds, *Her Own Life*.

19 Martin Ingram, *Church Courts, Sex and Marriage in England 1570–1 640* (Cambridge University Press 1987).

20 N. Bashar, 'Rape in England between 1500 and 1700', in London Feminist History Group, eds, *The Sexual Dynamics of History: Men's power, women's resistance* (Pluto Press, London 1983).

21 Hester, *Lewd Women and Wicked Witches*, 163.

22 J. A. Sharpe, *Crime in Seventeenth Century England* (Cambridge University Press 1983), 6.

23 Quoted in K. Wrightson, 'Infanticide in earlier seventeenth century England', *Local Population Studies*, 15 (1975), 11.

24 Nigel Walker, *Crime and Insanity in England* (Edinburgh University Press 1968), 126.

25 Macfarlane, *Witchcraft in Tudor and Stuart England*, 161; Thomas, *Religion*, 671.

26 Stearne, *A Confirmation and Discovery of Witchcraft*, 12.

27 P. Hoffer and N. Hull, *Murdering Mothers* (New York University Press 1981), 28.

28 L. Roper, *Oedipus and the Devil* (Routledge, London 1994), ch. 9.

29 Quoted in M. Macdonald (1986) 'The secularization of suicide in England 1660–1800', *Past and Present*, 111 (1986), 253.

30 See Graham, Hinds, Hobby and Wilcox, eds, *Her Own Life*, 165, for a discussion of the structure of the conversion narrative. A woman would be required to examine her experiences, looking for 'signs that God had destined her for heaven and to draw out broader theological lessons from things that happened to her'.

31   The study by Clive Holmes is Chapter 23 in this book. For Roper's analysis of
     the motives of mothers making witchcraft allegations, see her *Oedipus and the
     Devil*, ch. 9.
32   Hole, *A Mirror of Witchcraft*, 182.

PART NINE

The Decline of Witchcraft

IT IS IRONIC THAT THE EARLIEST BOOK on witchcraft printed in England, Reginald Scot's *The Discoverie of Witchcraft* (1584), is also the one sixteenth-century text on the subject that seems consistent with the dominant views about magic in our own age. Alone among sceptical writers in his lifetime, Scot not only rejected the notion of a pact between witches and the Devil, but also challenged the whole concept of sorcery. The effects of *maleficium* were, he asserted, no more than fables and delusions; and the misfortunes attributed to witches were incompatible with the orderly and immutable purposes of God:

> If all the devils in hell were dead, and all the witches in England burnt or hanged, I warrant you we should not fail to have rain, hail and tempests, as now we have, according to the appointment and will of God, and according to the constitution of the elements, and the course of the planets, wherein God hath set a perfect and perpetual order.[1]

Scot's impassioned attack on the 'fables of witchcraft' sought to expose what he regarded as the superstitious beliefs of most ordinary people, and to bring an end to the sporadic witch trials that had begun in his native Essex some twenty years earlier. It is arguable that his work had some influence on the treatment of witches in England in the late sixteenth century; but his arguments made little impression on European demonology as a whole. Indeed, James VI of Scotland denounced him as a deluded 'Sadducee' on the first page of his own work on witchcraft in 1597, and this view was endorsed by the major writers on the subject until the middle years of the seventeenth century.[2]

It is tempting to ascribe Scot's failure to the extraordinary, even 'far-sighted' nature of his thinking. But this is a temptation best resisted. While Scot was unusual among sixteenth-century writers in his emphasis on the 'natural causes' of phenomena, he belonged to a Renaissance tradition that dismissed most magical works as delusions inspired by the Devil, and his argument that God's power in the world rendered witchcraft impossible was a logical extension of conventional Protestant theology, which attributed all events to the ultimate designs of the Lord.[3] Potentially at least, the implications of this view were similar to the 'mechanical' model of the universe later accepted by many seventeenth-century intellectuals: in a world ruled by the 'perfect and perpetual order' of God, there was simply no place for miracles, magic or witchcraft. The eventual triumph of this view is often cited as a crucial factor in the decline of witch trials. But since Scot's position was already consistent with some of the most powerful currents in sixteenth-century theology, the truly remarkable aspect of his work was its failure to gain support among other intellectuals. To the extent that witch persecutions were inspired by the beliefs of educated men, this point is crucial to the debate about the decline of witchcraft in Europe.

One part of the solution to this puzzle seems obvious. It was not until the mid-seventeenth century that a new 'mental outlook' emerged that was more sympathetic to Scot's brand of scepticism. The key elements of this new outlook are described by Brian Levack in Chapter 27. Levack identifies the rise of empirical investigation as one critical development, since it undermined the kind of scholastic reasoning that had previously supported demonological writings. With this in mind, it is instructive to compare the arguments of early works on witchcraft like the *Malleus Maleficarum* (1486) with late publications such as Richard Baxter's *The Certainty of the World of Spirits* (1692). While Kramer and Sprenger were able to present a convincing case based largely on biblical and classical precedents, Baxter was forced to rely on empirical 'evidence' of witchcraft such as eyewitness accounts of *maleficium*. The result was a much less persuasive work, as Baxter's sources were open to question in a way that the 'authoritative evidence' of the *Malleus* was not. This new approach to evidence was also expressed in courts of law, where judges demanded increasingly high standards of proof in cases of alleged witchcraft. The empirical approach was complemented by a new emphasis on 'natural processes' as the causes of physical events. This provided alternative explanations for phenomena previously identified with harmful magic, such as epilepsy and mental illness; and it also discouraged belief in supernatural events that disturbed the mechanical order of the universe.

In some respects, the changed intellectual climate was sufficient in itself to explain the spread of doubts about witchcraft among educated men in the second half of the seventeenth century. The new emphasis on empirical investigation posed a methodological challenge to demonology that was generally lacking in the arguments of sixteenth-century sceptics. As Levack points out, however, other aspects of the 'new thinking' were present in sceptical texts during the worst periods of witch persecution. As early as the 1560s, Johann Weyer attributed *maleficium* to natural causes like melancholy and disorders of the uterus; and Reginald Scot argued that witchcraft was incompatible with God's orderly creation. What changes occurred to make these beliefs acceptable after 1660 when they had been widely rejected a hundred years earlier? It is difficult to explain the shift in terms of medical or scientific discoveries, since medical practice remained basically unchanged throughout the seventeenth and eighteenth centuries, and the major breakthrough in pure science, Newton's *Principia Mathematica* (1687), postdated the decline in European witch trials. It seems that we need to look beyond the world of ideas for a satisfying explanation of the rise of scepticism among educated Europeans, and consider changes in the wider social and political circumstances which allowed new attitudes to flourish. For Levack, the most important reason why the arguments of Weyer and Scot became acceptable in the late seventeenth century was that they 'no longer posed a threat to religion, philosophy or the social order'. This insight relates the decline of witch beliefs in learned circles to the wider phenomena of confessionalism and religious conflict, which had previously encouraged such beliefs among Catholic and Protestant elites. The religious warfare that had dominated western Europe in the first half of the seventeenth century ended with the Treaty of Westphalia in 1648, creating a climate in which the apocalyptic struggle between God and the Devil — and his various earthly allies — was a less pervasive political theme. At the same time, the declining threat of religious insurrection within most European states allowed the gradual and limited acceptance of toleration. This development relates to the argument of Stuart Clark in Chapter 12 that witch beliefs made sense only in the context of 'church-type' religious organisations which demanded universal conformity. As Clark suggests, one reason for the decline of witch persecutions 'was the coming of a religious pluralism that permitted the members of all types of churches to coexist and spelt the end of the confessional state'.[4]

These general factors go some way towards explaining the decline of witch beliefs among elite groups, but it is important also to recognise the particular circumstances of different European regions. In certain circumstances, it appears that the desire for religious conformity could actually encourage the suppression of witch beliefs, since they posed a threat to the state church. Gábor Klaniczay presents a fascinating example of this process in Chapter 28. He argues that popular anxieties about vampires in eighteenth-century Hungary compromised the status of holy objects in the Catholic church, as the bodies of vampires, like the uncorrupted relics of the saints, were believed to be immune from ageing and decay. Thus vampire beliefs provided an alternative — and wholly unacceptable — explanation for a phenomenon at the heart of official piety in the Habsburg state. It was the desire to eliminate this threat that led the government to condemn vampire lore as a form of vulgar superstition; and one consequence of this was the prohibition of witch trials in 1766, since witches were closely linked to vampires in popular culture. A similar process can be detected in England in the early seventeenth century, when witchcraft became entangled with the politically contentious subject of demonic possession. Following the trial of the puritan exorcist John Darrel in 1599, and the ensuing pamphlet war which identified Protestant nonconformity with belief in possession, the Church of England effectively banned the practice of exorcism.[5] This political act also undermined the idea of witchcraft, since possession was a common form of *maleficium*. In a recent study of the literature of English witchcraft, Marion Gibson has suggested that the controversy about possession discouraged the publication of witchcraft pamphlets, since the subject was tainted with official disapproval. She suspects that this development may explain the low level of witchcraft prosecutions in the decades before the civil war.[6] The experience of England and Hungary suggests that confessionalism could play a role in the decline of witch trials when this outcome coincided with the interests of the state church. In such circumstances, witch persecutions could end without the advent of religious toleration.

The discussion thus far has focused on the beliefs and actions of political elites, whose changing attitude towards witchcraft is traditionally cited as the major cause of the decline in persecutions. As Brian Levack notes, however, popular opinion was sometimes crucial in ending particular outbreaks of witch-hunting; and for historians like Wolfgang Behringer, who attribute witch trials primarily to popular fears of *maleficium*, the cessation of prosecutions was caused by new circumstances that alleviated these fears. Behringer suggests in Chapter 4 that the worst period of witch panics in Germany coincided with Europe's 'little ice age', and came to an end when weather patterns returned to normal. But while such factors probably contributed to the end of witch trials, it remains likely that the attitude of elite groups was more significant: the formal prosecution of witches depended on the support of the judiciary, and the withdrawal of this support made witch trials virtually impossible. There is, moreover, considerable evidence that witch beliefs survived in the general population long after they were abandoned in educated circles, and were eventually undermined by rather different factors. In Chapter 29, Owen Davies investigates the impact of urbanisation on the long-term decline of popular witch beliefs in England. He argues that the urban environement *per se* was not responsible for ending allegations of *maleficium*: indeed, such allegations were quite common in the London borough of Shoreditch until the early eighteenth century. A more crucial factor was the rapid turnover of population in some urban areas, as this disrupted the kind of neighbourhood relationships that were essential for witch beliefs to flourish. Davies notes that 'the reputation of a witch was usually generated and sustained through the long-term accumulation of supposed maleficent acts, held in the collective memory of the community'; and such reputations were hard to maintain in a largely transient population. Crucially, however, the effects of urban mobility did not undermine *all* magical beliefs: practices such as fortune-telling and the magical detection of thieves proved to be more enduring than the accusation of witches, since they did not depend on a stable social environment. Even some remedies against witchcraft remained widespread in London until the nineteenth century, as long as they did not involve a face-to-face confrontation with the alleged witch. Thus it was common to hang horseshoes on doors as a protection against *maleficium* until the 1830s.

As a corollary to Davies' thesis, we would expect to find that more personal kinds of witch belief survived in village communities where social mobility was more limited. While much work in this field remains to be done, the hypothesis is broadly supported by research from England and mainland Europe. In a classic study of folk religion in rural Lincolnshire, James Obelkevich has argued that *maleficium* still involved a personal relationship between a known suspect and her victim in the early decades of the nineteenth century, though the idea of witchcraft was gradually depersonalised during the Victorian age. The practice of 'scratching' alleged witches to remove their power continued long into the 1800s, and 'wise men' were still employed to combat the hurtful magic of individual witches.[7] Villagers continued to seek remedies against named witches in the early years of the twentieth century. When a man from Redmarley in Worcestershire was visited by a mysterious sickness in 1905, he accused a neighbouring woman of attacking him with the 'evil eye'.[8] It appears that similar attitudes survived elsewhere in Europe as late as the 1960s. Gustav Henningsen found a flourishing system of witch beliefs among the peasants and fishermen of Galacia in northern Spain during 1965–8: here the concept of witchcraft existed alongside conventional medicine as an explanation for disease, and both magic and psychiatry were employed to relieve the symptoms of mental illness.[9]

Notes

1   Peter Haining, ed., *The Witchcraft Papers* (Hale, London 1974), 67.

2   James Stuart, *Daemonologie* (Edinburgh 1597) preface, xi.

3   For another writer in this tradition, see H. C. Erik Midelfort, 'Johann Weyer and the Transformation of the Insanity Defence', in R. Po-Chia Hsia, ed., *The German People and the Reformation* (Cornell University Press, Ithaca, NY 1988). For a discussion of Protestant views of the power of Satan, see Jeffrey Burton Russell, *Mephistopheles: The Devil in the Modern World* (Cornell University Press, Ithaca, NY 1986), ch. two.

4   Stuart Clark, Chapter 12 in this collection.

5   See D. P. Walker, *Unclean Spirits* (Scolar, London 1981) for a full account of the controversy over possession and its aftermath.

6   Marion Gibson, *Reading Witchcraft* (Routledge, London 1999), 186–90.

7   James Obelkevich, *Religion and Rural Society* (Clarendon, Oxford 1976), 283–91.

8   Dorothy Amphlet, 'Worcestershire Folklore', in Francis Andrews, ed., *Memorials of Old Worcestershire* (George Allen, London 1911), 263.

9   Gustav Henningsen, *The Witches Advocate* (University of Nevada Press, Reno 1980), 12–13.

Chapter 27

Brian Levack

THE END OF WITCH TRIALS

DURING THE LATE SEVENTEENTH and early eighteenth centuries European witchcraft prosecutions declined in number and eventually came to an end. The decline did not occur simultaneously in all European countries and regions. In the Netherlands, for example, the decline became evident early in the seventeenth century, whereas in Poland prosecutions did not begin to drop off until after 1725. Despite these differences in timing, the decline of witchcraft was a European-wide phenomenon, and its occurrence within a one-hundred-year period in every country that had experienced witch-hunting suggests that there are general reasons for the end of the great witch-hunt, just as there were general reasons for its origin.

The decline of witchcraft prosecutions raises two major problems of interpretation. The first concerns the distinction between individual prosecutions and large hunts. There was a difference between the end of mass prosecutions that took scores if not hundreds of lives and the termination of all trials, no matter how small. The two developments are closely related, since many critics of witch-hunting opposed all trials, large and small, and because the negative reaction to some of the large panics contributed to the eventual termination of all witchcraft prosecutions. But the reasons for the decline of the two types of prosecution were not always the same. Large hunts came to an end as European communities, having experienced the social dysfunction that mass panics produce and having come to the conclusion that innocent people had suffered in the process, became determined to prevent the recurrence of such undertakings and establish legal procedures that would prevent the chain-reaction type of hunt from developing. These hunts also declined when the social, economic and religious conditions that helped to create a mood conducive to witch-hunting no longer prevailed. Individual witchcraft prosecutions, on the other hand, died out only after laws were passed prohibiting them or after the judicial authorities of a particular locality adopted a policy of refusing to try such cases. The decline of both types of witch-hunting required the emergence of a sceptical mentality, but the complete termination of witch-hunting was predicated upon a much more profound scepticism regarding the reality of witchcraft than that which caused the cessation of the large hunts.

The second problem of interpretation connected with the decline of witchcraft concerns the respective roles of the elite and the common people in the process. Traditionally historians have emphasized the part played by the ruling classes and the educated elite in bringing witch-hunting to an end. It was certainly within the upper levels of society that the new scepticism first took hold, and it was certainly these men who took the necessary political and legal steps to stop prosecutions completely. By way of contrast, popular witch beliefs showed little sign of changing at this time, and on numerous occasions members of the lower classes pushed for the prosecution of alleged witches, only to be frustrated by the refusal of a sceptical magistrate to countenance the prosecution. Nevertheless, the lower classes may have had much more to do with the decline of witchcraft than has been previously acknowledged. One scholar has argued that the hysteria manifested during the witch-hunts was mainly that of the bureaucratic class and that enlightenment came from the more rational common people.[1] It is true of course that the most extreme witch-beliefs, those most capable of sustaining a witch-hunt, came mainly from the upper classes and were shaped and disseminated mainly by them. It is also true that throughout the period of witch-hunting there was a tradition of lower-class scepticism that emerged when officials tried to obtain confessions. At the very peak of a major Scottish witch-hunt, for example, a woman from Newbattle in Midlothian challenged the entire theory of the Devil's mark, claiming that everyone had such bodily imperfections.[2] Even more important, the common people could and did play an important role in stopping large witch-hunts. Since they helped to sustain the mood of large witch-hunts, and since they also performed the essential judicial functions of denouncing and testifying against their neighbours, the common people had the capacity to bring witch-hunts to an end whenever they realized that the trials were doing more harm than good.

One of the best examples of the way in which the people of a community could take steps to stop a witch-hunt comes from the small German town of Lindheim, where in 1661 the magistrate, George Ludwig Geisz, executed a midwife and six other women for killing a child at birth and using the remains to concoct a magical ointment. He also arrested the mother and father of the child, who had testified that they did not suspect the midwife and had actually exhumed the baby's body to show that it was still intact. As the hunt developed (there were thirty executions in all) and when the father of the baby, a well-to-do miller, was tortured, sentiment in the town turned against the magistrate. The miller and a few other prisoners managed to escape and to present a counter-suit against Geisz at the imperial supreme court at Speyer, which ordered the witch-trials to cease. This action came too late to save the life of the miller's wife, but popular resistance to the trials became so strong that one man physically assaulted the judicial official who had come to arrest his wife, and Geisz himself was forced to flee.[3]

Although the lower classes did occasionally help to bring individual witch-hunts to an end, they cannot be credited with the primary responsibility for the long-term decline of witch-hunting. There is no evidence, for example, that European villagers of the late seventeenth and early eighteenth centuries gradually lost their magical beliefs and therefore became increasingly reluctant to accuse their neighbours of witchcraft. The number of formal accusations did in fact decline during these years, but this had nothing to do with popular scepticism or 'enlightenment'. Villagers made fewer witchcraft accusations against their neighbours either because they had little hope of prosecuting them successfully or because the conditions which encouraged them to do so no longer prevailed. In neither case could the villagers be considered to have actively caused the decline in accusations. Indeed, all the evidence regarding individual witchcraft prosecutions from the late seventeenth century until the end of the hunt suggests that they arose mainly in response to lower-class pressure and that any scepticism regarding the accusations came from the ruling classes and the educated elite.

It is tempting to claim that witchcraft prosecutions died of their own weight or that they contained the seeds of their own decline. To the extent that the conduct of the large hunts engendered criticism of the entire process of witch-hunting, this argument is certainly valid. But it would be misleading to assert that witch-hunts simply burned themselves out. The trials and even the large hunts went on long enough in the various regions of Europe to show that under certain circumstances the prosecution of witches could continue indefinitely. What brought the trials to an end was not simply a recognition that witch-hunting could get out of control, but a series of significant changes in European judicial systems, in the mental outlook of the educated and ruling classes, in the religious climate that prevailed throughout Europe, and in the general conditions in which people lived.

Judicial changes

In dealing with the decline of witchcraft it is appropriate first to discuss the various changes that took place in the operation of European judicial systems, both in general and with specific reference to witchcraft. These judicial changes deserve primary consideration because in most cases it was objections to witchcraft prosecutions on legal and judicial grounds that first led to their reduction in number. Indeed, some of the early critics of witch-hunting based their case solely on legal grounds, insisting that their scepticism was in no way philosophical.[4] These men actually facilitated the decline of witchcraft without abandoning the notion that witchcraft was possible or that witches did in fact exist.

There were three main judicial and legal developments that contributed to the decline of witchcraft: (1) the demand for conclusive evidence regarding *maleficium* and the pact; (2) the adoption of stricter rules regarding the use of torture; and (3) the promulgation of decrees either restricting or eliminating prosecutions for witchcraft. The first of these, the demand for more solid evidence of witchcraft, expressed itself in many different ways. It could take the form of a judicial decision that there was insufficient evidence to justify the use of torture, an investigation to determine whether *maleficium* might have had natural causes, an insistence on infallible proof of the demonic pact, or a more general plea for special caution in witchcraft cases.[5] Sometimes the sceptical demand for evidence would be based on the difficulty of establishing the actual commission of *maleficium*. In the late seventeenth century, for example, a number of judges became increasingly reluctant to accept the occurrence of misfortune shortly after the expression of hostility as proof that sorcery had in fact been practised. When we consider the fact that most charges of *maleficium* arose as attempts by neighbours to explain misfortunes that mysteriously beset them, the significance of this more demanding attitude becomes apparent. To prove the commission of *maleficium* one needed tangible evidence of magical intent, and without the actual instruments of magic (such as were often adduced in court against ritual magicians in the late Middle Ages) the case was difficult to prove. A similar scepticism arose regarding the demonic pact. Aside from confession itself, the main evidence regarding the pact was the Devil's mark. For more than one hundred years judges had accepted the mark as evidence of the pact, using it to allow torture and incorporating it into the libel or indictment. In the late seventeenth century, however, judges became increasingly reluctant to allow evidence of the Devil's mark to be admitted, thus making witchcraft prosecutions much more difficult to sustain.[6] A third type of evidence that was gradually excluded was spectral evidence, the testimony of an afflicted person that she could see the spectre or spirit of the offending party.

A second change in legal procedure that led to a significant reduction in witchcraft prosecutions and convictions was a growing reluctance to use torture as an instrument of judicial interrogation. The administration of torture had been criticized throughout the period of the great witch-hunt, both on humanitarian grounds and for the eminently practical reason that confessions adduced under torture were unreliable.[7] Nevertheless, the regular use of torture had persisted in most European jurisdictions, and it was because of torture, more than any other single factor, that large witch-hunts had been able to develop. During the seventeenth century, however, a number of European jurisdictions adopted much stricter rules than they had previously followed regarding both the application of torture and the admissibility of evidence obtained by it. Such rules were promulgated in Spain in 1614, in Italy in the 1620s and in Scotland in the 1660s.[8] Similar restrictions also emerged in various German principalities in the period after 1630, perhaps partially as a result of the publication of Friedrich Spee's *Cautio Criminalis,* a devastating critique of the procedures used in German witchcraft trials.[9]

Restrictions on the use of torture were followed ultimately by its complete abolition. This process, which was facilitated by the decline of non-capital punishments and a lower premium on confessions, occurred in Scotland in 1709, Prussia in 1740, Saxony in 1770, Austria in 1776, Belgium in 1787, Switzerland in 1803 and Bavaria in 1806. With the possible exception of Scotland, this final elimination of torture had little demonstrable effect on witch-hunting, if only because abolition came so late. Indeed, the desire to execute witches, which usually could not be accomplished unless confessions were forthcoming, was at least partially responsible for keeping the torture system functional. The abolition of torture became possible only when authorities no longer believed that witchcraft merited the death penalty.[10]

In addition to imposing restrictions on the use of torture, princes and legislative assemblies throughout Europe took deliberate steps in the late seventeenth and eighteenth centuries to reduce or eliminate witchcraft prosecutions. These proclamations often had a dramatic impact on the process of witch-hunting. An edict of Louis XIV of France in 1682, which prescribed only corporal punishment for acts of divination and classified the practice of magic as mere 'superstition', was largely responsible for bringing a virtual end to witch-hunting in France. One of the reasons it had such an effect was that it applied to the entire country and thereby greatly reduced the amount of judicial discretion that both local courts and the regional parlements had traditionally exercised in the treatment of witchcraft.[11] The same was true for the Prussian decrees of 1714 and 1721 against witchcraft prosecutions, and for the Polish prohibition of 1776.[12] We must not, however, assign too much significance to all such royal decrees and statutes, for some prohibitions of witchcraft trials were put into effect long after the trials had in fact ceased and therefore merely ratified an existing situation. The repeal of both the English and the Scottish witchcraft statutes by the Parliament of Great Britain in 1736 had very little practical effect and went virtually unnoticed by contemporaries because prosecutions in both countries had by that time long since come to an end. Nevertheless, in dealing with the decline of witchcraft, we must be aware of the fact that princes, central councils and representative assemblies very often did use their power to keep the prosecution of witches under control and in some instances effectively ended witch-hunting in their countries.

The new mental outlook

At the same time that judges and princes were creating new rules of evidence, restricting the use of torture, and banning witchcraft trials, changes were taking place in the mental world of European elites which made them sceptical regarding the reality of witchcraft. These changes were in fact closely related to the judicial changes we have just described, since judicial caution in handling witchcraft cases, the reluctance to use torture and the prohibition of trials were often based on a scepticism regarding the reality of the alleged crime. Although some magistrates and judges insisted that their scepticism was strictly legal and that witches did in fact exist, many harboured deep doubts about the reality of such phenomena and therefore were more inclined to insist upon complete proof or voluntary confession before conviction. Perhaps the best example of the combination and interaction of judicial and philosophical scepticism regarding witchcraft is the work of Christian Thomasius, a professor at the University of Halle who in the early years of the eighteenth century criticized both the system of judicial torture and prevailing witch beliefs.[13]

Although changes in mentality brought about a decline in witchcraft prosecutions only when they affected the magistrates and judges who were entrusted with criminal prosecutions, they were evident in a much broader cross-section of the European elite. Indeed, many of the early attacks on witch-beliefs were made by theologians, philosophers and scientists who had nothing to do with the prosecution of witches. Their ideas, however, gradually spread among educated Europeans and eventually penetrated the ruling and magisterial classes.

It is important to note that scepticism regarding witchcraft was not new to the seventeenth century. Throughout the period of the great witch-hunt there had always been a few individuals who questioned the reality of alleged acts of harmful magic and diabolism.[14] Indeed, many of the arguments against the reality of witchcraft that were advanced in the seventeenth and eighteenth centuries were the same as those used by Weyer, Scot and Montaigne in the sixteenth. The difference between the two periods is that whereas in the sixteenth century the views of the sceptics were refuted by such advocates of witch-hunting as Bodin and Erastus, in the late seventeenth and eighteenth centuries their views were widely and often warmly embraced. The reason for the change is that during the intervening period the entire mental outlook of educated Europeans had changed in such a way that the traditional arguments against the sceptics no longer had persuasive force. Even more important, there was no need to refute the sceptics, for their views no longer posed a threat to religion, philosophy or the social order.

The changes that took place in the mental outlook of educated Europeans, when taken together, amounted to an intellectual revolution that destroyed scholasticism as the predominant philosophical system of Europe and, among other things, dissolved many of the beliefs that lay at the basis of witchcraft prosecutions. The first and most basic of these changes – and at the same time the most difficult to trace – was a growing tendency in all fields of thought to reject dogma and inherited authority: to question everything, even the basic principles upon which one's world view is based. This tendency can be seen most clearly in the work of Rene Descartes, who in his search for certain knowledge abandoned reliance upon books, rejected the 'authority' of the ancients as well as of the scholastics, and built his philosophical system upon 'clear and distinct ideas'. Descartes denied that he was a sceptic, at least in the traditional Greek sense of doubting even that one could possess knowledge, since he arrived at a certain knowledge of his own existence and also that of God and the material world. But the process by which Descartes arrived at that certainty – the wholesale rejection of dogma and the systematic expression of doubt – became closely identified with him and with the Cartesianism that spread throughout Europe.[15]

Cartesianism as a philosophical system is important for our purposes, since it became the main rival of scholasticism in the seventeenth century, but the sceptical methodology that Descartes followed is even more important, for it reflects an attitude that was becoming increasingly prevalent in the seventeenth century. The seventeenth century, with all its religious intolerance and warfare, may strike us as a century of intense and uncompromising faith. In a certain sense it was. But within the literate elite, among university-educated men and especially among natural philosophers it was a period of profound and pervasive doubt. When specific witch-beliefs and the religious and philosophical systems that sustained them became the target of such doubt, the prosecution of witches became increasingly difficult to justify.

A second change in the mental outlook of educated Europeans in the late seventeenth century was the growing conviction that the universe functioned in an orderly, regular fashion, according to fixed laws. This belief found support in the scientific discoveries of Copernicus, Galileo, Kepler and Newton, all of whom contributed to the dethronement of the old Aristotelian-scholastic cosmology in which a stationary Earth remained at the centre of the universe, vulnerable to assault by all sorts of supernatural forces. The new mechanistic world view made the Earth part of a smoothly operating machine, and it drastically reduced, if it did not completely eliminate, the role of spirits and demons in this universe. Descartes, who was one of the leading exponents of the mechanical philosophy, did not deny the possibility of their existence, but he did deny that they had anything to do with the operation of the universe or that they could take on bodies. Once demons were denied these powers, of course, the entire cumulative concept of witchcraft came under attack.[16]

The mechanical philosophy represented a serious threat to current religious belief, since it could easily lead its advocates from the denial of the existence of spirits to a rejection of miracles, the efficacy of prayer, the operation of Divine Providence and even the existence of God. As Henry More warned in an attack upon the extreme materialistic version of the mechanistic philosophy, 'No spirit, No God'.[17] The implicit danger of atheism might have prevented the widespread acceptance of the mechanical philosophy had it not been for the determination of natural philosophers like Descartes to make it clear that there was a place for God in their universe and for the willingness of theologians and divines to accommodate the new philosophy. In England, for example, the Established Church and even the nonconformist sects proved to be surprisingly receptive to the new ideas. Latitudinarians rejected demonology, made every effort to reconcile faith with reason, and developed a sophisticated natural theology according to which God worked through the processes of nature.[18] Even biblical fundamentalists endorsed the denial of the power of demons on Earth, since the Bible, while making few references to witchcraft as such, claimed that God – the sovereign God of reformed Protestantism – had chained up the Devil in hell and had thereby prevented him from interfering in human affairs. Religion, therefore, did not prove to be a serious obstacle to the reception of the mechanical philosophy, nor did it prevent educated Europeans from abandoning their belief in demonic power. The Dutch Protestant minister and Cartesian philosopher Balthasar Bekker was representing a growing body of religious opinion when in 1691 he wrote that both scripture and reason prove that 'the Empire of the Devil is but a Chimera and that he has neither such a Power nor such an Administration as is ordinarily ascribed to him'.[19]

Closely related to the belief in a regular, orderly universe was the growing conviction among educated Europeans that there were natural explanations for mysterious or apparently supernatural phenomena. In the fifteenth and sixteenth centuries the natural world was rather narrowly defined. Any phenomena which could not be readily explained in fairly simple 'naturalistic' terms were attributed to supernatural intervention of some sort, a mode of thought that scholasticism encouraged. The first challenge to this scholastic outlook came not so much from the mechanical philosophy but from its rival, the magical cosmology of the neo-Platonists. It might seem surprising that neo-Platonism, a philosophy in which magic held such an important place, could be credited with uprooting a world view that was in many ways more realistic. But by emphasizing the fact that substances had natural sympathies and antipathies which explain why they act in a certain way, neo-Platonists discouraged a reliance upon supernatural explanations of extraordinary events and encouraged an exploration of the natural world in a genuinely scientific manner.[20] Even when Renaissance magicians felt compelled to supplement natural with spiritual magic they helped to undermine the scholastic cosmology, since in the neo-Platonic world the learned magician could compel spirits to respond to his commands and not therefore remain a victim of capricious demonic forces. In the long run the magical world view of the neo-Platonists was

successfully challenged by the other rival to scholasticism, the mechanical philosophy, according to which matter was completely inert and barren and incapable
therefore of accommodating any type of magic, natural or spiritual. During its
period of influence, however, neo-Platonism helped generations of intellectuals to
gain the confidence that extraordinary phenomena had natural causes. It is interesting to note that Reginald Scot, the most radical critic of witch-beliefs and
witchcraft prosecutions in the late sixteenth century, fully accepted the reality of
natural magic. His credulity may not have helped him respond to his critics, but
it does reveal how the theory of natural magic could lead to, or at the very least
accommodate, a naturalistic challenge to witch-beliefs.[21]

At the same time that educated Europeans were adopting world views that
encouraged them to attribute extraordinary occurrences to natural causes, they
were also beginning to discover that many of the unusual diseases and aberrant
forms of behaviour that were customarily attributed to witchcraft could be explained
without any reference to the supernatural. Beginning in the second half of the
sixteenth century, a number of learned men, especially trained physicians, began
to argue that many diseases which were allegedly caused by *maleficium* had natural
causes; that individuals who made free confessions to witchcraft were either under
the influence of drugs or suffering from some form of melancholy, depression or
mental disorder; and that persons who were possessed by the Devil had in fact
succumbed to some medical malady. The growth of such sentiment was by no
means steady, and the medical community itself was divided on these questions.[22]
Johann Weyer, whose views on the natural causes of alleged *maleficia* and the
melancholy of confessing witches have won him enduring fame as an early sceptic,
was effectively refuted by another physician, Thomas Erastus, while a doctor of
medicine from Provence, Jacques Fontaine of Maximin, later proved to be even
more credulous than Erastus.[23] It has even been suggested that doctors, finding
themselves unable to explain a rash of epidemic diseases, actually *caused* the witch-
craze.[24]

Nevertheless, doctors did eventually succeed in undermining witch-beliefs.[25]
The English doctor Edmund Jorden, in an attack upon popular witch-beliefs and
the activities of the cunning men, showed that many of the maladies allegedly
inflicted by witches were some form of what we would call hysteria, while John
Cotta attributed some of the same symptoms to epilepsy. It took some time before
a large proportion of educated Europeans became convinced that all diseases had
natural causes; even Cotta and Jorden were not willing to rule out certain supernatural maladies.[26] And since there remained a number of undiagnosed illnesses,
the temptation to attribute them to preternatural forces was strong. Even when
doctors were able to identify the natural causes of physical and mental disease, the
belief that witchcraft was involved did not evaporate, for it was perfectly plausible
to argue that the Devil worked *through* nature, just as the natural theologians made
the same claim with respect to God. By and large, however, the educated elite
became convinced that the diseases that witches were said to cause, the behaviour
that demoniacs manifested, and the wild confessions that some witches made, all
had natural causes and took place without any participation or cooperation of spirits
or demons. Even when the actual causes of the disease or exceptional behaviour
were not yet known, men were optimistic and confident that those causes would

eventually be discovered. By 1756 a Hungarian doctor was able to claim that 'these days physicians leave supernatural matters for the clergy'.[27]

The mental changes we have been describing – the growth of Cartesian doubt, the spread of the mechanical philosophy and the conviction that there were natural causes of supernatural phenomena – occurred primarily within the upper levels of European society. As far as we can tell, the witch-beliefs of the lower classes changed very little in the late seventeenth and eighteenth centuries. These were simply reclassified by the elite as 'superstition' and treated with contempt, a striking illustration of what Peter Burke has referred to as the withdrawal of the elite from popular culture.[28] Of course there was some inevitable percolation of upper-class ideas down to the lower levels of society, just as there had been in the fifteenth and sixteenth centuries when learned ideas of the demonic pact and the sabbat had been transmitted to the uneducated through the media of sermons, catechetical instruction, and even witchcraft trials themselves. It is possible that the two groups of educated or semieducated persons with whom the members of the lower classes had contact – the clergy and physicians – were able to weaken some popular witch-beliefs. The clergy may have been able to convince their parishioners that God worked through the processes of nature and that demons were not constantly threatening men with physical harm, while the doctors may have achieved some success in helping their patients to realize that their diseases were not caused supernaturally, as the cunning men had always argued.[29] It would be rash, however, to assume that these two groups of educated professionals achieved a great deal of success in changing popular attitudes. Scepticism regarding the supernatural is much more difficult to instil in people than credulity, and most local clerics and physicians were probably not confident enough in their scientifically based sceptical views to mount any sort of effective assault on lower-class credulity and superstition.[30]

The persistence of superstitious beliefs among the peasantry may have actually contributed, in a somewhat ironic way, to the triumph of scepticism among the elite. One of the tactics that sceptics like Nicolas de Malebranche, Laurent Bordelon and Cyrano de Bergerac used to win support for their views was to ridicule the beliefs of the silly rustic shepherds and other peasants who continued to claim that witches were active in their communities.[31] The same tactics of ridicule and satire, it should be noted, were later used by William Hogarth and Francisco Goya in the paintings and engravings they made on the theme of witchcraft and superstition. The effect of this ridicule was to encourage members of the upper classes, even those who were not well-educated, to give at least lip-service to the new scepticism so as to confirm their superiority over the lower classes. Scepticism, in other words, became fashionable. During the late seventeenth and early eighteenth centuries the barriers that separated the various social classes were raised and class divisions and conflicts became more acute throughout Europe. In order to put as much distance between themselves and the common people, the members of the landed and middle classes, especially those who were upwardly mobile, did all they could to prove that they shared nothing with their inferiors. Knowledge of the latest scientific discoveries may have been one way to establish one's social intellectual credentials, but scepticism regarding witchcraft, since it involved the expression of open contempt for the lower classes, was far more effective. The decline of witch-beliefs among the upper and middle classes may have had as much

to do with social snobbery as with the development of new scientific and philosophical ideas.

The new religious climate

The Reformation, while on the one hand serving to intensify the European witch-
hunt, on the other hand planted the seeds of its decline. The Protestant view of
the sovereignty of God worked against the very possibility of *maleficium,* and the
Christianization of the populace weakened the belief in magic; biblical fundamentalism led to a recognition of the Devil's impotence; and conflicts between Catholic
and Protestants over exorcism led many people to doubt the reality of possession,
the Devil and witchcraft. While each of these religious developments did make
some contribution to the end of the great witch-hunt, the most important religious
factor in the decline of witchcraft prosecutions was the change in the religious
climate that occurred in the late seventeenth century.

While it would be misleading to claim that Europe as a whole became more
religiously tolerant at this time,[32] there is plenty of evidence to show that religious
zeal and enthusiasm were waning in Europe after 1650. The clearest illustration
of this was the decline of religious warfare after the Peace of Westphalia in
1648. After that time international conflict had much more to do with national
self-interest and dynastic aggrandizement than with religious ideology. At the
national level the same tendency can be observed in the sources of domestic unrest:
after 1650 there were few religious wars in Europe. In theology the reaction to
enthusiasm and zeal is evident in the emphasis on the reasonableness of religion,[33]
while the most general indication of the new climate was the mistrust of men who
claimed to be directly inspired or directed by the deity.[34] All of this suggests that
the age of the Reformation, which had been marked by the intense expression of
religious zeal, by religiously inspired warfare, by a preference for the emotional
over the rational, and by the presence of ideologically inspired saints or fanatics,
was gradually coming to an end and that a more secular, more rational age was
dawning.

The decline of religious enthusiasm had a number of important effects on the
process of witch-hunting. Among theologians, as we have seen, the desire to accommodate religion to philosophy and science led churchmen like the Latitudinarians
in England to accept the mechanical philosophy and other cosmologies in which
Satan had very little power. The growing distrust of individuals who claimed to
have direct contact with the world of spirits made men sceptical of demoniacs,
which in turn led people to question the reality of the witchcraft that was so often
said to be its source. But the most important effect of the new religious outlook
was a decline in commitment of God-fearing Christians to purify the world by
burning witches. It is true of course that not all witchcraft prosecutions required
religious zeal or enthusiasm for their sustenance, especially those centring on the
alleged practice of *maleficia.* But many witchcraft trials and hunts were inspired by
the determination of magistrates, clergy and the entire community to purify the
world by waging war on Satan's confederates. As this type of militancy and millenar-
ianism declined, so too did the witchcraft prosecutions which they had encouraged.

Social and economic change

The effect of social and economic change on the decline of witchcraft prosecutions is extremely problematic. Part of the problem is that social and economic conditions had more of an impact on the original suspicions and accusations of witchcraft than on the actual prosecutions themselves, and it is difficult if not impossible to determine whether those accusations declined or whether officials simply refused to take action on the basis of them. The other part of the problem is that even if it could be shown that witchcraft accusations did decline in number in the late seventeenth and early eighteenth centuries, it would be difficult to identify those social and economic changes that made villagers and townsmen feel more secure and less vulnerable to the maleficent deeds of their neighbours. The effect of social and economic change on the decline of witchcraft is, in other words, very much a matter of speculation. Nevertheless, the fact that a number of social and economic conditions did play an important part in the growth of witchcraft prosecutions suggests that in corresponding fashion factors of this nature may have had something to do with their decline.

There are three different ways in which socio-economic change might have helped to bring the great witch-hunt to an end. The first is that a general improvement in living conditions in the late seventeenth and early eighteenth centuries may have reduced some of the local village tensions that lay at the basis of witchcraft prosecutions. During the final years of the great witch-hunt most Europeans lived in better economic circumstances than they had during its peak. The price revolution levelled off, wages stopped declining and in some countries actually rose, the population declined slightly and then grew at a more steady pace, and climatic conditions improved. These changes may have made life a little more comfortable for the lower classes, but it is unlikely that they could have significantly reduced or eliminated the specific social tensions that led to witchcraft accusations. Throughout the eighteenth century there was more than enough economically based conflict in village communities, more than enough poverty and hunger, and certainly more than enough misfortune in daily life to sustain frequent and intense witchhunting.

A second possibility is that villagers, while still having adequate cause to denounce neighbours as witches, no longer did so because the witches did not present the same type of threat that they had in the past. There may be some substance to this argument. Keith Thomas has shown, for example, that the full implementation of the poor-law system in England by the end of the seventeenth century eliminated some of the guilt that villagers experienced when they refused to dispense charity. In such circumstances they had less reason to relieve that guilt by accusing the poor of witchcraft.[35] In a more general sense, there was less reason to accuse solitary and isolated women of witchcraft as they became more familiar features of early modern European villages and towns. Instead of viewing such persons with suspicion and fear, people chose rather to ignore them. And as early modern European towns and cities grew in size, they lost their character as intimate, face-to-face societies, the very types of communities in which most accusations of witchcraft originate.

A third possible effect of social and economic change on the decline of witchcraft is more indirect but perhaps of greater importance than the other two. As we have seen, the tremendous economic and social turmoil of the early modern period, when compounded with the political and religious instability of the age, produced a mood of pessimism and deep anxiety that affected all social classes. It made villagers and magistrates, acting both as individuals and as members of the community, identify, accuse and prosecute witches as a means of relieving that anxiety. Witches, therefore, served as scapegoats, not simply for the daily misfortunes of village life but for the more general ills of society at a time of rapid and fundamental change. By the end of the seventeenth century, many of the conditions that had given rise to all of this unease and anxiety no longer existed. Not only was there a reduction of inflation and an overall improvement in living conditions, but the great pandemic of plague that had had such devastating social effects on European life during the past 300 years finally worked itself out and did not reappear again until the late nineteenth century. At the same time the religious turmoil of the Reformation period subsided, and the astonishing series of rebellions and revolutions that had occurred in the late sixteenth and early seventeenth centuries came to an end by 1660. Even international warfare, which had disrupted European society in countless ways during the period of witch-hunting, had somewhat less traumatic effects on European society after 1660.[36] European countries did not abandon warfare, but by 1700 they had virtually stopped the practice of sacking towns and villages.[37] The net effect of all this was that Europe after 1660 gradually entered a period of social, political, economic and religious stability, a period during which the absolutist states of Europe and the aristocracies that predominated within them discovered the means by which a more stable world could be maintained. In such an environment individuals and communities had less reason to accuse their helpless neighbours in order to relieve their general fears and even less reason to engage in a massive witch-hunt to eradicate an imaginary horde of Devil-worshippers who were threatening to turn the entire world and the social order upside down.

Notes

1   Wanda Baeyer-Katte, 'Die Historischen Hexenprozesse', in W. Bitter, ed., *Massenwahn in Geschichte und Gegenwart* (Stuttgart 1965), 220–31.

2   Scottish Record Office, CH2/276/4, Records of Newbattle Kirk Sessions, 31 July and 7 August 1661.

3   Kurt Baschwitz, *Hexen und Hexenprozesse* (Munich 1963), 302–4.

4   Keith Thomas, *Religion and the Decline of Magic* (London 1971), 576.

5   Barbara Shapiro, *Probability and Certainty in Seventeenth-Century England* (Princeton, NJ 1983), 194–226; Carlo Ginzburg, *The Night Battles*, trans. John and Anne Tedeschi (Baltimore, Md 1983), 126; Thomas, *Religion*, 574–5; Perry Miller, *The New England Mind* (Cambridge, Mass. 1953), 205.

6   George Mackenzie, *The Laws and Customes of Scotland* (Edinburgh 1678), 91.

7   Even those who urged the prosecution of witches recognized the problems inherent in torture. See Peter Binsfield, *De Confessionibus* (Treves 1596), 679–98.

8   Gustav Henningsen, *The Witches' Advocate* (Reno, Nev. 1980), 373; H. C. Lea, *Materials towards a History of Witchcraft* (New York 1957), ii, 960–1; *Register of the Privy Council of Scotland*, 3rd set, i, 187 and 210.

9   Bremen, where the first German translation of Spee's treatise was published, abandoned torture in witchcraft trials in 1640. For an English translation of sections of the *Cautio*, see A. Kors and E. Peters, eds, *Witchcraft in Europe* (Philadelphia, Pa 1972), 351–7.

10   Mirjan Damaska, 'The Death of Legal Torture', *Yale Law Journal*, 86 (1978), 873–8.

11   For the entire process of royal intervention in the provinces, see Robert Mandrou, *Magistrats et sorciers en France* (Paris 1968), 425–86.

12   W. Soldan and H. Heppe, *Geschichte der Hexenprozesse* (Munich 1912), ii, 265; Lea, *Materials*, iii, 1435. See Chapter 28 in this collection by Gábor Klaniczay for the restrictions on witchcraft prosecutions in Austria under Empress Maria Theresa.

13   Christian Thomasius, *Uber die Folter*, trans. R. Lieberwirth (Weimar 1960); *Dissertatio*, trans. Lieberwirth (Weimar 1967).

14   Lyndal Roper points out in Chapter 24 that scepticism could coexist with witch persecutions in Germany. See in particular note 21 to her chapter.

15   See R. H. Popkin, *The History of Scepticism from Erasmus to Descartes* (Assen 1960), 174–216, esp. 212–13.

16   On the attractions of the new philosophy, which allowed people to appropriate nature rather than to be victimized by it, see Brian Easlea, *Witch Hunting, Magic and the New Philosophy* (Brighton 1980), esp. 196–252.

17   Noel Brann, 'The Conflict between Reason and Magic in Seventeenth-Century England', *Huntington Library Quarterly*, 43 (1980), 114.

18   Some Latitudinarians, however, believed in witchcraft: see T. H. Jobe, 'The Devil in Restoration Science', *Isis*, 72 (1981).

19   Quoted in Easlea, *Witch Hunting*, 218.

20   H. R. Trevor-Roper, *The European Witch-Craze* (London 1969), 181.

21   Easlea, *Witch Hunting*, 23. Weyer also praised natural magic, although he was hostile to diabolical magic. See Lynn Thorndike, *A History of Magic and Experimental Science* (New York 1941), vi, 516.

22   Thorndike, *History of Magic*, vi, 533–4; E. W. Monter, ed., *European Witchcraft* (New York 1969), 61–3. On the credulousness of English physicians see Garfield Tourney, 'The Physician and Witchcraft in Restoration England', *Medical History*, 16 (1972), esp. 153–5.

23   L. Estes, 'The Medical Origins of the European Witch Craze', *Journal of Social History*, 17 (1984), 4–5.

24   Michael MacDonald, *Mystical Bedlam* (Cambridge 1979), 198–9.

25   For a list of physicians critical of witch-beliefs, see J. Nemec, *Witchcraft and Medicine, 1484–1793* (Washington, DC 1974), 4–5.

26   For the attempt of Cardinal Barberini to ascertain whether a disease had natural or supernatural causes see Ginzburg, *Night Battles*, 125–6.

27   Quoted in R. J. W. Evans, *The Making of the Habsburg Monarchy* (Oxford 1979), 405.

28   Peter Burke, *Popular Culture in Early Modern Europe* (London 1968), 270–81.

29   Jean Delumeau argues that the fear of the Devil diminished as the two Reformations filtered down to the parish level in the late seventeenth century: Delumeau, *Catholicism between Luther and Voltaire*, trans. J. Mosiser (London 1977), 174.

30   For the success of one cleric, using the tactics of disinterest rather than persuasion, see James Boswell, *Journal of a Tour of the Hebrides*, ed. R. W. Chapman (Oxford 1970), 266.

31   Monter, *European Witchcraft*, 113–26; Laurent Bordelon, *L'Histoire des imaginations* (Paris 1710).

32   A. L. Drummond and J. Bullock, *The Scottish Church, 1688–1843* (Edinburgh 1973), ch. 1.

33   G. R. Cragg, *From Puritanism to the Age of Reason* (Cambridge 1960).

34   Michael Heyd, 'The Reaction to Enthusiasm in the Seventeenth Century', *Journal of Modern History*, 53 (1981), 258–80.

35   Thomas, *Religion*, 581–2.

36   See J. Childs, *Armies and Warfare in Europe, 1648–1789* (New York 1982), 2.

37   Theodore Rabb, *The Struggle for Stability in Early Modern Europe* (New York 1975), 122.

Chapter 28

Gábor Klaniczay

THE DECLINE OF WITCHES AND
THE RISE OF VAMPIRES

THE DEMISE OF WITCH-HUNTING is generally hailed as the triumph of the modern rational mind over what has been labelled by various ages as 'superstition', 'witch-crazes', 'credulousness', or 'belief in magic'. The question of how a society crosses this watershed between traditional and modern mentality has always been rather a puzzle, and the answers given have depended on the explanations as to why witch-hunting had occurred at all, and what underlying causes might have occasioned its intensification. The other side of the story is, of course, the analysis of the intensification of scepticism, of how 'rational' arguments emerged that gradually dispelled the old system of explanation, and went on to assert themselves in the legal and the religious spheres. This chapter grew out of an attempt to shed some light on the measures adopted by Maria Theresa to outlaw witch-hunting in Hungary in the eighteenth century, by examining the precise circumstances of her initiatives. I intended to relate these initiatives to their intellectual background, to some of the major issues of eighteenth-century intellectual history. However, as so frequently happens, during my enquiries an unexpected problem arose: the discovery of the curious fact that the abolition of Hungarian witch-trials was related to the scandals concerning vampires.

Let me briefly outline the royal decrees and laws by which Maria Theresa followed the example of Louis XIV (1682) and Frederick William I (1728), who brought an end in their respective countries to widespread witch-hunting from above. The Empress, it is worth noting, was roused to action not by the persistence or re-emergence of witch-hunting in Hungary, but by the popular panic about a new kind of monstrous being, the vampire, whose frequent appearances in neighbouring Moravia had also aroused considerable interest in Vienna.

In 1755, in Hermersdorf, a village near the Silesian–Moravian border, the corpse of Rosina Polakin, deceased a few months previously, was exhumed by municipal decision, because people were complaining that she was a vampire and had attacked them at night. Her body was found to be in good condition (as befits vampires), without any signs of decomposition, and with blood still present in the veins. According to local custom, the poor family of the deceased was forced to drag the corpse, by means of a hook attached to a rope, through an opening made in the wall of the graveyard, to be beheaded and burnt outside.

After hearing of the Polakin affair, Maria Theresa sent two of her court doctors, Johannes Gasser and Christian Vabst, to Hermersdorf. When she received their report, she asked her principal court doctor, Gerard van Swieten (to whom we shall return later), to advise her as to what should be done. The two doctors and van Swieten counselled her to stamp out such repulsive 'superstitions' by legal measures, so she issued a *Rescriptum* in March 1755 forbidding any traditional measures connected with the so-called *magia pustuma*, and a few months later, in a circular letter to the parishes and legal courts of the various counties and cities of Hungary, she was already condemning other 'superstitions' beside the vampire beliefs and indicating that soothsaying, digging for treasure, divination and witch-persecution were also to be prohibited.[1]

This last issue, of course, proved to be the most important and far-reaching. In January 1756 the Empress ordered all material on current witchcraft trials to be submitted to her appeals court for examination by her experts before the execution of the judgements of the local courts. From this moment on, although witch-hunting could not be stopped immediately and although the county courts continued to hand down death sentences, the situation nonetheless became far more favourable for the accused. The experts of the appeals court overturned nearly all the sentences for witchcraft, using the most modern scientific and legal arguments to condemn the unfounded accusations and the 'ignorance of the brutish populace'. In vain did eleven counties protest against this interference in their legal rights, and in vain was the Empress's action opposed by Palatine Lajos Batthyany, who, while condemning the excesses of witch-hunting, had argued that witches existed, referring to Biblical injunctions for their punishment. A few years later, a commission was set up in Vienna, which by 1766 had drawn up a new law definitively forbidding any kind of witch-hunting.

The Imperial and royal law designed to uproot superstition and to promote the rational judgment of crimes involving magic and sorcery, which became part of the new *Constitutio Criminalis Theresiana* is an interesting early manifestation of so-called enlightened absolutism. Let me quote a few paragraphs that reveal the intellectual foundations of this legislation:

> it is well known to what intolerable extremes the craze concerning sorcery and witchcraft has lately extended. Its foundations were laid by the inclination of the stupid and vulgar crowd toward superstition.
>
> Silliness and ignorance, which gave rise to simple-minded amazement and superstitious practices, have finally led to a situation in which gullibility has gained ground everywhere among the people, who have become incapable of distinguishing reality from illusion. Any event which has seemed to them hard to explain (although caused merely by accident, science or speed), has been ascribed to the activity of sorcerers and witches. To these are attributed the causes even for natural events like tempest, animal disease, or human illness. And these fancies about the vicious herd of sorcerers and witches have been transmitted

from one generation to the next. The children have been infected from the cradle by terrible fairytales. Thus this craze has spread more and more widely, additionally distorting legal procedures in such matters.

The new law divided cases involving magic into four categories:

(1) witchcraft accusations originating from fantasy, imagination or fraud; (2) cases which derive from depression, madness or other kinds of mental illness; (3) cases when a person, renouncing God and his own salvation, has performed with serious intentions (although without result) the rituals and devices required for a pact with the Devil; (4) if there is infallible proof of some mischief or crime performed by real sorcery or devilish assistance.

According to the new law judges should always enquire whether the incidents mentioned in the accusation could have happened 'as a consequence of natural events': 'they should even consult experienced doctors and people acquainted with the natural sciences.' They should refrain from torturing the accused, searching for the so-called witch-mark or applying the spurious and archaic ordeal by water. As for punishments in accordance with the above-mentioned four categories: fraud was of course condemned, but so was defamation; mental illness was to be treated in hospital; blasphemy, even if harmless in its outcome, was still a major crime to be punished by banishment; and, as for 'real' devilish sorcery, the Queen declared that 'if such an extraordinary event should happen, We reserve to Ourselves the right to decide about its due punishment.' Thus it henceforth became virtually impossible in the Habsburg Empire to send anybody to the stake as a result of witchcraft accusations. In 1768 a series of royal proscriptions ordered the counties to refrain from initiating legal proceedings in cases of accusations of magical activity 'unless they have very clear proofs in the matter'.

It would be interesting to discuss how these 'enlightened' measures were received by the wider Hungarian population, how rapidly their 'mentality' changed in this respect. Unfortunately the documentation at our disposal is less plentiful than that available to Robert Mandrou and Alfred Soman, who tried to answer Lucien Febvre's analogous question concerning the end of persecutions in seventeenth-century France. What evidence we do have about eighteenth-century Hungary gives the impression that, after the initial grudging response of the fiercely independent and anti-centralist Hungarian nobility, the mass of the population accepted these measures with relief. Although before the royal proscription on witch-hunting there had not been much polemical writing in Hungary aimed at fighting legal abuses or popular superstitions, in the last decades of the eighteenth century they started to multiply, and at the beginning of the following century writers mentioning the matter demonstrated a total lack of identification with the 'superstitions' of their forefathers.

The fact that the ban on the persecutions came not only from above, but also from an external source, and the absence of previous internal debate on the whole matter make it interesting to enquire into the origins of the terminology we encounter in the new imperial law, which expresses a modern rational outlook and a conscious programme to 'reform popular culture'. Contemporaries ascribed the whole campaign against magic to Gerard van Swieten, the powerful court doctor of Maria Theresa. Istvan Weszpremi (1723–1799), one of the most outstanding doctors in eighteenth-century Hungary, wrote in 1778 with respect to the beliefs in vampires:

> This imaginary illness, due to perverted fantasy, was last analysed marvellously by the immortal van Swieten in his treatise on Vampires, published in Vienna in 1755. By dint of wise advice he managed to convince the queen to chase this illness from the mind of the uneducated and superstitious people, so since that time such absurdities cannot be heard about within the territories of our country.

It is worth taking a closer look at the activities and writings of van Swieten, a remarkable figure who was still venerated by Hungarians at the beginning of the nineteenth century. Through van Swieten we can locate this eighteenth-century campaign against magic within the broader currents of the Enlightenment. Before examining his two treatises on this subject (one on vampires, one on witches), here are a few brief details about his life.

Gerard van Swieten (1700–1772) was born in Leyden, where he studied medicine with one of the most outstanding professors of the time, Herman Boerhave (1668–1738). In 1743 he was invited to become *protomedicus* in the court of Maria Theresa; he accepted with some reluctance and a show of nonconformism (he refused, for example, to wear a wig). Within a few years he became one of the most powerful advisers to the Empress, not just in medical but also in much broader matters. He became the director of the Hofbibliothek, the organizer of the reform of the entire Vienna university, the administrator of hospitals, clinics and midwife education, the adviser on a series of measures that could be characterized as early examples of social welfare policy (asylums for the aged, widows, foundlings, orphans). He became one of the leaders of the Censorship Commission, where he earned fame for exercising a kind of countercensorship in the name of the new ideas of the Enlightenment: it was not Voltaire and Rousseau whom he put on index, but the literature of the esoteric, demonological and magical.

As we can see, van Swieten was just the person to take charge of the campaign for the elimination of magic beliefs. It is no wonder that (as I have already mentioned) the campaign was initiated on his advice. This advice was formulated in detail in his *Remarques sur le Vampyrisme* (1755). At first reading, the treatise surprises by its moderate tone: van Swieten starts his work by acknowledging the existence of miracles, of divine omnipotence and even of the power of Satan. He adds, however, that

> since the natural sciences have taken such a great upswing, many things formerly regarded as marvels have turned out to have natural causes . . . The eclipse for example, which produced such terror in olden times, does not frighten any more. We can contemplate calmly the omnipotence of the Creator, who can move these huge objects with such precision in such an infinitely vast space throughout so many centuries.

He refers further to gunpowder, electricity, optical reflection and other optical devices, which would all seem miraculous to the ignorant; jesters and charlatans, he says, had always exploited this ignorance.

He followed the same line of argument against the Moravian vampire beliefs. After describing in detail the story of Rosina Polakin, and some other eighteenth-century vampire cases, he sets out to find the natural causes of the extraordinary phenomena described in these accounts. He advances medical arguments for the existence of bodily fluids resembling blood in the corpse several weeks after death. He puts forward scientific arguments about chemical factors and the lack of air, which could result in the undecayed conservation of corpses for several months, years, even decades after death. He supports his argument by a series of famous cases that for him, show no traces of vampirism. As for the reported nightmares, which might, in fact, have a very powerful impact, he considers them to be the natural consequence of ignorance and lack of education, combined with a kind of indoctrination fostered by fairytales.

He also advances some legal arguments against exhuming corpses on suspicion of vampirism – sacrilegious profanation of the holy ground of the graveyard, violation of the rights of the relatives. He urges the Empress to take speedy measures against all these beliefs, on the plane both of law and of education.

Van Swieten's interest in magical matters did not stop here, but extended to embrace the whole problem of popular magic. While the royal campaign moved on to forbid witch-hunting as well, probably on his initiative, in 1758 he wrote a *Mémoire* on witchcraft, which shows very similar traits to the vampire treatise. It also relates to a concrete case – the trial of Magdalene Heruczina, a Croatian witch sentenced to death but liberated on the orders of Maria Theresa after her case was examined by van Swieten. Here, too, we encounter the formal acknowledgement of the existence of magic and of the workings of Satan, coupled with a scientific explanation of the actual events. Electricity and gunpowder are mentioned here too, and he also describes some 'scientific' experiments, where witches who claimed to have attended the witches' Sabbat were observed meanwhile remaining seated in their rooms, and were apparently only dreaming about their magical adventures.

The main attraction of van Swieten's treatise on witchcraft lies in his detailed enquiry into how the witchcraft accusation was constructed, and into how the distinctive Sabbat confession was obtained. He not only describes the terrible pain the old woman had to suffer under torture, but also how the judges put questions into her mouth, how the investigators took every item of hearsay as the truth, etc. His conduct in this case, where he personally supervised the medical treatment and the hospitalization of the poor woman, is a nice example of the unity of theory and practice in the time of the Enlightenment.

Van Swieten's ideas, which had such a revolutionary effect upon the entire body of legislation dealing with magic, were imported into Austria from other countries. It is evident that van Swieten's sceptical and rationalist approach must have evolved primarily out of his native Dutch culture. Indeed, if we examine the history of scepticism about witchcraft beliefs, and of the way in which criticism of such beliefs developed, Holland was one of the countries in the vanguard. It was in Holland that witch-hunting claimed the fewest victims (about thirty executions in total), and it was there, too, that this aberration of early-modern civilization was most rapidly corrected: the last known execution took place in 1603. It was probably this enlightened mentality which accounted for the surprisingly large number of critics of Dutch origin who attacked witchcraft beliefs.

In 1767, the same year that witch-trials were conclusively forbidden in the domain of the Habsburg monarchy, a vast synthesis on this theme was published in Vienna by Konstantin Franz von Cauz, a firm friend of most of the Italian leaders of enlightened thought. In this book, *De cultibus magicis*, we find a recap of the whole intellectual background to the Habsburg campaign against superstition: he praises the Queen, who could 'set an example to other sovereigns' in 'chasing this barbarian superstitious ignorance from the brains of the people'; he honours van Swieten for initiating the package of measures and contributing to their promotion with his treatises; and he bases his arguments mainly on Dutch and Italian polemicists.

We could end the description here of the intellectual background to Maria Theresa's enlightened legislation and that to van Swieten's treatises. But there is a way to proceed further with the present enquiry, as I have already indicated at the beginning of this chapter: to posit a problem on the basis of our new evidence that the sequence of legislation against magical practices arose from the scandals caused by the newly emerging belief in vampires, and, in consequence of this new type of scandal, moved on to forbid witch-hunting altogether.

Before trying to work through this problem, let me sketch the historical background of European beliefs in vampires.[2] Let us leave open the question as to whether Montague Summers was right, in *The Vampire, his Kith and Kin* (1928), in developing a universal category that included every variety of phenomena such as the returning dead, bloodsucking witches or cannibalistic killers from Antiquity to the Indians. I prefer a more specific definition that focuses mainly on the historically unified concept of the vampire that emerged in early-modern Central and Balkan Europe. According to the accounts of folklorists, the vampire synthesizes various traits from five different sets of magical beliefs: the revenants, the Alp-like nightly pressing spirits, the bloodsucking *stryx* of Antiquity, those witches from Slavic and Balkan territories who were said to persist in harmful activities after their deaths, and finally the werewolf, a person capable of adopting the form of a wolf in order to attack and devour humans.

After a few obscure mediaeval references, it was in the seventeenth century that the accounts of these monstrous beings started to multiply. The first clear vampire cases were reported from Silesia in 1591, from Bohemia in 1618, and there are some stories of *upierzyca* from Poland (near Cracovia) in 1624.[3] We can see here a remarkable geographical unity, which culminated in the second half of the seventeenth century with the Balkan (Greek, Bulgarian, Romanian and Serbian) stories of *Moroi* and *broucholachi*. Typically the stories describe cases of dead people, quite frequently deceased in irregular circumstances such as suicide, or dying unbaptised or excommunicated, or being deviant or abnormal in some other way, who return from the grave in human or in animal shape. They cause trouble or infestation, and kill men and beasts, until their undecayed bodies, still veined with blood, are exhumed and pierced by a pole, or beheaded, or have the heart extracted and burnt. Unfortunately, a more detailed analysis of these early cases is not possible, since the stories have been handed down by chronicles and other reports based upon hearsay, do not identify precisely the alleged vampire and say nothing about the 'victims' or the accusers.

Although vampire beliefs were basically of Slavic and Greek origin, eighteenth-century European public opinion nevertheless connected them mainly to Hungary, because nearly all the famous vampire cases of the eighteenth century occurred in the peripheral territories of the Hungarian kingdom. I shall review these cases briefly, not only because some of them are unknown to the vast literature about vampires, but also because of their relevance to the specific topic of this chapter. In 1706, the first widely read book on vampires was published, entitled *De magia postuma*. Written by Karl Ferdinand Scherz, the book describes vampire cases on the Moravian–Hungarian border. In 1707, the Lutheran synod of Rózsahegy (Ruzomberok) devoted time to a special discussion of the spreading custom of exhuming, beheading and burning corpses. In 1709, Samuel Köleséri, a Hungarian doctor, narrating the events of the plague in Transylvania, gave a shocked account of the number of corpses dug up and pierced by a pole or beheaded because they were considered responsible for spreading the plague.

One of the strangest events was recorded in 1718 in the town of Lublo on the Hungarian–Polish border. A certain merchant called Kaszparek, who stole the fortune of his Polish customer and died shortly afterwards, returned from the grave to be with his wife and to generate fear in other people. The panic led to a series of municipal investigations and hearings of witnesses' testimonies. Despite the resistance of Kaszparek's wife, there were several attempts to destroy the corpse, all of which were reported as unsuccessful, until eventually the entire body was burnt. The case became so noteworthy that not only did chroniclers describe it in great detail, but also it became the theme of a novel by the famous nineteenth-century Hungarian writer, Kalman Mikszath.

In the 1720s the vampire epidemic was further magnified by reports from Késmark in north Hungary and Brasso and Déva in Transylvania. The most famous instances occurred, however, in Serbia. For example, the case in 1730 of the *hajdu* Arnold Paul (a kind of peasant soldier) became the most widely known account of vampires, described in most European journals of the time and included ever since in every manual on vampires. This soldier, who came from Medvegia, a village near Belgrade, had always complained of being tormented by a Turkish vampire. Despite his attempts to cure himself (for example, by eating earth from the graves of presumed vampires), he died prematurely through an accident and became a vampire himself. According to the fable-like extremely confused account of this case, forty days after his death Paul was exhumed, found to have blood in his veins and was heard to emit a terrifying shriek when pierced by a pole. In the same period, from this same region, which must indeed have witnessed an intensive vampire epidemic, there were several testimonies to other, similar cases. The accounts of the persons involved are very imprecise and stereotyped, but remain as authentic testimonies to the spread of the belief. There even survived several brief medical reports by doctors of the Austrian imperial army who were present at exhumations carried out at the demand of local people.[4]

This series of cases signalled the start of the great debate of the 1730s about vampires. A long list of more or less scientific works discussed these phenomena, and in the 1740s continued to draw upon more recent vampire cases from

Transylvania, Serbia and Moravia. It therefore comes as no surprise that the contemporary authority in the field, the Benedictine abbot Dom Augustin Calmet, acknowledged this geographical specificity in his *Treatise on the apparitions, bad spirits and vampires of Hungary and Moravia* (1751). In consequence, the Hungarian word *vampyr* (itself derived from the Polish *upyr*) became the internationally recognized name for these monstrous beings.

However, it is not the folkloric or ethnic characterization of this belief that interests me here, but rather the question of how these few dozen stories about vampires attracted considerably greater attention in the Europe of the time than the burnings of several hundred alleged witches during this same period in Hungary, Poland, Austria and Germany. This shift of popular and intellectual interest to vampires, this 'vampire scandal', is worthy of attention, for it signals some of the essential contemporary preoccupations concerning magic. Although the witchcraft debate and the problem of witches were far from being completely resolved, in Western Europe this had begun to pale because witch persecution had long been in decline there. In these circumstances the more exotic East European bloodsuckers were bound to excite much greater popular interest.

The vampires provided doctors with a new and exciting riddle to be explained by the application of their newly elaborated system of scientific reasoning. P. Gabriel Rzaczynski was already puzzling over the question in describing the Polish accounts of vampires in his *Historia naturalis curiosa regni Poloniae* (1721). In polemical writings about vampires one meets similar kinds of historical examples and accounts by physicians (on the incorruptibility of corpses, on the characteristics of blood) to those found in van Swieten's treatise. The most detailed medical analysis of the period on vampires was prepared by a Hungarian doctor called George Tallar, who over several decades studied these phenomena among the Serbians and the Romanians. He not only observed the exhumation of corpses suspected of being vampires, but also examined people who complained of a certain illness accompanied by fever, digestive problems, pallor and sickness – which they generally attributed to having been bitten or touched by vampires. They tried to heal themselves by smearing their bodies with the blood of corpses exhumed from cemeteries, and by other magical devices. George Tallar had a different explanation of this illness: he attributed it to the extreme diets of the Orthodox church, which reached their peak in winter time, and resulted in digestive problems. He tried to heal these people accordingly, and – if we can believe his account – with considerable success.

As for the religious polemicists, vampire beliefs represented a serious challenge, for they were forced to recognize in them the blasphemous reversal of some crucial Christian dogmas and cults. The vampire belief touched upon Christian ideas about resurrection. The vampire, like the Christian saint, was also a 'very special dead', whose corpse resisted decay, whose grave radiated with a special light, whose fingernails and hair kept growing – like those of several mediaeval saints, e.g. Saint Oswald, Saint Edmund and Saint Olaf – thus demonstrating the persistence of vital energy beyond death. The apparitions of the vampires and the miracles connected with them were, in a way, negative reflections of the attributes of the saints. And as for the most haunting capacity of the vampire, the bloodsucking – not only can one account for it in terms of the history of sacrificial blood but also one could see it as a reversal of its Christianized version, the holy communion, which was depicted by late-mediaeval and early-modern mystics as a highly tangible bodily and material absorption of Christ's flesh and (more significantly) blood.

So here we are with this wicked, blasphemous belief, which had to be criticized and refuted in order to protect the holy model on which it was based. Calmet's chief intention in his book was to uphold the original Christian dogmas on resurrection, miracles and even the existence of Satan, as special signs of divine omnipotence (it was probably from this source that analogous passages of Swieten's treatises derived). At the same time, Calmet described all accounts of vampires and the witches' Sabbat as the consequences of 'illusion, superstition and prejudice', which could be explained either as natural phenomena or as fantasies on the part of the people concerned.

A similar view was expressed by Giuseppe Davanzati, bishop of Trani in southern Italy, who wrote his *Dissertation about Vampires* in 1739 on the basis of first-hand information given to him by Schrattenbach, Bishop of the Moravian town Olmutz. His explanation was partly geographical, partly social. According to him, the belief was gaining ground in Moravia and Hungary rather than in, say, Spain or France, because the inhabitants of these latter countries were less gullible. Moreover, it was current among 'the brutish, uneducated lower classes' and not among cultivated noblemen and scientists, because it was more difficult to deceive the latter. For this reason the educated should indeed consider it their duty to rid the ignorant of their 'superstitions'.

The extent to which this ecclesiastical fight against superstition served to maintain some basic Christian beliefs in magic is perhaps best illustrated by the fact that Pope Benedict XIV felt it necessary to refer to the 'vanity of the vampire beliefs' in his 1752 treatise on the canonization of saints. On the other hand, it was precisely this anomalous position adopted by the Catholic polemicists that gave Voltaire the opportunity, in writing about the absurdity of beliefs in vampires, to discuss in similarly sarcastic mode the Christian belief in miracles and in resurrection dogmas. Presenting the vampire stories in a mock-heroic style loaded with irony in his *Questions sur l'Encyclopédie* (1772), he went on to ask: 'Hearing all this, how could we cast doubt any longer on the stories about resurrected dead which our legends are so full of, and on the miracles described by Bollandus or by the sincere and very respectable Dom Ruinald?'

Alongside the medical view, the attempts of the Church to rescue basic dogmas by distancing itself from popular superstitions, and the sarcastic and rationalist critiques expounded by Enlightenment thinkers, we should make note of a fourth current that played an active part in the debates about vampires. It is tempting to call this tendency the occult revival of the eighteenth century, which developed as a kind of countercurrent to the rationalist, Cartesian mainstream of philosophical thought of the age. In the early eighteenth century a spate of literature attempted to explore the occult, mystical, spiritualist and psychic explanations for the 'forces of human fantasy'. It was not by chance that Muratori dedicated his first philosophical enquiry (mentioned above) to this subject, and in a much less dogmatic, dryly rationalist tone than Voltaire would have adopted. We should also bear in mind that the second half of the eighteenth century saw the emergence and triumphant success of Mesmerism, the 'magnetic, 'hypnotizing' method of healing.

We can now see fairly clearly the reasons for the popularity of vampires in the first half of the eighteenth century. But, apart from obscuring the popularity of the witch theme in public debate, how did all this contribute to the end of witch-hunting? In the first place, one could say that vampire beliefs provided an alternative explanatory system for persistent problems in the field of magic, so the contradictions of the previous explanations could be discussed more openly. This is the argument Keith Thomas advanced to explain the role of Renaissance neo-Platonism in the rise of doubt in witch-belief in sixteenth-century England. Unfortunately, this parallel is too remote to help us here – there are too many discrepancies: at that time the efforts to stop persecution were unsuccessful and the learned magical beliefs of the Renaissance caused no real scandals in their time, nor could they obscure in any way the popular tradition of belief in witches.

However, speaking of parallels raises the possibility of a more fruitful analogy: let us compare my account of the eighteenth century with what happened in France at the end of the seventeenth century, where, according to Robert Mandrou, witch persecutions were brought to an end partly as a result of public scandals inspired by famous cases of diabolical possession. This new type of magical phenomenon was exemplified by the spectacular and widely known cases of the Ursuline nuns of Loudun (1633) and Louviers (1643) who claimed to be possessed by the Devil, who had approached them through their confessors.

Of course I am not suggesting that there is any close resemblance between seventeenth-century French cases of diabolical possession and eighteenth-century Central European vampire scandals. There is obviously a difference between the two processes of 'decriminalizing' witchcraft. As Alfred Soman has shown, the growing doubts about witchcraft accusations and the stricter jurisdictional scrutiny in witchcraft cases started in France well before the possession cases, which acted only as catalysts to the existing public debate on the question. In the eighteenth-century Habsburg Empire, on the other hand, it was the vampire scandals that forced the initiation of the entire campaign to abolish persecution. Yet I think a meaningful analogy can be drawn in two respects: at the level of the internal logic of the historical evolution of the popular magical universe, and at the level of the effect that the emerging new beliefs had upon those held previously. More generally: at both levels these scandals presented the effects of harmful magical power in new and exciting terms for the people of that era. They thus contributed to the restructuring of witchcraft beliefs and to the reform of plurisecular judicial persecution in that domain. On the one hand, the seventeenth-century nunnery, diabolically possessed by a priest to the extent of transforming it into the sinister setting for perverted orgies; on the other hand, the monstrous bloodsuckers crawling out from their graves on the periphery of Europe – two extremes that first brought into play every existing belief in supernatural evils and terrors, and then, in the second phase, somehow provided illumination for contemporary thinkers trying to come to terms with these phenomena. It must have indicated how they could step out of the magic circle of witch-hunting.

In seventeenth-century France the theatrical appetite of Jesuit spirituality was obviously left unsatisfied by the conception of evil inherent in previous witchcraft accusations, which involved a secret crime and a hazy identification of the criminal with his or her satanic affiliations. The obscene spasms of the possessed nuns and the terrifyingly cruel rituals of exorcism placed Satan in centre stage much more efficiently. The traditional experts on sacred knowledge, the priests, were also quite logically destined to be the principal objects of suspicion and accusation (is it possible to imagine a more provocative and shrewd idea of the Devil than to pervert an entire monastery of nuns by means of their confessors?). However, the contradictions exposed by this extreme actualization of magical beliefs rapidly led to a kind of demystifying explosion. The accused, like Urbain Grandier of Loudun, defended themselves by the logical argument that one should not trust the voice of Satan speaking through the possessed nuns, for here again he is out to deceive and destroy the innocent.

Since this inner contradiction could no longer be resolved within the paradigms of witchcraft beliefs, the decisive role in the argument was very soon given over to the medical experts, with their dissertations on the psychic consequences of 'melancholy' and the mental effects of bodily *humeurs*. On the other hand, increasing numbers of people came to see the whole thing as pure deception and fraud, which view, though far from accounting for the complex psychological process of diabolical possession, had the beneficent effect of putting a speedy end to witch-hunting.[5]

As for eighteenth-century vampire beliefs, I have already attempted to explore their attraction for the people of that time. Here, too, the comparison with witchcraft could add a useful dimension. Vampire beliefs involved much more spectacular fantasies than traditional witchcraft accusations, by producing tangible proof not by means of the 'theatre of the Devil' but by the discovery of corpses showing unusual signs of life. At the same time, bloodsucking was a quasi-medical concept that appeared to explain magical aggression in terms more acceptable to the eighteenth-century mentality than the witches' invisible and unexplained power to cast spells. Another possible parallel between possession and vampire cases is that they both represented a more spiritualized conception of the workings of evil magic. Here I am thinking not only of demons, spirits and ghosts, but of the fact that, whereas witchcraft accusations were aimed at finding living scapegoats within the community – the witch was the 'traitor within the gates' – whereas they tried to account for misfortune by relating it to past human conflicts and present evil behaviour, the theory of diabolical possession shifted the focus of attention onto Satan and the devils, who used human beings only as passive media. Finally, vampire beliefs were shifted onto dead men returning from their graves, and increasingly explained the spreading of this evil as pure contagion, which naturally exculpated the living victims attacked by or related to vampires.

The vampire scandals also presented a more general paradigm for transcending the persisting belief in harmful magic. As we can see from contemporary opinion, this paradigm suggested the notion of civilizing the ignorant and superstitious East European savage (who was considered far from 'noble'). According to the intellectuals of that era, this mission of the Enlightenment, this civilizing process, could come only from 'above' in the social sense and from the 'west' in the geographical sense. This type of thinking was present not only in the royal decrees of Maria Theresa, but also in the descriptions by Hungarian doctors, who, like George Tallar, took pleasure in lamenting the ignorance of Serbian and Romanian peasants and the evil effects of the 'superstitious' Orthodox religion. It was this ideology that initiated the campaign against magical beliefs. And it was very soon generalized not only to the abolition of witch-hunting, but also to fighting any beliefs, practices and representatives of traditional popular culture.

Notes

1   For full citations of the sources used in this chapter, see the original version in Gábor Klaniczay, *The Uses of Supernatural Power* (Princeton University Press, Princeton, NJ 1990), ch. 10.

2   For an introduction to pre-industrial vampire beliefs, see Paul Barber, *Vampires, Burial and Death* (Yale University Press, New Haven, CT 1988). Also useful are Leonard Wolf, *A Dream of Dracula* (New York 1972), and Bernhardt Hurwood, *The Vampire Papers* (New York 1976).

3   The story from Silesia was described by Henry More in *An Antidote against Atheism* (1653). It concerns a shoemaker in Breslau who was reported to have haunted and harmed people after having committed suicide, and was exhumed and burnt by municipal decision.

4   The famous cases and the various European reports of them are reprinted in Dom Augustine Calmet, *Treatise on Vampires and Revenants* (1751; London 1850).

5   For detailed analyses of these events, see D. P. Walker, *Unclean Spirits* (London 1981), and Stephen Greenblatt, 'Loudun and London', *Critical Inquiry*, 11 (1985), 327–46.

Chapter 29

Owen Davies

URBANIZATION AND THE DECLINE OF WITCHCRAFT

An examination of London

HISTORICAL STUDIES OF EUROPEAN witchcraft have been remarkably quiet concerning the impact of urbanization on the structure of magical beliefs and practices. The work which has been done on witchcraft in urban areas of early modern Europe does suggest, however, that this would be a fruitful area for future study. Ruth Martin, for example, in her work on Venice, found an absence of 'traditional' *maleficium* associated with agricultural production. She also noted that much witchcraft activity centred instead 'on the main commodity of interest to an urban and a commercial society – money'.[1] Jens Christian Johansen also found that in Danish towns, witches were more often accused of bewitching trade and business than in rural areas. There was also less agriculturally related witchcraft. Rural witches, for example, were charged with souring milk three times as often as urban witches.[2] What these brief observations indicate is that the urban environment does seem to have had an effect on the nature of witchcraft accusations. This encourages one to look more closely at the possibility that as urban societies expanded and underwent profound economic and social change, so this wrought equally profound transformations in the structure of witchcraft accusations and beliefs.

As indicated by the title of this chapter, much of the following discussion will concentrate on evidence from London. As an urban centre spanning both pre-industrial and industrial ages, it provides a sense of continuity over a considerable period of time. A number of different urban contexts will also be introduced briefly when they represent substantially different models of urbanization. Instead of subscribing to the dogmatic idea that the spread of social and intellectual 'progress' led to the decline of witchcraft in urban society, this chapter will look at the relationship between urban community structures and the formation of witchcraft accusations.

We can gain some insight into the nature of witchcraft accusations in early modern London through an examination of the Surrey Assize records.[3] These allow us to compare indictments from urban Southwark with those from the rest of rural Surrey. Of the forty-two indictments which state the nature of the victims of witchcraft (whether human or animal), seven (16.6 per cent) came from Southwark, and in all seven indictments the victims were human. Of the thirty-five rural indictments, 31 per cent related to the bewitchment of livestock only, and, if we consider those cases involving both animals and humans, that percentage goes up to 43 per cent. The absence of agriculturally based accusations from Southwark is not surprising in itself, but when we consider that 43 per cent of the rural accusations involved livestock, then we have to ask ourselves what effect the divorce from livestock rearing had on accusations of witchcraft amongst the urban population. As Morgan's *London Map* of 1682 shows, Southwark was not completely divorced from rurality, showing considerable areas of adjacent open ground. Through much of the seventeenth century nearly half of the acreage of the parish of St George, Southwark, for example, consisted of St George's Fields, which was mostly agricultural land. From the Southwark witch indictments the occupational status of six of those involved directly or indirectly (husband of accused for instance) can be extracted. They show a strong non-agricultural bias: a butcher, joiner, blacksmith's apprentice, waterman, labourer, and yeoman. Statistical analysis of the baptism register of St Saviours, Southwark, 1618–25, further reveals that from a sample of 1,860 only 1.5 per cent of the working population were agricultural workers.[4]

Evidence that by the eighteenth century there was still a strong belief in witchcraft in London comes from the persecution and prosecution of Sarah Moredike in 1701. Richard Hathaway, a blacksmith's apprentice, accused Sarah Moredike, wife of a Southwark waterman, of having bewitched him on 1 April 1700, since when he had been terribly ill and was seen to vomit crooked pins and nails. What is significant is the large number of Southwark citizens who apparently believed Hathaway's imposture and took part in the mobbing of Moredike. Local pressure was so great that she removed herself to Paul's Wharf, only to be followed by Hathaway. Even after her acquittal she continued to be persecuted. A public collection was made for the bewitched Hathaway, and prayers were put up in the local churches.[5] Another late accusation brought before magistrates at the Surrey Quarter Sessions in 1699/1700 came from the neighbouring urban parish of Maria Magdelena, Bermondsey, when Thomas Watts, a scrivener, was accused by William Langham 'for being a sorcerer and using sorceries and witchcrafte'.[6] A pamphlet also records that in July 1704, Sarah Griffith of Rosemary Lane, was swum in the New River Head. She apparently swam like a cork, and was subsequently taken before Justice Bateman in Well Close, who committed her to the Bridewell, Clerkenwell.[7] After these last cases of the prosecution period I have not come across any other examples of witchcraft from urban London until 1818. That, of course, does not mean that none exists. I would be surprised if an exhaustive and systematic survey of eighteenth century London newspapers did not turn up a few relevant reports.

In 1818 one Michael Kenlish, an Irish shoemaker, was charged before the Bow Street magistrate with threatening to murder a woman.[8] Kenlish stated in evidence that the prosecutrix, and another woman, had bewitched him three years since, by means of some 'stuff' which they had put in his tea, after drinking which he was left in a trance for several days. They also bewitched him by means of a black cat and a 'pound of pins'. He was subsequently told by the two women that the only way he could rid himself of the spell they had put upon him was by 'crossing the sea'. He informed the court that he was shortly about to act on this advice and return to Ireland. Kenlish entreated the court not to suppose that he was deranged, but that his distracted state of mind arose wholly from his bewitchment, which had so disabled him that he was unable to work properly, and was, in consequence, so poor that he could not pay for the washing of his shirt. The prosecutrix denied any knowledge of the accusations made by Kenlish, but gave it as her opinion that his delusions resulted from his being a Roman Catholic and extremely superstitious. The charges against Kenlish were dismissed on condition that he keep the peace towards the prosecutrix prior to his leaving for Ireland.

The next piece of evidence for witch beliefs in London comes from the prosecution Sarah McDonald for 'obtaining the sum of 14s 6d, under the pretext of practising witchcraft', heard before Mr D'Eyncourt, at the Worship Street Police-Court, 3 September 1858.[9] The case resulted from a complaint made by Mrs Mary Ann Gable, 'a ladylike person', wife of a coppersmith, who resided in Russell Street, Stepney. She told the court that having had a great deal of trouble and illness lately, and fearing that a 'spell' was upon her, she paid a visit to Mrs McDonald, who lived in Cudworth Street, Bethnal Green. Gable suffered from 'frightful pains, cutting, shooting, pricking, and darting through' her head and body, for the relief of which she had consulted a Dr Ramsbotham. She had asked him if he thought they resulted from a 'spell', and he said he thought not. He gave her some medicine, and for a time she felt better. Subsequently she got worse again, and decided to consult McDonald. Gable stated in court that McDonald 'lays the cards and, indeed, is very clever with them. I had heard of that, but not that she possessed the power of relieving persons from torment by burning powders'. This suggests that unbewitching was a secondary and less employed aspect of McDonald's activities.

McDonald told Gable that a person was doing her an 'injury' and suggested as a remedy that she buy some of her powders for sixpence each. She bought ten powders, and McDonald proceeded to put each powder in the fire whilst inaudibly repeating an incantation – the object of this ritual being to 'torment' the person who was 'injuring' Gable. However, the substance of Gable's complaint against McDonald was not that she had defrauded her, but that whilst McDonald was being paid by her to do 'injury' to her tormentor, the very same tormentor – a relative who was coming into property – was, in turn, paying McDonald to burn powders against Gable.

Mr D'Eyncourt was obviously shocked to find such beliefs in urban London, and felt it necessary to inquire where Gable had been brought up, perhaps hoping to find that she was a country-woman, which would somewhat extenuate the circumstance of such beliefs being held in the neighbourhood. Unfortunately for D'Eyncourt's peace of mind Gable replied that she had been brought up in the parish of Bethnal Green, where her father was a timber merchant, and had possessed a large property. Furthermore, Gable's eighteen-year-old daughter, Eliza, 'a rather pretty healthy-looking girl', also stated her belief in such things: 'Oh I have suffered much from her spells, can't rest or sleep, and feel as though I could fly out of the place. I am sure she is a witch and has the power of making spells'. Police-Constable Horton, 37 K, gave evidence to the effect that a great number of people believed in McDonald, and he also suspected that she bribed several people to report her fortune-telling abilities. D'Eyncourt further inquired of Horton: 'You do not believe in it, I suppose?' 'Not a bit, sir. I offered to let her try her spells upon me, but she would not'.

D'Eyncourt in summing-up remarked 'how such absurd notions can be entertained I cannot comprehend', and had McDonald held on remand pending her being sent to the House of Correction. Looking back on the case eleven years later, the editor of *All the Year Round* expressed his dismay at the way in which the case had 'exhibited the metropolis in *nearly* [my italics] as unfavourable a light as the country districts'.[10]

Four years later, Charles Tilbrook, a discharged soldier, aged 27, was brought before the Bow Street magistrates charged with attempting to murder his grandmother, aged 75, residing in Charles Street, Westminster. On 13 April 1862, Tilbrook had attacked his grandmother with a razor, cutting her head and face, and then beat her head with a boiling stick. She was taken to Westminster Hospital where she recovered. When confronted with the evidence in court, the prisoner took exception to the claim that he had beaten her without any provocation:

> I have had enough provocation. Mr Corrie [magistrate] – Do you wish that to be taken down? Prisoner. – I wish it to be known that she is a very bad character, and not fit to live at all. She is a witch, in daily intercourse with the Devil. I know you don't believe in spirits, in what you call 'this enlightened age', but I don't call it enlightened. I call it a very dark age.[11]

Subsequently, when brought before the Central Criminal Court, Tilbrook explained sullenly that he had no intention of actually killing his grandmother:

> if I had wanted to take her life I should have locked the door; I merely intended to draw some of her blood, and that is the fact of the matter [sensation in court]. If she does not work at witchcraft or devilish arts I am willing to forfeit my life for her.[12]

He added that the reason why he shed her blood was so that 'she should not possess the power over him that she had done'.

The witchcraft beliefs expressed in these cases, and the behaviour of those concerned, certainly conform to the same patterns of accusation and counteraction which occurred in rural communities of the period. However, as will become apparent later, there are some indications that the urban social context, within which these accusations were generated, was having some effect on the nature of the accusations.

The anthropologist J. Clyde Mitchell put forward a theory concerning urban witchcraft which is based on the assumption that urban and rural social structures are completely separate. He suggested that unlike the latter, the former environment militated against witch-accusations because the social and administrative structure of the urban community allowed no direct retributive actions against witches. In response, Marc Swartz rejected this idea of structural cleavage, and warned:

so long as the town and the rural areas are considered separate structures and relationships are traced only within each, we are not likely
to raise questions which concern the organization and development of
the total social field surrounding processes such as changing rates of
witchcraft accusation and differences in rates, which may or may not
be real.[13]

A similar view, from a rather different academic quarter, has also been expressed,
albeit without reference to witchcraft, by Jeremy Boulton in his study of residential mobility in seventeenth-century Southwark: 'What is needed is a model which
might serve to embrace the experiences of both urban and rural inhabitants within
a common framework'.[14]

There are problems, alluded to, but not fully discussed by Swartz or Boulton,
with the gross generalizations inherent in the folk/urban dichotomy, which appor-
tions fundamentally different norms, values and behaviourial characteristics to each,
and which tend to mask the continuities, and more subtle social changes taking
place under the guise of urbanization. Crude folk-urban theory suggests that urbanization leads to social instability, and forced rejection of traditional communal
relations and beliefs. However, a number of in-depth case studies have revealed
that assimilation and adaption to urban life can occur with far greater ease than one
might expect, and without the abandonment of previously held social perceptions
and traditional practices. Oscar Lewis's study of peasants in Mexico City revealed
a remarkable level of continuity between rural and urban lifestyle. Herbalism,
animal rearing, belief in witchcraft, spiritualism, and public ceremony, were found
to be just as common among persons who had been in the city for over thirty years
as among recent arrivals. The primary group relations, which anthropologists have
often considered as exclusive to rural/folk societies, were just as psychologically
important for city people as for country people.[15] William Mangin also drew similar
conclusions from his study of peasant migration to Lima.[16] Research on migration
and community formation in the nineteenth century urban 'industrial villages' of
northern England has revealed a similar situation. Short-distance chain migration,
often undertaken in family groupings, led not only to the formation of tight kinship
groups, but also neighbourhoods where many of the people were from the same
rural region, creating a strong sense of continuity through association, and community through shared knowledge. These primary group relations were also
strengthened by the fact that neighbourhoods crystallized around individual factories, so that neighbours shared not only the same social space but also the same
working environment. As Ray Pahl noted, 'despite the census evidence there would
not be any great change in their way of living as a result of urbanization'.[17]

The question of the nature of urban communal relations is obviously a crucial
factor in the apparent decline of witch-accusations in the urban environment.
Historical thought on witchcraft has been heavily influenced by the work of Keith
Thomas and Alan Macfarlane, both of whom have stressed that the dynamics of
witchcraft were embedded in village communal relations. John Putnam Demos has
followed the same argument and has come to the conclusion that 'witchcraft
belonged, first and last, to the life of the little community'.[18] If this is the case,
then we might expect witchcraft accusations to decline as a result of the less close-

knit, more individualistic, ill-defined communities of the modern city, but be less affected by the community structure of 'industrial villages'.

Generalizations about urban social relationships are rightly open to criticism, and quantifying the strength and extent of communal relationships is incredibly difficult, whether in an urban or rural context, and more so over a period of time. One of the arguments against the sociological concept of 'urban villages', for example, is the high level of mobility of the urban population, which created instability within communal relationships. As Clark and Souden have pointed out though, mobility can be an important force for stability within the social system, as well as a dynamic and disruptive force for change.[19] In early modern England the flow of rural migrants to an expanding London did not necessarily lead to irrevocable breaks in social relations between village and city. Rural teenagers were apprenticed to urban relations or friends, and many townspeople returned to their village homes to help at harvest time, thus reinforcing those kinship links which geographical distance might otherwise have broken. Jeremy Boulton's work on seventeenth century Southwark has revealed just such a picture of a mobile but stable urban community. Boulton found that while there was a fairly high population turnover, much of this movement was localized. Householders 'moved from house to house and from street to street in response to social and economic forces but kept within the same familiar area'. In fact, the turnover statistics from the Boroughside of Southwark are not significantly higher than those from rural areas in the same period. Boulton remarks several times on the continuities of lifestyle between urban and rural living: 'As in English rural society, many Boroughside householders may have possessed geographically restricted social horizons, living out much of their lives within a local social system'.[20] This depiction of a seventeenth century urban community in Southwark helps explain the continued vigour of witch-accusations in the area until the early eighteenth century. There was sufficient residential stability for the formation of informal social networks based on neighbourhood ties, and in the sense that this fostered a level of communal interaction similar to that in the village, Southwark neighbourhoods, like the village unit, generated an environment conducive to witch-accusations.

Communities are not static, though, and as London continued to expand, especially in the nineteenth century, one might expect once stable, 'old' neighbourhoods to be overwhelmed by new immigrants, new housing, new industries, so that they lose their identity, and social networks are constantly undergoing a series of fluctuations. In this situation we might, if we follow the above argument, expect accusations to decline significantly. But we should be cautious in making gross generalizations about this process, since while some stable, cohesive communities disappear others are constantly being formed. The crucial factor is the frequency of these changes in comparison with the general long-term stability of villages. Peter Willmott's comparative study of mid nineteenth century Bethnal Green and Preston highlights the varying experiences of urban community formation.[21] Willmott found that mid nineteenth century Bethnal Green was characterized by rapid changes in the composition of its population, and reckoned that this hampered the formation of primary networks. In terms of family, only twenty-three households out of a thousand contained a relative of another household in the same neighbourhood. In contrast, the growth of Preston's textile industry led to chain migration, making the formation of extensive and tight-knit family networks possible, where newcomers could integrate.

As we have seen, the social environment of late sixteenth and seventeenth century Southwark was conducive to the making of witchcraft accusations. Communities remained relatively stable, as stable as many villages of the period, despite quite high levels of mobility, and it is quite likely that relations remained quite strong between migrants in urban Southwark and their relations in the rural home. Urban dwellers were still strongly bound to rural culture. Southwark was not so big that those who lived there were unaware of the agricultural rhythm of life, and many still returned to their rural home to help with harvesting or for village festivals. The complete divorce between urban and rural culture had not yet developed sufficiently to lead to potentially significant changes in the social organization and behaviour of urban dwellers, which could concomitantly affect the level of witchcraft accusations. The links with the rural home were firm but there was probably little thought of returning. Social mobility was high but the flow of people was not so much from Southwark to home village as from street to street. Thus resilient communities could form, firmly rooted through a level of social networking and interaction similar to that in the village community. In these circumstances, the victim's search for the person responsible for his or her misfortunes need not be sought back in the village community, since relations with fellow neighbours and colleagues were sufficiently personal and intimate for accusations to be levelled within the urban community. Witchcraft accusations have been seen by some as a response to communal insecurity and instability, but what this examination of urban witchcraft suggests is that the converse is also true. Witchcraft accusations may, in fact, be indicative of social stability. It is possible, therefore, that once that stability starts to break down, there might be a concomitant drop in the level of witchcraft accusations.

The rapid expansion of London during the nineteenth century led to quite significant levels of social instability (as seen from Willmott's work on Bethnal Green), resulting in the breakdown and swamping of existing communities. That is not to say that close-knit urban communities did not exist, but the intimacy of neighbourly relations and primary networks which fostered witchcraft accusations may not have been able to develop in this environment to the same extent as it had once done in early modern London, or as they continued to do in rural areas. As a result of this instability, it may be that some community-level social control mechanisms, such as witchcraft accusations, ceased to function properly, and declined. Without that depth of networking within a community, when suspicions of witchcraft were generated, a direct or public accusation was not made because the victim was uncertain as to how the people around would react to his or her claims. As J. Clyde Mitchell explained, to see the hand of witchcraft in misfortunes may be the first reaction of a townsman, but it is an interpretation which in terms of the social and administrative structure of the urban community allows him no direct retributive action.[22]

Another supernaturally inspired social control mechanism which does seem to have survived quite well within urban London was the use of the Bible-and-key for the identification of thieves and stolen property. In 1832, for example, Eleanor Blucher, a native of Prussia, was brought before the Thames Police-Court charged with assaulting Mary White, the wife of a mechanic. Both parties lived in the same court in Ratcliff. White, having recently lost several articles of value from her yard, assembled a number of other women to perform the Bible-and-key to find out the thief.[23] The key turned and it was unanimously agreed upon that Blucher was the thief, and it was accordingly given out in the neighbourhood that she had stolen two pairs of 'inexpressibles' belonging to Mrs White's husband. Blucher, incensed by the accusations, subsequently assaulted White. In court Blucher stated that 'the neighbours were always turning the key upon her'. White replied that the key and Bible was the surest way to discover a thief. In turn, Mr. Ballantine (magistrate) replied facetiously that he was sure 'the spell would be of great service to the police, who would be glad to avail themselves of it'. He also expressed surprise that 'such superstition should exist in the British metropolis in the 19th century'.[24] At the same police-court fifty-two years later, Ellen Lyons, twenty-seven, a married woman, residing at 18, Pell Street, St George's-in-the-East was charged with violently assaulting Sarah O'Brien after accusing her of theft. It transpired that Lyons had lost a shawl, and certain that it had been stolen she gathered several friends to her room where the Bible-and-key was performed. Lyons repeated several names to no effect until O'Brien's name was uttered and the key fell right out of the Bible. The same ritual was repeated to discover the name of the pawnbrokers where the shawl was pledged.[25]

The significance of the continued practice of the Bible-and-key in nineteenth-century London lies in the fact that, to gain legitimacy, the divination ceremony had to be performed in the presence of neighbours and friends (who, by inference, believed in the magic involved), who would then sanction the resulting accusation in the neighbourhood. For this control mechanism to operate, there had to be a certain level of communal integration, such as occurred in residential courts like those in Ratcliff. The crucial question this poses is whether witchcraft accusations were also generated in such enclosed London communities. Possibly, but not necessarily. Accusations concerning both types of social crime – theft and witchcraft – were usually based upon reputation, but the formation of reputation in each case was often different. Within the little community, complete strangers and new-comers were equally likely, if not more likely, to be potential petty thieves than long-term residents. One wonders, for example, if Blucher gained her reputation purely because she was a foreigner. Accusations of petty-theft were easily made and reputations easily gained. On the other hand, the making of the reputation of a witch was usually, but not always, based on certain traditional criteria such as visual appearance, gender, age, and position in the communal hierarchy. More importantly, the reputation of a witch was usually generated and sustained through the long-term accumulation of supposed maleficent acts, held in the collective memory of the community. So, it is possible that even in urban neighbourhoods where the Bible-and-key could operate effectively, a high population turnover could prevent the formation of the long-term reputations which led to public accusations.

There is some indication that in nineteenth century London, accusations of witchcraft were more likely to be made within the family group than in the wider community. The immediate family group was a social arena where relationships were still sufficiently intense, personal and long-standing to produce accusations. It is, perhaps, significant, therefore, that in all seven cases of witchcraft from early modern Southwark, the accusations were apparently generated outside the family group, whereas in two of the three nineteenth century cases conflict was located within the family. Irwin Press has also found that in non-western cities where witchcraft accusations do operate in the urban arena, they usually result from dyadic conflicts between individuals closely related to each other and particularly susceptible to mutual sanction: 'siblings, spouses, lovers, and rivals for mates are more common sources of supernatural attack than are business rivals, jealous neighbours, or generally antisocial acquaintances'.[26]

If, in nineteenth century London, social conditions were not so conducive to witchcraft accusations against neighbours and acquaintances as they were in rural society, and accusations were more likely to be made within the kin group, then another factor responsible for declining accusations may have been the weakening and dispersal of the traditional family group. As we have already seen, in the area of Bethnal Green, where Mary Gable and Sarah McDonald lived, only twenty-three out of a thousand households contained a relative of another household in the same neighbourhood. The potential weakening of the extended family group may have also been an influential factor in the decline of witch-beliefs as well as witch-accusations. Stories concerning witches and witchcraft, were primarily, though not exclusively, perpetuated through oral transmission, particularly within the family group – with perhaps the most influential flow of such information being from grandparent to grandchild. In urban environments, where communities are continually in a state of flux, where shared group knowledge is less intimate and the collective memory of the community is neither so broad nor so deep, the continued transmission of old traditions and beliefs through the family group becomes even more crucial. But as that pathway becomes increasingly interrupted and redundant, so the maintenance of those beliefs amongst subsequent generations can weaken. A folklore study of Humr communities in Khartoum, fifteen years after their migration there, has revealed just such a process. Out of thirty-two informants interviewed, only one reported that she had experienced story-telling during her stay. The rest of the informants stated that they had neither heard nor told any stories or riddles ever since they came to Khartoum.[27] This can be attributed to the break-up of the extended family system, which meant that the grandmother, who was the major story-teller in Humr society, was absent. That is not to say that folklore died in London, for while old folkloric traditions disappeared, new genres and new occasions for the exchange and performance of folklore were created. However, these were rooted in the new socio-economic conditions of the city rather than in the culture of the rural past.

The increasing separation from the vagaries of agricultural life must have also had an effect upon the relevance of witchcraft in an urban environment. Witchcraft accusations often stemmed from the inexplicable illness and death of livestock, or from problems associated with the processing of agricultural products. In early modern rural Surrey, nearly a half of all accusations involved livestock, and nearly a third related to livestock only. It was not only farmers who depended on livestock. Most members of rural society were involved in animal production in one way or another. The pig which many labourers fattened up in their backyards, for example, was an important economic and even psychological asset in a subsistence existence. In this context farm animals could almost be considered as an extension of the family group. As the importance of livestock rearing in the lives of urban dwellers diminished, then this, in the tong term, must surely have had a concomitant effect, not only on the pattern of witchcraft accusations, but also on the number of accusations, in that the range of potentially sensitive targets of witchcraft was narrowed. On a broader level, many magical operations involving farming practices, and rural flora and fauna, also became irrelevant and therefore redundant in the urban environment.

Where livestock still remained, then, even by the end of the century, we continue to find evidence of rural magical practices concerning them. As late as 1902, the folklorist, Edward Lovett, came across the case of a cowkeeper, a migrant from Devon, living in the north-east district of London, who, believing his cows were bewitched, removed the heart of one dead cow, stuck it full of pins and nails and hung it up in his chimney as a counter-charm.[28] The tradition of keeping a goat (sometimes a donkey) with cattle to prevent the latter from slipping their calves and to protect them from disease and bewitchment, was continued in the livery-stables of London. Many London carriers apparently kept them in their stables for the same purpose. A correspondent to *Notes and Queries* also recalled seeing the donkey charm for rickets being performed in Hoxton market-place in 1845, though the practice seems to have died out soon atter.[29]

Charles Phythian-Adams, in an innovative study of May Day rituals in London, has attempted to chart the process of London's growing detachment from that culture and economy. By the eighteenth century, the may-pole had fallen out of use in urban London. Instead, Londoners forsook the urban streets for the day, and went out to celebrate and join in festivities in the surrounding countryside, a move indicative of an increasing separation of rural and urban spheres. From the mid seventeenth to the late eighteenth century a contrary migration also took place, with milkmaids leading garlanded cows through the streets of London, bringing a breath of the country back into the city for the day. Around 1800 this last vestige of rural symbolism disappeared, partly as a result of the introduction of winter-feeding on oil cake in urban milk factories, but more significantly due to the appropriation of the festival by soot-blackened chimneysweeps. As Phythian-Adams concluded, 'what had originated in a largely rural society ended up in London as a strictly limited ritual dialogue between two separate urban "nations"'.[30] The irrevocable separation of London from traditional rural culture by the early nineteenth century has also been traced by Mark Judd through an examination of the city's fairs. The traditional function of fairs as markets for agricultural produce and hiring of labour had declined significantly by the early nineteenth century. The old seasonal basis for fairs had also lost much of its significance by this time.[31] Lynn Lees found that the initial impact of urban London on Irish migrants was to force them to abandon much of their rural lifestyle, a wide variety of cultural practices and communal rituals, as well as the use of the Irish language: 'Irish migrants abandoned a complex agricultural society for a complex urbanizing one'.[32] Not surprisingly, Lees has also suggested that the belief in witches and fairies amongst Irish immigrants declined in this environment, though no real evidence from London is cited.

It is quite clear that witch-believing rural migrants were not going to suddenly discard their beliefs and cultural baggage on entering their new home in the city.

The first time they were subjected to some unaccountable misfortune there might still have been a suspicion of witchcraft, even if that suspicion was not openly expressed. This begs the question whether the decline in urban accusations was actually indicative of a declining belief in witchcraft. Of course, one has to be extremely careful about extrapolating from individual accusations of witchcraft. Two of the three accusations of witchcraft I have found occurred within the family group. All we can infer from this is that the families concerned obviously believed in witchcraft, but we cannot conclude that the rest of the community they lived in were also believers. Conversely, an absence of accusations need not necessarily indicate an absence of belief.

An individual accusation of witchcraft within a rural context was usually representative of a communal expression of the belief in witchcraft. Most accusations may at first appear to involve only the accused and the accuser, but usually accusations were the culmination of a period of incubation during which the opinions of family, friends and neighbours were canvassed. Accusations were not usually made until the accuser was sure that those in his or her social group were convinced that there were grounds for the accusation. An accusation was, therefore, the legitimizing step towards the communal sanctioning of a direct action against a witch, whether that action be swimming, scratching, or prosecution prior to 1736. In nineteenth century London, public accusations of witchcraft seem to have been rare because direct action against a witch outside the family group was not certain to receive sanction by the community in which both actors lived.

There were other manifestations of the belief in witchcraft, however, which were not reliant on public accusations, face to face confrontation, or direct action. Private means of forcing witches to remove their spells were also employed. This could be achieved by supernaturally tormenting the witch: by burning powders, as Gable paid Sarah McDonald to do, by piercing a cow's heart as Lovett's cow-man did, or by employing a witch-bottle. One of the most common measures employed to prevent witchcraft was the displaying of horseshoes. It is the evidence of this expression of belief which provides us with the only indicator, albeit very basic, of the declining relevancy, if not the declining belief in witchcraft. Considering the paucity of information and lack of continuity of the other anti-witchcraft measures, the use and disappearance of horseshoes in London, from the late seventeenth to the early nineteenth century, provides us with at least some sense of change over time.

In the late seventeenth century John Aubrey commented that most houses in the west end of London had horseshoes on their thresholds to ward off witchcraft.[33] A hundred years later, in 1797, the antiquarian John Brand recorded that in Monmouth Street, in the West End, many horseshoes were still to be found nailed to the thresholds. In 1813 Sir Henry Ellis, editor of several editions of *Brand's Observations*, counted no fewer than seventeen horseshoes nailed against the steps of doors in Monmouth Street. However, when he surveyed the Street again in 1841, only five or six remained.[34] Up until at least the 1820s a famous horseshoe was to be found on the door of the one time residence of Lady Hatton, wife of Sir Christopher Hatton, in Bleeding Heart Yard. An inhabitant of the house in the early nineteenth century recalled how one old woman begged for admittance repeatedly to satisfy herself that the horseshoe was still secure in its place.[35] By the time of the First World War, the horseshoe was still to be found in London houses, but instead of being displayed on the threshold to ward off witchcraft, it was now to be found placed above the bed as a preventative against nightmares.

By the twentieth century, then, not only had the display of the overtly super-stitious horseshoe become a private affair, but its original purpose as a prophylactic against witches had been lost. This significant withdrawal of the horseshoe from public view seems to have occurred sometime during the 1820s and 1830s. This not only indicates the redundancy of the horseshoe in an urban environment where witchcraft was fast becoming an irrelevancy, but also reflects upon an increasing sense of public embarrassment concerning the visual display of anything supersti-tious. Such a date for the declining relevancy of witchcraft in London, fits well with the time-scale, posited above, for the declining relevancy of rural symbolism, traditional pastimes, and seasonal, agricultural dependency.

The reputations of rural cunning-folk were often built around their ability to unbewitch humans and livestock, and much of their business consisted of this activity. In London, though, cunning-folk such as Sarah McDonald were, it seems, more recognized for their prowess at fortune-telling and fortune-making than for their unbewitching skills. With the decline of this aspect of their business, many cunning-folk were, to all intents and purposes, little more than common fortune-tellers. Not surprisingly, then, the terms 'conjuror', 'wizard', 'white witch', 'wise-man' and 'wise-woman' all seem to have been uncommon but not unknown in London. McDonald, for example, was known as a 'wise woman', and the fortune-teller James Ball was popularly known as the 'wise man of Stepney'. Otherwise, though, 'fortune-teller' and 'astrologer' were the only epithets popularly used for occult practitioners. Similarly, a correspondent, writing of Bristol in the 1890s, remarked that the term 'white witch' had become obsolete in the city, and that 'planet-ruler' had become the popular term to describe such people.[36] Such shifts in popular terminology are not discernible in rural areas during the same period.

There has been a tendency amongst historians of witchcraft and magic to see the belief in witchcraft and other expressions of popular magic as a single cultural phenomenon. Because of this assumption, it has been taken for granted that the social and economic factors which affected the belief in witchcraft also similarly affected the belief in other aspects of popular magic. What this study of witchcraft in London indicates, however, is that different expressions of popular magic decline and survive at different rates depending on particular socio-economic changes. Thus the divorce from rurality and changing urban community structures seem to have led to a decline in the expression of witchcraft beliefs in London, but did not simi-larly affect the belief in fortune-telling, divination and love magic. While the modem urban environment militated against the expression of personal misfortunes and tensions in terms of witchcraft, the same insecurities were still able to find relief in the fortune-teller's assurance of better things to come, and in the resort to magical manipulation of the future.

Notes

1   Ruth Martin, *Witchcraft and the Inquisition in Venice 1550–1650* (Oxford 1989), 241–4.

2   Jens Christian V. Johansen, 'Denmark: The Sociology of Accusations', in Bengt Ankarloo and Gustav Henningsen eds, *Early Modern European Witchcraft: Centres and Peripheries* (Oxford 1990), 30.

3   J. S. Cockburn ed., *Calendar of Assize Records: Surrey Indictments Elizabeth I* (London 1980); *Calendar of Assize Records: Surrey Indictments, James I* (London, 1982). For an examination of seventeenth century witchcraft beliefs in another part of London see Robert Higgins, 'Popular Beliefs about Witches: The Evidence from East London, 1645–60', *East London Record* 4 (1981), 36–41.

4   Jeremy Boulton, *Neighbourhood and Society: A London Suburb in the Seventeenth Century* (Cambridge 1987), table 3.3.

5   See *A Full and True Account of the Apprehending and Taking of Mrs. Sarah Moordike* (London 1701); *The Tryall of Richard Hathaway* (London 1702).

6   Surrey Quarter Sessions Roll, Epiphany 1699/1 700 (m117).

7   *A Full and True Account of the Discovery, Apprehending, and Taking of a Notorious Witch* (London 1704).

8   *The Times*, 21 October 1818; *Westmorland Gazette*, 7 November 1818.

9   *Somerset County Herald*, 4 September 1858.

10 *All The Year Round*, 6 November 1869.

11 *The Times*, 2 June 1862.

12 *Somerset County Herald*, 21 June 1862.

13 J. Clyde Mitchell, 'The Meaning in Misfortune for Urban Africans', and Marc J. Swartz, 'Modern Conditions and Witchcraft/Sorcery Accusations', both in Max Marwick ed., *Witchcraft and Sorcery* (London 1970).

14 Jeremy Boulton, 'Residential Mobility in Seventeenth-century Southwark', *Urban History Yearbook* (1986), 1–14.

15 Oscar Lewis, 'Further Observations on the Folk–Urban Continuum and Urbanization with Special Reference to Mexico City', in Philip Hauser and Leo Schnore eds, *The Study of Urbanization* (New York 1965), 500.

16 William Mangin, 'Mental Health and Migration to Cities', in Paul Meadows and Ephraim Mizruchi, eds, *Urbanism, Urbanization, and Change: Comparative Perspectives* (Boston, Mass. 1969).

17 Ray Pahl, *Patterns of Urban Life* (London 1970), 30–1. Robin Pearson has identified a process of active reassertion of communal identity in the out-townships of Leeds during the second half of the nineteenth century, with local traditions and customs being actively revived; Robin Pearson, 'Knowing One's Place', *Journal of Social History* 26 (1993), 221–44.

18 John Putnam Demos, *Entertaining Satan: Witchcraft and the Culture of New England* (Oxford 1982), 275.

19 Peter Clark and David Souden, *Migration and Society in Early Modern England* (London 1987), 22.

20 Boulton, *Neighbourhood and Society*, 291.

21 Peter Willmott, *Kinship and Urban Community: Past and Present* (Leicester 1987).

22 Mitchell, 'The Meaning in Misfortune', 389.

23 In this instance the ritual involved the street-door key being placed on the 50th Psalm, the Bible being closed and fastened tightly with a woman's garter, and then suspended from a nail. Blucher's name was then repeated three times by one woman, while another recited the following words: 'If it turns to thee, thou art the thief, and we are all free'.

24 *The Times*, 17 June 1832.

25 *The Times,* 17 April 1884.

26 Irwin Press, 'Urban Folk Medicine: A Functional Overview', *American Anthropologist* 80 (1978), 73–83; 76.

27 Sayyid H. Hurriez, 'Folklore, Urbanization and Modernization in Contemporary Africa', in Szilárd Biernaczky ed., *Folklore in Africa Today* (Budapest 1984), 619–63.

28 Lovett, *Magic in Modern London,* 67. Areas of north-east London like Walthamstow and Wanstead still backed onto agricultural areas by 1902.

29 *Notes and Queries,* 6 October 1855, 260. The charm involved passing the afflicted child over the back and under the belly of the donkey eighty-one times.

30 Charles Phythian-Adams, 'Milk and Soot: The Changing Vocabulary of a Popular Ritual in Stuart and Hanoverian London', in Derek Fraser and Anthony Sutcliffe eds, *The Pursuit of Urban History* (London 1983), 104.

31 Mark Judd, '"The oddest combination of town and country": popular culture and the London fairs, 1800–1860', in John Walton and James Walvin eds, *Leisure in Britain 1780–1939* (Manchester 1983), 11–30.

32 Lynn Hollen Lees, *Exiles of Erin: Irish Migrants in Victorian London* (New York 1979), 247.

33 John Aubrey, *Miscellanies* (London 1696), 148.

34 John Brand, *Observations on Popular Antiquities,* revised with additions by Henry Ellis (London 1849), 17.

35 Charles Mackay, *Extraordinary Popular Delusions and the Madness of Crowds* (New York 1932; first published 1841), 558–9.

36 *The Spectator,* 17 February 1894, 231.

PART TEN

A New Witch-Hunt?

I N 1602 HENRI BOGUET DESCRIBED a dramatic and tragic encounter between a father and his child. The man, Guillaume Le Baillu, was accused by his 12-year-old son of attending the witches' sabbat at the nearby village of Coirieres, where 'his father had urged him to give himself to the Devil'. Boguet himself attended the meeting between the alleged witch and his child, and recalled it with unusual feeling in his treatise on the philosophy and procedure of witch trials:

> It was a strange and harrowing experience to witness these confrontations. For the father was emaciated through his imprisonment, he had fetters on his hands and feet, he wailed and shouted and threw himself to the ground. I remember too that, when he became calmer, he sometimes spoke kindly to his son, saying that whatever he did he would always own him as his child.

Despite the boy's allegations, the accused man never confessed to the 'secret abominations' with which he was charged. He died in prison before his case reached the court.[1]

It is hard for anyone reading this account in the early twenty-first century to ignore the echoes of Le Baillu's fate in the allegations of satanic child abuse in Britain and North America during the 1980s and 1990s. Beginning in 1980 with the publication of *Michelle Remembers*, a 'survivor's testimony' of life in a clandestine organisation of Devil-worshipping child-killers in Montreal, a series of reports concerning satanic abuse were made to police and social workers in North America and the United Kingdom. Many of these, like *Michelle Remembers* itself, came from adult survivors of abuse that had apparently occurred in childhood. Other allegations, including most of those in Britain, were made by children taken into care on suspicion of abuse. Some of these disclosures resulted in the removal of children from other families, and the prosecution of adults for alleged partici-pation in abusive rites. The British experience of satanic abuse culminated in 1990, when the children of two families were removed from their parents on the Orkney Islands in Scotland. Amid a storm of media interest, the children were returned when a judge ruled that there was no case to answer. This episode prompted a government inquiry into eighty-four cases of alleged child abuse in a ritual context, which concluded that there was no evidence of organised satanic abuse in the UK.[2] There is, nonetheless, a continuing debate about the existence of the phenomenon, which has inspired passionate contributions from therapists, police officers and academics.[3]

Given the apparent similarities between early modern witch persecutions and contemporary prosecutions for satanic crime, it is not surprising that the spectre of 'witchcraft' has been evoked by the critics of ritual abuse allegations. Some historians have compared witch trials to the twentieth-century 'demonology' of satanic abuse. In the conclusion to an article on the trial of child witches in early modern Germany, Robert Walinski-Kiehl noted that historians can no longer 'console themselves with the comforting knowledge that satanic scares involving children have been banished from the historical stage never to return'.[4] More boldly, Robin Briggs has asked how long it will be 'before the renewed enthusiasm for the death penalty in the United States leads to someone being executed for, in all but name, being a witch?'[5] It is more surprising, perhaps, to find that some supporters of the existence of satanic abuse have also referred to early modern witchcraft. Both Brett Kahr and Martin Katchen have suggested that child-killing sects did indeed exist in the pre-industrial period.[6] For Katchen, there are clear parallels between the prosecution of witches and the pursuit of modern-day satanists:

> The inquisition comes to be seen as a police force, perhaps no worse than the KGB, attempting to investigate and bring to justice criminals, some of whom were not only criminals under the laws of the mediaeval church, but under the laws of any modern society. The problems that the inquisition faced, of reliability of evidence, overzealousness, and political pressures, are also the problems of modern police forces and serious investigators of contemporary satanism.[7]

In his enthusiasm to identify historical precedents for satanic abuse, Katchen comes close to endorsing the views of Montague Summers, who argued in 1925 that witches were guilty of many of the crimes of child murder and cannibalism for which they were condemned.[8]

The willingness of both sides to refer to witchcraft in the debate about satanic abuse suggests that there are strong connections between the two phenomena. This is only partially true, however. Modern accounts of satanic crime contain relatively few references to harmful magic, which was the most widely accepted aspect of pre-industrial witchcraft. While the testimonies of alleged survivors often mention supernatural events – such as flight, bodily transformations or the physical appearance of the Devil – these details are generally dismissed by therapists and social workers, whose cultural background does not permit them to accept the reality of such occurrences. In effect, the theory of satanic abuse is a secularised version of the sabbat: the secret gathering of satanists to perform obscene acts of worship, indulge in unlawful sexual acts and murder young children.[9] This image was already well established in the fifteenth-century texts described by Norman Cohn in Chapter 2, and can be traced back further to allegations against early Christians and mediaeval Jews.

There are also some procedural similarities between the investigation of witches' sabbats and satanic abuse. Both crimes involve members of the same family or community, who conspire to keep their activities hidden. As Boguet remarked in 1602, 'they always commit their crimes and abominations in the night and in secret, so it is only their kindred who are able to give evidence against them'.[10] In such circumstances, it is necessary to attach enormous importance to the confessions or testimonies of supposed members of the group, which often provide the only evidence that secret meetings have taken place. At a different level, the attempts of historians to identify the social reality behind the idea of the sabbat raise similar questions to those posed by investigators of satanic abuse. How much weight can be attached to uncorroborated descriptions of clandestine meetings? Are some confessions more reliable than others? Which elements of the confessions – if any – can be attributed to folk beliefs or personal experiences, and which elements were probably imposed by those conducting the interrogations?

One obvious insight that witchcraft scholars have provided is that allegations of collective satanism can be entirely fictitious. No serious historian since the 1950s has argued that those accused of witchcraft were genuine Devil-worshippers, though Carlo Ginzburg and Éva Pócs have suggested that some of those accused were involved in cultic activities of some kind (see Chapters 8 and 9). The confessions of many witches were demonstrably false, a fact that was sometimes recognised by contemporary investigators.[11] In Chapter 30, Philip Jenkins and Daniel Maier-Katkin offer compelling evidence that many survivors' accounts of satanic abuse – including the seminal testimony of Michelle Smith in *Michelle Remembers* – cannot stand up to empirical scrutiny. In some cases, reliable alternative sources contradict the stories told by alleged survivors; in others, there is a complete lack of corroborative evidence in sources where one could reasonably expect to find it. As Jenkins and Maier-Katkin point out, the allegations made by Smith and others conform to a stereotype of 'secret crimes' attributed to various minority groups in American society in the last two hundred years. In each of these earlier cases, it appears that the allegations were equally unsubstantiated.

The fact that very few allegations of ritual abuse can be verified, and some have been disproved, does not mean that the crime has *never* taken place. It does suggest, however, that a large number of accusations must be treated with considerable scepticism. If many of these accusations are false, it appears that the fantasy of a secret community of sexually transgressive, child-killing diabolists is as compelling today as it was in the sixteenth century. Why is this myth so enduring? One possibility, which is touched on by Lyndal Roper in Chapter 24, is that the idea of satanic witchcraft appeals to unchanging human experiences and needs, rooted in basic relationships between parents and children. Such trans-historical factors may shed light on the recurring elements in accounts of secret satanic crimes, but they cannot explain why such fantasies surface in particular societies at particular moments. The reasons why false allegations of murderous Devil-worship occurred in North America and Britain in the 1980s are probably as complex as those behind the similar phenomenon in early modern Europe, and cannot be explored fully here. But one helpful concept, which has been employed by both witchcraft historians and critics of satanic abuse, is the idea of 'moral panics'. A moral panic occurs when members of a community perceive a real or imagined threat to their fundamental values, and respond with a disproportionate effort to destroy that threat. Such panics are often associated with periods of insta-bility or change, when traditional assumptions need to be reaffirmed.[12] Historians like Larner and Walinski-Kiehl have argued that the Reformation stimulated concerns about the family in the early modern period, providing the impetus for moral panics about witches. Similarly, David Bromley has suggested that changing patterns of employment in 1980s America inspired anxieties about the care of minors, as more and more families were obliged to leave their children with profes-sional carers as they went to work. He points out that many allegations of satanic abuse involved day care centres, and argues that this reflected the unease of parents forced to leave their children in the hands of strangers.[13] If Bromley is correct, the desire to defend an idealised concept of the family in a time of social change was an important element in the satanic abuse scare, just as it probably contributed to the witch persecutions of the pre-industrial age.

On the other side of the debate, those authors who accept the existence of satanic abuse rely largely on the testimonies of alleged cult survivors. For coun-sellors such as George Greaves and Valerie Sinason, the failure to secure convictions for satanic crimes lies in the different methodologies adopted by psychotherapists and lawyers. The kind of evidence required to secure a criminal conviction is very different to that needed to establish the validity of their patients' disclosures.[14] In many instances, the crimes they describe took place in the distant past, or in places they can no longer locate. Furthermore, Greaves suggests that in some cases there *is* corroborative evidence, but this is apparently insufficient to satisfy the courts.[15] It is useful, perhaps, to balance this perspective with that of Kenneth Lanning, an FBI agent with experience of investigating satanic crime. Lanning notes that 'many of those not involved in law enforcement do not understand that, while it is possible to get rid of a body, it is much more difficult to get rid of the physical evidence that a murder took place, especially a human sacrifice involving sex, blood and mutilation'. In the course of more than a hundred investigations into such alleged crimes, Lanning has never found evidence of a satanic murder, though this is one of the acts most frequently described in survivor accounts.[16]

Ultimately, the debate about satanic abuse presents readers with very different interpretations of the same body of limited and problematical evidence. In this, it resembles the debate between historians about the meaning of the sabbat in early modern Europe. Some details of the sabbat were undoubtedly false: witches did not fly through the air or transform themselves into animals; nor did they murder children or worship the Devil. Many witchcraft confessions were heavily influenced by the expectations of demonologists; but some included details that had no obvious source in learned theory, and possibly reflected the existence of local fairy cults or shamanistic practices. Likewise, it appears that many allegations of satanic abuse include wildly implausible elements, and some accusations are demonstrably untrue. It is possible, nonetheless, that some testimonies contain accurate descriptions of abuse; and this places therapists, social workers and police officers in the testing position of separating fact from fantasy in the statements of alleged survivors. It is relatively easy for historians to discuss these issues in the context of sixteenth- and seventeenth-century witchcraft; but they involve more immediate and serious consequences when the supposed satanists, and their alleged victims, are people living today.

One consequence of satanic abuse is that it makes us appreciate the appalling problems involved in dealing with secret crimes that, if they are real, involve terrible acts of brutality. However sceptical we might be in the face of apparently outlandish accusations, we find it hard to dismiss them completely. This problem is summed up eloquently by Patrick Casement in Chapter 31:

> What if some of these accounts *are* true? Not to believe someone who has actually been a victim of such abuse leaves that person still alone in the torment of their own experiences, and leaves the perpetrators free to continue these practices undeterred. At the very least, I believe we must keep an open mind when we begin to hear of such things: some- times we may be hearing the truth – as far as these victims are able to risk telling that truth to anyone.

It is Casement's view that the horrific nature of allegations of satanic abuse means that most people are reluctant to believe them. It is tempting, however, to argue that precisely the reverse is true: the awful content of these disclosures puts a high price on scepticism, since to disbelieve the alleged victim is to allow the atrocities to go on. Once the idea of the witches' sabbat was widely disseminated in Renaissance Europe, those concerned with the threat of satanic witchcraft faced a similar dilemma. Indeed, their situation was more difficult than our own, since their belief system did not allow them to dismiss the physical reality of the Devil, and their authoritative sources of information – the Bible and the church fathers – clearly endorsed the existence of witches. It is hardly surprising that many educated Europeans came to believe in a satanic conspiracy. In our own time, when some highly qualified professionals believe in essentially the same thing, we can perhaps begin to understand why.

Notes

1   Henri Boguet, *An Examen of Witches*, trans. Montague Summers (John Rodker, London 1929), 160–2.

2   Jean La Fontaine, *The Extent and Nature of Organised Ritual Abuse* (HMSO, London 1994).

3   For a collection of essays supporting the existence of satanic abuse, see Valerie Sinason, ed., *Treating Survivors of Satanist Abuse* (Routledge, London 1994). A critique of satanic abuse allegations, and the related subject of recovered memories of abuse, can be found in Hollinda Wakefield and Ralph Underwager, *Return of the Furies* (Open Court, Illinois 1994).

4   Robert Walinski-Kiehl, 'The Devil's Children: Child Witch-Trials in Early Modern Germany', *Continuity and Change*, 11(2), (1996), 186.

5   Robin Briggs, *Witches and Neighbours* (HarperCollins, London 1996), 411.

6   Brett Kahr, 'The Historical Foundations of Ritual Abuse', in Sinason, ed., *Treating Survivors*, 52–3; Martin Katchen, 'The History of Satanic Religions', in David Sakheim and Susan Devine, eds, *Out of Darkness: Exploring Satanism and Ritual Abuse* (Lexington Books, New York 1992), 1–19.

7   Katchen, ibid., 7.

8   Montague Summers, *The History of Witchcraft* (1925; repr. Studio Editions, London 1994), 160–2.

9   The prevalence of allegations of child killing is noted in the La Fontaine report, 22. For a detailed survivors' account from America making similar allegations, see Linda and David Stone, 'Ritual Abuse: the Experiences of Five Families', in Sakheim and Devine, eds, *Out of Darkness*, 175–83.

10   Boguet, *Examen*, 162.

11   For an exceptionally well-documented account of contemporary scepticism, see Gustav Henningsen, *The Witches' Advocate: Basque Witchcraft and the Spanish Inquisition* (University of Nevada Press, Reno 1980).

12   For a sociological introduction to this concept, see Kenneth Thompson, *Moral Panics* (Routledge, London 1998).

13   David Bromley, 'Satanic Abuse: The New Cult Scare', in J. T. Richardson, J. Best and D. G. Bromley, eds, *The Satanism Scare* (Aldine De Gruyter, New York 1991), ch. 4.

14   George Greaves, 'Alternative Hypotheses Regarding Claims of Satanic Cult Activity', in Sakheim and Devine, eds, *Out of Darkness*, ch. 3; Sinason, *Treating Survivors*, ch. 1.

15   Greaves, 'Alternative Hypotheses', 66–7.

16   Kenneth Lanning, 'A Law-Enforcement Perspective on Allegations of Ritual Abuse', in Sakheim and Devine, eds, *Out of Darkness*, 130.

Chapter 30

Philip Jenkins and Daniel Maier-Katkin

OCCULT SURVIVORS

The making of a myth

'Proofs of a conspiracy'

IN THE LATE 1980s, it was frequently alleged that the United States faced a serious crime-wave associated with the occult or satanism.[1] However, the lack of solid corroborating evidence has caused many critics to dismiss these claims.[2] In response, believers in a satanic menace suggest various reasons why proof is not forthcoming. The authorities might fail to note evidence through ignorance or more sinister motives; or else the satanists demonstrate extreme cunning in concealing evidence of their crimes. Without material evidence, the focus of inquiry must shift to the first-hand testimony of witnesses and participants. These are the occult 'survivors', alleged former cult members or victims, whose evidence thus attains unique significance.

There are now hundreds of individuals who claim to be 'survivors' and they even maintain a self-help group, 'Overcomers Victorious', led by Jacquie Balodis. Survivor accounts have become a mainstay, and almost a cliché of media investigations of satanism. Typically, the survivor is a woman in her thirties or forties, who tells of confronting her satanic past, usually during intensive therapy. Sometimes, she will also have had a 'born-again' conversion experience. Her recollections may date back to early childhood, or be limited to recent events. At a minimum, reported experiences are likely to include cult worship, blood drinking, and ritual sexual acts, often involving children and pornography. Most stories also involve ritual murder and cannibalism. One of the best-known survivors, Lauren Stratford, is the major source for the idea of 'breeders', women who deliver children solely for the purpose of sacrifice. She claims to have had three of her own babies taken in this way.[3]

The reality of the occult threat seems to be confirmed by the similarity of accounts presented by survivors from different regions of the country. Claims-makers like Bob Larson and Ted Gunderson make extensive use of such testimony to support apparently outlandish claims about satanic crime. For example, it is the statements of 'the few survivors' which prove that 'a large number of missing children are victims of human sacrifice cults'.[4] At every point, survivors' testimony allows the claims-makers to confound their critics. For example, ritual child abuse cases had usually foundered when children's testimony proved to be inaccurate and unreliable; but now this could be explained. To quote fundamentalist writer Johanna Michaelsen,

> in the past few years, adult survivors, defectors from satanist camps, and investigators have begun to shed some light on the satanists' tactics. Animals are indeed killed and buried, but are later dug up and disposed of elsewhere. The children are frequently given a stupefying drug before the rituals so that their senses and perceptions are easily manipulated in the dim candlelight of the ritual scene.[5]

Perhaps most valuable for the claims-makers was the lengthy history that the survivors gave to contemporary charges of 'ritual abuse'.[6] This offence is essentially undocumented before the 1980s, but now the survivors were offering accounts of such acts being performed in the 1950s or before. If accepted, this would add plausibility to the charges of cult involvement in contemporary mass abuse cases.

Assessing the objective reality of these survivor accounts is difficult. They appear wildly implausible, but that is not necessarily damning in itself. It is also likely that the individuals themselves believe firmly in the reality of their experiences, and would probably pass a test like a polygraph examination. Some appear to be reliable witnesses; but close examination of the most influential and widely publicized cases suggests numerous problems that cast doubt on the whole 'survivor' genre. Most commonly, the difficulties arise from history and logic: witnesses are depicting events that almost certainly could not have happened in that particular time and place.

The fictional elements in these stories can be attributed partly to the fundamentalist religious agendas of many of those creating and publicizing the accounts. In addition, the role of the therapeutic and psychiatric procedures used to elicit much of the supposed evidence needs to be examined closely. Whatever the reasons, the whole subculture of survivor tales must be viewed as thoroughly tainted. Given the central place of the survivors in the whole structure of beliefs and myths about diabolism, the consequence must be to weaken still further the claim that society faces a real satanic danger.

A historical context

The stories of satanic survivors fit well into long-established traditions that have become distinctively American, above all the radical Protestant idea of conversion and the inner experience of rebirth. The saved sinner denounces and probably exaggerates former misdeeds, in order to emphasize the miraculous role of divine arbitrary Grace. This is often undertaken as an evangelistic duty, the confession being presented in a public context where others can learn from the experience. This sense of salvation from the forces of sin and the Devil led many to write and publish accounts of their redemption, sometimes full autobiographies. Bunyan's title, *Grace Abounding to the Chief of Sinners*, could serve as the subtitle of any of them.

Parallel to this religious genre, we also find a secular political tradition that is particularly associated with conservative and nativist sentiment. America has experienced many previous panics directed against 'dangerous outsiders', from Catholics and Freemasons in the nineteenth century to communists and the mafia in the twentieth century. In each of these cases, opposition to the supposed alien conspiracy has drawn largely on the testimony of survivors or defectors, former members of the deviant movement, who subsequently exposed the misdeeds of their colleagues.[7] In the Jacksonian era, a major issue for the powerful anti-masonic movement was the apparent murder of one such Masonic defector, who had been on the verge of exposing the secrets of the craft.

Anti-Catholicism, meanwhile, flourished on the testimony of the 'survivor' nun Maria Monk, who portrayed convents in terms of frequent casual sexuality between priests and nuns. In a striking parallel to more recent charges, Maria claimed to know from personal experience that children born of such unions were murdered:

[The Mother Superior] gave me another piece of information which excited other feelings in me . . . Infants were sometimes born in the Convent, but they were always baptized, and immediately strangled. This secured their everlasting happiness; for the baptism purifies them from all sinfulness, and being sent out of the world before they had time to do any wrong, they were at once admitted into heaven . . . How different did a Convent now appear from what I supposed it to be![8]

Throughout the nineteenth century, Protestant activism was regularly stirred by lectures and testimony from ex-priests and nuns, real or feigned; and the tradition survives today. The fundamentalist publisher 'Chick' distributes not only occult survivor stories, but also harrowing memoirs and conspiracy tales by purported former Catholic priests and Jesuits.[9]

In the mid-twentieth century too, the validity of such defectors' evidence would again be a prime political issue with the numerous exposes of the American Communist movement by its former supporters. Figures such as Whittaker Chambers and 'red spy queen' Elizabeth Bentley became national heroes, at least for the political right. When attention turned to the alleged alien conspiracy known as the Mafia or *La Cosa Nostra*, the most powerful evidence was again believed to come from former members of the group, such as Joseph Valachi and Jimmy Fratianno. To some extent, occult survivors are but the latest manifestation of an ancient tradition, and there are many resemblances between satanic defectors and earlier Mafia or communist witnesses. All seek to emphasize their own importance in the conspiracy and the depths of its wrongdoing, from which they were in due course converted.

Assessing the evidence

Most tales by occult survivors diverge from historical precedent in their approach to evidence. In the earlier cases, charges could be debated and rebutted, either by members of the accused groups themselves or by critical observers. Corroboration could be sought in the form of supporting testimony or material evidence, as both accusers and 'conspirators' attempted to present a coherent and plausible case that could convince the uncommitted. None of these considerations seems to be highly valued when assessing the testimony of current occult survivors. It is difficult even to extract specific dates and places from most accounts, often because the witnesses wish to remain anonymous. Corroboration is rarely claimed or (apparently) sought.

Survivors appear to be treated according to a wholly different set of evidentiary criteria that effectively invert normally accepted principles. The guiding principle resembles the statement attributed to the early Christian, Tertullian, 'I believe because it is impossible.' Such a statement may be of great value in the history of religious faith, but modern accounts of occult crime offer what can only be described as a similar irrationalism in their approach to matters of evidence. Not only do they admit that the claims they report are quite outrageous, they actually cite the improbability to support the truth of the charges. Larson is typical in suggesting that, 'satanic cults deliberately fabricate preposterous forms of child victimization, knowing that the more unbelievable their atrocity, the less likely the victim will be believed'.[10]

The concept that cults deliberately attempt to provoke incredulity can be traced to the influential television journalist, Kenneth Wooden, who originally based the idea on his observations of Jim Jones' People's Temple. Wooden has been well placed to promote this view, and to publicize material that might otherwise have been thought too shocking or outre. He was an investigator or producer for many of the network documentary reports on satanism during the decade, most significantly for Geraldo Rivera's *Devil Worship* (1988). Wooden appears in 'survivor' Lauren Stratford's autobiography as a major force in persuading her to write the book.[11]

Wooden and Larson may or may not be correct in their view of cult tactics, but the practical effect of their beliefs is to remove plausibility as a criterion for assessing evidence. Quite the contrary, it seems that survivors must tell fantastic tales to be credible. In the Rivera television special, perhaps the most controversial material involved interviews with women who claimed not only to have bred children for sacrifice, but to have seen them flayed. In only one recent case has a sacrifice allegation drawn forth the public outcry that it deserved, when an alleged survivor reported on national television about the prevalence of ritual infanticide among American Jewish families.[12] The story, clearly absurd, drew massive criticism from a variety of groups; but most of these outrageous allegations are allowed to pass without comment.

Survivors' accounts are valued despite apparent flaws that would *ipso facto* discredit them in a normal criminal case. Alleged adult survivors of ritual abuse often appear badly disturbed, and it is soon admitted that they do in fact have lengthy records of serious psychiatric disorders, often combined with substance abuse. Nevertheless, believers in ritual abuse argue that the severity of the disorders is itself testimony to the extent of the traumatization. In almost every case, survivors are said to have no conscious memory of the abuse until it is released in therapy. In recent years, it has even been explained why the witnesses are so often multiple personalities: they were deliberately brainwashed into this condition by satanic psychiatrists: 'Every adult [survivor] that I have dealt with is a multiple personality. That behavior, doctors believe, can be induced by mental cruelty and drugs'.[13] Jacquie Balodis makes a similar point about multiple personality, and notes a link to traditional ideas of possession.

If these views are accurate, little is gained by conventional criticism of survivor accounts. Almost any logical flaw or contradiction could be explained within this belief system, while skepticism could be rejected as demonstrating a lack of sympathy for victims, who are usually thought to be abused children. Personal conviction, rather than evidence, would determine one's attitude to this growing corpus of stories.

Analyzing survivor stories

In reality, conventional methods of criticism can still be used to analyze survivor tales, even within the limits set by their advocates: in this light, the accounts demonstrate fundamental flaws and contradictions. One critical approach is through a painstaking analysis of individual cases, a necessarily laborious procedure that effectively means dissecting the whole life history of the claimant. However, the method can yield rich rewards, as suggested by the impressive demolition of Lauren Stratford's memoirs by a team of researchers reporting in the Christian magazine, *Cornerstone*. The investigators reconstructed Stratford's life history and undertook extensive interviews among her family and friends. *Cornerstone* noted Stratford's many contradictions and falsehoods, too numerous to report here, and generally suggested a consistent pattern of wild fantasies on her part. Her book was unreliable about matters as basic as her family structure, and her accounts of her parents and siblings have been subject to kaleidoscopic changes over the years. Her claims of abuse had similarly changed frequently, and satanism had only appeared as a claim as late as 1985, in the aftermath of the McMartin case (in which she claimed a direct role). The physical scars that she attributed to satanic abuse appear in fact to have been self-inflicted.[14]

Of her most dramatic charge, about 'breeding' and sacrificing three children, the story noted that she had variously claimed:

> she's sterile/had two children killed in snuff films/three children killed, two in snuff films, one in satanic ritual/says she had children during teenage years/her twenties/lived two years in a breeder warehouse. In reality, there is no evidence that she was ever pregnant.

The most remarkable conclusion was neither that the charges were unsupported, nor that they frequently contradicted known events; it was that virtually no outlet for these claims had undertaken any serious verification. 'The most stunning element . . . is that no one even checked out the main details'.[15] In early 1990, it was reported that *Satan's Underground* had been withdrawn by the publisher; but a number of distributors continued to circulate it.

Michelle and Jenny

Ideally, all survivor series should be subjected to such a searching individual analysis, but more general principles of evaluation can be formulated, that cast doubt on survivor stories as a category. This can be illustrated from a critique of two similar autobiographies that are among the most important sources for contemporary ideas about satanism. Both are pseudonymous recollections of ritual abuse suffered during early childhood, and both are presented in what appears to be a critical and indeed clinical style, which apparently lends substance to their argument.

The pioneering account of 'Michelle' effectively shaped the whole survivor genre.[16] It takes the form of a recollection during months of intensive psychotherapy in 1977–8, with the subject recalling elaborate rituals she believed to have occurred in her childhood. Over a 12-month period, she recalled what had happened to her on the corresponding dates in 1954–5, when she was 5 years old. The traumatic memories were at their strongest on the days of great satanic rituals. Her account is so important because it incorporates virtually all the major charges that would become popular in the 1980s – satanic worship, ritual child abuse, blood sacrifices of animals and perhaps babies, mock burials, and defecation on crucifixes. Obviously, she could not have been influenced by the later storm of publicity surrounding ritual abuse, so her account, whatever its possible flaws, is at least an independent source.

Michelle's story has achieved considerable acceptance, as has the similar account of 'Jenny', described by Judith Spencer (1989) in the best-selling mass-market paperback, *Suffer the Child*. This book includes a scholarly apparatus and some 40 citations, often to respectable psychiatric journals; and the author made an admirable effort to confirm the subject's sense of recall by checking biographical details. Jenny's story was hailed in reviews from therapists as well as child abuse support groups; author Larry Kahaner called the book 'the best account' of its kind that he had encountered. Jenny's experiences were almost identical to Michelle's. Initiated into her mother's cult at the age of 5, 'the rhythms of Satan worship permeated her childhood'. She 'stood boldly to see other dogs, and then cats, chickens, squir-rels, rabbits, and goats killed. She watched the amputation of fingers and nipples, and sometimes, penises'.[17] The religious life described here suggests a large and influential cult, with frequent rituals including as the centerpiece a classical Black Mass.

Both accounts include the idea that the abused child was being prepared for a special role as a 'Devil's Bride', a common theme in the genre. The notion of special mission is in the context almost a logical necessity, required to resolve a paradox in the narrative. The survivors wish to describe cults as homicidal groups that regularly kill children; and yet the narrators, by definition, survived. Election as a 'bride' explains this contradiction. However, the conflict is never quite resolved, and satanists are depicted both callously killing children and painstakingly brainwashing them over years. This has led writers into real confusion. Larson, for example, writes that 'children are abducted and subjected to the terrible intimi-dation of drugs and brainwashing before being sacrificed'.[18] Brainwashing a person one intends to kill anyway seems a waste of time and energy; but the dilemma is explained if we understand the ambiguous nature of the 'survivor' accounts.

Neither Michelle nor Jenny inspire confidence as witnesses. 'Michelle's' psychi-atric problems were apparent, to the point of demonstrating classic hysterical symptoms. She is reported to have developed physical stigmata that supposedly recalled her suffering. Moreover, the book demands belief in objective supernatural forces: Michelle's torment culminates with a dramatic purgation not unlike an exorcism, in which a spirit or apparition was photographed by the participants. Despite the 'therapeutic' format, *Michelle Remembers* is not a standard psychiatric case study. It is also interesting to read the ambiguous commendation that a Catholic bishop provided for the book, stressing that 'for Michelle, this experience was real'.[19]

Suffer the Child lacks the spiritual trappings, but it depicts an even more disturbed individual. Jenny had been hospitalized for mental illness at the ages of 14 and 21, with schizophrenia a possible diagnosis. She was believed by the author to have several hundred distinct personalities, 35 of whom are named in a glossary. If one accepts this as a true case of multiple personality disorder, then obvious questions arise about the causation of the illness. The author believes that Jenny evolved new personalities to help her cope with her childhood experiences. These characters included witches, sorcerers, and demons, in keeping with the ritual nature of the abuse. In contrast, we might argue that Jenny developed the personalities from reasons other than actual experience. Her mind then contained a whole cast of *dramatis personae*, such as 'Sandy' the witch and 'Mindoline' the demon, for whom Jenny created appropriate myths and histories.

Such criticisms would readily be countered by those who believe the survivors. In this case, though, we can seek historical confirmation for the truth of the stories, and the implied chronology of events is critical. Allegedly, both girls were introduced to satanic cults around the age of 5, and they spent several years in a continuing nightmare of ritual abuse and bloodshed. These events can be dated with fair confidence to almost exactly the same time: Michelle suffered during 1954 and 1955, while Jenny's cult experiences must have begun about 1954. The suggestion is that quite sophisticated clandestine cult satanists must have been firmly established by the early 1950s – Michelle's group in British Columbia and Jenny's group in an unspecified area of rural Dixie. The presence of many children already born into the movement means that the satanists must have long remained as a secret alternative religion in these widely separated areas. We would have to hypothesize local traditions dating back for decades. In addition, this early to mid-1950s chronology is frequently presented in the accounts of less celebrated survivors, such as Heather Cambridge or Casandra Hoyer.[20] Lauren Stratford's cult experiences are presumably set about 1960, as are the memoirs of the pseudonymous 'Elaine', recounted in yet another book.[21] Most occult survivors are baby-boomers.

There are some today who claim that North American Devil worshippers run into the millions, and that cult satanists are engaged in a wholesale assault on society; but these charges are paltry besides the implications of Michelle and *Suffer the Child*. These survivor tales require us to believe that the sophisticated satanic rituals of 1890s Paris or 1970s California were commonplace in remote rural or suburban communities during the Eisenhower era. The regularity of blood sacrifices implies that the cults were so powerful as to have no fear of legal intervention. They could abduct and kill with impunity in a time of far lower homicide rates, when missing persons were likely to attract more law enforcement concern than today. Further, no individual from such a cult ever betrayed its secrets or ever revealed its existence to a local church or newspaper. No religious revival ever forced a defection or an investigation, and no local politician sought celebrity by exposing such heinous crimes. This calls less for a suspension of disbelief than a complete rewriting of the history of the United States and Canada. One even older survivor reported the near total involvement of the entire village where she grew up on the affluent North Side of Chicago, Illinois, during the 1930s. Her parents 'as well as Christian ministers, policemen, lawyers and socialites were involved' in a cult active in human sacrifice and Black Masses.[22] The only contemporary parallel to such a picture comes from popular Gothic fiction by authors such as Robert Bloch or H. P. Lovecraft, whose protagonists so often stumbled across diabolical secrets shared by remote communities. As a portrait of the reality of rural or suburban American in mid-century, the survivors' reminiscences are monstrously improbable.

The news media

If cults of this sort existed at all, to say nothing of the vast scale required by the accounts proliferating today, we would expect some trace in the news media — some rumor, scandal, or investigation. This should have reached a crescendo about 1954, which modern sources claim witnessed a 'Feast of the Beast', with sacrifices in unprecedented numbers. We might expect increased reports, however speculative, on ritual killings, child abductions, church desecrations, or cult activity. In order to test this, we searched the index volumes of the *New York Times* between 1948 and 1960. Key words used included crime and criminals, cult, Devil, kidnapping, murder, occult, religion and churches, ritual, ritual murder, sacrifice, Satan, and witchcraft. Witchcraft and ritual murder provided by far the richest material. Every year produced three or four stories, which did indeed depict powerful secret cults involved in black magic, ritual human sacrifice, and even the abduction and brainwashing of children. However, virtually every one of these stories occurred in Africa, as traditional cults became politically active in the last days of European colonial rule. Other Third World countries provided for most of the remaining tales, for example the 1955 lynching of an alleged witch in Guatemala.

Within North America, only three such stories were found. One concerned the efforts of the modern citizens of Salem to clear retroactively the victims of the great trials. In 1951, a semi-humorous story told of a court case where a Hispanic resident of the Bronx accused a neighbor of using a 'voodoo hex' (September 15). Finally, in 1959, an Alabama teacher was dismissed for a sympathetic classroom discussion of voodoo beliefs (January 6). This last story illustrates that an occult case was seen as sufficiently weird and novel to attract national attention, even without criminal or sensational elements. The implication is that a real 'Feast of the Beast' would have caused a flood of media attention, if it had ever occurred, but the overwhelming evidence is that it did not.

It is useful here to compare media attitudes toward the real occult practices found in many remote communities about this time, the magical healing practices and witch beliefs associated with the Pennsylvania Dutch country or parts of the Appalachians. Though these customs were almost always benevolent in intent, the communities usually attempted to keep them secret, largely through fear of ridicule. However, they were bound to fail on occasion, and the slightest rumor of occult-related crime drew widespread attention. The most celebrated instance occurred in York County, Pennsylvania, in 1928–9, when three boys were implicated in murdering a reputed local wizard for his magical 'Pow-wow Book'. The case earned national and international coverage as 'the witch murder', attracting comment from celebrities such as Clarence Darrow. The media sensation was such that throughout the 1930s, journalists regularly read 'hex' and ritual elements into ordinary murder cases in the area, even when the motive was clearly personal or financial. There is no reason to believe that the media of the 1950s were any more reluctant to seek a sensational story than their predecessors.

Real satanic groups

The question might be placed in another way. Devil-worshipping groups have unquestionably existed in twentieth-century America, but how does our knowledge of them fit the cults described by the survivors? Michelle's biographer attempts to link her mid-1950s persecutors to known movements, specifically the 'Church of Satan', an organization 'actually older than the Christian Church . . . There's a lot in the psychiatric literature about them'.[23] Despite this claim, no satanist group has even a tenuous organizational continuity dating before the [twentieth] century; and the Church of Satan to which this appears to refer is the American movement of that name founded by Anton LaVey in 1966. Michelle's biographer, Lawrence Pazder, also attempted to corroborate the presence of occultists in the Vancouver area, and includes as an appendix a news story about modern-day witch activity in the area. However, this only supports the possible existence of witchcraft in 1977, which is irrelevant to the situation in the 1950s.[24]

We know of no evidence from any source of cult activity of this sort in North America before 1960. Most American satanism can be traced to the late 1960s. LaVey's group was the most celebrated, but the following years saw the creation and growth of several movements: the Process, the Solar Lodge, the Temple of Set. There was also some development of local groups out of the whole subculture described by Mike Warnke; and a proliferation of individual satanic believers, partly inspired by media depictions in films such as *Rosemary's Baby* and *The Exorcist*.

Before 1965, however, the religious fringe was more sparsely populated. The closest approximations to 'Devil-worship' were strictly confined to geographic areas far removed from the locales of Michelle and Jenny above all, to California. The Agape Lodge in 1930s Hollywood had been associated with wealthy decadence; by the 1940s, Jack Parsons transformed it into the Crowleyite Church of Thelema, based in Pasadena. At least in rumor, this group was active in orgies and sacrifice, but the tiny cult was moribund by the mid-1950s. In addition, Aleister Crowley had a handful of American followers of his OTO lodge, *Ordo Templi Orientis*, some dating back to the Magus' sojourn in New York during the First World War.[25] However, no informed Crowleyan would have been associated with the inverted fundamentalism of Michelle's group; and the chants recalled by Jenny fit no known magical tradition. Finally, none of the new satanic movements of the 1960s demonstrated any influence from or contact with any older American Devil cults of the sort recorded by the survivors.

We cannot prove a negative. We are unable to show that organized cult satanism was wholly unknown in America before about 1966, or that there might not have been one or two isolated cults on the lines described by Michelle and Jenny. On the other hand, the evidence they present contradicts what we know from many other sources, it is wholly unconfirmed, and inherently improbable, and it fits poorly with the historical context. Similar objections would apply to any other conceivable account of ritual abuse or satanic crime in America before the mid-1960s — and that includes a large majority of all survivor stories.

The therapeutic process

Most accounts of survivors essentially consider the role of one protagonist, the woman herself. However, even those who accept these stories as true admit that the accounts are not presented spontaneously. They are drawn out gradually in a lengthy therapeutic process in which there are at least two actors. Understanding the stories therefore requires knowledge of the process and its underlying assumptions.

One central idea is that early childhood trauma can cause the mind to bury painful memories that lie dormant until revived by therapy such as hypnotic age regression. This may not be controversial as such, but it is questionable whether the memories will come back in an accurate and unadulterated form, untainted by images or fantasies acquired at a later date. Again, early trauma might lead to later psychiatric disorders; but these same complaints could also have other origins, including biological and biochemical dysfunctions. European psychiatrists in particular would be skeptical of the unreconstructed Freudianism of some of their American counterparts. There might be cases where childhood sufferings could be reconstructed during therapy; but it would seem rash to insist on their objective reality, without extensive corroboration.

It would not be hard to suggest why survivors might formulate stories of satanic rituals, especially when their accounts were collected during the [1980s]. Patients under therapy in the 1980s might have heard and internalized the kind of charges initially made in *Michelle Remembers*, and subsequently repeated in child molestation cases such as McMartin, Jordan, or Bakersfield. Jenny herself appears to have begun therapy in 1984, just as these allegations were reaching their height; Lauren Stratford's tales of cults and sacrifices began about 1985. Ritual abuse became a major topic in the mass media, with new survivors regularly appearing on television talk shows and in the pages of the *National Enquirer*. Their stories involved powerful images of the sort often found in mythology and dream imagery, stories and symbols with a universal Jungian relevance. In addition, there might have been specific issues such as guilt or internal conflict about the issue of abortion that might go far towards explaining the 'breeder' tales. As Gordon Melton suggests, 'satanism has emerged as a reflecting board on which people have projected a wide variety of fantasies'.[26]

Images and speculations then reappear as fantasies, which the patient increasingly holds to as literally true — especially if the therapist is supportive and encouraging. In this context, it is intriguing that Michelle's analyst, Dr Lawrence Pazder, came from a rather unusual background. He practiced medicine in West Africa in the early 1960s, at the height of widespread public concern there over the activities of cults and secret societies active in blood sacrifice, cannibalism, and child maltreatment.[27] Dr Pazder makes no secret of this background, to which he frequently makes reference; and we must obviously accept his assurance that he 'never told Michelle about the correspondences he sometimes saw between her experiences and the things he had studied'.[28] On the other hand, the 'cult' described in Michelle is in fact very close to the notorious African 'leopard societies' to which Pazder specifically refers. African memories might have made him more prepared to accept the literal truth of Michelle's account, far more so than the majority of his North American colleagues.

We must therefore know what a therapist will be prepared to believe or accept and how directive the therapist is in the therapy setting. Observations of the profession in general suggest that these expectations have changed substantially in recent years. The alleged consistency of accounts across the nation might therefore reflect no more than the dissemination of ideas across the therapeutic disciplines. Dr Frank Putnam of the National Institute of Mental Health has pointed to the influence of seminars on ritual abuse, and to published memoirs such as those of Lauren Stratford and Michelle. He remarks, 'There is an enormous rumor mill out there. Patients pick up stories, and therapists trade stories'.[29] We may therefore see survivor stories as the product of the dynamic process between patient and therapist.

Crucially, large sections of the therapeutic profession are now prepared to credit charges that would once have been dismissed as fantasy, and 'ritual crimes' have become an issue in several ongoing debates. For example, extreme abuse during childhood was believed to contribute to multiple personality disorder, a condition hitherto viewed as a peripheral and rather faddish notion. In the 1980s, however, it has become more widely accepted as a respectable issue for therapists, with occult survivors providing important case studies. One serious scholarly text on multiple personality notes cases of 'forced participation since childhood in satanistic cult worship entailing ritual sex, human sacrifice and cannibalism'. The author claims to know of some 60 such cases, and has also stated that his attempts to help these patients have led to threats from satanic groups.[30]

Another debate concerns the frequency of early childhood abuse, and the veracity of accounts purporting to describe it. A bitter controversy of the 1980s involved the charge that Sigmund Freud had suppressed his seduction theory, bowing to the outcry that arose when he had originally suggested the prevalence of child molestation and incest. His revised form of the theory had portrayed memories of abuse or incest as mere fantasies or wish-fulfillment. In the political and social context of the 1980s, this approach seemed a callous betrayal of the powerless, of women and children, of victims. In the new view, it was almost an article of faith that such accounts were rarely invented, even when they involved grotesque 'ritual' elements, and even when the memories appeared to come from the deepest levels of the subconscious. To reject Jenny might be to question the bona fides of any abuse victim.

But this reaction in favor of the victim may well mean a refusal to doubt even the most absurd allegation about early experiences. It is controversial whether therapists might encourage the actual creation of an idea of early abuse; but even well-founded memories might be distorted and elaborated into grand ritualistic fantasies. A medical practice specializing in ritual abuse – and these are proliferating – is likely to be receptive to these purported memories, and the therapist might shape, even if unintentionally, the patient's narrative by asking questions that support an occult context. One Texas clinic that advertises its treatment of satanic survivors from all parts of the country now reports dealing with 'many women', whose early ritual abuse led to pregnancy, with the children subsequently sacrificed.

Conclusion: a new mythology

One of the recent studies of the occult threat bears the title *Satanism: Is Your Family Safe?* and the authors would certainly answer in the negative. Their conclusion is based partly on a case study of a bloodthirsty California cult allegedly operating from the early 1950s, whose members would indirectly be connected with major criminal acts. These included the 1970 Fort Bragg murders allegedly blamed on Jeffrey MacDonald. It is possible to proceed far in this narrative before noticing that virtually every detail and accusation is taken from the purported memories of survivor (multiple personality and 'Devil's Bride') Heather Cambridge. Her memoirs are subject to all the criticisms made above against works such as *Michelle Remembers,* and we would suggest that her account is not likely to be reliable as literal truth.

But what is most interesting here is the use of evidence. The survivor accounts are seen as credible first-hand testimony, and they are beginning to be drawn together to create a new synthetic history of cults and satanic activity in the United States. The MacDonald case is only one example of a controversial or mysterious case where survivors have offered testimony in support of an occult interpretation; and other instances might well occur in the near future. If it is objected that Michelle portrays diabolical cults of the sort that never existed in the 1950s, it will soon be answered that in fact they did, and that there are dozens of survivor accounts to confirm it. Far from being an innovation of the 1960s, American satanism is likely to be portrayed by the claims-makers as having real historical roots. Overall, a golden age of myth-making seems imminent.

We can already discern the early stages of a troubling process that permits the almost unlimited 'manufacture' of survivors and their grisly tales. Ideological and theoretical changes within the therapeutic community have contributed to a dramatic increase in the numbers of self-described occult survivors. These individuals may find themselves interviewed and promoted by exponents of the 'satanic threat', including occult experts from religious groups and law enforcement. In turn, these accounts gain widespread publicity in the mass media, especially on sensationalistic talk shows. Accounts appear in book form, which owe their commercial success in large part to a prurient interest in the detailed descriptions of sadism and perversion – an appeal far removed from the intentions of the original authors. As these stories appear ever more frequently in television and published accounts, so survivors and 'ritual crimes' increasingly permeate the public consciousness, providing a vocabulary for disturbed individuals to recount in therapy. The process thus becomes self-sustaining, and it is difficult to see how the cycle could be broken in the foreseeable future.

Notes

1   The American literature warning about satanic cults is very extensive. Illustrative texts include: Bob Larson, *Satanism: The Seduction of America's Youth* (Thomas Nelson Press, Nashville, Tenn. 1989); Jerry Johnston, *The Edge of Evil: The Rise of Satanism in North America* (Word Publishing, Dallas, Tex. 1989); Kevin Marron, *Ritual Abuse* (Seal Books, Toronto 1988); Pat Pulling, *The Devil's Web* (Huntington House, Lafayette, La 1988); and Larry Kahaner, *Cults that Kill* (Warner, New York 1988).

2   See, for example, Ann Rodgers-Melnick, *Rumors from Hell* (University of Pittsburgh Press, Pittsburgh, Pa 1989), and K. V. Lanning, 'Satanic, Occult and Ritualistic Crime: A Law Enforcement Perspective', *Police Chief* 56 (October 1989), 62–85.

3   Lauren Stratford, *Satan's Underground* (Harvest House, Eugene, Oreg. 1988).

4   Larson, *Satanism*, 125.

5   Johanna Michaelsen, *Like Lambs to the Slaughter* (Harvest House, Eugene, Oreg. 1988); cf. Stratford, *Satan's Underground*, foreword.

6   Marron, *Ritual Abuse*; Paul and Shirley Erble, *The Politics of Child Abuse* (Lyle Stuart, Secaucus, NJ 1986).

7   For examples of this process, see Richard Hofstadter, *The Paranoid Style in American Politics* (University of Chicago Press 1979), and Seymour Lipset and Earl Rabb, *The Politics of Unreason* (University of Chicago Press 1978).

8   *The Awful Disclosures of Maria Monk; and the Mysteries of a Convent Exposed* (Philadelphia, Pa 1865), 39.

9   For example, Rebecca Brown, *He Came to Set the Captives Free* (Chick Chino, Calif. 1986).

10 Mike Warnke, *The Satan-Seller* (Logos International, Plainfield, NJ 1972), 195; Larson, *Satanism*, 126.

11 Stratford, *Satan's Underground*, 165.

12 Jeremy Gerard, 'Winfrey Show Evokes Protests', *New York Times*, May 6, 50. For allegations of ritual murder against Jews in the mediaeval and early modern period, see R. Po-Chia Hsia, *The Myth of Ritual Murder* (Yale University Press, New Haven, Conn. 1988).

13 Kahaner, *Cults*, 237.

14 Gretchen Passantino and Jon Trott, 'Satan's Sideshow', *Cornerstone* 18 (90) (1989), 23–8.

15 Ibid., 27.

16 Michelle Smith and Lawrence Pazder, *Michelle Remembers* (Congdon and Lattes, New York 1980).

17 Judith Spencer, *Suffer the Child* (Pocket, New York 1989), 14, 15.

18 Larson, *Satanism*, 125.

19 Smith and Pazner, *Michelle Remembers*, foreword.

20 Pulling, *The Devil's Web*, 66; Ted Schwarz and Duane Empey, *Satanism: Is Your Family Safe?* (Zondervan, Grand Rapids, Mich. 1988).

21 Brown, *He Came to Set the Captives Free*.

22 Alan H. Peterson, *The American Focus on Satanic Crime* (American Focus Publishing, South Orange, NJ 1988), 28.

23 Smith and Pazner, *Michelle Remembers*, 117.

24 Ibid., 299–300.

25   For Crowley's career, see John Symonds, *The Great Beast* (Mayflower, London 1973).
26   Cited in Rodgers-Melnick, *Rumors*.
27   See Edward Parrinder, *Witchcraft: European and African* (Faber, London 1963), and Alastair Scobie, *Murder for Magic: Witchcraft in Africa* (Cassell, London 1965).
28   Smith and Pazner, *Michelle Remembers*, 140 n.
29   Cited in Rodgers-Melnick, *Rumors*.
30   B. G. Braun, *The Treatment of Multiple Personality Disorder* (American Psychiatric Press, Washington, DC 1986).

Chapter 31

Patrick Casement

THE WISH NOT TO KNOW

WHEN CONFRONTED BY SOME PAINFUL or disorienting truth, one possible defence is that of wishing not to know. As Laub and Auerhahn have said: 'To protect ourselves from affect, we must, at times, avoid knowledge'.[1] Some people, for example, when faced by symptoms that might indicate cancer, choose to increase the risk of death through delaying appropriate investigation rather than possibly have their fears confirmed by proper diagnosis. They prefer to prolong the time of not knowing even though this could be lethal. It is more usually those who can bear to know the truth, whatever that might be, who take the course of insisting upon early investigation. It is this defence of not wanting to know that has also operated, until recently, in relation to the sexual abuse of children.

Society has however come to recognise that *some* children *are* abused, even in their own homes. The former wish of not knowing has therefore shifted, and in some cases it has swung too far the other way into a salacious wish to seek out further abuse even where it may not exist. And that over-zealous interest has rightly created a new caution about such things. But there are yet other children who continue to be abused, some of them in ways so horrifying that most people are unprepared to consider that the emerging accounts could possibly be true. Most often, people who are told of such things have difficulty in believing what they hear, preferring to dismiss it in exchange for some other more comfortable theory.

For some time, evidence has been coming to light that indicates the existence of some adults, and groups of adults, who appear to be addicted to extremes of sexual perversion and corruption that defy imagination. 'These activities include rituals of all sorts, imaginable and unimaginable, which serve a dual purpose: to increase sexual excitement because of the dangers and risk, and to terrify the victims into silence'.[2] Because these rituals and practices are so evil in their nature they are sometimes described as 'satanic'. For instance, we hear of such outrageous practices as the use of young children in ritual abuse and even the ritual slaughter of babies before the eyes of children, who are forced to witness these acts and to take part in them.

These accounts are so horrifying, it is no wonder that most people wish not to believe them to be true. Therefore, any therapist who begins to hear about such things from a patient is confronted by a very serious dilemma. What if some of these accounts are true? Not to believe someone who has actually been a victim of such abuse leaves that person still alone in the torment of their own experiences, and leaves the perpetrators free to continue with these practices undeterred. At the very least, I believe we must keep an open mind when we begin to hear of such things: sometimes we may be hearing the truth — as far as these victims are able to risk telling that truth to anyone.

We should also bear in mind that the telling of these experiences is usually the last thing these victims wish to do. They are always terrified of telling: terrified of the consequences of telling and of not being believed. And these victims often behave as if they have been hypnotically programmed not to remember or, if they do remember, to be either too terrified to tell or unable to tell much that can be verified. For this reason they are most often not believed.

I will give just one example from those that have come to my notice.[3] A child, suspected to have been the victim of incest, and then taken into care, told her therapist that she had seen babies murdered and buried. She eventually took the police to where she said they would find the bodies; but no body was found. Had she made all this up? Had she been witness to something else that was to be concealed, but duped into believing that there had been real murders when perhaps there had not been? For sure, if there had been 'satanic' abuse, a false account reported to others would certainly reduce the chances of this patient being believed with regard to anything else that she had witnessed and experienced.

Similarly, might this patient have been hypnotically programmed not to be able to identify where these events had taken place? Or might she have remained unable to risk exposing the perpetrators, amongst whom she claimed had been her own father? (Her mother had already left the home, unable to stay, so this child had no other parent to turn to.) To succeed in bringing her remaining parent to justice would have risked her finally losing the illusion that he could, under some other circumstances, still be a valid parent to her. Or should we put this down to psychosis and/or revenge against the father? I think that an open mind to these different possibilities is essential.

For those who hear such accounts, the wish not to believe them is often very acute. To believe what one is being told by a victim of 'satanic' abuse would mean facing something for which one has no adequate means to deal with or to explain. It means accepting that there could be human beings capable of behaving in ways so evil that we cannot bear to conceive of such a possibility. It means facing an outrage to all that we have come to regard as human. It means facing such degrees of deception and corruption of young children that one would no longer know what to believe. It is much less disorienting to think that these accounts could not be true.

In addition, if these things are true, it means facing that we are being told of things that go beyond anything that our familiar theories of personality are able to grasp. No wonder, therefore, that we prefer to keep to the more usual ways of trying to understand such things; in particular, in terms of familiar psychiatric disorders. For it is far less uncomfortable for us to assume that we are merely being lied to, or that the person who dares to tell us such things must be deluded and therefore victim to his or her own psychotic processes, rather than being a victim of something so very much more sinister. We can then dismiss all else that we may hear as phantasy, hallucination or delusion, and we need not have our own sleep too much disturbed by what we have been privy to.

But there is a disturbing degree of consistency in these reports that cannot be so easily explained away. And these accounts are from people who are afraid to tell, and they themselves do not want them to be true. But when memories of 'satanic' abuse are eventually recovered by a patient, in the presence of a therapist able to give sufficient security so that the barriers to remembering can then be lifted, the process of remembering is very similar to that which takes place in the course of any analysis: it has all the signs of being authentic. But the patient is then caught between the terrors of telling (against an inner voice that threatens dreadful consequences against telling) and the fear of not being believed and being treated instead as mad. But the patient desperately needs not to remain so isolated with what cannot be borne alone.

It may be that some accounts which are reputed to be of 'satanic' abuse are delusional, and the narrators may indeed be psychotic in some cases. Then at least our theories, and our more usual views and beliefs, are not necessarily going to be challenged. But we must still face the awful fact that if some of these accounts are true, if we do not have the courage to see the truth that may be there (amidst however much confusion that may also be there), we may tacitly be allowing these practices to continue under the cover of secrecy, supported also by the almost universal refusal to believe that they could exist. We may then continue safe in our wish not to know whilst others are still left exposed to those abuses which we, for our own peace of mind, prefer to think could not possibly happen.

When such a patient, claiming to be the victim of 'satanic' abuse, eventually finds the courage to tell someone who is trusted enough to be told, I believe that we owe it to the patient to consider the possibility that there may be truth in the patient's account, even at the risk of this disturbing much of our usual ways of thinking about mental disturbance. The alternative is for us to remain cut off from what could be the kernel of truth that seems repeatedly and uncomfortably to be there, leaving the victim feeling mad because of the isolation from anyone else who will believe what they are trying to tell. Such a person may then have to remain defended by insanity, because it is not possible to maintain the threatened self in an integrated state without the support of another person who is prepared to share the experience of facing what cannot be faced alone.

And when a therapist does have the courage to listen with an open mind, balancing his or her understanding between the more familiar view of this as a patient's phantasy or delusion, and the awful possibility that some truth may actually be contained in these accounts, then clinical experience shows that the victim of 'satanic' abuse can be helped. But the traditional approach, of treating these accounts as psychotic phantasy, is likely to do nothing other than drive that person further into a state of isolation and madness.

In therapy, with a therapist who is prepared to accept that there could be truth in what is being told, a 'satanically' abused patient can gradually recover from the nightmare of those memories from which there had seemed to be no escape except perhaps into insanity. But to enable this kind of patient to recover, the therapist has to take risks with his or her own more usual sense of sanity – and often without the security of having colleagues prepared to understand the nature of this work or prepared to support it.

It can be a very lonely business when a therapist is prepared to believe that a patient's account of 'satanic' abuse may actually be true. Colleagues are more likely to criticise the therapist than be willing to believe what they themselves have not yet encountered, or dare to consider with an equally open mind. Professional colleagues will often continue to protect themselves with this wish not to know, leaving the therapist who has been exposed to the trauma of 'knowing' terribly isolated, somewhat as the victim had been isolated from anyone else prepared to know.

It is essential, therefore, that therapists who encounter 'satanically' abused patients should be able to get support from others who have had similar experience of working with this kind of patient.

Notes

1   D. Laub and N. C. Auerhahn, 'Knowing and not knowing massive psychic trauma: forms of traumatic memory', *International Journal of Psycho-Analysis*, 74 (1993), 288. This article offers an important discussion of the defence of not knowing.
2   Dr Judith Trowell, personal communication to the author.
3   Names, identities and background details have been changed wherever necessary to protect confidentiality.

Index

abductions 129, 130–1
abuse *see* satanic abuse
Aconcio, Giacomo 175
Adamo, Donna Laura de 100
agrarian cults 8–10
Agrippa, Henry Cornelius 113
Albert V, Duke of Bavaria 80
Alexander V, Pope 41
Anabaptists 163, 164, 172, 176, 177, 189–92,
    197–8, 238; and accusations against accusers
    196; in authorities' perspective 192–5; and
    baptism 191, 192–3, 195–6, 197, 198;
    common views on 190; executions of 190, 194;
    fear of 193; own perspective 195–7; views on
    Catholicism 197
Ancel, Catherine 59
Anderson, Sir Edmund 220
Angelo of Poli 45–6
animals 64–6, 90, 111, 308; as familiars 314, 319;
    riding on 124, 126; transformation into 122–3,
    124, 126, 127, 131–2, 184
Anne of Denmark 210
anti-church, fear of 163–4
Antichrist 170, 172, 177, 190
antinomianism 28
Antoine, Barbelline 64
Antonio of Sacco 46
Apuleius 155
Ardent, Rudolf 50
Arminians 176
Armitage, Mary 292
art, Satanic depictions 233, 234–5
Artisson, Robert 27

Ashby, Anne 296
Asseau, Claude 140
Aubrey, John 409
Augustine, St 235, 236
Austin, J.L. 150, 158
Austria 248, 251

Baile, Jean, Archbishop 41, 43
Bale, John 161
Balfour, Alison 219
Ball, James 410
Balthasar, Bekker 379
Balthasar von Dernbach, Prince Abbot 114
'barbes' 42
Bardel family 90–1
Bartholome, Regina 324, 325, 329–40
Bashar, N. 359
Batthyany, Lajos 388
Bauthumley, Jacob 176
Bavaria 12, 76, 81, 205, 251
Baxter, Richard 14, 368
Becon, Thomas 228
Beelzebub *see* Devil, the
Behmenism 177
Behringer, W. 134
Bekker, Balthasar 379
Belcher, Elizabeth 312
beliefs *see* folk beliefs/traditions
benandanti of Friuli 7, 122–3, 124
Benedict XI, Pope 395
Benedict XII, Pope 28, 41
Bennet, Elizabeth 283
Bennet, Isobel 62

Bennett, J. 284–5
Bentley, Elizabeth 421
Bergerac, Cyrano de 381
Bergier, George Colas 68
Bernard of Bergamo 44–5
Bernard family 91
Bernard, Richard 170, 280, 316
Bernardino da Siena, St 127
Bernardo da Como 121
Berquin, Louis de 263
bewitchment 275, 281, 345, 400; and accidents
   66–7; accusations of 62; and animals 64–6; and
   childbirth 63–4; discouragement of ideas
   concerning 59–60; and entrancement 129; and
   ill-health 57–9, 61–2, 64; and wealth/poverty
   67–8, 103
Bideford, Thomas 309
Binsfield, Peter 76
Bithner, Jakob 162–3, 180–7
Black Masses 426
Blair, Magdalen 62
Bloch, R. 426
Blucher, Eleanor 405–6
Blum, Pastor Nicolaus 250
Bodenham, Ann 297–8
Bodin, Jean 5, 88–9, 109, 149, 150, 256
Boerhave, Herman 390
Bogomiles of Thrace 50
Boguet, Henri 5–6, 11, 13, 66, 90, 413
Boissonnet, Laurent 260
Bombastus von Hohenheim, Theophrastus
   (Paracelsus) 113
Bonham, John 346, 349
Bordelon, Laurent 381
Boucher, Jean 172
Boulton, J. 403, 404
Bourbon, Louis de 258
Bradwell, Dr Stephen 312
Brand, John 409
Brant, Sebastian 242
Bregille, Leonard 89
Brenner, Martin 186
Brigs, Prissilla and Abigail 355
Briscoe, Mary 298
Brome, Richard 155
Brossier, Marthe 256, 260
Buhon, Claude 91
Burke, P. 75, 97, 381
Byrom, Margaret 313

Cabinet du roy de France (1581) 236
Calmet, Dom Augustin 394, 395
Calvin, John 172, 233, 235, 238, 263

Calvinists 168–9, 172, 176, 187, 239, 263
Canisius, Peter 80
Canne, John 164
cannibalism 48, 49, 63–4, 109, 120
Capetian dynasty (France) 25–6
Carena, Cesare 98
Carlier, Marguerite 67
Carolina see Constitutio Criminalis Carolina (1532)
Carpocratians 49
Carrozzo, Giacomo 105–6
Cason, Joan 295
Cathars 22, 28, 30, 48, 50–1, 126
Catherine of Palumbaria 46, 47
Catholic/Protestant witchcraft 161, 230, 237;
   countermeasures for maleficium 161–2, 167–9;
   depictions of 169–72; difference/consensus
   165–7; joint accusations 171; and moral system
   of confessional state 162, 172–3, 177; and
   possession 257–8, 262–3; and prosecution of
   witches 163; and religious identity 162, 169,
   173–5
Catholicism between Luther and Voltaire (Delumeau)
   186
Cattaneo, Albert 41, 43
Cauz, Konstantin Franz von 392
Celichius, Andreus 244
Certainty of the World of Spirits, The (1692) 368
Chambers, Whittaker 421
Charles, Archduke of Styria 180, 181, 182
Charles IX, King 256
Charles V, Emperor 116, 140, 191, 207
Charles of Valois 26
Chaundler, John 281
Chaunu, P. 137
children: as accused 66, 83, 90, 117, 413; as
   accusers 65, 90, 117–18, 119, 143; demonic
   possession of 249, 260, 296; eaten 48, 49,
   63–4, 109, 120; illness/deaths of 63–4, 83,
   309; language/behaviour of 313; murder of
   109, 120, 184, 360–1, 414; trial/execution of
   139, 142; visions of 345, 347
Chretien, Colas 66
Christina, Queen of Sweden 118, 209
Church of Thelma 427
Clarskon, Lawrence 176
Claudon, Claudon Jean 66
Claudon, Curien 66
Claverie, E. 147
Clement V, Pope 26
Clement VI, Pope 41
Clerc, Merzine 94
Clerk family 9
climate 11–12, 54, 67; interference in 155; Little

Ice Age 11–12, 71, 74–5, 83, 84; magic associated with 69–71, 73, 83, 110, 184, 185; patterns 71–2; as unnatural 71; and witch-hunts 69, 73–5

Coccioli, Abbot Filippo 105

Cockburn, J.S. 317

Cocke, Joan 312

Cohn, Mengeon and Agathe 64

Cohn, N. 120, 136, 141, 242, 278

Collegiants 176

Collit, Priscilla 359

Colonna family 45

Condé, Louis de Bourbon, Prince of 263

confessions 5–7, 8, 55, 100, 104, 107, 132, 133, 180–1, 345–6; as collective psychosis 332; as conversion narrative 357–8; cultural context 325–6, 357; and decline in trials 370; as fantasy 324, 332–40; logic of 323–4; as means of seeking revenge 334; past/present relationship 324–5; process of 354–6; and unfulfilled promises 359–60; as voluntary 354, 364; and witch beliefs 326

Conrad of Marburg 37, 39, 51

Consigli, Niccolö 31

Constitutio Criminalis Carolina (1532) 116, 117, 207, 222

Constitutio Criminalis Theresiana 388–9

Conti, Count Stefano di 45

Cooper, Thomas 280, 282

Coritzen, Adam 81

Cornfoot, Janet 206

Cotta, Dr John 312

Cotton, Margaret 309

Council of Basle 121

Council of Trent 99, 107, 167, 168, 185

Counter-Reformation 172, 210, 211, 221, 234, 236, 239, 251, 275

Crab, Nathan 14

Crespet, Pierre 151, 168, 172

crime: abstract 202; central/local activities against 217–24; inquisitorial procedure against 217–19; and judicial revolution 207–8; and possession 247; redefinition of 206; secular/religious identification 214; state view of 206; and witchcraft 205–6, 210

Crowley, Vivianne 2

Crucible, The (Miller) 2

Crutch, Alice 310

Cullender, Rose 309

Dabo, Claudette 66

Daemonolatria 72

Daemonologie (1597) 153

Dale, Antonius van 176

Dalton, M. 280, 316, 363

dancing 101, 157, 184

Daneau, Lambert 154, 165

Dannhauer, Johann Conrad 243, 244, 248

Darcy, Brian 308, 315

Darling, Thomas 312

Darrel, John 13, 369

Darrow, Clarence 427

d'Aubigne, Agrippa 256

Davanzati, Giuseppe, Bishop of Trani 395

David of Augsburg 37

Davis, N.Z. 152, 330

Davy, Sarah 358

De Crimine Magiae (1701) 118

De la dimonomanie des sorciers (1580) 149

De Lancre, Pierre 133–4, 149, 150, 153, 155, 156

De Praestigiis Daemonum (1563) 113, 244, 245

Deekes, Elizabeth 361

Del Rio, Martin 172, 186

Delcambre, E. 93–4, 95

Delphy, C. 281

Delumeau, J. 165, 167, 186, 210–11, 233, 234

Demenge, Claudon Grand 60

demonology 97, 131, 137; accusations of 99–102; causal mechanics 166; and female possession 5, 103–6, 221; and folk beliefs 110–11; incredulity concerning 116

demons 235–6, 242

Denmark 12, 118, 139, 223

Dent, Arthur 177

Descartes, René 378

d'Etaples, Lefevre 262

Deutel, Jan Jansz 176

Deux Livres (1590) 168

Devil, the: and Anabaptists 194–5, 196; conversations with 243–4, 362; depictions of 101, 227, 228–30, 234–5, 242; Germanic possession by 241–52; as God's jailer 247; impotence of 382; legends concerning 238; and magic 163, 184; marriage to 323; and mimicry of the liturgy 153; Oedipal relationship with 329–30, 333, 336–8; pacts with 100–1, 116, 132, 154, 183, 211, 314–15, 348, 359–60; possession by 239; as real 331; religious beliefs concerning 233–4, 238–9; role of 335–6; and sabbat 124, 141; style of rule 153–4; as symbolic 176; theatrical presentations of 236–7; as threatening 228; transformation of 311; women's allegiance/attraction to 103–6, 115, 280; worship of 164, 239

Devil's mark 141, 219, 374; searching for 290–3, 303, 313–17

D'Eyncourt, Mr 401–2

diabolism 28; and conspiracies 189–97; in mediaeval Europe 27, 29–32, 33–5; and possession 311; textual 242, 243

Diamond of Devotion 176

Dick, John 217

Diefenbach, Johann 165

Dietrich, Veit 249

Diez, Jean 67

Diggers 176

Dircxdochter, Lysbet 195

Directorium Inquisitorum (*c*. 1368) 39

Discourse of the Damned Art of Witchcraft, A (1610) 170

Discoverie of Witchcraft, The (1584) 176, 367

Displaying of supposed witchcraft, The (1677) 177

Disquisitonum Magicarum Libri Sex 186

Donatino, Antonio 103, 104, 105

dreams 347–8

Driver, Ellen 323

Dualists 49, 50, 51

Duny, Amy 309

Durent, Dorothy 309

Durkheim, E. 207

Earle, Katherine 291, 292

East Anglia 9, 11, 12, 314, 344, 353

economic factors *see* socio-economic factors

Edward II of England 27

Edward III of England 28

Edwards, Charles 170

Egmond, Karl van, Duke of Guelders 193

Ehrenberg, Bishop Philipp Adolf von 114

Eisengrein, Dr Martin 251

El Sadawi, N. 282

Eliade, M. 104, 137

Elizabeth of Schonau 262

Ellinger, Johann 170

Ellis, Ann 357

Ellis, Sir Henry 409

Elsas, M.J. 76

England, witchcraft and state power 219–20

Esienne, Henri 239

Essex (1645) 109–10

Eugenius IV, Pope 4

Europe's Inner Demons (Cohn) 120

Evans-Pritchard, E.E. 82, 347

evil eye 141

exorcism 101, 185–6, 228, 235, 243, 255, 259–60, 397

Eymeric, Nicolas 39, 51

Fairfax, Edward 307

fairies 9–10, 103, 110, 133, 134, 233

fairy-tales 125–6

Familism 176

Family of Love 176

fantasies 331, 341, 349; of death/poverty 345, 349; emergence of 333–6; judicial reactions to 338–40; Oedipal elements 336–8

fantasy 429

Feast of Fools 151, 237

feasts/feast days 101, 134, 168

Febvre, L. 233, 389

Fellow, Joan 15

Ferdinand, Duke of Bavaria 73, 74, 77

Ferdinand, Emperor 180

Ferdinand Maria, Duke of Bavaria 81

Ferry, Claudatte 65

fertility cults 8, 10

festivals 111

Field, Elizabeth 295

Fillet, Elizabeth 363

films 427

Fleming, Abraham 176

flying 101, 122–4, 127, 129, 131–2, 135, 184

folk beliefs/traditions 3, 5, 102–3, 105–6, 110–11, 112, 123, 124, 126, 138; and the Devil 228–9; Satanic 238; scepticism concerning 381–2

folk-urban theory 403; communal relations 403–4; and rural beliefs 408–9; and separation of agricultural/town life 407–8; social changes 404–5; and town beliefs 409–10

Fontaine, Jacques 380

Formicarius (1437) 33, 121

Forner, Friedrich, Bishop of Bamberg 168–9

Fort Bragg murders 430

Fortescue, Sir John 221

France 4, 5, 6, 30, 41–3, 140, 167, 206, 221–2; demonic possession in 256–63; depictions of the Devil in 237–8

Francesco, Matteuccia di 127

Francis of Assisi, St 22, 36, 43

Francis of Girundino 42

Francis of Maiolati 45, 46, 47

Franciscans 38, 39, 43–4, 186

Francys, Agnes 309

Franz Wilhelm of Wartenberg 77

Fratianno, Jimmy 421

Fraticelli 22, 43–8

Frederick II, Emperor 37, 41

Frederick William I 387

Free Spirit, Brethren of 48–9

Freud, Sigmund 429
Friedrich, Johann, Archbishop of Bremen 118
Fründ, John 31
Fuchs von Dornheim, Bishop Johann Georg II 114–15
Fugger, Philip Eduard 78

Gable, Mary Ann 401, 407, 409
Gaeledochter, Claesken 195–6
Galen, Christoph Bernhard von, Prince Bishop 118
Gallero, Gratia 100–1
Galosna, Antonio, of Monte San Raffaello 40, 42
Gandillon, Perrenette 66
Gardner, Gerard 2, 3
Garini, Massetus 34
Garrison, Ellen 316
Gaste, Mayette 65
Gaule, John 170
Geisslbrecht, Appolonia 250
Geisz, George Ludwig 374
Gemes, Mrs Gyorgy 133
gender relations 280–6, 289, 326, 356–8
Geneva, *engraisseurs* at 87, 88, 89–95
Georg Friedrich of Greiffenclau, Prince-Bishop 78
George, Claude 58
Géraud, Hugo, Bishop of Cahors 26
Germany 4, 10, 30, 33, 145, 172, 173, 206; central/local prosecutions 222; crop failures in 73; demonic possession in 241–52; and end of witch-hunts 374; inflation in 76; Waldensians in 39–40; and witch-burnings 82–3; witch-hunts in 69–70, 74, 77–8, 80, 114–17; witchcraft as social offence 114
Ghisleri, Cardinal Michele 105
Gifford, George 177
Gillat, Zabel and Demenge 67–8
Gillies, E. 82
Ginzburg, C. 3, 102, 104–5, 134–5, 137, 138
Glanvill, Joseph 314
Glover, Mary 57, 296
Gloxinus, Pastor Caspar 240
Goeury, Didier 64
Golden Legend 236
Goodcole, Henry 297
Gooderidge, Alice 61, 312
Goody, E. 209
Gouge, William 10, 360
Goya, Francisco 381
Greenblatt, S. 330–1
Gregory IX, Pope 37, 41, 49
Grien, Hans Baldung 116
Griffiths, Sarah 400
Grindletonians 177

Gui, Bernard 51
Gulyas, Mrs Andras 131
Gunter, Anne 221, 313
Gunter, Brian 221
Guyart, George 63

Habsburgs 180–1, 186
Haizmann, Christoph 250
Hale, John 317
'Hammer of Witches, the' *see Malleus Maleficarum* (1486)
Hampa, Erzsébat 132
Hanry, Meline 64
Hansen, Joseph 29
Harley, D. 316
Harmansdr, Volckgen 197
Harvey, Elizabeth 292
Harvey, William 313
Hathaway, Richard 295, 400
Hatton, Sir Christopher 409
Hauldecoeur, Anne 139
health 15–16, 53, 57–8; and appearance of the Devil 361; illness/death due to bewitchment 57–9, 61–2, 64; and possession 229, 248
Heard, Annis 308
Heerbrand, Jacob 170
hell/underworld 133–4, 156, 175, 237
Hemmingsen, Niels 165, 170
Henningsen, G. 7, 103, 110, 134
Henry, Claude 64
Henry, Marion 64
Henry of Schonberg 37
heresy/heretics 21–2, 28, 120, 163, 168, 171–2, 190, 195, 278; demonization of 36–51
Herteman, Georgeatte 59
Herwarth, Hans Friedrich 73
Heywood, Thomas 155
Hildegard of Bingen 262
History of Witchcraft (Summers) 1
Hobbes, Thomas 150
Hobert, Elizabeth 360
Hogarth, William 381
Hole, C. 354, 364
Holland, Henry 155, 170
Holmes, C. 280, 282, 355
Hopkins, Matthew (Witchfinder General) 220, 280, 292, 311, 344, 346, 353, 363
horseshoes 409–10
Hos, Anna 129
Hugonid, Stephan 34
Huguenots 172
Hungary 5, 167, 387

Hus, Jan 172, 191
hysteria 2–3, 57, 374

idolatry 167, 168
infanticide 14, 48, 49, 202, 208, 210, 286, 360–2, 363, 374
Innocent VIII, Pope 33, 41
Inquisition, Roman 98, 223; Schongau 73–4; Spanish 98
inquisitors 2–3, 51, 90, 100–1, 102, 103, 121, 122, 180, 197, 218–19, 220
Institoris, Heinrich 33, 70, 115, 116
inversions see ritual inversion
Italy 5, 7, 31, 32, 40, 223

Jackson, Elizabeth 57
Jacopo, Pietro de 42
James VI of Scotland 5, 8, 13, 153, 205, 217, 218, 219, 280, 315
Japnuel, Jennon 59
Jeffries, Judge 294–5
Jesuits 170, 186, 396
Jetherell, Perry 345
Jews 121, 330, 332, 334, 338
Joan of Arc 33
Johann VII, Archbishop of Schwarzenburg 76
John of Ojun 47, 50
John of Winterthur 38, 39
John XXII, pope 26–7, 28, 37, 44, 45
Joliet, Mongeatte 66
Joly, Marie 91–2, 94
Jones, Jim 422
Jorden, Edmund 380
Joris, David 176
Journal, Humbert 58
Judd, M. 408
judicial system 97–101, 106–7; central/local relationship 216–24; changes in 375–7; ecclesiastical courts 293, 298; effect of print technology on 201; female involvement in 310; officialisation of power 214, 219; secular criminal law courts 290–8; and treatment of women 289–90
Junius, Johannes 3, 115
Jura region witches (1571–2) 88, 89–95

Kahr, B. 414
Kamen, H. 84
Karlstadt, 172
Katchen, M. 414
Kemp, Ursley 308, 314
Kempe, Margery 227
Kenlish, Michael 400–1

Kephart, M.J. 3
Kerbl, Hans 73
Kieckhefer, R. 99, 242
Kincaid, John 217
Kint, Kortrijk Joos 197
Klaniczay, Gábor 3
Klatten, Judith 240–1, 243, 251
Klein, M. 337
Knights Templars 22, 26, 27
Kornmann, Heinrich 241
Kramer, Heinrich 4, 78, 267
Kyteler, Dame Alice 4, 27

Labanchi, Bishop 98
Lamothe-Langon, Etienne-Léon de 29, 31
Landish, Margaret 295
Langin, Georg 165
Langton, Walter, Bishop of Coventry 27
language 125, 165
Larner, C. 165, 166, 276, 281
Late Lancashire Witches, The (1634) 155
Lauderdale, Duke of 13
Laurence, Ann 357
LaVey, Anthony 427
Law of freedom in a platform, The (1652) 177
Le Baillu, Guillaume 413
Le Roy Ladurie, E. 152
Lea, Henry Charles 49
Leipzig, David 113
Lenman, B. 207
Leon, Lucrezia de 262
lepers 121
Lepzet of Cologne 49–50
L'Estrange Ewen, C. 353
Levack, B. 190
L'Hullier, Didelon and Bietrix 62
Lieb, Jeremias 78
Liegey, Margueritte (la Geline) 58, 65
Lienard, Mengeatte 62
literature 17–18, 33; demonic associations in 228, 235, 242, 243
Lloyd, Temperance 295, 309
Lodi, Bishop of 99
Löher, Hermann 77
London: accusations of witchcraft in 406–7; Bible-and-key identification 405–6; expansion of 405; witchcraft in 399–410
Lorichius, Jodocus 166
Louis X of France 26
Louis XII of France 43, 237
Louis XIV of France 387
Lovecraft, H.P. 426
Lovett, E. 408

Lucifer *see* Devil, the
Luciferans 28, 29, 38–9, 49–50, 51
Luckison, William, of Stirling 62
Luther, Martin 12, 16, 161, 172, 190, 191, 192, 235, 247
Lutherans 172, 180, 185, 187, 189, 191–2, 251

Macarella, Antonia 105–6
Macbeth (Shakespeare) 157
MacDonald, Jeffrey 430
MacDonald, Michael 312
McDonald, Sarah 401, 407, 409
McDougall, J. 334
Macfarlane, A. 75, 361, 403
Mackenzie, Sir George 217, 219
MacMurdoch, Janet 274–5
Mafia 421
magic 16–17, 22, 26, 28, 53, 54, 55, 56, 100, 110, 115, 131–2, 168, 348, 367–8, 390, 409–10; belief in 189; and climate 69–71, 73; demonic/non-demonic 163, 183, 184; harmful/harmless distinction 116, 117; linked to heresy 171–2; loss of belief in 374; and revenge 146–7; use of superstitions/spells 143–4
magicians 101, 113, 379
Magny, Oliver de 234
Magus, Simon 172
Maietta, Cinzia 100, 101
Maillard, Olivier 236
Maillat, Humberte and Claude 11, 15
Maillat, Loyse 5, 6
Maldonado, Juan 168, 172
Malebranche, Nicolas de 381
maleficium 5, 6, 10, 11, 12, 14, 15, 16, 17, 100, 109, 155, 270, 367, 369, 370; allegations of 53–4, 183; criminal aspects 208; diagnosis of 55–6; individual 70; physical/social reality of 54; and possession 256–7; religious reactions to 168; understanding of 154–5
Malleus Maleficarum (1486) 1, 4, 16–17, 23, 33, 63, 69, 87, 115–16, 143, 149, 173, 239, 267, 277, 368
Mandrou, R. 389, 396
Mangin, W. 403
Mann, M. 220
Marchal, Claudon 62
Maria Theresa, Empress 387, 388, 390, 392, 397
Marigny, Enguerrand 26
Marriott, M. 152–3
Masini, Eliseo 98
Massé, Pierre 172
Mather, Cotton 312
Maximilian, Duke of Bavaria 81

Maximilian I, Emperor 113
Mayhew, Robert 361
Maynes, Thomas 344
medicine 60–2, 380–1
Mengin, George 63
Mennonites 176, 190, 194, 195
Mer, Albrecht 116
metamorphosis *see* transformations
Methodus civilis doctrinae seu Abissini regis historia (1628) 81
Michaelis, Sebastien 172
Michaelsen, J. 420
Middleton, C. 283
Midelfort, E. 87, 173, 208, 230
midwives 63–4, 90, 193, 292
Miette, Pentecost 62
Mikszath, Kalman 393
Miller, Arthur 2
Millini, Cardinal Giovanni 98–9
Mingolla, Leonarda 104
Miracle of Laon 158, 256
Mitchell, J.C. 402
Moats, Ann 353
Molitor, Ulrich 69, 70
Mongenot, Didier 58
Monk, Maria 421
Monter, E.W. 109, 166, 190, 208
Montmorency, Marechal de 258
Moore, Margaret 344–50
moral panics 207, 210
Morand, Bénigne 143
Morduck, Sarah 295
More, Henry 379
Morel, Bastienne 59
Morphology of the Folktale (Propp) 125–6
Morton, Margaret 317
Muchembled, R. 211, 214, 221, 242
Muggleton, Lodowick 176
Munnings, Philippa 306
Müntzer, Thomas 175
Murray, M. 2, 3, 7, 8, 152, 355
Muschamp, Margaret 297
mystics 105, 262

Nadel, E. 209
Naogeorgus, Thomas 70
Napier, Richard 15
nation-state 201–2; and church–state relationship 214; development of 201, 213; and judicial/administrative centralisation 213, 219, 220–3; link with witch-hunting 215–24; officialisation of judicial power 214, 219; and reform of society 214, 224

Netherlands 4, 5, 140, 145, 167, 172
Neukirch, Melchior 248–9
Newman, Ales 283
Newton, Isaac 369
Nicholas of Massaro 45, 46, 47
Niclaes, Hendrick 176
Nider, Johannes 33, 121
Nix, Thomas 344–5, 346
Nodé, Pierre 172
Nogent, Guibert de 47
Noirot, Claude 152
Norway 139–40
Norwood, Robert 176
Notwendige Erinnerung Von des Sathans letzten
   Zornsturm (1594, 1595) 244
Nowell, Roger 307–8

O'Brien, Sarah 406
Obry, Nicole 229–30, 239, 254–63
Oecolampadius, 172
Olah, Mrs Mihaly 133
Onerdamme, Hans van 196
orgies 42, 48, 120, 427
Ovid 155

Pacy, Samuel 309
pagan cults 2–3, 236
Pahl, R. 403
Palingh, Abraham 176
Palladius, Peder, Bishop of Sealand 118
panics 54, 119; in Denmark 223; in East Anglia
   11, 12, 314, 344; in Germany 69–70, 74,
   77–8, 80, 114–17; in Jura 88, 89–95; in Salem
   2, 4, 220–1; in Scotland 210, 215, 216, 222; in
   Styria 182–3
Panneguin, Antoinette 67
Paracelsus 241
Pare, Ambroise 259
Parker, G. 207
Parsons, Jack 427
patriarchy 274, 279, 325
Patrimia, Caterina 107
Paulicians 47, 50
Paulus, Nikolaus 165
Pazder, Dr Lawrence 427, 428
Pelletier, François 66–7
Pendle witches 269–70, 308
People's Temple 422
Perkins, William 154, 170
Perry, William 312
Persijn, Hippolitus 193
Peter of Greyerz 31
Peterson, Joan 297

Petit, Jennon 64
Philip II of Spain 172, 193
Philip III of France 26
Philip V of France 121
Philip VI of France 28
Philips, Dirck 176
Philips, Mary 292
philosophy 60, 378–81
Phythian-Adams, C. 408
Pickering, Thomas 170
Pico della Mirandola, Gianfrancesco 97
Pilgram, Kunigunde von 248
pilgrimages 62, 142
Piver, Mongeotte 65
pixies/elves 240–1
plague 76, 87, 121
Plan, Raoul du 94
Plouvier, François 43
Polakin, Rosina 387–8
Poland 5, 206, 373
Pölnitz, Götz von 80
possession 5, 103–6, 221, 227, 239, 396; and
   accusations of witchcraft 311–13; of adolescents
   296–7; and anti-Protestant manifestations 230;
   characteristics of 257–8; of children 296;
   demonic 355; deviation from official
   expectations 247–50; and exorcism 235;
   Germanic reactions to 241–52; and illness 229;
   not a crime 247; of nuns 396–7; preconditions
   for 247; rise in 245; spirit 254–63; theological
   aspects 258–9, 262–3; with/without maleficium
   256–7
Postel, Guillaume 256
Prat, Thomas 281
Press, I. 407
Principia Mathematica (1687) 369
printing see literature
Process, the 427
Propp, V. 125–6
prostitutes 100, 261
Pruystinck de Schaliedecker, Loy 192
Psellos 50
psychoanalytic notions 329–31, 334, 336–8
Purston, Alice 291

Quaife, G.R. 103
Quakers 179
Quaranta, Giustina 106
Questions sur l'Encyclopédie (1772) 395

Rabb, T. 84
Rabelais, François 233, 234, 235, 236, 237
Raemond, Florimond de 256

Ralph of Coggeshall 21–2
Ratcliffe, Thomazine 355, 359
Recordi, Peter 27
Reformation 12, 14, 71, 161–2, 167, 210–11, 236, 275, 283, 382
Reidler, Michael 329, 333
religion 16, 210–11; conflicts in 230; and demonic beliefs 233–4, 238–9; effects of division in 12–15; general ideas on witchcraft 166; and identity 169; increase in toleration 382; and Marian state-programme 80; and mechanical philosophy 379; pessimism of 81–2; power/influence of 60–1, 174; second Reformation 81–2; see also Catholic/Protestant witchcraft
Religion and the Decline of Magic (Thomas) 169–70
Remarques sur le Vampyrisme (1755) 390–1
Rémy, Dion 63
Rémy, Nicolas 13, 72, 149, 155
Rémy, Zabel 63
Renaissance 4, 22, 233, 235, 252, 379
Renauldin, Claudon 62
Reynolds, Bridget 292, 316
Reyte, Hellenix le 67
Rheims 21–2
Rice, Thomas 308
ritual inversion 101, 151–3, 156, 248
Rivera, G. 422
Robinson, Arthur 291
Robinson, Joan 308
Rodes, Dorothea 291
Romaine, Claudon la 59
Roots (Propp) 126
Roper, L. 263, 363
Roschmann, Anna 250
Ross, Balthasar 114
Roy, Nicole le 260, 263
Rummel, Walter 70
Russell, J.B. 106

sabbat 10, 14, 109, 110, 111, 112, 116, 162–3, 183, 413; as alien notion 137; Catholic/Protestant attitudes towards 166–7; common genetic source 125; as cultural phenomenon 120; and diabolization of the night 141–2; diffusion hypothesis 124–5, 127; elements of 141; and fairies 133; and fairy-tales 125–6; and feasts 134; and flight/metamorphosis 100, 122–4, 127, 129, 131–2, 135; as liturgy of fear 138; myths concerning 136–40; origins of 134–5; scenes of 130–1; shaping of 121–2; societies of 132–3;

stereotype image of 120–1, 126–7, 184; theologian's creation 136–7, 144; underworld/hell 133–4
Sabean, D. 330
Sabie, Adam 348–9
sacrifice 10, 22, 109, 152, 426, 427
Sacro Arsenale (1625) 98
Salazar, Alfonso 7–8
Salem (New England) 2, 4, 220–1, 245, 311
Salimbeni, Fulvio 105
Salinaro, Mario 101, 103, 104
Salter, Joan 292
Sandeswell, Anne 309
Satan see Devil, the
satanic abuse 428; belief/scepticism in 433–6; and use of therapy 434–6
satanic rituals 414–17; evidence of 421–30; historical context 420–1; and news media 426–7; proofs of conspiracy 419–20; real groups 427–8; survivor stories 423–6; therapeutic process 428–30
satanism 16–18, 22, 23, 109, 111, 163; myths of 136–40, 144
Saulnier, Demenge 65
Savory, Anne 292
Savron, Jean 152
Sawyer, Elizabeth 291, 297, 316
Scandinavia 118–19, 139–40
Scherz, Karl Ferdinand 393
Schiller, Regina 339
Schilling, H. 181
Schlutterbaurin, Anna 245
Schmidt, Hans 250
Schonborn, Johann Philipp von, Archbishop of Mainz 118
Schormann, G. 77
science 378–9
Scot, Reginald 165, 176, 354, 367
Scotland 4, 5, 10, 11, 13, 154, 167, 203, 206, 210, 315, 374; central/local prosecutions 216–17; inquisitorial procedures 217–19; secular prosecutions 216; witch-hunt panics 210, 215, 216, 222; witchcraft statute (1563) 215
Scrutton, Mary 361
Secretain, Françoise 5–7, 9, 11
sectaries 175–7
sects 173–5
Segersz, Jeronimus 196
Seiler, Tobias 243, 244
Setto, Antonio di, of Savigliano 40
sex 14, 28, 48; and demonic possession 261–2; and the Devil 103–6; double standard of 278;

female power 267; and promiscuity 155;
related to witchcraft 208, 209
Shakespeare, William 157
shamans 123
Short, Mercy 312
Sicily 9, 110, 134
Sigismond of Tirol 33
Sikes, Mary 291
Simmenthal (Switzerland) 31
Simon, Catherine 33–4
Simon, Jacotte 61
Simons, Menno 176, 190, 193
Skinner, Q. 150
sleep paralysis 16, 129, 240
Sloman, A. 221–2
Smith, Mary 310
Smith, Susanna 361, 363
Smithe, Elleine 281
socio-economic factors, changes in 283–6, 383–4,
407–10; and class/ideology 79–82; crop
failures 70, 72, 73, 76–7, 83, 185;
famine/malnutrition 75, 76; inflation 75–6, 78;
and mentality transformation 78–82; plagues
76, 87; and quality of life 79; and rise in witch-
hunts 75–8; and social relationships 82–4
Solar Lodge 427
Soldan, Wilhelm Gottlieb 165
Soman, A. 389, 396
sorcerers 170
sorcery 25–6, 101, 139, 147, 161, 172, 182
Sotterel, Marye 64
Spaans, Joke 197
Spain 4, 5, 7, 16–17, 30, 222–3
Spencer, J. 424
spirit travel 110, 112
spirits 241–2, 345; possession by 254–63
Sprenger, Jacob 4, 33, 115, 116, 267
Sprot, Jean 275
Stampken, Appolonia 248–9
Stanton, Margery 305
Stapleton, Thomas 171
Starkey, Nicholas 313
state see nation-state
Staunton , Mother 281
Stearne, John 220, 344, 346, 354
Stegold, Susanna 358–9
Steiner, Veronica 248
Stratagematum Satanae (1555) 175
Stratford, Lauren 419, 423, 429
Striglin, Barbara 184
Strix (1523) 97
Stubbes, Philip 151
Styria 180–7

suicide 362–3
Summers, Montague 1, 392, 414
superstitions 233–4, 238, 381
Swartz, M. 402–3
Sweden 140
Swettson, John 309
Swieten, Gerard van 390–1
Switzerland 4, 30–1, 33, 38, 71, 87, 89–95, 114,
315

Tableau de l'inconstance des mauvais anges et demons,
Le (1612) 156
Taillepied, Noel 259
Tallar, George 394
Tardea, Rosa 104
Taylor, Lidea 362–3
Teall, J.L. 166
Tedeschi, J. 98
Tempest, Henry 291
Temple of Set 427
Teresa of Avila 262
Tertullian 422
Teufelbucher 228, 242, 248
Teutonic Order 114
theatre 236–8
Third Order of Saint Francis 40
Thomas, K. 87, 152, 169–70, 276–7, 281, 361,
383, 403
Thomasius, Christian 118, 377
Tilbrook, Charles 402
Tinctor, Johann 155
Titelmans (inquisitor) 197
Tixerand, Jacquotte 63
Torpietto, Francesca Antonia di 104
torture 118–19, 132, 195, 218–19, 221, 224,
346, 377
Tractatus de Officio Sanctissimae Inquisitionis (1655)
98
traditions see folk beliefs/traditions
transformations 33–4, 66, 111, 122–3, 124, 126,
155, 184, 235
Trapnel, Anna 295
Treatise on the heresy of the poor of Lyons (1265) 37
Trevor-Roper, H.R. 165, 209, 210, 211
trials 4–7, 22, 23; and allegiance with the Devil
280; central/local prosecutions 114, 203,
215–24; chain-reaction/panic 114–16, 117,
119, 182–3; and charges of diabolism 27,
29–32, 33–5; and charges of sorcery 25–6, 33,
101; decline/demise of 373–84, 392;
disappearance of 117–19; and gender 269; and
idea of sabbat/magic merger 127; increase in
29–31; inquisitorial 218–19; linked to

judicial/literary developments 33; management of 205; mildness of allegations 27–9; monocausal explanations 269; and night-time amusements 142; pattern of 138–9; and persecution of unorthodox religious groups 163; persecution/gender relationships 356–8; political character of 25–8; records 99–100, 101, 131, 282–3; religious division 12–15; secularisation of 207, 216; sentences 139; social/political contexts 11–15; of unknowns 28–9

Trier (1587–93) 12, 70, 71, 72, 74, 76, 109, 114, 172

Trithemius, Johannes, Abbot of Sponheim 113

Troeltsch, E. 173, 174, 175

troop flags 132

underworld *see* hell/underworld

Urban VIII, Pope 81

Vagnier, Claudon Didier 66

Valach, Joseph 421

vampires: beliefs concerning 392–3, 394–5; ecclesiastical views on 394–5; medical views on 394; popularity of 396; rise of 387–98; scandals of 397–8; stories of 393–4

Van der Camere, Charles 145

Vannier, Mesenne 62

Vatable, François 263

Vaughan, Joan 312

village inquisitions 70–1

Villon, François 234

Viragos, Mrs Marton 131

Viret, Pierre 239

Virgin Mary 80, 104–5, 234, 236

Visconti, Matteo and Galeazzo 26

visions 13–14, 62, 104–5, 262; Christian 129–30; of the dead 345, 347; and enchantment 129

Voltaire, François Marie Arouet de 395

'Voodoo death' 58

Vox in Rama (1233) papal bull 37, 38, 50

Wagner, Tobias 250

Walby, S. 284

Waldensians 28, 30, 36–43, 51, 126, 172

Walker, Joan 293

Walther, Georg 249

Walz, R. 75

warlocks 121

Warnke, M. 427

Watson, William 346

Watts, Thomas 400

weather *see* climate

Webb, Robert 309

Webster, John 177

Weller, Hieronymus 248

Welsford, E. 152

Wenham, Jane 295, 306

werewolves 66, 123, 124, 135

Weruick, Peter van 196–7

Wesxpremi, Istvan 390

Weyer, Johann 71, 113, 149, 176, 244, 245, 368

Whishall, Margery 298

White, Mary 406

Wicca: The Old Religion in the New Age (Crowley) 2

William V, Duke of Bavaria 80, 81

Willmott, P. 404

Willoughby, Elizabeth 295

Winne, Cicely 298

Winstanley, Gerrard 176, 177

witch cults 7–10, 110, 111–12; credibility of 17–18

witch-finders *see* inquisitors

witch-hunts: Christian aspects 278; decline in 157, 211, 387; end of 373–4; gender aspects 276, 277, 281; and growth of state power 217–24; major 69–70, 74, 76–8, 114–17, 219; and peasant involvement 142, 144, 145–6; as sociological phenomenon 144–8, 211; as woman-hunting 273–5, 326

witchcraft: anxieties concerning 205–6; artistic representations of 116; attitude of suspects 55; beliefs concerning 15–18, 307, 314, 318; centred within women's community 283; collective 54, 55, 109, 110, 111; control of 206; as crime 15, 116; as *crimen exceptum* 205, 206, 207–8, 210; cultural context 53–6; decline in 368–71; depersonalisation of 371; as disordered 156–7; explanations of 206–7; and female lust 115, 116; and hysteria 2–3; individual 54; interpretations of 149–51; as inversion of the norm 151–3, 156; judicial reactions 106–7; kinship patterns 55; learned vs popular 242–3; meanings of 153–6; mediaeval origins 21–3; and new mental outlook on 377–82; ordinances against 139–40, 146; as pagan cult 2–3; physical/spiritual difference 190; as political dissent 215; and popular culture 102–3; popularity of 1–2; religious reactions to 168; as secret crime 355; as social offence 114; as special case 205; victims of 296, 318, 344; *see also* Catholic/Protestant witchcraft

Witchcraft, Oracles and Magic amongst the Azande (Evans-Pritchard) 82

witches: alleged intentions of 155–6; burning of 82–3, 274; defiance in courtroom 295–6; as the 'evils' 132; execution of 206, 220, 295–6, 297–8; experiences of 270; as female 87–9, 115, 142–3, 157, 182–3, 202, 208; lynching of 206, 278; as male 208; persecution of 144–8, 202; as poor 11, 87, 89, 101, 115, 283; power of 57–8; prepared for death 297–8, 299; prosecution of 318–19; as scapegoats 384; and searching for the mark 290–3; sex-related, not sex-specific 268–9, 277–9; as solitary 114; stereotypes of 87–9, 208–9, 273, 276–7, 279, 280, 357; and troop flags 132

witnesses 345; and experience of *maleficium* 304; local aspects 73–4, 306, 307–11, 344–50; male 309; as possessed victims 303, 311–13; as reporters of physical searching 303, 313–17; sources of 304; women as 299, 303–19

Wittgenstein, L. 123, 150

wizards 138, 143, 426

Wollar, Ulrich, of Krems 37

women: and the brewing industry 284–5; characteristics of 245–6, 357; courtroom experiences 294–5; criminalization of 208–9, 274; culpability of 268; demonic possession of 260–1; deviant behaviour of 260–1; economic position 283–5, 357; and encounters with witches 269–70; hostility towards 209; impact of witch-hunts on 363–4; patriarchal attitude/responsibility for 274, 279; personified as Deadly Sins 236; and possession 246; power of 267, 344–5; psychic identity of 341; as searchers 290–3, 303, 313–17, 355; sexuality of 267, 280; status of 209–10; weaknesses of 245; wife/mother relationship 358–63; as witches 87–9, 115, 142–3, 157, 182–3, 202, 208, 245–6, 268, 340; as witnesses 293–4, 295, 299, 303–19, 340, 355–6

Wooden, K. 422

Wootton, D. 176

Wright, Ann 298–9

Wright, Katherine 313

Wurzlburger, Augustin 164

Wyclif, John 172

Wyne, Benjamin 345

Zabey, Jennon 62

Zelanti (or zealots) 81